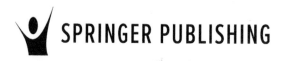

GET THE MOST FROM YOUR BOOK

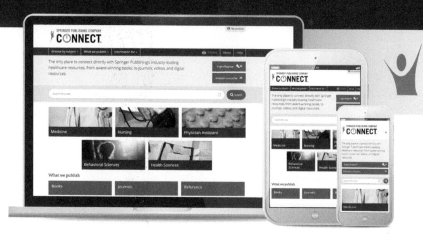

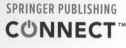

VOUCHER CODE:

FK9X1P1H

Online Access

Your print purchase of *Advanced Health Assessment of Women, Fifth Edition,* includes **online access via Springer Publishing Connect**™ to increase accessibility, portability, and searchability.

Insert the code at http://connect.springerpub.com/content/book/978-0-8261-7963-0 today!

Having trouble? Contact our customer service department at cs@springerpub.com

Instructor Resource Access for Adopters

Let us do some of the heavy lifting to create an engaging classroom experience with a variety of instructor resources included in most textbooks SUCH AS:

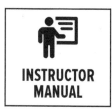

INSTRUCTOR MANUAL

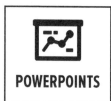

POWERPOINTS

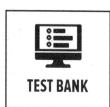

TEST BANK

Visit **https://connect.springerpub.com/** and look for the **"Show Supplementary"** button on your **book homepage** to see what is available to instructors! First time using Springer Publishing Connect?

Email **textbook@springerpub.com** to create an account and start unlocking valuable resources.

Advanced Health Assessment of
WOMEN

R. Mimi Secor, DNP, FNP-BC, FAANP, FAAN, is an NP, national speaker/educator, media ambassador, international best-selling author, and health and fitness advocate. She has worked for 45 years as a family nurse practitioner specializing in women's health and more recently in health/fitness. In 2015, Dr. Secor earned her doctorate in nursing practice degree from Rocky Mountain University of Health Professions (RMUoHP) in Provo, Utah, and now serves on their Board of Trustees.

Dr. Secor is senior faculty at Advanced Practice Education Associates (APEA) in Lafayette, Louisiana, and guest lecturer at NP programs around the country. She is a fellow in both the American Association of Nurse Practitioners (AANP) and the American Academy of Nursing (AAN).

She has also published extensively, including her 2018 coauthored text, *Advanced Health Assessment of Women: Clinical Skills and Procedures, Fourth Edition*, her 2018 coauthored book, *Fast Facts About the Gynecologic Exam: A Professional Guide for NPs, PAs, and Midwives, Second Edition*, as well as two internationally acclaimed health and fitness books.

Dr. Secor has received several awards for her contributions to the NP profession, including the 2013 Lifetime Achievement Award from the Massachusetts Coalition of Nurse Practitioners (MCNP) and the 2019 Outstanding Alumnae Award from Rocky Mountain University. In addition to her nursing work, Dr. Secor and her daughter help women, especially NPs, become healthy and fit, offering a variety of virtual programs as "Coach Kat and Dr. Mimi."

Aimee Chism Holland, DNP, WHNP-BC, FNP-C, FAANP, FAAN, is globally recognized as a women's health expert, NP educator, leader, and policy advocate. Dr. Holland is known for the global impact of the Gynecology Procedures Workshop that she envisioned, created, and disseminated. She has prepared over 4,000 providers through live courses and virtual workshops. Her unique workshop includes five interactive educational videos demonstrating step-by-step how to perform essential gynecology clinical procedures. The videos are published with peer-reviewed journal articles in women's health journals that have received over 25,000 views around the world.

Dr. Holland is the Associate Dean for Graduate Clinical Education and a Professor at the University of Alabama at Birmingham (UAB). Her faculty practice at the UAB Student Health and Wellness Center is the primary platform for her scholarly work focused on office gynecology procedures, contraception, vaginal infections, and gynecologic cancer prevention. She was elected to the Board of Directors for the National Association of Nurse Practitioners in Women's Health (NPWH) in 2013 and served a 6-year term as the Chair-elect (2016-2017), Chair (2018-2019), and Past Chair (2020-2021). She is the inaugural 2016 NONPF Rising Star Faculty award recipient and a current member of the NONPF Board of Directors. Her service on key national policy bodies include LACE, the National Task Force (NTF) on Quality Nurse Practitioner Education, and the ASCCP Risk-Based Management for Abnormal Cervical Cancer Screening Results Guidelines Workgroup. Dr. Holland is a past Ambassador and NP for the National Health Service Corps (NHSC). She is a primary contributor to the Eighth Edition of the WHNP Guidelines for Practice and Education and a member of the Editorial Board for *Women's Healthcare.*

Dr. Holland was inducted as a Fellow of the American Association of Nurse Practitioners (FAANP) and the American Academy of Nursing (FAAN) for distinguished leadership contributions to NP education, practice, and policy. Other distinguished accolades received for her sustained contributions to nursing include the Top Twenty Outstanding Professors of Women's Health Nursing Award, NPWH Inspiration Award for Policy, AANP State Award for Excellence, NP Alliance of Alabama Outstanding Educator Award, the Vanderbilt University Alumni Award for Healthcare Innovation, and the UAB School of Nursing Visionary Leader Award.

Advanced Health Assessment of WOMEN

SKILLS, PROCEDURES, AND MANAGEMENT

Fifth Edition

R. Mimi Secor, DNP, FNP-BC, FAANP, FAAN

Aimee Chism Holland, DNP, WHNP-BC, FNP-C, FAANP, FAAN

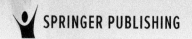

SPRINGER PUBLISHING

Springer Publishing Company, LLC
11 West 42nd Street, New York, NY 10036
www.springerpub.com
connect.springerpub.com/

Executive Acquisitions Editor: Joseph Morita
Senior Content Development Editor: Lucia Gunzel
Compositor: Exeter Premedia Services Private Limited

ISBN: 978-0-8261-7962-3
ebook ISBN: 978-0-8261-7963-0
DOI: 10.1891/9780826179630

A robust set of instructor resources designed to supplement this text is located at **http://connect.springerpub.com/content/book/978-0-8261-7963-0.** Qualifying instructors may request access by emailing **textbook@springerpub.com.**

Instructor Manual ISBN: 978-0-8261-7964-7
Instructor PowerPoints ISBN: 978-0-8261-7965-4
Instructor Test Bank ISBN: 978-0-8261-7966-1

Qualified instructors may request supplements by emailing textbook@springerpub.com.

23 24 25 26 27 / 5 4 3 2 1

The author and the publisher of this Work have made every effort to use sources believed to be reliable to provide information that is accurate and compatible with the standards generally accepted at the time of publication. Because medical science is continually advancing, our knowledge base continues to expand. Therefore, as new information becomes available, changes in procedures become necessary. We recommend that the reader always consult current research and specific institutional policies before performing any clinical procedure. The author and publisher shall not be liable for any special, consequential, or exemplary damages resulting, in whole or in part, from the readers' use of, or reliance on, the information contained in this book. The publisher has no responsibility for the persistence or accuracy of URLs for external or third-party Internet websites referred to in this publication and does not guarantee that any content on such websites is, or will remain, accurate or appropriate.

Library of Congress Control Number: 2022952354

Publisher's Note: **New and used products purchased from third-party sellers are not guaranteed for quality, authenticity, or access to any included digital components.**

Printed in the United States of America.

Contents

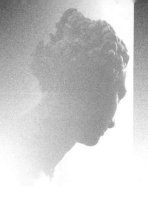

UNIT X   ADVANCED SKILLS

UNIT XI   PHARMACOLOGIC MANAGEMENT (ONLINE ONLY)

(The eChapters can be accessed at http://connect.springerpub.com/content/book/978-0-8261-7963-0)

UNIT XII   SUPPLEMENTAL CHAPTERS (ONLINE ONLY)

(The eChapters can be accessed at http://connect.springerpub.com/content/book/978-0-8261-7963-0)

Contributors

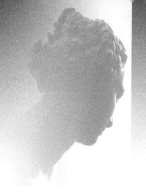

Ivy M. Alexander, PhD, APRN, ANP-BC, FAANP, FAAN
Clinical Professor; Director, Adult-Gerontology Primary Care Nurse Practitioner MS Track;
University of Connecticut School of Nursing, Storrs, Connecticut

Hannah E. Bergbower, MSN, MPH, CNM, WHNP-BC
Nurse-Midwife, Emory University - Grady Memorial Hospital, School of Medicine, Department
of Obstetrics and Gynecology, Atlanta, Georgia; Adjunct Associate Professor, Tufts University,
School of Medicine, Department of Public Health and Community Medicine, Boston,
Massachusetts

Nancy R. Berman, MSN, ANP-BC, NCMP, FAANP
Nurse Practitioner, Michigan Healthcare Professionals, Farmington Hills, Michigan

Kelley Stallworth Borella, DNP, MSN, WHNP-BC
Assistant Professor; Co-Specialty Track Coordinator MSN Women's Health Nurse Practitioner
Track; Family, Community, and Health Systems; School of Nursing; The University of Alabama at
Birmingham, Birmingham, Alabama

Paula Brooks, DNP, FNP-BC, MBA, RNFA
Director of Advanced Practitioners, Baystate Health System, Springfield, Massachusetts

Teri Bunker, MS, DNP, FNP
Family Nurse Practitioner, Bridge City Family Medical Clinic, Portland, Oregon

Helen A. Carcio, MS, MEd, ANP-BC
Director and Founder, The Health and Continence Institute of New England, South Deerfield,
Massachusetts

Lisa Astalos Chism, DNP, APRN, BC, CSC, NCMP, FAAN, FAANP
Oakland Macomb Center for Breast Health, Rochester Hills, Michigan

Kim Choma, DNP, APN, WHNP-BC
School of Nursing, Rutgers University-Camden, Camden, New Jersey

Barbara Dehn, RN, MS, NP
Nurse Practitioner, El Camino Women's Medical Group, Mountain View, California

Kahlil A. Demonbreun, DNP, RNC-OB, WHNP-BC, ANP-BC, FAANP
Women's Health Medical Director, WJB Dorn VA Medical Center, Orangeburg, South Carolina

Marcia Denine, MSN Ed, NP
Staff Nurse Practitioner, Island Health Care, Edgartown, Massachusetts

Whitney Taylor Eriksen, PhD, MSN, WHNP-BC
Department of Obstetrics and Gynecology, Thomas Jefferson University Hospital, Philadelphia,
Pennsylvania

Katharine Green, PhD, CNM, FACNM
Clinical Assistant Professor, Elaine Marieb College of Nursing, University of Massachusetts-Amherst, Amherst, Massachusetts

Hanne S. Harbison, MHSPH, MSN, WHNP-BC
Senior Lecturer; Director, Women's Health Gender Related Nurse Practitioner Track; Penn Nursing, University of Pennsylvania, Philadelphia, Pennsylvania

Kathleen Haycraft, DNP, FNP/PNP-BC, DCNP, FAANP
Kathleen Haycraft, LLC; Hannibal, Missouri

Aimee Chism Holland, DNP, WHNP-BC, FNP-C, FAANP, FAAN
Professor and Interim Associate Dean for Graduate Clinical Education, University of Alabama at Birmingham School of Nursing, Birmingham, Alabama

Samantha Debra Iervolino, BSN, RNC-OB, C-EFM, WHNP-S
SUNY Downstate Health Sciences University, Brooklyn, New York

Debra Ilchak, DNP, RN, FNP-BC, CNE
Clinical Associate Professor, Edson College of Nursing and Health Innovation, Arizona State University, Phoenix, Arizona

Karen A. Kalmakis, PhD, MPH, FNP-BC, FAANP
Associate Professor; Director, DNP Program, Elaine Marieb College of Nursing, University of Massachusetts Amherst, Amherst, Massachusetts

Cathy R. Kessenich, PhD, ARNP
Nurse Practitioner, DaVita Medical Group, New Port Richey, Florida

Rebecca Koeniger-Donohue, PhD, APRN, FAANP
Professor of Practice, Simmons College, Boston, Massachusetts

Annette Jakubisin Konicki, PhD, APRN, ANP-BC, FNP-BC, FAANP
Clinical Professor; Interim Associate Dean for Graduate Studies; Director, Family Nurse Practitioner Program, University of Connecticut School of Nursing, Storrs, Connecticut

Shelagh B. Larson, DNP, APRN, WHNP-BC, NCMP
Acclaim Physician Group, Fort Worth, Texas

Timothy Legg, PhD, PsyD, MSN, MPA, MSc
Clinical Assistant Professor; P.M.H.N.P Track Director, Nursing; University of North Dakota, Grand Forks, North Dakota

Carol Lesser, NP
Nurse Practitioner, Boston IVF, Beth Israel Deaconess Medical Center and Harvard University's School of Medicine, Waltham, Massachusetts

Deborah A. Lipkin, MSN, FNP
Family Nurse Practitioner, Harvard Vanguard Medical Associates, Vulvovaginal Services, Burlington, Massachusetts

Elisabeth J. Maher, MSN, PMHNP-BC
Montefiore Medical Center, Bronx, New York

Patrice C. Malena, MS, BSN, APRN, FNP-BC
Women Veterans Program Manager, Family Nurse Practitioner (retired), Hampton VA Medical Center, Department of Veterans Affairs, Hampton, Virginia

Amy Mandeville O'Meara, DNP, WHNP, AGNP
Assistant Clinical Professor, University of Vermont, Burlington, Vermont

Christy Martin, DNP, FNP-C
University of Alabama at Birmingham, Birmingham, Alabama

Randee L. Masciola, DNP, APRN-CNP, WHNP-BC, FAANP
Associate Professor of Clinical Nursing; Director, DNP Program – Clinical Expert Track, The Ohio State University College of Nursing, Columbus, Ohio

Nicole Metcalf, DNP, FNP-C, RN, MSN
Provider, Student Health Services, The University of Alabama at Birmingham, Birmingham, Alabama; Adjunct Didactic Instructor, The University of Alabama at Birmingham School of Nursing, Birmingham, Alabama

Ginny Moore, DNP, WHNP-BC
Associate Professor and Academic Director WHNP Specialty, Vanderbilt University School of Nursing, Nashville, Tennessee

Shawana S. Moore, DNP, MSN, CRNP, WHNP-BC
Associate Professor, Clinical Track; DNP Program Director, Nell Hodgson-Woodruff School of Nursing, Emory University, Atlanta, Georgia

Tonia Moore-Davis, MSN, SNM, FACNM
Instructor of Nursing, Vanderbilt University School of Nursing, Nashville, Tennessee

Jamille Nagtalon-Ramos, EdD, WHNP-BC, IBCLC, FAANP
Assistant Professor, Rutgers University, Camden, New Jersey; Women's Health Nurse Practitioner, Department of Obstetrics and Gynecology, Penn Medicine, Philadelphia, Pennsylvania

Samantha E. Nobeljas, BS, BSN, RN, C-EFM
Women's Health Nurse Practitioner Student, University of Pennsylvania School of Nursing, Philadelphia, Pennsylvania; Co-Adjutant Instructor, Rutgers University-Camden, Camden, New Jersey

Diane Todd Pace, PhD, APRN, FNP-BC, NCMP, IF, FAANP, FAAN
Professor and Director, Special Academic Programs, College of Nursing; Associate Professor, College of Medicine/Department of OB/GYN, University of Tennessee, Memphis, Tennessee

Lisa S. Pair, APRN-Faculty, DNP, WHNP-BC
Assistant Professor, Co-Coordinator of the WHNP Track, School of Nursing, The University of Alabama at Birmingham, Birmingham, Alabama

Komkwuan P. Parachabtr, DNP, FNP-BC, WHNP-BC, CNM, FACNM
Family Medicine Residency Site Director in the Department of OB/GYN, Fort Belvoir Community Hospital, Fort Belvoir, Virginia

Sarah L. Pederson, BSN, RN, SANE-A, SANE-P
Georgia Statewide Sexual Assault Nurse Examiner (SANE) Coordinator, Marietta, Georgia

Nancie Petrucelli, MS, CGC
Director, Cancer Center Counseling Service, Karmanos Cancer Institute, Detroit, Michigan

Yvette Marie Petti, PhD, ANP-BC
VA Ann Arbor Healthcare System/ Lt Col Charles S. Kettles VA Medical Center, Ann Arbor, Michigan

Richard S. Pope, MPAS, PA-C
Rheumatology Physician Assistant, Western CT Health Network, Department of Rheumatology, Southbury, Connecticut

Kathleen Pridgen, MD
Associate Medical Director, Student Health Services, The University of Alabama at Birmingham, Birmingham, Alabama

Heather Quaile, DNP, WHNP-BC, CSC, IF CEO
The SHOW Center; Clinical Lead Wellspring Living, Receiving Hope Center, Kennesaw, Georgia; Laura Reed, DNP, APRN, FNP-BC Assistant Professor and FNP Concentration Coordinator, College of Nursing, University of Tennessee, Memphis, Tennessee

Constance A. Roche, MSN, ANP-BC
Nurse Practitioner, Advanced Practice Nurse in Genetics, Avon Comprehensive Breast Center, Massachusetts General Hospital, Boston, Massachusetts

Frances M. Sahebzamani, PhD, ARNP, FAANP
Team Member Medical Clinic, H. Lee Moffitt Cancer Center and Research Institute, Healthy Weight and Cardiovascular Risk Reduction Program, Tampa, Florida

R. Mimi Secor, DNP, FNP-BC, FAANP, FAAN
Senior Faculty, Advanced Practice Education Associates/ATI, Onset, Massachusetts

William E. Somerall, Jr., MD, MAEd
Associate Professor of Nursing, School of Nursing, The University of Alabama at Birmingham, Birmingham, Alabama

Beth R. Steinfeld, DNP, WHNP-BC, FYNAM
Assistant Professor, Track Director WHNP Program, Chair of Advanced Level Programs, SUNY Downstate Health Sciences University, Brooklyn, New York; BoroPark OB/GYN, Brooklyn, New York

Iris Stendig-Raskin, MSN, CRNP, WHNP-BC
Women's Center at Nazareth-Red Lion Road, Philadelphia, Pennsylvania; St. Mary Physician's Group, Langhorne, Pennsylvania

Ashton Tureaud Strachan, DNP, FNP-C, WHNP-BC, APRN
Women's Health Nurse Practitioner, George Institute of Technology, Atlanta, Georgia

Kathryn Trotter, DNP, CNM, FNP, FAAN
Associate Clinical Professor, Duke University School of Nursing, Durham, North Carolina

Caitlin M. Vlaeminck, MSN, RN, FNP-BC
Bone Health Nurse Practitioner, Beacon Bone and Joint Specialists; Clinical Associate Professor, Indiana University of South Bend; CAPNI Past President, South Bend, Indiana

Meghan M. Whitfield, DNP, CRNP, ANP-C
Nurse Practitioner, UAB Student Health and Wellness, The University of Alabama at Birmingham, Birmingham, Alabama

Leslie Saltzstein Wooldridge, GNP-BC, CUNP
Director, Mercy Health Bladder Clinic, Muskegon, Michigan

Alit Yousif, MD
Oakland Macomb Center for Breast Health, Karmanos Cancer Institute, Wayne State University, Detroit, Michigan

INSTRUCTOR RESOURCE AUTHORS

Karen M. Coles, DNP, RN
Assistant Professor; Family, Community, and Health Systems; School of Nursing; The University of Alabama at Birmingham, Birmingham, Alabama

Shannon R. Hall, MSN, RN, AGPCNP-C APP
Wellness Champion for Staff Neurosurgery, Adjunct Clinical Instructor, The University of Alabama School of Nursing, UAB Neurosurgery at Greystone, Birmingham, Alabama

Karen Harris, DNP, RN, CNML
Nurse Manager, Head and Neck, Plastics, and Urology; The University of Alabama at Birmingham Hospital, Birmingham, Alabama

Sabrina Dollar Kopf, DNP, ACNP-BC, CRNP
Assistant Professor, Acute, Chronic and Continuing Care, UAB School of Nursing, Nurse Practitioner, Division of Infectious Disease, The University of Alabama at Birmingham, Birmingham, Alabama

Gary W. Milligan, DNP, MHSA, RN, CNE
Assistant Professor of Nursing, Nursing Acute, Chronic, and Continuing Care, Nursing Academic Affairs, The University of Alabama at Birmingham, Birmingham, Alabama

Laura Steadman, EdD, CRNP, MSN, RN
School of Nursing, The University of Alabama at Birmingham, Birmingham, Alabama

Preface

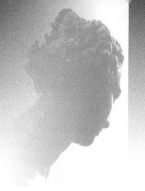

This fifth edition of *Advanced Health Assessment of Women: Skills, Procedures, and Management* is a comprehensive, user-friendly, clinically focused resource for busy clinicians, advanced practice students, and faculty. Previous editions focused on the assessment of women and related women's health skills and procedures. This fifth edition continues to provide updated skills and procedures, along with enhanced tables and figures, to help clearly describe these basic and advanced skills. Responding to reader requests, chapters now include (if appropriate) management/pharmacology summary charts and case studies. Instructor guides that include key statistics/epidemiology, learning objectives, suggested student activities, and self-assessment questions are available at www .connect.springerpub.com/content/book/978-0-8261-7963-0.

In this fifth edition, as we expanded into management of various women's health conditions, the need to include additional topics became apparent. This led to 14 new chapters written by content experts. These chapters include Chapter 4, "Telehealth in Women's Health"; Chapter 6, "Vaginal Microscopy and Vaginal Infections"; Chapter 11, "Mental Health Screening; Anxiety, Depression, Eating Disorders, PTSD, Substance Abuse, Suicide, Dementia"; Chapter 12, "Preconception Care"; Chapter 13, "Complementary and Alternative Medical Therapies"; Chapter 15, "Adolescent Health"; Chapter 16, "Lactation Assessment and Management"; Chapter 20, "Female Veterans: When the Woman Was a Warrior"; Chapter 21, "Male Sexual and Reproductive Health"; Chapter 29, "Amenorrhea"; Chapter 30, "Premenstrual Syndrome and Premenstrual Dysphoric Disorder"; Chapter 33, "Sexual Health and Related Problems"; Chapter 36, "Human Trafficking"; and Chapter 40, "The Contraceptive Consult."

Here are a few personal statements from health experts supporting the addition of the new chapters:

Chapter 4: Telehealth in Women's Health
"This chapter explores the basics of telehealth in women's healthcare. Telehealth in women's health is essential to providing accessible, innovative, and equitable healthcare services to the women's health gender-related population. In an ever-evolving healthcare landscape, understanding key components of telehealth service in women's health is critical to ensuring patients receive optimal care and health outcomes." — Shawana S. Moore, DNP, WHNP-BC (Chair, National Association of Nurse Practitioners in Women's Health and DNP Program Director for the Nell Hodgson Woodruff School of Nursing at Emory University)

Chapter 6: Vaginal Microscopy and Vaginal Infections
"Vaginitis is one of the most common reasons people seek gynecologic care. This chapter provides up to date assessment and management guidelines incorporating the 2021 CDC STD Treatment Guidelines. It also includes step-by-step instructions for microscopy as an aid for busy clinicians." — Hanne S. Harbison, MHSPH, MSN, WHNP-BC (WHNP Track Director for the University of Pennsylvania)

Chapter 11: Mental Health Screening
"Primary care is often the first point of contact for patients with concerns about their mental health. This chapter will help give a brief overview of common diagnoses and how to manage these conditions while within the setting of primary care. Mental health and mental illness can feel overwhelming, but the information and tools can help a clinician provide care not only for the physical health of a patient but also their mental health." — Elisabeth Maher, PMHNP-BC (Montefiore Medical Center)

Chapter 12: Preconception Care

"Preconception care is essential to increase chances of conception, prevent unintended pregnancies, and reduce risk factors that negatively impact maternal and fetal health. Clinicians should approach ALL patient encounters of all genders with reproductive potential as an opportunity to counsel regarding current holistic wellness and healthy habits which may improve reproductive and obstetric outcomes if their intent is to plan a future pregnancy." — Komkwuan Paruchabutr, DNP, CNM, WHNP-BC, FNP-BC, FACNM (Army Nurse Corps combat veteran, Operation Iraqi Freedom from 2003–2004)

Chapter 13: Complementary and Alternative Medical Therapies

"Many individuals are now utilizing and seeking out complementary/alternative practices as adjunct therapy to their medical care. Many have also chosen to discard traditional Western practice and solely rely upon nonmainstream therapies. While there exists a plethora of information available on the web, it is our responsibility and obligation to provide the most up-to-date and clinically relevant, evidence-based information to those we care for." — Iris Stendig-Raskin, WHNP-BC (Trinity Health Mid-Atlantic)

Chapter 15: Adolescent Health

"This chapter addresses the specific sexual and reproductive health needs of adolescents including care for common gynecologic conditions in adolescence as well as pregnancy. There is also information about mental health, suicide prevention, bullying, sexting, and age specific vaccination recommendations." — Hanne S. Harbison, MHSPH, MSN, WHNP-BC (WHNP Track Director for the University of Pennsylvania)

Chapter 16: Lactation Assessment and Management

"It is important for clinicians to provide women with the benefits and importance of breastfeeding, while understanding the barriers and factors that exist while counseling and educating. Women who identify with racial and ethnic minority groups that have shown lower rates of breastfeeding initiation and continuation, especially African American women, may benefit from targeted education, support, resources, and enhanced breastfeeding programs." — Jamille Nagtalon-Ramos, EdD, WHNP-BC, IBCLC, FAANP (Assistant Professor, Rutgers University)

Chapter 20: Female Veterans: When the Woman Was a Warrior

"This chapter provides the basics of identifying which of your patients are veterans, or have served in the armed forces, and how to care for them with dignity and respect, emphasizing trauma-informed care. Resources for women veterans' healthcare through the Veterans Health Administration are provided. The needs of women veterans are often challenging, but the rewards for the nurse practitioner and veterans can be gratifying." — Patrice Malena, MSN, WHNP-BC (Retired Women Veterans Program Manager at Hampton Veterans Administration Medical Center)

Chapter 21: Male Sexual and Reproductive Health

"This chapter examines normal and abnormal aspects of male sexual and reproductive health. Male sexual health has a significant impact on female health, relationships, family, and mental and physical health outcomes." — Randee Masciola, DNP, WHNP-BC, FAANP (Director, Doctor of Nursing Practice Program, The Ohio State University-College of Nursing)

Chapter 29: Amenorrhea

"There are various potential impacts of amenorrhea, including infertility, osteoporosis, metabolic disorders, emotional health issues, and depression." — Shelagh Larson, DNP, WHNP-BC, NCMP (AANP Texas Representative)

Chapter 30: Premenstrual Syndrome and Premenstrual Dysphoric Disorder
"It estimated that, at some point during a woman's life, nearly 75% will experience PMS-like symptoms." — Shelagh Larson, DNP, WHNP-BC, NCMP (AANP Texas Representative)

Chapter 33: Sexual Health and Related Problems
"Sexual health is a state of physical, emotional, mental, and social well-being in relation to sexuality; not merely the absence of disease, dysfunction, or infirmity." — Shelagh Larson, DNP, WHNP-BC, NCMP (AANP Texas Representative)

Chapter 36: Human Trafficking
"Human trafficking, also known as trafficking in persons or modern-day slavery, is a crime that involves compelling or coercing a person to provide labor or services or to engage in commercial sex acts."—Heather Quaile, DNP, WHNP-BC, CSC, IF (The SHOW Center in Kennesaw, Georgia)

Chapter 40: The Contraceptive Consult
"Shared decision-making with the patient is important with all factors considered when performing a contraceptive consult. Providing resources for patients to make informed choices is imperative." — Komkwuan Paruchabutr, DNP, CNM, WHNP-BC, FNP-BC, FACNM (Army Nurse Corps combat veteran, Operation Iraqi Freedom from 2003–2004)

This comprehensive manual contains essential content focused on improving the quality of healthcare provided to women/persons with a vagina across the life span. Today's women/persons with a vagina are empowered and proactive, actively seeking access to high-quality and sensitive care, which is a key component in the prescription for women's health equity. The majority of individuals who seek healthcare are women/persons with a vagina. In addition, as baby boomers age at record numbers, an increasing number of women are seeking professional care.

In today's rapidly changing healthcare climate, advanced practice clinicians are well positioned and qualified to care for the unique healthcare needs of women/persons with a vagina. In addition, the scope of their practice is expanding to include more advanced clinical skills, procedures, and management. *Advanced Health Assessment of Women: Skills, Procedures, and Management, Fifth Edition* provides clear and concise, factual information related to the health assessment and management of women/persons with a vagina. This text provides an enhanced definition of the role and clinical skills of providers, including physicians, physician assistants (PAs), certified nurse midwives (CNMs), and nurse practitioners (NPs). These practitioners play a vital role in managing the health of women/persons with a vagina in a variety of settings, including internal medicine and primary care; family practice; and specialty areas such as women's health, urogynecology, pelvic health, aesthetics, fertility, and obstetrics and gynecology.

Some of the procedures described in this manual are more advanced and are appropriate only within certain practice settings. It must be emphasized that advanced practice clinicians are under a mandate to practice within their legal and professional scope of practice, as well as within their personal comfort level. This is especially important when considering performing advanced techniques and procedures. Consult your state association and/or licensing board if you are uncertain about the legality of performing any of the procedures described in this text. The scope of practice varies among NPs, PAs, MDs, and CNMs in relation to educational programs, practice settings, geographical location, and state laws and regulations. This text provides guidance so that each practitioner may become increasingly aware of when to practice independently, when to co-manage, when to consult, and when to refer.

Many of the assessment skills, techniques, and procedures described are becoming integrated into the advanced practice clinician everyday practice. Advanced practice clinicians (NPs, PAs, midwives, physicians) are educated in a variety of different ways, with differing approaches within today's nursing and medical models. Master's-level and doctoral-level (DNP, PhD, EdD) curricula provide basic content for the advanced practice clinician (NP, CNM, MD, and PA), but may not provide sufficient education and training regarding advanced women's health skills and procedures. This text is designed to fill that gap.

The assessment of many aspects of care related to women/persons with a vagina is outlined, with sample assessment forms, such as the Assessment of Sexually Transmitted Infections, integrated throughout. In addition, many educational handouts—including a bladder-tracking diary and information on how to perform Kegel exercises—further enhance the educational aspects of the text. An outline format was chosen because this clear and concise layout allows the information to flow in a logical sequence without one having to wade through unnecessary jargon. When techniques are explained, a comprehensive list of equipment necessary for each technique or procedure is given as well as information on patient preparation and recommended follow-up. The entire text is enhanced with a plethora of boxes, figures, and tables. The practical format offers easy access to pertinent information.

The different techniques and procedures were selected because they are within the expanding scope of the practitioner's experience but are often not included in the advanced practice clinician's curriculum or described in assessment books. This manual delineates strategies that are on the leading edge in the expanded role of the advanced practice clinician. Obviously, one cannot expect to learn the technical aspects from simply reading about them. This manual provides a foundation for, and an understanding of, the rationale behind the assessments and procedures described. Please note that it is a good idea to observe a new procedure first and then be supervised for as many times as it takes to feel comfortable performing that procedure. Always carefully read manufacturers' recommendations that accompany any instrumentation you might use in addition to the information found in this text. This manual is not meant to dictate how procedures should be performed or to supply a strict recipe for techniques and procedures. It does, however, provide a clear starting point for developing practice guidelines specific to each individual's clinical scope, expertise, and practice setting.

All chapters have been updated and expanded to reflect current research, evidence-based clinical guidelines, and new technologies. The text begins with a comprehensive review of the basic anatomy and physiology of women/persons with a vagina. A complete understanding of the complexities of the menstrual cycle and normal vaginal flora, examined at the cellular level, is imperative for accurate understanding and diagnoses of conditions that affect this community.

Chapter 3, "The Health History," discusses elements of a comprehensive, developmentally relevant health history with a unique approach to the physiological, psychological, and sociocultural components involved. Advanced health history techniques are detailed in the context of an equal partnership between provider and patient. Critical issues related to the assessment of HIV infection are summarized. The basic techniques of the physical examination—with a focus on the gynecologic examination—are outlined, with possible clinical alterations listed for each area assessed. Evaluation of the breast includes basic techniques with a section on how to examine the augmented breast (an explanation not commonly found in traditional health assessment books).

Chapter 26, "Assessment of Vulvar Pain and Vulvodynia," addresses the diagnoses and management of vulvodynia and vestibulitis, including a new treatment summary table. Chapter 19, "Transgender Healthcare," has been updated with changing healthcare trends and increased recognition of the unique needs of special populations. Chapters on menopause (Chapter 22), cervical cancer screening (Chapter 45), and osteoporosis (Chapter 23) have also been extensively updated to reflect the most recent evidence-based clinical practice guidelines. Additional topics are explored; for example, the assessment of skin is described in Chapter 8, lesbian health in Chapter 18, pelvic pain in Chapter 25, abnormal uterine bleeding in Chapter 28, and polycystic ovarian syndrome (PCOS) in Chapter 27. PCOS, which is associated with serious cardiometabolic sequelae and other risks, is increasingly common and clinicians need to know how to assess, diagnose, and manage this condition. A new treatment summary table is also included in this updated chapter.

The chapter on lesbian health addresses critical aspects of taking a history and special considerations essential for all clinicians. Pelvic health issues are more evident as the population of women ages. Unique chapters include the investigative procedures and advanced skills sections as an adjunct to Chapter 3, describing pelvic organ prolapse, and Chapter 32, which explores treatment for urinary incontinence and includes information about pelvic floor electrical stimulation, pelvic floor rehabilitation, and percutaneous tibial nerve stimulation. Information provided in Chapter 6, "Vaginal Microscopy and Vaginal Infection," is the most comprehensive description of the interpretation and evaluation of the wet mount available in any current text. Chapter 45, "Cervical Cancer Screening and Colposcopy," covers the Pap test and human papillomavirus (HPV) and recommendations for interpretation and follow-up of an abnormal Pap test, reflecting the new American Society of Colposcopy and Cervical Pathology (ASCCP) guidelines for screening and follow-up. The new recommendations for HPV testing are also included.

Chapter 47, "Urinalysis and Urinary Tract Infections," offers a fresh look at an old test. The differential diagnosis of gynecologic versus urologic conditions is always challenging in women/persons with a vagina. This chapter contains an in-depth analysis of the components of urinalysis, and a step-by-step explanation of urine microscopy—a skill with which every advanced practice clinician should feel comfortable. Concerns of older women/persons with a vagina are addressed in the comprehensive new sections on menopause and urinary incontinence. Mastering the technique of acrochordonectomy, or the removal of skin tags, described in Chapter 50 will please many patients bothered by skin tags. New information on how to perform a simple cystometrogram, provided in Chapter 57, is important in diagnosing the cause of urinary incontinence. Two newly emerging techniques that are becoming an integral part of assessment of women are sonohysteroscopy and bone densitometry. The various machines used are described and interpretation of results is clearly explained.

Up-to-date information on emerging topics such as *BRCA* gene testing is provided. Content on *BRCA* gene testing in Chapter 46 will help identify those women at risk and provide the clinician with skills necessary to help a woman choose whether or not to be tested. Chapter 37, "Initial Evaluation of Infertility," has been updated and presents guidelines for the assessment, evaluation, and management of the woman/person with a vagina who is unable to conceive. Controversies and clinical dilemmas are explained. Techniques for evaluation of the infertile woman/person with a vagina and intrauterine and donor insemination are clearly delineated. In Unit VI, there is critical information regarding women at risk including a new important chapter on human trafficking. A nationally tested questionnaire is included to help identify the victims of violence and abuse. Management guidelines and follow-up of the rape victim are also included.

Another unique section of this text is found in Chapter 53, "Pessary Insertion." Such descriptive information is not found in any comparable text. As baby boomers age, the incidence of genital prolapses, often accompanied by incontinence, is increasing. A decade ago, use of pessaries was replaced by surgical alternatives, which were not risk free. Today pessaries offer a viable conservative alternative to urologic surgery. The fitting of pessaries requires patience, knowledge, and experience. Advanced-level clinicians are in a key position to assume care of this rapidly expanding population of women. Emphasis is now appropriately placed on the broader issue of pelvic health and wellness and away from specific entities such as urinary incontinence.

Technical skills related to insertion of various contraceptive devices are outlined in Unit VIII. Characteristics, such as the advantages and disadvantages, mechanisms of action, and contraindications of each device, are necessary to educate the woman/person with a vagina in making an informed decision regarding their contraceptive management. The techniques of fitting contraceptive devices and follow-up care are outlined in detail. In Chapter 42, information on the technique of insertion and removal of Nexplanon and use of the FemCap are clearly described, with figures supplied for clarification. Chapter 43, "Intrauterine Contraception," has been expanded to include not only the levonorgestrel-containing Mirena, but also the new, smaller Kyleena and Skyla devices.

In Unit X, the more advanced techniques are explained. Performing an endometrial biopsy requires skill and practice. It is also important to understand the indications for biopsy, its implications, and interpretation of the results. Chapter 49 describes the necessary equipment required and walks the practitioner through each step.

SUMMARY

Advanced Health Assessment of Women offers a variety of clinical tools to enhance content. Feel free to use any information provided and adapt it to your organization. Readers have access to online step-by-step videos of five office gynecology simulations: treatment of condyloma with trichloro-acetic acid (TCA), endocervical polypectomy, vulvar biopsy, endometrial biopsy, and incision and drainage of a Bartholin glad abscess with Word catheter placement (https://www.uab.edu/nursing/home/technology-innovation/faculty-clinician-resources/gyn-procedures). These videos are the intellectual property of the University of Alabama at Birmingham and are available in the public domain for educational purposes only.

Many chapters, when appropriate, now include management/treatment summary sections at the end of each chapter. Students and busy clinicians alike will welcome the addition of these treatment summaries. **Qualified instructors may obtain access to ancillary instructor manual, instructor test bank, and PowerPoints by emailing textbook@springerpub.com or by going to connect .springerpub.com/content/book/978-0-8261-7963-0.** This text offers practical guidance to help advanced practice students, preceptors, faculty, and clinicians. The content reflects an extensive review of current literature integrated with our authors' extensive years of clinical experience and teaching. In addition, we welcome our expanded panel of advanced practice clinicians from a wide variety of women's health specialties who have generously shared their expertise as contributing authors and reviewers.

R. Mimi Secor
Aimee Chism Holland

Acknowledgments

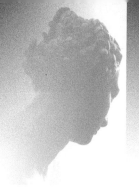

Thanks to my new co-editor, Dr. Aimee Chism Holland, for her expert help and support throughout the lengthy process of updating the fifth edition of our textbook. You've been a pleasure to work with and I'm very grateful for our new partnership. Together, with your creative ideas and suggestions, we've added 14 new chapters, many new authors, and several new sections. I also want to thank my nursing colleagues and friends; husband, Mike; and daughter, Katherine, for their understanding and support throughout this extensive process. Finally, I'd like to thank my mom, who recently passed, for always believing in me (often before I believed in myself) and encouraging my career ambitions.

—*R. Mimi Secor*

Dr. Mimi Secor, you have been a wonderful co-editor! Thank you for inviting me to take this journey with you and for mentoring me. I appreciate the opportunity to join you for this important work and for the sincere respect and kindness you have continuously demonstrated each step of the way. You are the real deal and you make the world a better place! I also want to thank my precious, supportive family: my husband, Tim Holland; my parents, Billy and Mary Dell Chism; and my sweet furbabies. I am grateful for my colleagues at the University of Alabama at Birmingham School of Nursing, the University of Alabama at Birmingham Student Health and Wellness Clinic, and the National Association of Nurse Practitioners in Women's Health (NPWH) for their continuous support of my passion for women's health! Finally, I acknowledge my faith in Jesus Christ who sustains me daily and gives me incomparable joy, hope, and peace (Philippians 1).

—*Aimee Chism Holland*

The preparation of this fifth edition of *Advanced Health Assessment of Women* was exciting, challenging, and, as usual, a lot of hard work, which we could not have managed without the many people who helped make it all happen.

We are ***enormously grateful*** to Lucia Gunzel, our Senior Content Development Editor, for her excellent work organizing our textbook project so we could successfully complete this enormous task efficiently and while minimizing our stress. Her organizational skills and upbeat "can do" attitude helped us meet our deadlines and maintain momentum throughout the project.

We also acknowledge and thank Elizabeth Nieginski, VP/Publisher; Joe Morita, Executive Acquisitions Editor; and Diana Osborne, Production Manager, for their support and assistance through the lengthy publication process.

We are so thankful to all our contributing authors for accepting our invitation, and for including the most current content, following the format guidelines, and meeting the deadlines for submission. We are grateful for their outstanding contributions to our new edition.

Finally, we thank Springer Publishing Company for their dedication to educating advanced practice clinicians (NPs, PAs, CNWs, and physicians) and for their commitment to promoting excellence in women's healthcare.

Teamwork truly made this dream work, and we are grateful for each member of this amazing team who contributed to the firth edition of *Advanced Health Assessment of Women*!

Instructor Resources

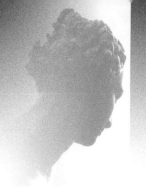

A robust set of instructor resources designed to supplement this text is located at http://connect .springerpub.com/content/book/978-0-8261-7963-0. Qualifying instructors may request access by emailing textbook@springerpub.com.

Instructor resources include:

- Instructor Manual
- PowerPoint Presentations for each chapter
- Instructor Test Bank
- Mapping to AACN Essentials: Core Competencies for Professional Nursing Education

FEMALE REPRODUCTION

1

ANATOMY AND PHYSIOLOGY OF THE URINARY AND REPRODUCTIVE SYSTEMS

WILLIAM E. SOMERALL AND HELEN A. CARCIO

GENERAL OVERVIEW

A. The female urinary and reproductive systems are near to, but separate, from each other, unlike the male.
B. The internal female reproductive organs are located in the lower pelvis inside the bony pelvis, behind the pubic bone.
C. The external genitalia collectively include the mons pubis, the labia majora, the labia minora, the vestibule, the clitoris, and the vaginal orifice (Figure 1.1).
D. The structures of the peritoneum are listed and compared in Table 1.1.

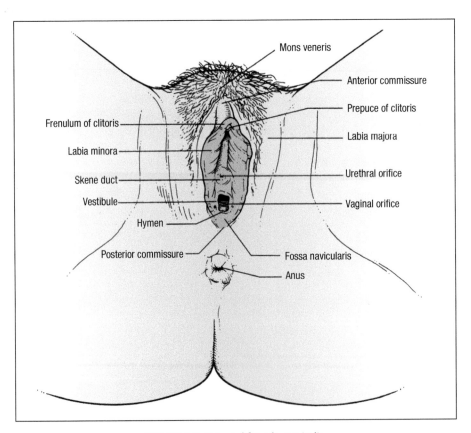

FIGURE 1.1 External female genitalia.

TABLE 1.1 Structure, Functions, and Purposes of the Organs of Female Reproduction

STRUCTURE	FUNCTIONS	PURPOSES
External genitalia	Sensitive to touch and external stimulation	Sexual arousal and sensation of orgasm
Vagina	Passage for intercourse Provides space for containment of sperm Excretory outlet for the uterus Becomes birth canal during the birthing process	Organ of copulation
Cervix	Fibrous, muscular band that holds the bottom of the uterus closed and keeps the fetus inside the uterus during pregnancy	Major source of mucus production during the menstrual cycle
Uterus	Organ of menstruation	Fertilized egg implants here Maintains and protects developing fetus until birth Contracts during labor to birth the neonate
Fallopian tubes	Transport of sperm upward Transport of the egg downward	Location of fertilization of the egg Carries the egg to the uterus
Ovaries	Maturation and development of eggs Release of eggs Secrete hormones, including estrogen, progesterone, and small amounts of testosterone	Produce eggs during ovulation

OVARIES

A. Description
   1. Each ovary lies behind the broad ligament on either side of the uterus.
   2. Ovaries vary considerably in size among women, but usually measure between 3 and 5 cm long, 1.5 and 3 cm wide, and 1 and 1.5 cm thick.
   3. Ovaries are pinkish white to gray.
   4. They are not directly attached to the uterus or fallopian tubes. The ovaries lie suspended by the broad ligament, a thin peritoneal film attached to a flexible structure called the *round ligament.* The round ligament is a suspensory ligament that helps anchor the uterus in the mid-pelvis.
   5. The fallopian tubes, also called oviducts, are attached to the fundus of the uterus. They are not directly connected to the ovaries but open into the peritoneal cavity near the ovaries.
B. Function
   1. The ovaries house the female sex gametes.
   2. The ovaries secrete the female sex hormones, estrogen and progesterone. A small amount of testosterone is also produced.
   3. The ovaries produce an ovum (egg) during ovulation in response to hormonal stimulation.

FALLOPIAN TUBES

A. Description
   1. The fallopian tubes extend outward from both sides of the uterus and act as a connecting conduit between the ovary and the uterus.

2. Fallopian tubes are approximately 13 cm (5 in.), rubbery, and less than half the diameter of a pencil (0.05–1.0 cm).
3. They have two layers—inner and outer serous layers—that surround the layers of involuntary muscle.
4. Fallopian tubes are narrow and muscular and lined with cilia.
5. Fallopian tubes consist of four sections.
   a. Interstitial section, which lies within the uterine wall
   b. Isthmus
      (1) The isthmus is the narrowest section closest to the uterus.
      (2) The isthmus opens into the cavity of the uterus.
      (3) It has a thick muscular wall.
   c. Ampulla
      (1) The ampulla is the longest section.
      (2) It widens progressively to the wide distal opening in the infundibulum.
      (3) It is thin walled.
      (4) Fertilization of the egg occurs in the ampulla.
   d. Infundibulum or fimbria
      (1) The infundibulum is the fimbriated end that lies in close proximity to the ovary.
      (2) Finger-like projections at the ends of the tubes are the *fimbriae*. The fimbriae, which sweep over the ovary, grasp the egg and transport it toward the inner ampullae.

B. Function
   1. Transports the sperm and the egg (Box 1.1).
      a. The inner wall of the fallopian tubes is lined with hair-like projections called cilia.
      b. The peristaltic motion of the cilia transports the fertilized egg through the tube to the uterus, where a fertilized egg may be implanted.

BOX 1.1 Transport of the Egg by the Fallopian Tubes

Egg is released during ovulation
↓
Egg is picked up by petals of fimbriae
↓
Egg enters the fallopian tube at the infundibulum
↓
Fertilization occurs in the ampulla
↓
The ampulla transports a fertilized egg (ovum) in the direction of the uterus (tube progressively narrows from the flared tips)
↓
Muscle contractions and ciliary action in the tube help propel the egg
↓
The egg enters the uterus from the isthmus
↓
Implantation of the egg in the wall of the uterus
↓
Pregnancy

      c. Muscle contractions in the fallopian tube assist in moving the egg along its journey, much as in intestinal peristalsis.

      d. Fallopian tubes have the unique ability to transport the egg in one direction and the sperm in the opposite direction.

  2. Collects the egg.

      a. The cilia on the fimbriae have adhesive sites that help draw the egg into the fallopian tube.

      b. Near the time of ovulation, the fimbriae bend down in proximity to the ovaries.

      c. The sweeping motion of the fimbriae locates and transports the egg.

THE UTERUS

A. Description of the uterine corpus, or uterine body

  1. The uterus is shaped like an inverted pear.

  2. The uterus is a hollow, thick-walled muscle located posterior to the bladder and anterior to the rectum.

  3. The size and the shape of the non-pregnant uterus vary.

      a. Length—7.5 cm (3 in.)

      b. Width—5 cm (2 in.)

      c. Depth—2.5 cm (1 in.)—a little smaller than a fist

  4. The uterus consists of two sections, roughly divided in the middle at the isthmus.

      a. Upper portion

         (1) The corpus—the main body

         (2) The fundus—the dome-shaped portion located at the point at which the fallopian tubes enter the uterus

      b. Lower, narrower portion—the cervix

  5. The uterus is mobile and expands readily to accommodate a developing fetus.

  6. The uterine artery is the main blood supply to the uterus.

  7. The uterus is supported by the levator ani muscle and eight ligaments.

  8. Major ligaments that help the uterus remain supported in mid-position are the elastic broad ligaments, which act as "guide wires."

  9. The position of the uterus within the pelvis varies (Figure 1.2).

      a. Anteverted/anteflexed—tilted toward the bladder

      b. Retroverted/retroflexed—tilted toward the rectum

      c. Mid-position—found less frequently

      d. Positions do not affect fertility

 10. Relationship of the uterine body to the cervix

      a. Anteflexed—the anterior surface bends toward the cervix

      b. Retroflexed—the posterior surface bends toward the cervix

 11. The uterus is a freely movable organ suspended in the pelvic cavity and actual placement varies as the woman changes position.

 12. The wall of the uterus consists of three layers.

      a. Perimetrium—the serosal external peritoneal covering

      b. Myometrium—the middle muscular layer

      c. Endometrium—the inner glandular layer of the cavity

         (1) The function of the endometrium is controlled hormonally.

         (2) It is involved with menstruation or implantation of the placenta.

B. Description of the uterine cervix

  1. The uterine cervix is visible and palpable in the upper vagina and is a knob-like structure.

  2. It is smooth, shiny, and pink.

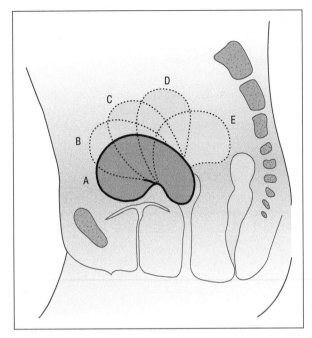

FIGURE 1.2 Positions of the uterus: (A) anteflexion; (B) anteversion, the normal position; (C) midposition; (D) retroversion; (E) retroflexion.

3. It is firmer to palpation than the uterine corpus because it contains more connective tissues. (It feels like the dense cartilage of the nose.)
4. The cervix is covered by two types of epithelium
   a. Squamous epithelium
      (1) The squamous epithelium is pink and shiny and is contiguous with the vaginal lining.
   b. Columnar epithelium
      (1) The columnar epithelium is deep red and is an extension of the lining of the endocervical canal.
5. The cervical opening, the *external os*, connects the vagina to the endocervical canal, which connects to the body of the uterus.
6. The size of the external os varies.
   a. The external os is a very small, round opening in women who have not given birth vaginally.
   b. The external os is more open, slit-like, and irregular in women who have had children vaginally.
   c. The os becomes tight and very small in postmenopausal women because of a decrease in estrogen levels.
C. Description of nabothian cysts
   1. The surface of the cervix normally has glands that secrete mucus in response to hormonal stimulation.
   2. The ducts can become obstructed and cystic.
   3. The extent of obstruction varies from a few tiny cysts to large cysts covering the entire cervix.
   4. Nabothian cysts are common; however, infection may increase their number.
D. Description of endocervical canal
   1. The endocervical canal is open at both ends, connecting the external os to the internal os.

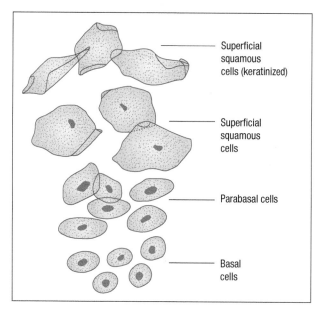

FIGURE 1.3 Layers of squamous epithelium.

2. The os is about 2 to 2.5 cm (1 in.) and is lined by columnar epithelium.
3. The *ectocervix* is the cervical portion extending outward from the external cervical os.
   a. Anterior lip—the portion above the cervical os
   b. Posterior lip—the portion below the cervical os
4. The *endocervix* is a narrow column, extending upward from the external os to the internal os of the uterine endometrium.

E. The cervical epithelium is composed of squamous and columnar epithelia.
   1. Squamous epithelium
      a. Squamous epithelium is smooth, shiny, pink, and covers the ectocervix.
      b. It has four main layers, similar to the skin (Figure 1.3).
         (1) Basal layer—lies within the thin basement membrane. This layer is one or two cells thick. All ectocervical cells arise from the basal layer.
         (2) Parabasal layer—this layer has three or four cell layers.
         (3) Intermediate layer—this layer is thicker than the parabasal and basal layers.
         (4) Superficial layer—this layer is composed of mature cells that continuously shed. It is the thickest layer.
   2. Columnar epithelium
      a. The columnar epithelium is dark red and granular.
      b. Columnar epithelium lines the endocervical canal and secretes mucus.
   3. Squamocolumnar junction or transformation zone
      a. This junction is the boundary between the squamous and columnar epithelia.
      b. Squamous metaplasia occurs naturally as columnar epithelium is changed to squamous epithelium. (It is differentiated.)
      c. The area of metaplasia is the area of endocervical cells, which is critical to sampling during the routine Pap test because it is particularly susceptible to neoplastic changes.
      d. The location of the squamocolumnar junction varies with hormonal variation.
         (1) In adolescents, the junction is visible on the external cervix.

TABLE 1.2 Comparison of Fertile and Non-Fertile Cervical Mucus	
OVULATORY FERTILE MUCUS	**NONOVULATORY MUCUS**
Clear to slightly cloudy	Opaque
Abundant	Scant
Stretchy, like raw egg white	Non-stretchy
Slippery	Rubbery
Dries without residue	Leaves white flakes when dry

    (2) The squamocolumnar junction extends up the canal as estrogen levels decrease and is termed *eversion, ectropion,* or *ectopy* if visible on the ectocervix as a granular, red, well-circumscribed area.

F. Cervical mucus—changes in response to hormonal variations (Table 1.2).

VAGINA

A. Description of the vaginal canal
1. The vaginal canal is a fibromuscular canal approximately 7.5 cm (3 in.) long located between the rectum, posteriorly, anterior to the urethra.
2. The vagina is lined with squamous epithelia arranged in folds called *rugae,* extending from the cervix to the vestibule.
3. The vagina extends from the vaginal *introitus* on the outside of the body to the uterus.
4. The muscular coat of the vagina is much thinner than that of the uterus.
5. The uterine cervix protrudes into the upper vagina, causing the formation of deeper rings around the cervix, called *fornices.*
6. The vagina can stretch and contract easily during intercourse or delivery.
7. It is usually pink-red.
8. The vagina does not contain mucous-secreting glands.
    a. It is moistened by cervical secretions.
    b. Additional fluids percolate into the vagina from other fluid compartments during sexual arousal.
9. The blood supply of the vagina is supplied by the vaginal branches of the uterine artery.

B. The vagina serves as a passageway for:
1. Menstrual blood flow from the uterus
2. Expulsion of a fetus from the uterus
3. Sperm to travel toward the egg

C. Vaginal ecology
1. The vaginal epithelium contains large amounts of glycogen.
2. Normal bacterial florae of the vagina consist of:
    a. *Lactobacillus,* which metabolizes the glycogen and produces lactic acid which helps maintain the vaginal pH as acidic, thus decreasing bacteria.

D. Hymen
1. The hymen is a folded membrane of connective tissue located at the outer opening of the vagina.
2. The hymen may nearly occlude the vaginal opening in women who have never had sexual intercourse or who have never used tampons.

E. Bartholin glands
1. The Bartholin glands are two small, bean-shaped glands and are located on either side of the vagina, deep in the labia minora.
2. The glands secrete a mucosal substance that helps lubricate the vaginal canal.
F. Fornix
1. The fornix is a deep ring that posteriorly surrounds the cervix where it protrudes through the upper vagina.
2. It is comparatively thin walled and allows palpation of the ovaries and the uterus.
3. Following ejaculation during intercourse, semen pools in the fornix. This provides a time-release effect as the sperm intermittently swim through the cervix.

PELVIC SUPPORT

A. All the internal reproductive organs are supported in a sling-like fashion by ligaments that are covered by peritoneal folds.
B. The pelvic and urogenital diaphragms provide support for the perineum (Figure 1.4).
1. The pelvic diaphragm
   a. The pelvic diaphragm is also known as the *pelvic floor.*
   b. It forms an occlusive bowl-shaped muscular sheet that supports the abdominal and pelvic organs and that:
      (1) Stabilizes and protects them during periods of increased intra-abdominal pressure such as coughing or heavy lifting.
      (2) Controls and tightens the sphincters around the urethra and anal canal to maintain continence.
   c. These muscles work differently from most other muscles in the body, which are usually in a state of relaxation unless performing a task.
      (1) In contrast, pelvic floor muscles continuously maintain a low level of contraction that allows them to continuously stabilize and support the pelvic organs in proper position.
      (2) The normal resting tone of the muscles squeezes the rectum, vagina, and urethra closed by compressing them against the pubic bone.
   d. The pelvic diaphragm rests at the bottom of the pelvis and is primarily formed by the levator ani muscle group, consisting of the pubococcygeus muscle.

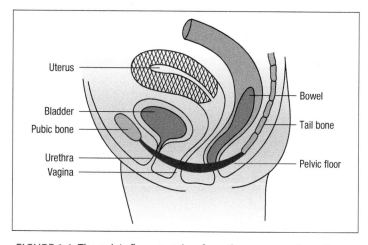

FIGURE 1.4 The pelvic floor stretches from the coccyx to the tailbone.

     (1) The pubococcygeus muscle, as the name implies, stretches like a muscular trampoline from where it arises at the pubic bone to where it inserts in the coccyx.

     (2) It forms the anterior portion of the levator ani and is mainly responsible for maintaining continence.

     (3) There are three holes that open to and through this muscular band. These structures are the urethra, vagina, and anal canal, which open and close to allow urine and feces to flow out of the body.

    e. The pubic portion of the pelvic diaphragm is a 2- to 2.5-cm band. The fibers pass backward from the pubis to encircle the rectum where fibers pass behind the vagina and support the lateral wall of the vagina.

    f. The muscles and ligaments within the pelvis support the bladder, uterus, urethra, and rectum—they also hold the pelvic organs in position and help them function properly.

  2. The urogenital diaphragm

    a. The urogenital diaphragm is the triangular area between the ischial tuberosities and the symphysis pubis. It contains the urethral striated sphincter muscles, trigone fascia, and the inferior urogenital trigone fascia.

    b. It provides support for the lower urethra and the anterior wall of the vaginal canal.

UTERINE LIGAMENTS

A. Broad ligaments
  1. The broad ligaments are two thin, film-like structures extending from the lateral margin of the uterus to the pelvic walls, dividing the uterine cavity into anterior and posterior compartments.
  2. Cardinal ligament
    a. The lower portion of the cardinal ligament is composed of dense connective tissue that is firmly joined to the supravaginal portion of the cervix.
  3. The cardinal ligaments support the vagina and prevent uterine prolapse.

B. Round ligaments
  1. The round ligaments are fibrous cords.
  2. They attach to either side of the fundus, just below the fallopian tubes and extend through the inguinal canal and attach in the upper portion of the labia minora as an aid in holding the fundus forward.

C. Uterosacral ligaments (two)
  1. The uterosacral ligaments are dense, cord-like structures that extend from the posterior cervical portion of the uterus and attach to the sacrum.
  2. The uterosacral ligaments help support the cervix.

D. Uterovesical ligament
  1. The uterovesical ligament is a fold of peritoneum that passes over the fundus, extending to the bladder.

E. Rectovaginal ligament
  1. The rectovaginal ligament is a fold of peritoneum that passes over the posterior surface of the uterus.

ASSOCIATED PELVIC ORGANS

A. Bladder (see Chapter 32, "Urinary Incontinence"). The lower urinary tract system (LUTS) consists of the bladder and urethra.
  1. Location of the bladder
    a. The bladder is located anteriorly in the pelvis, immediately posterior to the pubic symphysis.
    b. The bladder has three layers (Figure 1.5).

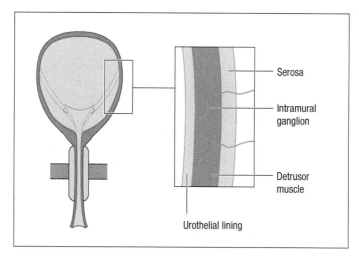

FIGURE 1.5 Bladder wall.

    (1) Outer layer—an adventitious layer of connective tissue that is covered by the peritoneum of the anterior wall of the pelvis.
    (2) Middle layer—consists of the detrusor muscle, which facilitates bladder emptying.
    (3) Inner layer—lined with uroepithelium (transitional epithelium).
  c. When the bladder is empty, it is flatter and tucked securely behind the pubic bone.
  d. The bladder fills from the bottom, where the ureters insert on either side of the trigone (forms the three angles that consist of the orifice of the two ureters and the urethra) of the bladder. As urine accumulates in the bladder, the dome of the bladder stretches and fills, rising above the symphysis pubis (Figure 1.6).

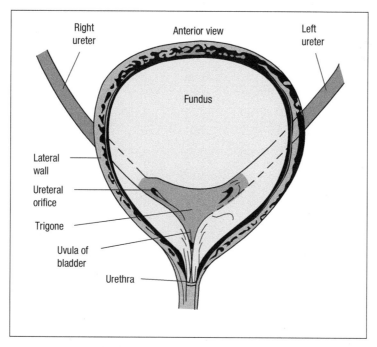

FIGURE 1.6 The trigone, the triangular region between the bilateral ureters and the urethra. (Note how the urine enters the bladder from the bottom and as it fills the distensible fundus rises and enlarges.)

e. The bladder fills at about 1 mL/min.

f. The sympathetic nervous system controls detrusor relaxation and urethral and bladder neck contraction.

g. The parasympathetic system stimulates bladder contraction that empties the bladder when intravesical pressure exceeds the bladder sphincter pressure.

h. The somatic nervous system controls the external sphincter and the pelvic floor via the pudendal nerve.

i. The bladder is also supported in proper position by the pubococcygeus muscle.

B. Urethra

1. Description

a. The urethra is a small tube, 2.5 to 5.0 cm long.

b. It is 2 to 8 mm wide.

2. The orifice lies between the labia minora, anterior to the vagina, approximately 2 cm posterior to the clitoris.

BIBLIOGRAPHY

Ashton-Miller, J. A., Howard, D., & DeLancey, J. O. (2001). The functional anatomy of the female pelvic floor and stress continence control system. *Scandinavian Journal of Urology and Nephrology, 2001*(207), 1–7. https://doi.org/10.1080/003655901750174773.

Bharucha, A. E. (2006). Pelvic floor: Anatomy and function. *Journal of Neurogastroenterology and Motility, 18*(7), 507–519. https://doi.org/10.1111/j.1365-2982.2006.00803.x

Bickley, L. (2021). *Bates' guide to physical examination and history taking* (13th ed.). Wolters Kluwer.

Blumenthal, P. D., & Berek, J. C. (2013). *A practical guide to office gynecologic procedures*. Lippincott Williams & Wilkins.

Pair, L. P, & Somerall, W.E., Jr. (2018). Urinary incontinence: Pelvic floor muscle and behavioral training for women. *Nurse Practitioner, 43*(1), 21–25. https://doi.org/10.1097/01.NPR.0000527571.66854.0d

Schuiling, K.D., & Likis, F.E. (2022). *Women's gynecologic health* (4th ed.). Jones & Bartlett Learning.

Secor, M., & Fantasia, H. (2018). *Fast facts about the gynecologic exam: A professional guide for NPs, PAs, and midwives* (2nd ed.). Springer Publishing.

2

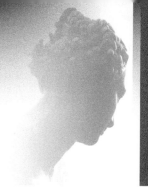

THE REPRODUCTIVE CYCLE

TONIA MOORE-DAVIS, GINNY MOORE, AND HELEN A. CARCIO

REPRODUCTIVE CYCLE

A. The female reproductive cycle is regulated through highly coordinated functions of the hypothalamus, the pituitary gland, the ovaries, and the uterus.
B. Each component must be in communication with the others to stimulate or suppress one of the other hormones.
C. Communication among the component organs is accomplished through various positive and negative feedback mechanisms.
D. Under the influence of these hormonal signals, the ovaries and uterus function in cyclical patterns that intimately parallel each other.

HORMONAL INFLUENCES EXPLAINED

A. Hypothalamus
   1. The cells of the hypothalamus produce gonadotropin-releasing hormone (GnRH).
   2. GnRH regulates the release of hormones from the anterior pituitary gland.
      a. Increases in the pulsatile secretion of GnRH are responsible for the initiation of puberty.
      b. Timing of puberty is regulated by genetic factors and is highly sensitive to nutritional status, environmental factors, and socioeconomic conditions.
B. Pituitary gland
   1. Under the influence of GnRH from the hypothalamus, the pituitary gland secretes two hormones: follicle stimulating hormone (FSH) and lutenizing hormone (LH)
   2. FSH and LH affect the female reproductive tract. These hormones are directly concerned with gonadal function and, therefore, are classified as gonadotropic hormones.
      a. FSH stimulates the development of the follicles in the ovary, which leads to the ripening of the follicle, ovulation, and the secretion of estrogens.
      b. LH stimulates the maturing follicle before its rupture and is directly responsible for the release of the ovum during ovulation.
      c. FSH stimulates the first part of the ovarian cycle; LH, together with FSH, influence pre-ovulatory enlargement, ovulation, and development of the corpus luteum (Box 2.1).
C. Ovaries
   1. Under the influence of gonadotrophic hormones from the pituitary gland, the ovaries secrete two hormones: estrogen and progesterone.
      a. Basic functions of estrogen
         (1) Produces all the physical characteristics of a mature female.
         (2) Helps prepare the endometrium of the uterus for implantation by a fertilized egg.
         (3) Helps regulate the production and release of FSH and LH by the pituitary gland.
         (4) Intensifies the effects of progesterone.
         (5) Together with FSH, helps promote the growth and development of the primary follicle.

BOX 2.1 Hormonal Influences in the Reproductive Cycle

Oocytes recruited and mature in the follicular phase
(under influence of FSH)
↓
Dominance of one follicle
↓
Grows and matures while others regress
↓
Final maturation and release of dominant follicle (under influence LH)

Ovarian Cycle	**Endometrial Cycle**
↓	↓
Ovulation occurs	Estrogen increases
↓	↓
Egg fertilized in fallopian tube	Endometrium proliferates
↓	↓
Egg transported to uterus	Secretory endometrium forms (under progesterone influence)

↓
Implantation of the embryo
↓
Secretion of hCG
↓
Stimulates corpus luteum
↓
Increases production of estrogen and progesterone
↓
Maintains pregnancy

FSH, follicle-stimulating hormone; hCG, human chorionic gonadotropin; LH, luteinizing hormone.

    b. Basic functions of progesterone
      (1) After ovulation, progesterone prepares the uterus for pregnancy by promoting the growth of secretory endometrial cells.
      (2) If pregnancy occurs, progesterone acts to maintain the placenta and inhibits uterine contraction to prevent abortion of the embryo.

(3) The corpus luteum forms from the residual parts of the ruptured ovarian follicle and is the main source of progesterone in the second half of the reproductive cycle.

D. Uterus
1. The endometrium undergoes cyclic changes in response to ovarian hormones.
2. Estrogen promotes growth of the endometrial lining and spiral arteries.
3. Progesterone stabilizes and maintains the endometrial lining by promoting maturation of endometrial glands and blood vessels.

THE OVARIAN CYCLE

A. Basics of the ovarian cycle
1. During hormonal stimulation, the ovary undergoes many changes that result in the development and release of an ovum and formation of a corpus luteum.
2. The ovarian cycle consists of three distinct phases: the follicular phase, ovulation, and the luteal phase.
  a. Follicular phase explained
    (1) At birth, each ovary contains about 400,000 primordial egg cells (oocytes).
    (2) These oocytes have a large nucleus with clear cytoplasm surrounded by theca and granuloma cells.
      • Oocytes secrete fluid to create the ovarian blister.
      • Theca cells are the primary source of circulating estrogens.
      • Granuloma cells are the source of estrogens in the follicular fluid.
    (3) A *primordial follicle* comprises an egg cell and its surrounding cells.
      • The production of primordial follicles stops around the time of birth of the fetus.
      • The primordial follicles are considered permanent cells.
      • Additional eggs are not produced throughout the woman's life cycle.
    (4) At the time of puberty, about 30,000 primordial follicles remain, which will either mature into eggs or disintegrate in the approximately 30 years of active ovarian activity between puberty and menopause.
    (5) In normally ovulating women, one egg will mature within a follicle each month, totaling between 300 and 400 eggs during the reproductive years.
  b. Ovulation explained
    (1) As the egg matures and the fluid pressure increases, the egg and the follicle are naturally moved toward the outside of the ovary.
    (2) The mature egg and the follicular fluid are now called a *graafian follicle.*
    (3) At some point, the graafian follicle thins to the outside edge of the ovary and ruptures into the area outside of the ovary.
    (4) The fimbriated edges of the fallopian tube draw the egg toward the tube.
  c. Luteal phase explained
    (1) Development of the corpus luteum
      • After ovulation, the spot at which the egg ruptured transforms itself.
      • Cells remaining in the follicle become filled with yellow-colored lutein material, and the follicle is now referred to as the *corpus luteum.*
    (2) The development of the corpus albicans
      • Approximately 8 days after ovulation, the corpus luteum reaches full maturity.
      • It slowly begins to evolve into a white body called the *corpus albicans.*
    (3) If conception and pregnancy occur, the corpus luteum increases in size and governs hormonal requirements during gestation, particularly for the first 4 months.
    (4) The principal hormone secreted by the corpus luteum is progesterone.
    (5) If conception does not occur, the progesterone secreted by the corpus luteum controls the postovulatory phase of the menstrual cycle for approximately 2 weeks.

THE ENDOMETRIAL CYCLE

A. Basics of the endometrial cycle
   1. Hormonal stimulation from the ovary stimulates simultaneous cyclical changes in the lining of the uterus (endometrium).
   2. These cycles correspond directly to phases that are occurring in the ovary (Table 2.1).
   3. The endometrial cycle is broken into three phases: proliferative, secretory, and menstruation.
      a. The proliferative phase explained
         (1) At the end of menstruation, the endometrium is thin and considered ischemic.
         (2) Within the second week of the cycle, hormonal production of estrogen increases, and the endometrium becomes thicker.
         (3) The cells undergo proliferative growth and become taller as the glandular cells become deeper and wider.
         (4) This thickness can increase up to eight times.
         (5) Glands of the endometrium become more active, secretory, and nutritive.
         (6) At the same time, the follicles (i.e., theca cells) are producing more follicular fluid containing estrogen, which further primes the uterine lining.
         (7) The proliferative phase of the endometrium is also called the *follicular phase* or *estrogenic phase* (to signify that the predominant hormone at this time is estrogen).
      b. The secretory phase explained
         (1) The secretory phase comprises the last 2 weeks (days 14–28) of the cycle.
         (2) After the egg is released from the follicle, the cells of the corpus luteum secrete progesterone, which governs the second half of the endometrial cycle.
         (3) Under the influence of progesterone and estrogen, the endometrial glands grow even more fluid filled and congested.
         (4) The blood supply of the endometrium increases, and the lining becomes filled with vacuoles and reservoirs that contain nutrient fluids.
         (5) The vascular arterioles become more spiral, twisted, and looped back, allowing for a nutritive layer if conception should occur.
         (6) Other names for this phase are *luteal* (referring to the ovary), *progestational* (referring to the dominant hormone), and *premenstrual* (see Table 2.1).
      c. The menstrual phase explained
         (1) If conception does not occur, the function of the corpus luteum wanes and levels of progesterone and estrogen decrease.
         (2) The lining of the endometrium becomes ischemic and cell degeneration occurs.
         (3) As further cell degeneration occurs, the cells rupture, bursting small arterioles.
         (4) The deteriorated endometrium sloughs off the uterine wall and passes through the vagina.
         (5) Menstruation allows the endometrial wall to be rebuilt with each monthly cycle, ensuring a fresh new lining for each possible conceptus.
         (6) This phase is called the *ischemic phase* or *menstruation.*

TABLE 2.1 Comparison of Nomenclature for the Various Phases of the Reproductive Cycle

DAY	PREDOMINANT HORMONE	OVARIAN CYCLE	ENDOMETRIAL CYCLE	MENSTRUAL CYCLE
Days 1–14	Estrogenic phase	Follicular phase	Proliferative phase	Menstrual phase (days 1–7)
Days 14–28	Progestational phase	Luteal phase	Secretory phase	Premenstrual phase (days 21–28)

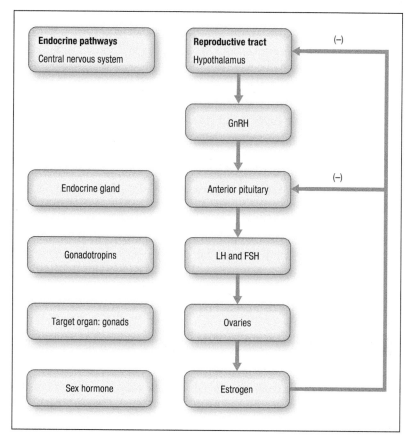

FIGURE 2.1 Feedback mechanism of the hypothalamic–pituitary–ovarian axis. Estrogen inhibits both the hypothalamus and the anterior pituitary.

FSH, follicle-stimulating hormone; GnRH, gonadotropin-releasing hormone; LH, luteinizing hormone.

HORMONAL REGULATION AND FEEDBACK MECHANISMS (FIGURE 2.1)

A. Each ovarian and endometrial cycle is regulated through the complex interaction of hypothalamic, pituitary, and ovarian hormones secreted in varying concentrations throughout the cycle.

B. To integrate the system, various feedback mechanisms organize the sequencing of hormones.

C. Within the hypothalamus, which is connected to the pituitary by a network of vessels called the *hypothalamic–hypophyseal (pituitary) portal system,* GnRH is secreted.

D. GnRH moves down the portal system to control the secretion of FSH, LH, and gonadotropin from the anterior pituitary.

E. FSH is active in the early and mid-cycle and controls the growth of the ovarian follicle; LH is most active in the mid- to late cycle (luteal phase) and controls the release of the ovum and promotes the secretion of progesterone from the corpus luteum.

F. The hypothalamus is influenced by the changes in neural and cerebral environments.

G. Prostaglandin also influences the cycle by influencing receptors in the hypothalamus.

H. At the start of each menstrual cycle, the pituitary secretes larger amounts of FSH, which, together with LH, promotes the maturation of several ovum follicles.

   1. The emission of LH and FSH in combination promotes the secretion of estradiol, the most active estrogen and the primary estrogen of younger women.

   2. Blood levels of estradiol begin to increase, and these increasing levels of estradiol provide negative feedback on the hypothalamic–pituitary secretion of FSH.
   3. The level of FSH begins to decrease, but FSH continues to work on the follicle in combination with LH to ripen one follicle.

I. On approximately day 12 (about 2 days before ovulation), most of the follicles that have ripened—except one—begin to degenerate or undergo atresia.

J. The follicle that is most mature continues to grow and, in turn, estrogen activity increases markedly.

K. Increasing amounts of estrogen secreted at this time promote secretion of GnRH (positive feedback), which causes LH to be released from the pituitary.

L. This LH spike provides the final stimulus for maturation of the follicle, and ovulation takes place within 1 to 2 days.

M. Changes in estrogen levels before ovulation prepare the cervical mucus to allow sperm to migrate up the reproductive tract.

N. Changes in mucus
   1. During the period immediately after menstruation, the mucus in the cervix is thick, scanty, and slightly opaque.
   2. Around the time of ovulation, the mucus becomes much thinner, clear, and stretchable to allow the passage of sperm.
   3. *Spinnbarkeit,* or stretchability of midcycle mucus, provides a good clinical assessment of cyclic changes.

O. After ovulation
   1. The ruptured follicle becomes a corpus luteum, which is supported by LH.
   2. The corpus luteum begins to secrete progesterone, and by cycle days 19 to 21, progesterone secretion is at its maximum to prepare for implantation.
   3. Increased progesterone levels after ovulation inhibit the secretion of FSH and LH (negative feedback).

P. If implantation occurs, another hormone produced by the chorionic villi of the conceptus/trophoblast called *human chorionic gonadotropin* (hCG; the hormone assayed in pregnancy tests) converts the corpus luteum into a corpus luteum of pregnancy to maintain its function to support the developing pregnancy.

Q. If pregnancy does not occur, the corpus luteum deteriorates, progesterone levels decrease markedly, and, without hormonal support, the endometrium begins to degenerate and sloughs off as menstrual flow.

BIBLIOGRAPHY

Allshouse, A., Pavlovic, J., & Santoro, N. (2018). Menstrual cycle hormone changes associated with reproductive aging and how they may relate to symptoms. *Obstetrics & Gynecology Clinics of North America, 45*(4), 613–628. https://doi.org/10.1016/j.ogc.2018.07.004

American College of Obstetricians and Gynecologists. (2015 December). *Menstruation in girls and adolescents: Using the menstrual cycle as a vital sign* (Committee Opinion No. 651). Reaffirmed 2020. https://www.acog.org/clinical/clinical-guidance/committee-opinion/articles/2015/12/menstruation-in-girls-and-adolescents-using-the-menstrual-cycle-as-a-vital-sign

Bickley, L. S. (2021). *Bates' guide to physical examination and history taking* (13th ed., pp. 697–705). Wolters Kluwer.

Rankin, J. (2017). *Physiology in childbearing with anatomy and related biosciences* (4th ed., pp. 33–42). Elsevier.

Schuiling, K. D., & Likis, F. E. (2022). *Gynecologic health care* (4th ed., pp. 94–98). Jones & Bartlett Learning.

Silverthorn, Dee U. (2019). *Human physiology: An integrated approach* (8th ed., pp. 815–823). Pearson Education.

Sultan, C., Gaspari, L., Maimoun, L., Kalfa, N., & Paris, F. (2018). Disorders of puberty. *Best Practice & Research Clinical Obstetrics & Gynaecology, 48*, 62–89. https://doi.org/10.1016/j.bpobgyn.2017.11.004

Taylor, H. S., Pal, L., & Seli, E. (2020). *Speroff's clinical gynecologic endocrinology and infertility* (9th ed.). Wolters Kluwer.

Valsamakis, G., Choruses, G., & Mastorakos, G. (2019). Stress, female reproduction and pregnancy. *Psychoneuroendocrinology, 100*, 48–57. https://doi.org/10.1016/j.psyneuen.2018.09.031

Unit II

HEALTH ASSESSMENT

3

THE HEALTH HISTORY

PAULA BROOKS AND HELEN A. CARCIO

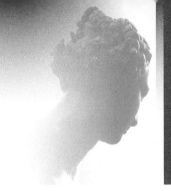

DEFINITION OF *SEXUAL HEALTH*

A. *Sexual health* is defined as the integration of somatic, emotional, intellectual, and social aspects of sexual beings in ways that are positively enriching and that enhance personality, communication, and love.

B. It is multidimensional and involves sexual attitudes, behavior, practices, and activity.

C. Its definition incorporates the whole person, including sexual thoughts, experiences, and values about being male or female. The three key elements of sexual health include:

1. A capacity to enjoy and control sexual and reproductive behavior in accordance with a personal and social ethic

2. Freedom from fear, shame, guilt, false beliefs, and other psychological factors that inhibit sexual response and impair sexual relationships

3. Freedom from organic disorders, diseases, and deficiencies that interfere with sexual and reproductive functions

ELEMENTS OF A COMPREHENSIVE, DEVELOPMENTALLY RELEVANT SEXUAL HEALTH ASSESSMENT

A. Interviewing to gather information regarding a patient's sexual history is an art requiring grace and skill that can only come with practice.

B. Sexuality underlies much of who and what a person is, and it is an inherent, ever-changing aspect of life from birth to death.

C. The sexual assessment must include a physiologic, psychological, and sociocultural evaluation, as well as elements that focus on age-related issues.

1. **The physiologic component:** Data should be gathered regarding the client's sexual response cycle (i.e., excitement, plateau, orgasm, and resolution) and any alterations in those phases. Also ask about:

   a. Attempts to conceive
   b. Previous high-risk pregnancies
   c. Previous postpartum difficulties
   d. Contraceptive choices and any associated problems
   e. Data relating to past and present illnesses, surgeries, and medications

2. **The psychological component:** A woman's view of herself as female incorporates concepts of gender identity; the sense of having characteristics customarily defined as feminine, masculine, both, or other gender (transgender or non-binary); and body image. Data should include:

   a. The client's self-concept and body image
   b. Client's view of the self as a sexual being (what pronoun they prefer)
   c. Level of confidence in ability to function sexually

      d. Past and current psychiatric problems or illnesses, including anxiety and depression

      e. Information about the use of psychotropic medications

      f. Satisfaction with current relationship

      g. History of sexual abuse

  3. The sociocultural component: A woman's view of herself as female can be defined by her sociocultural upbringing and environment. Data should include:

      a. Information about the client's perceptions of gender-appropriate roles for men and women in relationships and her perception of her ability to fulfill those roles competently

      b. Information about the client's religious affiliation and beliefs

      c. Information about the client's ethnic and cultural belief system

      d. The woman's sources of sexual education, when she received it, and her reactions to the information; it is always important for the healthcare provider to assess whether the information that the client received was correct and accurate.

D. Age-related issues

  1. Toddler and preschool child: Toddlers are able to identify themselves as "I'm a girl" or "I'm a boy," but they cannot integrate gender identity into their self-concept until they are 3 or 4 years of age, when they are able to understand that gender is a permanent condition.

      a. Children at this age are extremely curious. Assist parents in giving children the message that they and their bodies—including its sexual parts—are valuable and important.

      b. Family is the most important source of learning about sexuality issues in this age group, and the parents' attitudes and behaviors begin to shape feelings about sexuality.

      c. Provide parents with information about "normal" sexual behavior and emphasize which developmental tasks are expected at approximate ages.

      d. Assist the parents in defining limits of appropriate and inappropriate behavior (e.g., it is not acceptable for a 3-year-old girl to discuss with a stranger on the bus the fact that she and her mother have vaginas, but that her father and brother have penises).

      e. Stress the importance of teaching the child about appropriate and inappropriate touching from other people.

      f. Always assess for sexual abuse in all children in any health assessment.

  2. School-age child: School-age children continue to have a high level of curiosity about sexuality, their bodies, and their environment, and, because they are aware of the pleasure stimulation gives, may actively seek sexual arousal.

      a. By the time a child reaches school age, or about 8 years of age, they begin to understand the significance of sexuality. This is an important time for the clinician to start discussing pubertal changes with parents and to encourage parents to discuss these changes with their child.

      b. The same principles of inclusiveness and freedom from assumptions apply when taking a family history of a pediatric patient. A mother or father may be part of the LBGTQIA community. The parent or parents may live alone, in a group house with other men or women, with the family of origin, with a partner, or may be homeless.

      c. Children are now experiencing sexual activity at a younger age. Assess the child's understanding and activity. Begin to address these issues as you would during adolescence (see the following text).

      d. As in any age group, assess for sexual abuse.

  3. Adolescence: Sexual awareness and changes in sexual feelings occur during adolescence.

      a. Adolescence is a time to develop a capacity for sexual intimacy, sexual curiosity, and experimentation.

      b. Adolescents are adapting their sense of sexual being into their evolving self-image and personal identity.

c. They are learning about their bodies' sensual and sexual responses to stimulation and are developing a sense of the moral significance of sexuality. The sexual history that is gathered from adolescents is designed to:
   (1) Collect information
   (2) Give the adolescent permission to ask questions and receive reliable information regarding issues of sexual concern
      • Reinforce privacy and confidentiality.
      • Communicate an aura of comfort with the client; create an atmosphere that is free of prejudice; and avoid imposing one's values.
      • Assist the adolescent in feeling validated and comfortable revealing concerns and asking questions.
      • Ask questions that give the message that you expect the client is changing and is aware of and curious about these changes (e.g., "How are you feeling?" "How's your body?" "Do you notice that you are getting taller?").
      • Ask questions to give the message that you care about the client's feelings ("How does that make you feel?" "Do you wonder sometimes about what is happening to your body?").
      • Always listen thoughtfully and carefully to the client's comments and respond positively by answering the client's questions as fully as possible while being calm, friendly, and open.
   (3) Incorporate sexuality-specific education as a normal component of anticipatory guidance.
      • Always give appropriate and factual information.
      • Offer complete, accurate information conveyed in an open, professional manner.
      • Assist the adolescent in understanding the physical, emotional, and psychological changes of puberty, and inform the client of the true risks associated with premature sexual activity.
      • Ask questions to give the message that sexual changes are as expected and normal as other body changes ("Have you noticed your breasts getting any bigger?").
      • Sexually transmitted infections (STIs) and vaginitis occur most frequently during the reproductive years and reach peak incidence during adolescence and young adulthood. For this reason, it is necessary for a healthcare provider to offer services, education, and counseling.
      • Reinforce that sexual activity under the influence of alcohol or drugs can lead to unsafe sexual practices and the risk of unwanted intercourse, pregnancy, STIs, and even inappropriate sexual assault and rape.
   (4) The American College of Obstetricians and Gynecologists (ACOG) recommends that the first visit to the OB/GYN for screening and preventive services occur between the ages of 13 and 15 years.
      • The focus of this visit is education and does not include a pelvic examination unless indicated. The primary goal of the initial reproductive health visit is to provide preventive healthcare services, educational information, and guidance, in addition to problem-focused care
4. **Early adulthood and the reproductive years (21–40 years of age):** This is a critical period during which developmental tasks include achieving maturity in a sexual role and in a relationship, tasks started in adolescence.
   a. Many of the problems experienced by this age group in terms of sexual relationships involve poor communication between partners.
   b. Major concerns in this age group include:
      (1) Balancing careers
      (2) Raising children

(3) Nurturing and maintaining relationships

(4) Experiencing pregnancy, the postpartum period, and lactation

(5) Dealing with infertility

(6) High stress and managing multiple stressors

  c. Assess the use of safe sexual practices (monogamy, condom use), discuss family planning and contraceptive choices, and address fertility concerns.

  d. Assist in facilitating communication between sexual partners, teach clients about sexuality, and clarify any misconceptions by providing information about sexual behavior, sexual activity, and sexual response.

  e. Provide information about intercourse, good hygiene practices, and foreplay, and to reinforce the practice of health-promotion activities (i.e., breast self-examinations, yearly Pap tests).

5. **Middle adulthood (41–65 years):** This is a critical period for expanded sexual freedom and major physiologic changes.

  a. The primary tasks of midlife and later years are

(1) Reappraisal, which includes a review of past and present accomplishments

(2) Reassessment of goals and life direction

(3) Redirection of energies or rededication of life's goals

  b. Most women have established their careers and families by midlife.

  c. During this period, women experience menopause (around the age of 50–52 years in the United States).

  d. Health problems of either partner can be a major source of concern during these years.

ADVANCED HEALTH HISTORY TECHNIQUES

A. **The interview:** The gynecologic interview is primarily intended for gathering information. For many women, this may be the woman's sole source of preventive healthcare. Therefore, the purpose of this visit is fivefold.

1. Provides information to identify potential health problems/diagnoses that may become the basis for the development of management plans.

2. Screens for other existing or potential health problems

3. Provides general health maintenance and prevention of illness

4. Establishes a relationship between the care provider and the patient

5. Sets a tone for the visit and for subsequent visits

B. Patient–practitioner interaction is an equal partnership.

1. Each partner contributes expertise.

2. The provider has knowledge about health and healthcare in general.

3. The patient has knowledge about their history and their body.

4. When a practitioner expresses respect for what the patient brings to the encounter, shared decision-making and implementation of common goals become possible.

  a. Express respect through verbal communication. This begins with the introduction.

(1) When possible, go into the waiting area to call the patient rather than have the medical assistant bring the patient into the examination room. This allows the patient to meet the practitioner for the first time while the patient is fully dressed. This also sets a more personal tone and promotes a feeling of equality in the patient–practitioner relationship. Another option is to take the history when the patient is dressed.

(2) Determine how you as the clinician want to be addressed. Many practitioners establish relationships with patients on a first-name basis. This is both equal and personal. Ask the patient how they want to be addressed (e.g., first name, last name, Ms., Mrs., or Miss).

Some practitioners are most comfortable being called Ms., Mrs., Miss, Mr., or Dr. (if DNP or PhD); consequently, consider addressing the patient in an equivalent manner).

    (3) Ask the patients for their gender pronoun preference simply by inquiring, "What name and pronouns would you like me to use?" or "I would like to be respectful—how would you like to be addressed?" In addition, providers can ask what terms they use for their bodies or specific body parts.

  b. Express respect through nonverbal communication, including facial expressions, eye contact, posture, and, when appropriate, touch.

    (1) **Smiling:** When appropriate, smiling conveys warmth and caring.

    (2) **Eye contact:** Maintaining eye contact by frequently looking up from the computer/EMR. Waiting until the end of the conversation to document findings sends a message of interest to the patient. Continuously looking at the computer to chart can be seen as disrespectful to the patient.

    (3) **Posture:** Sitting up in one's seat or leaning toward the patient shows interest in the patient.

    (4) **Touch:** Touching may or may not be appropriate. Be aware that touch has meaning; use it to instill trust rather than distrust. In our culture, a handshake is generally a respectful form of physical contact although if infectious diseases are prevalent then this may not be appropriate. However, some cultures consider touching intrusive. Be aware of cultural norms/and patient preferences to guide your practice.

  c. Express respect through the environment.

    (1) Use round tables or couches and chairs rather than sitting behind a desk to conduct the interview. Interviewing the patient from behind the desk can be interpreted was having authority over the patient.

    (2) Ensure privacy by shutting the doors and pulling the curtains. If this is not possible, at least ensure "psychological privacy" by using a soft voice and avoid excessive interruptions.

5. Be aware of your own sexual biases. To provide adequate sexual healthcare, the healthcare provider should:

  a. Be aware of their own sexual biases.

  b. Be comfortable with their sexuality.

  c. Have a genuine desire to help the client.

  d. Understand that personal barriers may prevent clinicians from comfortably addressing sexual issues.

    (1) It is critical to address any barriers and not make assumptions about a woman's sexual identity, behaviors, feelings, or attitudes.

  e. Continuously self-monitor personal responses to detect negative feelings that may be conveyed to the client.

6. Set the stage.

  a. Choose a private location where the client is comfortable and assure them that the information they share will be held in strict confidence.

  b. Sufficient time must be given to build trust and develop a rapport (at least a few minutes) before soliciting information that the client may consider highly personal or intimate.

  c. Avoid obtaining a sexual health history when the client is experiencing an acute health problem.

  d. Obtain permission to ask questions in this potentially sensitive area: "I would like to ask you some questions about your sex history. I don't mean to embarrass you and it's okay if you'd rather not answer some of these questions. May I begin?"

7. Begin with open-ended questions. Ask open-ended questions at the beginning of the interview and at the beginning of each section.

    a. This gives the practitioner a chance to assess the language used by the patient and reveals the concerns that are most important to the patient.

    b. More pointed questions can then be asked to specify the conditions that are important for the practitioner to know about.

    c. For transgender patients, younger patients, and women who have sex with women, open-ended questions may elicit more accurate information and may help the patient feel more comfortable.

8. Avoid using excessive medical terminology. Language must be understood clearly by both the provider and the client.

    a. Make sure that both you and the client know the meaning of the terms used.

    b. Sometimes it may be helpful to use technical and nontechnical words in the same question: "Have you ever had hypertension, or high blood pressure?"

9. Avoid euphemisms. Inclusive language should be used while taking the patient history and going through the review of systems.

    a. Follow a standard procedure, ask every patient the same questions, and make no assumptions.

    b. Avoid wording such as *slept with*.

    c. Use gender-neutral terms to refer to significant others, such as *partner* or *spouse*.

    d. Frame inclusive questions when asking about sexual activity, but when the questions are pertinent to the complaint or workup, make inclusive questions about the sexual activity as specific as possible.

    e. Rather than using the words *coitus* and *intercourse*, or the even more vague *sexual activity* or *sexual relations*, inquire about oral sex, anal sex, and vaginal intercourse (or) sex.

    f. If the client does not understand, describe the behavior being asked about (e.g., "Have you ever taken a man's penis into your rectum or mouth?").

    g. Many practitioners are uncomfortable discussing sex, particularly specific sexual acts. The only way to overcome such discomfort is through repeated practice.

10. Universalizing should be used only in appropriate situations.

    a. Prefacing questions with phrases such as *many people* or *research shows that,* may make the client feel more comfortable when answering sensitive questions.

    b. Do not presume a client is heterosexual because the patient discusses an opposite-sex spouse or has children.

    c. Sexual orientation and sexual behaviors encompass a broad spectrum; the astute clinician recognizes that outward appearances may not be accurate.

    d. Do not assume that a woman who identifies herself as a lesbian is having sex only with women.

    e. Avoid labels that the patient does not use. For example, a client who might acknowledge same-sex sexual behavior may not identify themselves as homosexual/gay/lesbian.

11. Move from simple to complex items. Always begin the interview with least threatening material and explain to clients the purpose of the questions. This approach will help build trust and rapport.

    a. A general guideline is to begin with questions about the individual's sexual learning history, such as childhood sexual education, then proceed to personal attitudes and beliefs about sexuality, and finally, assess actual sexual behaviors.

SPECIAL APPROACHES TO SEXUAL HEALTH HISTORY

A. A thorough sexual health history is the cornerstone of making an accurate diagnosis identifying health risk factors and lays the foundation for providing health promotion guidance. There are three basic types of sexual health histories:

1. **Initial or comprehensive history:** A comprehensive sexual history is a detailed history that encompasses all aspects of sexual information about the individual, as well as their family of origin, siblings, and significant relationships.
   a. The initial or comprehensive history includes information concerning
      (1) Each phase of sexual development
      (2) Body image
      (3) Learned attitudes
      (4) Feelings relating to sexuality
      (5) Sexual debut
      (6) Sexual orientation
      (7) Range of sexual behaviors
         - Keep in mind that transgender individuals differ in hormone use, history of gender-affirming surgical procedures, and patterns of sexual behavior. Avoid making any assumptions about presence or absence of specific anatomy, sexual orientation, or sexual practices.
         - Anatomy and behavior may change over time in the transgender individual. It will be important to periodically assess for changes that may impact care.
   b. The purpose of this type of history is to document an accurate and complete account of the patient's health status.
   c. It is a lengthy process that may not be accomplished at the first visit or with a single interview.
2. **A well-interim history:** This history focuses on in-depth family and lifestyle information and is used to form the basis of health maintenance and health promotion.
3. **A problem-focused history:** This type of history is obtained when the patient presents with a specific symptom. The focus is to gather information regarding the patient's current health problems and any confounding health factors.
   a. The systematic history focuses on the presenting symptom or assessment of specific behaviors, such as the risks for becoming pregnant or the acquisition of STIs.
   b. **Problem-oriented sexual histories:** This type of history is shorter, more direct, and specific to the immediate issue.
      (1) Indications that make it necessary to conduct the problem-focused pelvic examination
         - Information obtained from the history, with or without symptoms
            - Maternal diethylstilbestrol (DES) exposure
            - Multiple (contemporaneous or serial) sexual partners
         - New or recurrent sentinel symptoms
            - Change in character, frequency, regularity, or duration of menses
            - Midcycle, postcoital, or postmenopausal vaginal bleeding
            - Lower abdominal pain or swelling, especially when it is unilateral
            - Painful sexual intercourse (dyspareunia)
            - Vulvar or vaginal pruritus
            - Change in quantity or character of vaginal discharge
            - Urinary incontinence
            - Burning, frequency, or pain on urination (dysuria), with or without diagnosed urinary tract infection
            - Lower back pain or any symptoms that bear a consistent relationship to menstrual cycle
            - Unexpected onset of menarche or menopause
            - Bilateral lower limb edema (unexplained)

THE REPRODUCTIVE HEALTH HISTORY

A. **Preconception care and counseling:** The goal of preconception counseling is to optimize the health of the woman and the health of her potential infant. To reach this goal, the National Institutes of Health expert panel recommends that preconception counseling begin prior to 1 year before conception of a planned pregnancy (see Chapter 12, "Preconception Care" and Chapter 14, "Assessment of the Pregnant Woman").

1. Preconception assessment data: Include history, physical examination results, and laboratory data

   a. History
      (1) A complete medical, social, reproductive, and family history must be obtained.
      (2) Information should be specific to the client's family, medical, reproductive, and drug histories, and HIV risk factors.
      (3) Nutrition and lifestyle choices should also be evaluated. Per the Centers for Disease Control and Prevention (CDC), use of folic acid should be assessed and encouraged.
      (4) The use of a comprehensive screening tool, such as the sample prenatal genetic screen, can be useful (see Appendix 3.1).

   b. Physical examination
      (1) Should include screening, evaluation and counseling, and immunizations based on age and risk factors.
      (2) A complete physical examination, including a possible breast and pelvic assessment, should be considered, along with a cervical cancer screening test per guidelines, cultures for gonorrhea and chlamydia/and other STIs as indicated, and possible vaginitis evaluation (pH, amine/whiff test, possible microscopy) depending on the patient's age, sexual activity, past medical history, and symptoms.
         • ACOG recommends that the annual pelvic examination should be considered for patients aged 21 years or older and include cervical cancer screening according to the latest guidelines.
         • Data do not support the necessity of performing a pelvic examination prior to initiating oral contraceptives in an otherwise healthy, asymptomatic patient younger than 21 years.
         • Women may stop cervical cancer screening after age 65 years if the woman:
            ▪ Does not have a history of precancer.
            ▪ Has no history of cervical cancer.
            ▪ Has three negative cervical cancer screening tests in a row, or two negative results within the past 10 years, with the most recent test performed within the last 5 years.

   c. Laboratory testing
      (1) Rubella titer and antibody screen
      (2) Serology for syphilis
      (3) Complete blood count (CBC) with indices
      (4) Blood type and Rh
      (5) Blood sugar screening by either random blood sugar, fasting blook sugar (FBS), or hemoglobin A1C
      (6) Urinalysis
      (7) If sickle cell disease or thalassemia is a concern, hemoglobin electrophoresis should be performed.
      (8) Screening should be considered as appropriate for: viral infections, such as HIV, human papillomavirus (HPV), hepatitis, cytomegalovirus (CMV), or toxoplasmosis.
      (9) For those younger than 21 years, nucleic acid amplification testing of urine samples or self-collected vaginal swabs is acceptable for gonorrhea and chlamydia, yeast, trichomoniasis, and bacterial vaginosis infections.

2. Client education and counseling
   a. **Menstrual cycles and basal body temperature (BBT):** Advise client to keep accurate records of her menstrual and ovulation cycles to help establish gestational dating (see Chapter 38, "Methods to Detect Ovulation").
   b. Exercise and nutrition
      (1) Vitamin and mineral supplements
      (2) Folic acid supplementation (per CDC, 0.4 mg/400 mcg pre-pregnancy)
      (3) Ideal weight before conception
      (4) Exercise program to improve cardiovascular status and to facilitate health/well-being
      (5) Balanced diet
   c. **Avoidance of teratogens:** Warn the client that potential teratogens can be related to occupation and lifestyle (see Appendix 3.2). Teratogens may include:
      (1) Cleaning solutions
      (2) Hair coloring and permanents
      (3) Photography solutions
      (4) Radiation
      (5) Chemicals used in processing food and textiles
      (6) Drugs, including prescription, over-the-counter, and recreational
   d. **Affirmation of pregnancy decision**: Stress that a couple may need time to affirm the decision to attempt pregnancy.
   e. **Readiness for parenthood:** Assess the couple's social, financial, and psychological readiness for pregnancy and commitment to parenthood.
   f. **Identification of unhealthy behaviors:** Assist the couple in identifying and reducing unhealthy behaviors, such as:
      (1) Smoking
      (2) Alcohol consumption
      (3) Drug use—prescription, over-the-counter, recreational, and illegal
   g. **Treatment of medical conditions:** Ensure that medical conditions that may jeopardize the pregnancy outcome are evaluated. Refer the couple to specialists as needed.
   h. Identify genetic risks (Appendix 3.1).
      (1) Indications for genetic counseling
         • Women who are pregnant or are planning pregnancies and will be 35 years of age or older at delivery (i.e., advanced maternal age)
         • Couples or individuals who have had a previous fetus/baby or child with a genetic disorder, birth defects, or mental retardation
         • Individuals who have or are suspected to have a genetic disorder
         • Individuals who have a parent with a genetic disorder
         • Couples or individuals with a family history of a genetic disorder, birth defects, mental retardation/developmental disability, learning disabilities, cancer, or other conditions
         • Families with members who have been diagnosed with the same mental or physical condition
         • Couples or individuals with a history of pregnancy loss, miscarriages, or with unexplained infertility
         • Individuals who are known carriers of a genetic disorder
         • Couples or individuals of specific ethnic backgrounds known to have a higher incidence of certain disorders
         • Women who were exposed during or before pregnancy to teratogenic drugs, infections, x-ray studies, radiotherapy, or occupational hazards
         • Couples who are first cousins or close blood relatives
         • Women planning to undergo amniocentesis or chorionic villus sampling

- Women with abnormal findings on fetal ultrasonography
- Women with abnormal results on prenatal screening tests

i. **Preconception classes:** When appropriate, refer the couple to community adult educational resources for preconception classes, such as

(1) March of Dimes

(2) Prenatal, pregnancy, birth, and after-childbirth classes

(3) Parent training and sibling relations classes

(4) Cardiopulmonary resuscitation (CPR) classes

(5) Couple to Couple League

(6) Pursuing Parenthood class

(7) Parent Encouragement Program, which offers classes on parenting, marriage, and families

j. **Laboratory tests:** Order all appropriate laboratory tests, evaluate the results, and discuss the findings and implications with the client.

k. Appropriate vaccinations (CDC, 2016)

(1) **Rubella (live attenuated):** If the client is not immune, administer the measles, mumps, rubella (MMR) vaccine, and advise the client to wait 28 days before attempting conception.

(2) **Tetanus, diphtheria, pertussis (Tdap):** CDC recommends administration of Tdap vaccine during the 27th to 36th week of pregnancy to protect the newborn.

(3) **Hepatitis B:** The CDC recommends pregnant women who meet the risk for HBV infection during pregnancy should be vaccinated. Risk includes more than one sexual partner within the last 6 months, history of or treatment for (STI, past or previous injection drug use, or having a partner who test positive for HBs Ag.

(4) **Influenza vaccine (inactivated):** Administer during flu season; can be administered during any trimester.

(5) **COVID-19 vaccine:** The CDC recommends completing the initial series and updating with booster vaccines when recommended for women who are pregnant or may become pregnant. The mRNA COVID-19 vaccines (Pfizer-BioNTech or Moderna) are the preferred choice for initial series and boosters (CDC, 2022)

l. **Special dietary needs:** If the client has special dietary needs (vegetarian, cultural restrictions, diabetes, overweight, underweight, gluten-free, lactose intolerant), refer to a dietitian. Women are often highly motivated to improve their nutritional status when planning a pregnancy.

m. CDC recommends all women of reproductive age take over-the-counter folic acid 400 mcg (0.4. mg) daily.

TECHNIQUES FOR SCREENING FOR SEXUAL ABUSE

A. Screening for sexual abuse is an important component of any health assessment (see Chapter 34, "The Sexual Assault Victim" and Chapter 35, "Intimate Partner Violence").

THE SEXUAL HISTORY OF THE LGBTQIA PATIENT

A. Ask about sexual orientation and gender identity.

1. Put patients at ease by ensuring confidentiality and routine practice

2. Ask about sexual partners and orientation: Do you have a partner? When you have sex, do you do so with men, women, or both? How do you identify your sexual orientation?

3. Open room for discussion: Do you have any concerns or questions about your sexuality, sexual orientation, or gender?"

4. Keep in mind that identity, behavior, and attraction are fluid and can change over time.

5. Sexual orientation and gender identity/expression are influenced by cultural norms, environmental factors, societal and/or familial pressures.
6. Healthcare disparities vary by identity, attraction, and behavior.
7. Always let people self-identify sexual orientation and gender identity.

B. LGBTQIA health screening/prevention
1. Healthcare and screening are based on the organs present and hormonal status.
   a. Transwomen who have undergone male-to-female sex reassignment surgery still have a prostate gland. Provider must still screen for BPH, prostate cancer, prostatitis, and so forth.
   b. Transmen who have undergone female-to-male sex reassignment surgery with breast reduction still retain breast tissue. Providers must still screen for breast cancer.
   c. Providers must screen for adverse effects of hormone replacement surgery.
2. Prevention strategies
   a. **Sexual protection (dental dams, condoms, etc.):** Condoms have been shown to be reduce risk of STIs including HIV, gonorrhea, chlamydia, trichomoniasis, and HPV.
   b. **Vaccines:** According to the CDC: "Among gay and bisexual men, hepatitis A can be spread through sexual activity or contact with fingers or objects that have the virus on it." Thus, the hepatitis A vaccine is given as two shots, 6 months apart.
   c. Consider healthcare risk factors and disparities that are applicable to your patient.

HIV RISK ASSESSMENT

A. HIV is transmitted through the exchange of infected bodily fluids, including blood and semen. High-risk behaviors include:
1. Sexual activity: Unprotected intercourse with multiple partners
2. Intravenous (IV) drug use
3. Persons who received blood products before 1985. Highest risk is for those who received blood transfusions between 1975 and March 1985.
4. Hemophiliac clients who have received pooled plasma products
5. Children of HIV-infected women
6. Healthcare workers (e.g., those at risk for accidental needle sticks)

B. Questions to consider
1. Are you a healthcare worker? Have you ever been stuck by a contaminated needle?
2. Do you have sex with men, women, or both?
3. How many partners have you had in the past year?
4. Have you had intercourse without a condom? When did you start using condoms?
5. Have you performed oral sex on a man or a woman without a barrier (such as a dental dam, plastic wrap, or a condom)?
6. Have you been treated for an STI? Include the date and treatment received.
7. Do you smoke cigarettes, drink alcohol, or use other drugs?
8. Have you had unprotected sex while under the influence of alcohol or other drugs/substances?
9. Have you had sexual partners who are at high risk for HIV?
10. Do you now or have you ever injected drugs?
11. Have you shared hypodermic needles, other drug equipment, or other skin-piercing or cutting instruments with another person (for injection drug use, steroid use, vitamin injection, tattooing, body piercing, or scarification)?
12. Do you use crack cocaine? If yes, have you had sex in crack houses?

13. Have you received a tattoo from an unlicensed tattoo artist or when you were not sure that the needle used had been properly sterilized?

14. Have you received any blood transfusions, or have you undergone surgery (most important between 1975 and 1985)?

C. Components of the history when assessing an HIV-positive individual (see Appendix 3.3): The patient with HIV infection requires an initial evaluation, ongoing psychosocial support, and medical assessment. A complete history is needed, and questions should be directed to gather information specifically about HIV-related illnesses, vaccination history, history of STIs, and assessment of HIV transmission category. The history should include:

1. Medical history that includes information on cardiovascular disease; pulmonary disease; gastrointestinal disease; renal disease; neurologic disease; cancer; endocrine disease; ear, nose, and throat disease; liver disease; skin disease; chickenpox or shingles; viral hepatitis; bacterial infections; gynecologic problems; exposure to tuberculosis; and psychiatric treatment (outpatient or inpatient treatment)

2. Current medications and treatments: Over-the-counter drugs, vitamins, and, especially, immunosuppressive therapy (e.g., in an asthmatic patient who intermittently requires corticosteroids)

3. Identify when a patient's acute HIV illness occurred, as this may be helpful in determining the patient's prognosis.

   a. At least half of all HIV-positive patients may report a history of acute HIV infection, which presents clinically as a mild to severe mononucleosis-like illness lasting 1 to 2 weeks.

   b. The incubation period (time from exposure to onset of illness) for the acute syndromes may range from 5 days to 3 months but is usually 2 to 4 weeks.

   c. Symptoms include fever, diaphoresis, malaise, myalgia, arthralgia, pharyngitis, retro-orbital headaches, and, in some patients, lymphadenopathy or aseptic meningitis.

   d. Other less common manifestations of acute HIV infection include polyneuropathy, brachial neuritis, and odynophagia with esophageal ulcers.

4. **HIV-related opportunistic infections:** Oral candidiasis (thrush), persistent diarrhea, varicella zoster (shingles), oral hairy leukoplakia, *Pneumocystis jirovecii* pneumonia, recurrent bacterial pneumonia (in 12 months), cryptococcal meningitis, toxoplasmosis, Kaposi's sarcoma, candida esophagitis, disseminated *Mycobacterium avium* complex (MAC), cytomegalovirus (CMV) infection, and tuberculosis

5. **HIV-related symptoms:** Malaise, fever, night sweats, changes in sleep pattern, changes in appetite, weight loss, abdominal pain, vomiting, diarrhea, skin rashes or lesions, oral candidiasis or ulceration, odynophagia, lymphadenopathy, unusual headaches, nuchal rigidity, difficulty thinking, chest pain, cough, shortness of breath, paresthesia in hands or feet, muscle weakness, changes in vision, and changes in neurologic function or mental status

6. **Vaccination history:** Measles, mumps, rubella (MMR); last tetanus booster; HPV; hepatitis B; pneumococcal vaccine; zoster vaccine; influenza vaccine; and COVID-19 vaccine.

   a. Tuberculosis history should include information on any known exposure to tuberculosis, international travel to area endemic of tuberculosis, date of last purified protein derivative (PPD) test, and history of positive PPD test result. If prior positive PPD, was any treatment administered? If yes, what was the duration and type?

7. **STIs:** Information about possible exposure to syphilis, gonorrhea, genital herpes, chlamydia, condyloma (warts), HPV, hepatitis, and trichomoniasis. The history should also include:

   a. Questions about where the patient has lived and traveled

    b. Questions about current sexual practices (gender and number of sexual partners), specifically, a sexual history should be taken to assess the patient's current sexual practices and to determine whether sexual partners are aware of the patient's possible HIV status and if they have been tested for HIV

    c. Questions about the types of contraception used and consistency using contraception

    d. Questions about past or present IV drug use

    e. Questions about behaviors that might lead to further transmission of HIV

8. **Drug use:** Ask about current IV drug use including drug-using practices, source of needles, if they share needles and, if so, with whom.

9. Psychosocial history

    a. Depression is common among HIV-infected patients, and the history should include questions that focus on changes in

      (1) Mood

      (2) Libido

      (3) Sleeping patterns

      (4) Appetite

      (5) Concentration

      (6) Memory

    b. Patients should also be asked specifically about whom they have informed of their HIV status, how they have been coping with the diagnosis of HIV infection, and what types of support they have been receiving.

    c. It is important to know about the patient's living situation, family and work environment, and how these have been affected by the diagnosis of HIV infection.

10. Assess the patient's level of awareness about HIV infection and treatment

    a. Evaluate the patient's educational needs and determine specific information/support that might be needed.

    b. Assessment of patient education should include information on safer-sex guidelines, use of condoms and spermicide, and safe versus unsafe practices.

    c. Drug use and abuse must be discussed and include issues of needle sharing, the use of bleach to sterilize needles, and drug treatment options.

SAMPLE QUESTIONS AND SCREENING TOOLS

A. General initial history

1. **Sexual activity:** When were you last sexually active? Have you had sex in the past few months?

2. **Sexual orientation:** Are you intimate with males, females, or both?

3. **Number of partners:** How many sexual partners do you or did you have? How long have you been with your current partner? Quantify the number and gender of your sexual partners over the past few months and/or years.

4. **Types of sexual activity:** Do you or did you have vaginal, anal, or oral sex? If anal or oral, ask, "Do you give it or receive it, or both?"

5. **Pregnancy and contraception:** Do you desire to become (make your partner) pregnant? Is it possible that you are (they are) pregnant now? What are you doing to prevent pregnancy?

6. **STIs:** Do you have abnormal vaginal discharge, itching, or pain on urination? Do you have any sores or lumps? Have you or any of your partners ever been treated for an STI? Which STI? How long ago? Do you or any of your partners have risk factors for HIV or AIDS, such as blood transfusions, IV drug use, frequent sex with multiple partners or strangers, sex in exchange for money or drugs?

7. **Protection from STIs:** Do you or did you use a condom or other protection during sex or when you have had sex in the past? If not, why not? Do you ever have sex without protection? How recently?

8. **Violence and abuse:** Have you ever been hurt or abused by your partner? Have you ever been raped? If the answer is yes, assess the situation.

9. **Satisfaction:** Is sex satisfying for you? If not, why not?

10. **Sexual concerns:** Do you have any problems with or concerns about your sexual function?

B. Comprehensive adolescent sexual history

1. **Background data:** Age (birth date), parents' ages, parents' religion, parents' educational levels, parents' occupations, parents' marital status, amount of affection in relationship (parent to parent), feelings toward parent or parents

2. **Childhood sexuality:** What were your parents' attitudes about sexuality when you were a child? In what way did your parents handle nudity? Who taught you about sex? From whom did you learn about sex play, pregnancy, intercourse, masturbation, homosexuality, STIs, childbirth? When do you first recall seeing a nude person of the same sex? Of the opposite sex? How often did you play doctor–nurse or engage in other sex play with another child? Tell me about any other sexual activity or experience that had a significant impact on you.

3. **Adolescent sexuality:** How old were you when you had your first period? How old were you when you noticed breast development? When did pubic hair appear? What were the characteristics of onset of menstruation (age, regularity of periods, initially, now)? What hygienic method do you/did you use (pads, tampons)? How were you prepared for menstruation? By whom? What were your feelings about early periods? Later periods? Have you had unusual bleeding?

4. **Body image:** How do you feel about your body? What about your breasts and genitals?

5. **Masturbation:** Do you masturbate? How old were you when you began masturbating? What were others' reactions to your masturbation? What methods do you use? What are your feelings about masturbation?

6. **Necking and petting:** How old were you when you began? How often? How many partners do you currently have?

7. **Intercourse:** How often do you have intercourse? How many partners?

8. **Contraceptive use:** What kind of contraceptives have you used? Did you have side effects? What are you using now? Do you consistently use contraception?

9. **STIs:** How old were you when you learned about STIs? Have you ever had a an STI? What infections have you been diagnosed with? When? Did you receive treatment? Did your partner receive treatment?

10. **Pregnancy:** Have you ever been pregnant? How many times? At what age(s)? Were there any complications?

C. Content areas of reproductive health history for adolescent females

1. Menarche

   a. Age of onset

   b. **Duration of flow:** How many days do your periods usually last?

   c. **Frequency:** How often do you have your period? Do you keep track of them by using a calendar/app?

   d. **Date of last normal menstrual period (LNMP):** When was the date of your LNMP?

   e. **Dysmenorrhea:** Do you have cramps with your periods? If so, does it affect your activities or school attendance? Do you use any remedies and/or medications? What is the name of the drug, the dosage, and the frequency of ingestion? Do you get relief?

2. Sexual activity
   a. **Age of sexual debut (first penile–vaginal sex, versus first intimacy with or without penile–vaginal sex):** In the past, have you had or are you currently having sex? If so, at what age did you have your first sexual experience? Has anyone ever touched you on any part of your body where you did not want to be touched? Issues of past sexual abuse or date rape by an acquaintance may be important areas of discussion.
   b. **Sexual orientation:** Are you attracted to men, women, or both? Have you ever had sex or been sexually intimate with a person of your same sex?
   c. **Frequency of coitus:** How often do you have sex? Once a month? Once a week? Twice a week? When was the last time you had sex/intercourse (penile–vaginal sex)?
   d. **Number of sexual partners:** How many partners have you had in the past 2 months? How many in the past year? How many since you first started having sex?
   e. **Sexual practices:** Include questions that involve a full range of sexual expression, including activities such as kissing, touching, and masturbation. To counsel youth regarding safer sex practices, the clinician must be aware of the teen's entire repertoire of behaviors.
   f. **Sexual pleasure:** Is having intercourse or sex pleasurable for you? Are you satisfied with your sexual life the way it is now? Do you think your partner is satisfied?
3. Contraceptive use
   a. **Current method of birth control:** It may be helpful to list the choice of specific methods (e.g., foam, condoms, withdrawal or "pulling out," birth-control pill, implant, patch, intrauterine contraceptive [IUC]). Ask the teen the frequency with which they use a method (e.g., never, sometimes, always). Ask whether they have any real side effects from using a specific method. Ask whether condoms are used with partners especially new partners. What percent of the time are condoms used (25%, 50%, 75%, 100%)?
   b. Communication skills regarding use of contraception: Are condoms or other barrier methods used as a method of fertility control or to prevent the transmission of STIs?
4. Obstetric and gynecologic considerations
   a. **Number of pregnancies:** List the exact number and outcome, including number of live births and spontaneous and therapeutic abortions (medical vs. surgical).
   b. **Recent gynecologic procedures:** Dilation and curettage (D&C), recent abortion, and any complications after the procedure?
   c. **History of pelvic inflammatory disease:** When and how was it treated. Did you have inpatient or outpatient management? Any complications such as continued pelvic pain and/or infertility?
5. STIs
   a. **History of previous STIs:** Specific STI, date, treatment, any complications?
   b. Was your partner treated?
6. Drug use
   a. **Onset, duration, and frequency of use:** Ask about the use of cigarettes, alcohol, or illicit drugs. Ask about IV, inhalation, or injection drug use. Including this information is essential for the assessment of behaviors that may place the client at risk for HIV/hepatitis infection.
7. Partner
   a. **Partner involvement:** Is the adolescent female's partner involved in the visit today? Was there prior discussion regarding contraception or other topics?
   b. **Male partner STI assessment:** Ask whether the male partner has any symptoms of infection. Include symptoms of urethritis (discharge or dysuria), any open sores, or warts in the genital area.
8. Support system
   a. **Parents and friends:** Who is aware of your sexual activity? Have you experienced any potential negative effects regarding disclosure of your behavior to parents or friends? Have you received support? If so, from whom?

D. Adolescent sexual problem history
1. Ask the adolescent to describe the sexual concern, problem, issue, or difficulty: How do you feel about discussing this problem? How long have you had it? When did this problem begin? What do you think caused you to have this problem? What might be contributing to this problem? How have you tried to treat or solve this problem? What health professionals have you seen? What, if any, medications have you taken or are you taking? Have you talked to a friend or relative? Have you gone online to explore solutions to your problem? Have you tried anything? Did it help?

BIBLIOGRAPHY

The American College of Osteopathic Family Physicians. *The Sexual History Examination and the LGBT Patient – ACOFP*. Retrieved from https://www.acofp.org/acofpimis/acofporg/PDFs/OFP/Articles/MODULE_Sexual_History _Examination_LGBT_Patient.pdf

Bickley, L. S., Szilagyi, P. G., Hoffman, R. M., & Soriano, R. P. (2020). *Bates' guide to physical examination and history taking* (13th ed.). Wolters Kluwer.

Centers for Disease Control and Prevention. (2015). *2015 sexually transmitted diseases treatment guidelines*. Retrieved from https://www.cdc.gov/std/tg2015/default.htm

Centers for Disease Control and Prevention. (2016). *Guidelines for vaccinating pregnant women*. Retrieved from https:// www.cdc.gov/vaccines/pregnancy/hcp-toolkit/guidelines.html#tdap

Centers for Disease Control and Prevention. (2021). *AIDS and Opportunistic Infections*. Retrieved from https://www.cdc. gov/hiv/basics/livingwithhiv/opportunisticinfections.html

Centers for Disease Control and Prevention. (2022). *Safety and effectiveness of COVID-19 vaccination during Pregnancy*. Retrieved from https://www.cdc.gov/coronavirus/2019-ncov/vaccines/recommendations/pregnancy.html #anchor_1628692520287

Committee on Gynecologic Practice. (2012). Committee opinion no. 534: Well-woman visit. *Obstetrics and Gynecology, 120*(2 Pt. 1), 421–424. https://doi.org/[0-9A-z]0.1097/AOG.0b013e3182680517

Deutsch, M. B. (Ed.). (2016). *Guidelines for the primary and gender-affirming care of transgender and gender nonbinary people* (2nd ed.). Retrieved from http://www.transhealth.ucsf.edu/guidelines

Division of HIV/AIDS Prevention, National Center for HIV/AIDS. (2020). *Viral Hepatitis, STD, and TB Prevention, Centers for Disease Control and Prevention*. Retrieved from https://www.cdc.gov/hiv/clinicians/transforming-health/ health-care-providers/sexual-history.html

MacLaren, A. (1995). Primary care for women. Comprehensive sexual health assessment. *Journal of Nurse-Midwifery, 40*(2), 104–119. https://doi.org/[0-9A-z]0.1016/0091-2182(95)00010-H

Nelson, R. (2017). *USPSTF has new draft guidance for cervical cancer screening*. Retrieved from https://www.medscape. com/viewarticle/885542

Secor, M., & Fantasia, H. (2018). *Fast facts about the gynecologic exam: A professional guide for NPs, PAs, and midwives* (2nd ed.). Springer Publishing.

APPENDIX 3.1: SAMPLE PRENATAL GENETIC SCREEN

1. Will you be 35 years or older when the baby is due?	Yes ❏	No ❏
2. Have you or the baby's father or anyone in either of your families ever had any of the following disorders?		
Down syndrome (mongolism)	Yes ❏	No ❏
Other chromosomal abnormality	Yes ❏	No ❏
Neural tube defect, spina bifida (meningomyelocele or open spine), anencephaly	Yes ❏	No ❏
Hemophilia	Yes ❏	No ❏
Muscular dystrophy	Yes ❏	No ❏
Cystic fibrosis	Yes ❏	No ❏
If yes, indicate the relationship of the affected person to you or to the baby's father.		
3. Do you or does the baby's father have a birth defect?	Yes ❏	No ❏
If yes, who has the defect and what is it?		
4. In any previous marriages, have you or has the baby's father had a child, born dead or alive, with a birth defect not listed in question 2?	Yes ❏	No ❏
If yes, what was the defect and who had it?		
5. Do you or does the baby's father have any close relatives with mental retardation?	Yes ❏	No ❏
If yes, indicate the relationship of the affected person to you or to the baby's father. Indicate the cause, if known.		
6. Do you or does the baby's father or a close relative in either of your families have a birth defect, any familial disorder, or a chromosomal abnormality not listed previously?	Yes ❏	No ❏
If yes, indicate the condition and the relationship of the affected person to you or to the baby's father.		
7. In any previous marriages, have you or the baby's father had a stillborn child or three or more first-trimester spontaneous pregnancy losses?	Yes ❏	No ❏
8. Have either of you undergone a chromosomal study?	Yes ❏	No ❏
If yes, indicate who and the results.		
9. If you or the baby's father is of Jewish ancestry, have either of you been screened for Tay–Sachs disease?	Yes ❏	No ❏
If yes, indicate who and the results.		
10. If you or the baby's father is Black, have either of you been screened for the sickle cell trait?	Yes ❏	No ❏
If yes, indicate who and the results.		
11. If you or the baby's father is of Italian, Greek, or Mediterranean background, have either of you been tested for beta thalassemia?	Yes ❏	No ❏
If yes, indicate who and the results.		

(continued)

12. If you or the baby's father is of Philippine or Southeast Asian ancestry, have either of you been tested for alpha thalassemia?	Yes ❏	No ❏

If yes, indicate who and the results.

13. Excluding iron and vitamins, have you taken any medications or recreational drugs since being pregnant or since your last menstrual period? (Include nonprescription drugs.)	Yes ❏	No ❏

If yes, give name of medication and time taken during pregnancy.

APPENDIX 3.2: ENVIRONMENTAL EXPOSURE HISTORY FORM

1. Have you ever worked at a job or a hobby in which you came in contact with any of the following by breathing, touching, or ingesting (swallowing)? If yes, please place a check beside the name.

Acids	Ethylene dibromide	Phenol
Alcohols (industrial)	Ethylene dichloride	Phosgene
Alkalies	Fiberglass	Radiation
Ammonia	Halothane	Rock dust
Arsenic	Isocyanates	Silica powder
Asbestos	Ketones	Solvents
Benzene	Lead	Styrene
Beryllium	Manganese	Toluene
Cadmium	MDI (methylenediphenyl diisocyanate)	Toluene diisocyanate (TDI)
Carbon tetrachloride	Mercury	Trichloroethylene
Chlorinated naphthalenes	Methylene chloride	Trinitrotoluene
Chloroform	Nickel	Vinyl chloride
Chloroprene	Polybrominated biphenyls (PBBs)	Welding fumes
Chromates	Polychlorinated biphenyls (PCBs)	Xrays
Coal dust	Perchloroethylene	Other (specify)
Dichlorobenzene	Pesticides	

2. Do you live next to or near an industrial plant, commercial business, dump site, or nonresidential property?   Yes ☐   No ☐

3. Which of the following do you have in your home? *Please circle those that apply.*

Air conditioner	Electric stove (gas or oil?)
Air purifier	Wood stove
Central heating	Humidifier
Gas stove	Fireplace

4. Have you recently acquired new furniture or carpet, refinished furniture, or remodeled your home?   Yes ☐   No ☐

5. Have you weatherized your home recently?   Yes ☐   No ☐

6. Are pesticides or herbicides (bug or weed killers, flea and tick sprays, collars, powders, or shampoos) used in your home or garden, or on pets?   Yes ☐   No ☐

7. Do you (or any household member) have a hobby or craft?   Yes ☐   No ☐

8. Do you work on your car?   Yes ☐   No ☐

9. Have you ever changed your residence because of a health problem?   Yes ☐   No ☐

10. Does your drinking water come from a private well, city water supply, or grocery store?   Yes ☐   No ☐

11. Approximately what year was your home built?   _____

If you answered yes to any of the questions, please explain.

APPENDIX 3.3: SUMMARY OF CRITICAL ISSUES IN THE HIV INITIAL HISTORY

HIV Testing

When did the patient first have a positive test result for HIV?

Where was the first test conducted that resulted in positive HIV status?

What was the reason for being tested?

Does the patient have documentation of a positive enzyme-linked immunosorbent assay (ELISA) and Western blot test results?

Has the patient ever had a negative HIV test result?

What is the patient's usual source of healthcare?

What is the patient's most recent CD4 cell count (if known)?

Medical History

Cardiovascular disease

Pulmonary disease

Gastrointestinal disease

Renal disease

Neurologic disease

Cancer

Endocrine disease

Ear, nose, and throat disease

Liver disease

Obstetric and gynecologic illness

Skin disease

Chickenpox or shingles (varicella)

Psychiatric treatment

HIV-Related Illnesses

Oral candidiasis (thrush)

Diarrhea

Varicella zoster (shingles)

Oral hairy leukoplakia

Pneumocystis jiorvecii pneumonia (PJP)

Recurrent bacterial pneumonia (in 12-month period)

Cryptococcal meningitis

Toxoplasmosis

Kaposi's sarcoma

Candida esophagitis

Disseminated *Mycobacterium avium* complex (MAC)

CMV infection

Tuberculosis

Invasive cervical cancer

Other HIV-related illnesses

Vaccination History

MMR vaccine

Last tetanus booster

Hepatitis B

Hepatitis A

Pneumococcal vaccine
Influenza vaccine
COVID-19 vaccine
HPV vaccine (Gardasil)

Tuberculosis History

Any known exposure to *Mycobacterium tuberculosis?*
Date of last purified protein derivative (PPD) test?
History of positive PPD test result?
    If yes, was prophylaxis given?
    If yes, duration and type?

Sexually Transmitted Infections

Syphilis
Gonorrhea
Genital herpes
Chlamydia (nongonococcal urethritis [NGU] or cervicitis)
Condyloma (warts)
Hepatitis B
Trichomoniasis
Pelvic inflammatory disease (PID)

Gynecologic History

Has the patient ever been pregnant?
    If yes, how many:
    Full-term pregnancies
    Premature births
    Miscarriages or abortions
    Living children
Have there been any pregnancies since the patient has learned of their HIV status?
What was the beginning date of the client's last menstrual period?
Was the last menstrual period normal?
Is the patient pregnant now?
    If yes, was a prenatal care referral made?
Does the patient use a birth-control method?
    If yes, specify what type.
When was the patient's last Pap test? Was it normal?

Medication

Current medications and treatments (include over-the-counter drugs and vitamins)

Habits

Does the patient smoke or has the patient smoked in the past? (Inquire about quantity.)
Does the patient use alcohol or has the patient used alcohol in the past? (Inquire about quantity.)
Does the patient use drugs or has the patient used drugs in the past? (Specify what type and the quantity used.)

HIV Transmission Category

Homosexual contact
Heterosexual contact
Injection drug use

Transfusion recipients (dates and location)
Hemophilia
Unknown

Patient Education

Safe-sex guidelines (condoms, spermicide); safe versus unsafe practices. Is the patient sexually active?

    If yes, is the partner (or partners) aware of the patient's status?
    Has the partner (or partners) been tested for HIV?
    If so, were the results positive? (Inquire about drug use [needle sharing, bleach].)
    Was a treatment referral offered?

Review of Systems

Has the patient had any of the following symptoms in the past 3 months?
    Unexplained weight loss
    Swollen lymph nodes
    Night sweats
    Fevers
    Unusual headaches
    Changes in appetite or sleep pattern
    Trouble thinking
    New skin rash or spots on the skin
    Sores or white spots in the mouth
    Pain when swallowing
    Chest pain, cough, or shortness of breath
    Stomach pain
    Vomiting or diarrhea
    Numbness or tingling in the hands or feet
    Muscle weakness
    Changes in vision

4

TELEHEALTH IN WOMEN'S HEALTH SETTINGS

SHAWANA S. MOORE

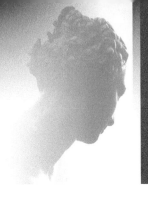

TELEHEALTH

A. Telehealth is a term that has been used interchangeably with telemedicine. It is defined as the use of medical information exchanged from one site to another through electronic communication to improve a patient's health.

B. Telehealth technology was introduced into healthcare in the late 1960s due to the needs of the National Aeronautics and Space Administration (NASA) and the Nebraska Psychology Institute.

C. It is estimated that 76% of U.S. health systems connect healthcare providers and patients remotely via telehealth visits, up from 35% a decade ago (Harvard Health Publishing, 2020).

D. Goals of telehealth include the following:

   1. Enhance overall patient outcomes

   2. Make healthcare accessible to individuals in rural or isolated communities

   3. Allow services to be more readily available for people with limited mobility, time, or transportation options

   4. Lower healthcare costs

DELIVERY OF TELEHEALTH

A. Telehealth services can be delivered in women's health settings in the following four ways.

   1. Synchronously

     a. When the healthcare provider communicates with the patient in real-time via computer, telephone, tablet, or smartphone.

   2. Asynchronously

     a. The data, images, or messages are recorded to share with the healthcare provider later.

   3. mHealth

     a. Occurs when mobile phones or tablet devices are used for self-managed patient care and do not necessarily require involvement monitoring by the healthcare provider (e.g., appointment medication/reminders, patient education self-care steps).

   4. Remote patient monitoring

     a. Measurements, such as weight or blood pressure, are sent to provider.

ADVANTAGES AND DISADVANTAGES OF TELEHEALTH

A. There are benefits and challenges with telehealth services in any setting.

B. Here are some pros and cons for the use of telehealth services.

   1. Pros

     a. Convenience

     b. Cost savings

   c. Limit exposure to potential infections such as COVID-19 and influenza
   d. Increase accessibility to healthcare services
2. Cons
   a. Limitations in types of visits (e.g., pelvic examinations, cervical cancer screenings, and clinical breast examinations)
   b. Insurance coverage
   c. Some concerns with the security of personal healthcare data

EQUIPMENT INVOLVED WITH TELEHEALTH DELIVERY

A. Equipment utilized for the delivery of telehealth services may vary among practice settings. The appropriate equipment to use for your clinical site should be customized to your clinical and patient needs. Here are some recommendations to consider:
1. Computers with or without additional monitoring screens
2. Tablet devices
3. Smartphone devices
4. Headphones
5. Microphones
6. Speakers
7. Docking stations
8. Internet accessibility

TIPS FOR FACILITATING TELEHEALTH VISITS

A. Patients and healthcare providers need to be adequately prepared to communicate during the visit.
B. Tips for patients and providers to consider when preparing and facilitating a telehealth visit
1. Patient
   a. **Test technology:** Provide patients with the opportunity to test their technology before the visit via the option to arrive 15 to 30 minutes before the start of the visit.
   b. **Optimize the location:** Encourage patients to select a quiet and private space to conduct the telehealth visit.
   c. **Have a backup plan:** Advise patients to have a backup plan if the technology they planned to use does not function properly at the time of their visit; this may include switching to a telephone to complete the visit.
2. Healthcare provider
   a. **Look, listen, and observe:** Maintain good eye contact during the visit. Listen carefully to the patient as they speak and avoid interrupting them. Observe facial expression and body language, as this may be helpful with overall assessment of the reason for seeking care.
   b. **Convey empathy:** Use facial expression to convey empathy during the visit. Be sure to explore any strong emotions expressed by the patient and provide validation.

TYPES OF TELEHEALTH SERVICES FOR WOMEN'S HEALTHCARE SETTINGS

A. Increased use in nearly every aspect of women's healthcare, including the following services:
1. Consultations for specialty services
   a. Reproductive endocrinology and infertility
   b. Prenatal genetic screening

    c. Urogynecology

    d. Gynecology/oncology

2. Remote observation of ultrasound recordings by maternal/fetal medicine and reproductive endocrinology experts

    a. Allows for a detailed review of findings on imaging and developing a plan of care in collaboration with the patient.

3. Bladder diary tracking with smartphone applications

    a. Enables patients to monitor their urinary patterns on smartphone devices and report to a healthcare provider during visits to determine the best plan of care.

4. Postpartum blood pressure monitoring with WIFI-connected devices

    a. Allows patients and healthcare providers access to current blood pressure readings and develop a plan of care or intervention when needed.

5. Remote provision of medication abortion

    a. Enables healthcare providers to provide optional medication abortion care for patients.

6. Fertility tracking with patient-generated data

    a. Enables patients to enter fertility information to support themselves and the healthcare provider in developing the best plan of care to optimize fertility.

7. Contraceptive counseling

    a. Enables patients and healthcare providers to discuss birth control options.

8. Screenings for sexually transmitted infections (STI)

    a. Allows for screening for routine STIs and thorough assessment of patient's sexual practices and risks for STI exposures.

9. Vaginitis or STI exposure

    a. Enables patient to connect with healthcare providers who will complete a thorough medical history and history of present illness to determine if presumptive treatment care can be initiated along with ordering of lab tests.

10. Follow-up on lab or imaging results

    a. Allows patients and healthcare providers to discuss results related to STI screenings, abnormal uterine bleeding, or cervical cancer screenings and develop a plan of care.

BILLING AND CODING

A. Billing and coding uniquely designed for telehealth are constantly evolving. Two Healthcare Common Procedure Coding System (HCPCS) codes (Table 4.1) and Current Procedural Terminology (CPT) codes (Table 4.2) for telehealth services were added in 2019.

TABLE 4.1 Overview of Two New Healthcare Common Procedure Coding System (HCPCS) Coding for Telehealth

HEALTHCARE COMMON PROCEDURE CODING SYSTEM (HCPCS) CODES	INDICATION FOR USE OF CODE
HCPCS code G2010	Remote evaluation of recorded video or images submitted by a patient with established care
HCPCS code G2012	Brief communication using technology-based services (5–10 minutes)

TABLE 4.2 Overview of Three New Current Procedural Terminology (CPT) Coding for Telehealth

CURRENT PROCEDURAL TERMINOLOGY (CPT)	INDICATION FOR USE OF CODE
CPT code 99453	Initial set-up and patient education on equipment include remote monitoring of physiologic parameters (e.g., weight or blood pressure).
CPT code 99454	Remote monitoring of physiologic parameters (weight or blood pressure) device supplies daily recordings or programmed alerts transmission every 30 days.
CPT code 99457	Remote physiologic monitoring treatment management services; 20 minutes or more of clinical staff time in a calendar month requires interactive communication with the patient and caregiver during the month.

BIBLIOGRAPHY

American College of Obstetricians and Gynecologists. (2020). Implementing telehealth in practice: ACOG Committee opinion summary, number 798. *Obstet Gynecol, 135*(2), 493–494. https://doi.org/10.1097/AOG.0000000000003672

American Hospital Association. (2021). *Fact sheet: Telehealth*. Retrieved from: https://www.aha.org/factsheet/telehealth.

Davis, T. M., Barden, C., Dean, S., Gavish, A., Goliath, I., Goran, S., ... & Bernard, J. (2016). American telemedicine association guidelines for TeleICU operations. *Telemedicine and e-Health, 22*(12), 971–980. https://doi.org/10.1089/tmj.2016.0065

DeNicola, N., Grossman, D., Marko, K., Sonalkar, S., Butler Tobah, Y. S., Ganju, N., Witkop, C. T., Henderson, J. T., Butler, J.L., & Lowery, C. (2020). Telehealth interventions to improve obstetric and gynecologic health outcomes: A systematic review. *Obstetrics and Gynecology, 135*(2), 371–382. https://doi.org/10.1097/AOG.0000000000003646.

eVisit. (2021) *How does telemedicine work?* Retrieved from https://evisit.com/resources/how-does-telemedicine-work.

Harvard Health Publishing. (2020) *Telehealth: The advantages and disadvantages*. Retrieved from https://www.health.harvard.edu/staying-healthy/telehealth-the-advantages-and-disadvantages.

Jewell T. (2020) *The best telemedicine apps of 2022. Healthline*. Retrieved from https://www.healthline.com/health/best-telemedicine-iphone-android-apps.

LeRouge, C., & Garfield, M. J. (2013). Crossing the telemedicine chasm: Have the U.S. barriers to widespread adoption of telemedicine been significantly reduced? *International Journal of Environmental Research and Public Health, 10*(12), 6472–6484. https://doi.org/10.3390/ijerph10126472

Mayo Clinic. (2020). *Telehealth: Technology meets health care*. Retrieved from: https://www.mayoclinic.org/healthy-lifestyle/consumer-health/in-depth/telehealth/art-20044878#:~:text=Telehealth%20is%20the%20use%20of,or%20support%20health%20care%20services.

Medscape. (2021). *Setting up a telemedicine program in your practice*. Retrieved from: https://www.medscape.com/courses/section/921364.

Saldivar, R. T., Tew, W. P., Shahrokni, A., & Nelson, J. (2021). Goals of care conversations and telemedicine. *Journal of Geriatric Oncology, 12*(7), 995–999. https://doi.org/10.1016/j.jgo.2021.02.016

Tuckson, R. V., Edmunds, M., & Hodgkins, M. L. (2017). Telehealth. *New England Journal of Medicine, 377*(16), 1585–1592. https://doi.org/10.1056/NEJMsr1503323

5

THE PHYSICAL EXAMINATION

HELEN A. CARCIO AND R. MIMI SECOR

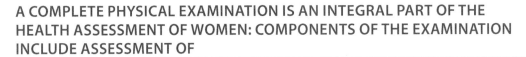

A COMPLETE PHYSICAL EXAMINATION IS AN INTEGRAL PART OF THE HEALTH ASSESSMENT OF WOMEN: COMPONENTS OF THE EXAMINATION INCLUDE ASSESSMENT OF

A. Body habitus, including fat and hair distribution

B. Thyroid gland

C. Heart and lungs

D. Breast examination (see Chapter 9, "Assessment of the Female Breast")

E. Abdominal examination

F. Pelvic examination

G. Rectal exam (may be part of the pelvic exam especially if uterus is retroverted)

H. Skin

EXAMINATION OF THE THYROID GLAND: THYROID DYSFUNCTION CAN CAUSE IRREGULAR MENSES, ANOVULATION, AND INFERTILITY

A. Anterior approach
1. Examiner stands in front of the patient.
2. The woman is asked to extend her head and neck slightly.
3. As the woman swallows, using your finger pads, palpate below the cricoid cartilage for the isthmus of the thyroid.
4. Ask the woman to flex her head and neck slightly forward to her right. This relaxes the sternocleidomastoid muscles, enhancing palpation.
5. Place right examining thumb on upper portion of the left lobe and displace the gland to anatomic right while hooking the tips of the index and middle fingers of the left hand behind right sternocleidomastoid muscle and palpate deeply in front of the muscle with the left thumb for the right lobe.
6. Reverse and repeat the procedure on the left side.
7. The isthmus may be palpable, but the thyroid gland itself is usually not visible or palpable.

B. Posterior approach
1. Examiner stands behind the patient, who is seated.
2. Instruct patient to slightly flex her chin toward her chest.
3. Place finger pads of both hands around the patient's neck.
4. Palpate the isthmus by placing finger pads in the midline of the neck, below the cricoid cartilage.
5. Compare the right and left lobes by sliding your finger pads laterally, below the cricoid cartilage, on either side of the tracheal rings.
6. Ask the patient to tilt her head to the left as you displace the right lobe to the left (medially) with the right hand.

7. Palpate the left lobe as patient swallows, using the finger pads of the left hand.
8. Reverse the procedure to examine the right lobe.

C. Thyroid-stimulating hormone (TSH) testing is indicated if
   1. Anomaly of the thyroid gland is palpated
   2. In the presence of associated signs or symptoms
   3. During an infertility workup, as indicated
   4. If galactorrhea is present or hyperprolactinemia is suspected (hypothyroidism is present in 3%–5% of women with hyperprolactinemia)

D. Note
   1. Motion of isthmus as the woman swallows. Thyroid tissue rises with swallowing; this movement is noticeable with an enlarged gland.
   2. Compare lobes for contour, consistency, or tenderness as the patient swallows.

E. Normal findings
   1. The thyroid gland is usually not palpable.
   2. The isthmus may be felt as a band of tissue that obliterates the tracheal rings.
   3. No nodules or enlargement of the lobes should be felt.

BREAST EXAMINATION (See Chapter 9, "Assessment of the Female Breast")

ABDOMINAL EXAMINATION

A. A thorough abdominal examination should precede the gynecologic examination and include assessing any palpable masses or tenderness, including inguinal lymph nodes.

B. Conducting the abdominal examination before the gynecologic examination often helps reduce some of the anxiety associated with having the gynecologic examination and may serve to "break the ice." Make sure hands are warm. NOTE: This may not be the case if the woman has a history of physical assault involving the abdominal area.

C. Position
   1. Patient should be in the supine position with examiner standing at the patient's side.
   2. Closely monitor the woman's expressions for signs of discomfort.

D. If the woman is ticklish, begin examination with her hand under the examiner's hand.

E. Inspect the abdomen for diastasis recti.
   1. Is there a separation of the abdominal rectus muscles from pregnancy, multiparity, congenital weakness, or marked obesity?
      a. Ask the patient to raise her head and hold it above the pillow for 5 seconds, tensing the abdominal muscles.
      b. Note the location, width, and length of any midline separation between the contracted muscles.
      c. Abdominal muscles should be tight together.

F. Inspect the contour and shape of the abdomen.

G. Observe for the presence of striae (i.e., lines seen after the normal skin has been excessively stretched)
      a. Linea alba from the stretching of the skin from pregnancy
      b. Purple lines associated with Cushing's disease

H. Palpate the lower abdomen for tenderness in the presence of pelvic pain.

I. Palpate the inguinal lymph nodes.
   1. The nodes may be enlarged in the presence of herpes simplex virus, other sexually transmitted infections (STIs), or pelvic inflammatory disease (PID).

  a. Note the size, shape, mobility, consistency, temperature, and tenderness of the nodes. Refer for any hard, immobile nodes.
  b. Nodes may be enlarged and tender in a patient with PID or other STIs.

PELVIC EXAMINATION EXPLAINED

A. The approach
  1. The approach to the gynecologic examination must be systematic, thorough, and carried out in a calm, relaxed manner. Encourage the woman to give verbal feedback throughout the examination.
  2. The pelvic examination should follow other parts of the physical examination to allow the woman time to become comfortable with the examiner. However, sometimes the woman is so anxious that it is best to proceed with the examination first to "get it over with." The preferred order of the exam should be negotiated with the patient.
  3. Ask the patient to empty her bladder before the examination.
  4. Determine if this is her first pelvic examination. A woman undergoing a first pelvic examination is usually more anxious than a woman who has undergone the examination previously. (Also remember that anxiety can be more significant if any previous pelvic examination was not a positive experience or if the woman has a history of sexual abuse or sexual trauma/assault.)
  5. Observe for signs that indicate increased anxiety as the client assumes the supine position. For example, if the patient:
     a. Holds or wrings her hands
     b. Covers her eyes or has her eyes shut
     c. Places her hands on shoulders
     d. Places her hands over pelvis
     e. Places her hands on thighs
     f. Holds onto the exam table
  6. Explain each aspect of the examination thoroughly before it is performed in order to reduce the woman's level of anxiety. Always be as gentle as possible.
     a. Explain the rationale for each aspect of the examination and provide information about what a woman might feel during the examination (e.g., "You might feel some pressure when I insert my fingers into your vagina.").
     b. Suggest coping strategies to deal with any stress the woman may be experiencing.
     c. Encourage the patient to progressively relax different body parts or to try taking deep breaths and exhaling slowly at any point during the examination when she might feel tense.
     d. Teach her how to use statements to herself, such as "I know this is uncomfortable, but I will be fine."
     e. Reassure her that you will stop anytime she becomes uncomfortable.
  7. Before performing the examination, it is often a good idea to offer an "educational" pelvic examination by explaining about the techniques used, the sensations that the patient may feel, and the function of body parts examined.
  8. Consider offering the patient a mirror (a telescoping-handled type is best that can be purchased at an auto parts store) so she can view her vulvar area and if she chooses to observe during the cervical cancer screening procedure. Such measures help patients feel more in control at a time when they may feel especially vulnerable and apprehensive.
     a. Some women are very interested in seeing their cervix, whereas others are not interested or may even be "turned off" by the suggestion.

9. The woman should be encouraged to give verbal feedback throughout the examination so that the examiner can be informed of any maneuvers that cause discomfort. This feedback will help maximize the client's cooperation and minimize anxiety regarding the examination.
10. Explain that the entire examination should take no longer than a few minutes.
11. Acknowledge that the woman may feel rather awkward, but she should not experience any pain unless certain conditions are present, such as STIs, PID, or certain gynecological conditions such as dyspareunia, vulvodynia, an ovarian cyst, ectopic pregnancy, or endometriosis.
12. The examiner may offer an alternative to the traditional pelvic examination (Table 5.1).
13. Table 5.2 summarizes common pelvic examination problems.
14. It is recommended having a chaperone/observer present during the gynecologic examination.

B. Draping
1. Draping can be negotiated between the clinician and patient based on the woman's preference. Some patients prefer draping, and some do not.
2. If draping is used, the drape should cover the patient's lower abdomen and upper thighs and should be depressed in between the knees to allow for eye contact between the examiner and patient.

C. **Position:** The patient should be asked to assume a comfortable lithotomy position on the examination table.
1. For some women, the semi-sitting position (semi-Fowler's) is often preferable to the supine position. Advantages are summarized in Box 5.1.
2. Position the patient's legs in the stirrups, with buttocks slightly overhanging the end of the table. Note: This may be difficult for older women or those with physical challenges.
3. The patient should be asked to keep her knees widely separated and her buttocks flat on the table. Women tend to push against their heels in the stirrups, unknowingly raising their buttocks off the table and tightening their pelvic floor muscles. Remind the patient to drop her hips, slide down (if she has slid up), and take some slow deep breaths.
4. The woman's hands should be relaxed at her sides. This helps enhance abdominal relaxation. In contrast, gripping the side of the examination table increases anxiety and tension.

D. Equipment
1. A good light, either freestanding or attached to a plastic speculum

TABLE 5.1 Alternatives to the Traditional Pelvic Examination	
ALTERNATIVE EXAMINATION	**REASON**
Bimanual examination without the use of speculum	Only indicated for patients at low risk Perform a bimanual examination Digitally locate cervix Slide cotton swab adjacent to finger Rotate the swab over cervix several times Preliminary data support efficacy despite lack of endocervical component
Ultrasound	Virginal women at low risk Can identify other problems such as uterine fibroids or ovarian cysts
Sedation	Recommended for women who have a disability and cannot tolerate the examination; may use 2–8 mg/kg ketamine, 0.2–0.4 mg/kg midazolam

TABLE 5.2 Common Pelvic Examination Problems and Interventions

PELVIC EXAMINATION PROBLEM	INTERVENTIONS
Extreme anxiety	Step-by-step desensitization, relaxation techniques, deep breathing, have the patient do a Kegel then bear down as the speculum is inserted, antianxiety medications, counseling, consider hypnosis or EMDR especially if anxiety is secondary to sexual assault/PTSD
Inability to insert speculum due to discomfort	Use Pederson or small speculum, or use a small swab to collect samples for Pap, STIs, wet mount; encourage deep breathing Consider urine testing for STIs Consider performing the bimanual before the speculum exam
Inability to insert speculum due to dryness	Palpate introital tissues or palpate cervix before speculum insertion Apply scant lubricant to tip of speculum
Inability to insert speculum due to small and/or tight introitus	Use small, Pederson speculum or nasal speculum, have patient do a Kegel and bear down or use a Dacron swab, encourage deep/slow breathing If virginal, a bimanual is not necessary; pregnancy and STI testing can be done using urine or vaginal samples
Inability to visualize cervix	Palpate cervix before speculum examination, move speculum side to side (shimmy), change angle slightly, instruct patient to bear down, try larger speculum, open speculum wider
Vaginal walls impede visualizing cervix	Apply condom over speculum (cutoff tip) Use larger blade speculum such as Graves or Clinton, open-wide Guttman, or "Snowman" lateral vaginal wall
Inability to view cervix because of extreme posterior position	Use large, extra-long speculum, such as "Clinton Pederson" and open wide Palpate cervix before Push down on suprapubic area Instruct patient to bear down Lift hips, spread thighs, use knee stirrups
Speculum comes out unless clinician holds it	While holding the speculum, take samples, remove speculum, then prepare samples for lab testing (cervical cancer screening, STI testing) Seek an assistant to hold the speculum while you collect specimens; remove speculum, then prepare tests
Patient unable to tolerate speculum in situ secondary to anxiety and/or pain	Collect samples, remove speculum, then prepare tests Remember, samples are stable on sampling tools
History of sexual abuse and extreme phobia of pelvic examinations—with or without vaginismus	Co-manage with a specialized counselor Consider hypnosis, and/or EMDR Use step-by-step desensitization program May not be able to complete a pelvic examination for several visits (may take months or years)

EMDR, eye movement desensitization reprocessing; STI, sexually transmitted infection.

Source: R. Mimi Secor © 2021

2. Vaginal speculum (metal or plastic)
3. Water-soluble lubricant (not always necessary)
4. Supplies for the cervical cancer screening test and cultures/STI testing as indicated. NOTE: Gloves should be worn throughout the examination and afterward when handling any samples, equipment, or supplies.

BOX 5.1 Advantages of the Semi-Sitting Position During a Pelvic Examination

- More comfortable for the patient
- Relaxes the rectus and abdominal muscles
- Increases eye contact
- Allows the woman to hold the mirror to more easily view her anatomy while the examination is conducted
- Enables the patient to feel less vulnerable

INSPECTION OF THE EXTERNAL GENITALIA

A. Some comments
   1. Examination of the external genitalia is conducted before the internal speculum and bimanual examinations.
   2. The examiner should sit on a stool at the end of the table facing the patient.
   3. Position the light to achieve maximum illumination of the external genitalia.
   4. Inspection begins by viewing the suprapubic and inguinal regions superiorly and then progressing inferiorly to include the clitoral hood, clitoris, urethral meatus, vaginal introitus, fourchette, and posteriorly, the anal and sacral areas.
   5. Visual inspection of the genitals is also conducted in a medial to lateral fashion, from the vaginal introitus laterally to the labia minora, labia majora, and upper and inner thigh regions. A thorough visual inspection also includes gentle palpation as needed to view overlapping tissues.
   6. A saline-moistened cotton or Dacron swab may also be used to separate overlapping skin surfaces (and to assess for areas of tenderness) and is particularly helpful in examining the labia, introital, and hymenal structures.
   7. Always remember to touch the thigh gently before actually touching the genitals. Ask permission before touching/palpating and tell the woman when she will feel your touch.
   8. For physical changes related to genital atrophy, see Chapter 24, "Genitourinary Syndrome of Menopause and Vulvovaginal Atrophy," which includes genital atrophy/atrophic vaginitis.
   9. For assessment of pelvic organ prolapse, see Chapter 31, "Pelvic Organ Prolapse."
B. Assess the mons pubis.
   1. Note general hygiene, hair distribution, and any lesions.
   2. **Normal findings:** Clean, coarse pubic hair extending in an inverse triangle, with the base over the mons pubis. No lesions should be present.
   3. Clinical alterations
      a. "Dirty-appearing" hair shafts from pediculosis
      b. Localized inflammation at the base of the hair shaft caused by folliculitis
      c. Scaly epidermal plaques from psoriasis
      d. Sparse hair associated with hormonal problems or advancing age
      e. Racial variations
         (1) **Blacks:** Shorter hair that is more tightly coiled.
         (2) **Asians, Native Americans, and Alaskan Natives:** Hair is generally sparser.
      f. *Phthirus pubis* (lice) or their eggs (nits). Bites appear as small, red maculopapules.
C. Tanner staging (Figure 5.1)
   1. Pubic hair growth begins between 8 and 14 years of age.

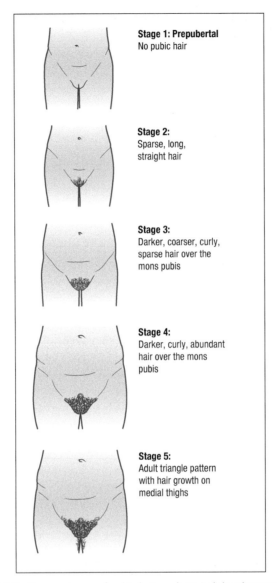

Stage 1: Prepubertal
No pubic hair

Stage 2:
Sparse, long,
straight hair

Stage 3:
Darker, coarser, curly,
sparse hair over the
mons pubis

Stage 4:
Darker, curly, abundant
hair over the mons
pubis

Stage 5:
Adult triangle pattern
with hair growth on
medial thighs

FIGURE 5.1: Tanner stages of pubic hair and genital development in girls.

Source: From Chiocca, EM. (2019). Ad*vanced Pediatric Assessment,* Third Edition. Springer Publishing Company.

2. Staging should be assessed in adolescent girls as an assessment of the maturity of the pituitary–ovarian axis. It should be performed as routinely as possible.

D. Quantify the signs of androgen excess.

1. *Hirsutism* is defined as the presence of hair in a location where hair is not commonly found in women. The extent of hair distribution varies among ethnic groups.

2. Hair morphology and distribution should be graded. The most functional and widely used instrument is the Farriman–Gallwey (F–G) scale, which semi-quantitatively grades hair growth in nine body areas.

3. Clinical alterations

a. More than 10% of adult women have hair that extends up the abdomen to the umbilicus. This distribution is usually associated with ethnic/racial variations.

b. Absent or scant hair distribution may indicate endocrine dysfunction or post-menopause.

    c. Hirsutism may be associated with polycystic ovarian syndrome (sideburns, chin, chest, and lower abdomen) or other endocrinopathies like Cushings syndrome, Cushings disease, or late onset congenital adrenal hyperplasia.

E. Inspect the vulva for genital lesions.

  1. Note cysts, warts, chancres, ulcerations, and areas of hypo- or hyperpigmentation.

  2. **Normal findings:** Labia majora are hair-covered epidermal surfaces; labia minora are pink, glistening mucosal surfaces. Hart's line is the mucocutaneous border between the labia minora and labia majora.

  3. Clinical alterations

    a. Nontender, firm nodules of sebaceous cysts

    b. Micropapillomatosis labialis is a normal variant but can be confused with condyloma accuminata. Normal micropapillomatosis are single stalk papillations.

    c. In contrast, condyloma (genital warts) are characterized by multiple papillae extending from a single base. Wart-like protrusion singly or in clusters from condyloma acuminatum or condyloma latum.

    d. Round, clear umbilicated vesicles of molluscum contagiosum

    e. Nontender chancre with a well-demarcated border from primary syphilis

    f. Chancroid

    g. Single or clustered tender vesicles or ulcerations of genital herpes

    h. Irregular, nontender hyperpigmented lesions related to carcinoma of the vulva

    i. Genital mutilation associated with certain cultural practices

    j. Varicosities associated with pelvic congestion (pregnancy)

F. Inspect the vulva for discoloration and pigmentation.

  1. **Normal findings:** Pink with varying shades of white, brown, and red, depending on racial characteristics

    a. Usually, the same color as the skin covering the external parts of the rest of the body.

  2. Clinical alterations

    a. Redness or erythema occurring in response to inflammation

      (1) A reddened vulva is a dermatologic condition such as psoriasis, seborrheic dermatitis, lichen sclerosis, or vulvitis/vulvovaginitis (*Candida*).

    b. Dark or pigmented lesions usually caused by an increase in the amount or concentration of melanin

      (1) Dark lesions require biopsy to exclude malignant melanoma and clarify the nature of such lesions.

      (2) Most dark lesions are either harmless freckles or nevi.

      (3) Routinely monitor nevi because of their potential to develop into melanoma.

    c. White lesions are related to:

      (1) Decreased vascularity

      (2) Depigmentation (decrease in melanocytes in the basal layer)

      (3) Changes in the keratin in the presence of moisture (presence of water turns the keratin white, as if a hand or foot was soaked in water for 10 to 20 minutes.)

      (4) Common conditions associated with white lesions/lichenification are lichen sclerosus, squamous cell hyperplasia (also known as *lichen simplex chronicus*), psoriasis, eczematous vulvitis, and vitiligo (lacking lichenification).

G. Examine the external genitalia for any bruises or injuries that might suggest sexual assault.

H. Examine the clitoris.

  1. Note the size.

  2. **Normal findings:** Round, pink erectile tissue under the fourchette. Approximately 2 cm (0.75 in.) in length and 0.5 cm in width.

  3. Clinical alterations

      a. Enlargement in masculinizing conditions, excess testosterone, and use of testosterone-containing medications

      b. Atrophy to the point of disappearance with late-stage lichen sclerosis

I. Inspect the urethral orifice.

  1. Note erythema or purulent discharge

  2. **Normal findings:** Pink tissue without discharge

  3. Clinical alterations

      a. A caruncle is associated with estrogen deprivation and appears as a small, red protrusion through the urethral orifice. It often resembles a polyp.

      b. Prolapse of the urethral mucosa, which forms a swollen red ring around the urinary meatus. This condition is often associated with post-menopause.

      c. Leakage of urine is associated with stress incontinence and post-menopause, lack of muscle tone, obesity, and advanced age.

J. Examine the vaginal orifice.

  1. Note the presence of discharge, intact hymen or hymenal remnants, and bulging of vaginal tissue or cervix through the orifice.

  2. Normal findings are a small amount of white to clear discharge, intact hymen or hymenal remnant surrounding the orifice, no bulging.

  3. Clinical alterations

      a. Discharge secondary to vaginitis or cervicitis

          (1) Perform wet mount evaluation and other diagnostic testing as appropriate on any discharge present.

      b. Thick, pink membrane overlying the vaginal orifice from an imperforate hymen; vaginal insertion of a swab rules out an imperforate hymen

      c. Anterior bulging of vaginal tissue through the orifice from a cystocele

          (1) A cystocele is the downward prolapse of the bladder against the anterior (upper) vaginal wall.

          (2) It is generally related to weakening of vaginal and pelvic support due to childbirth or obesity.

          (3) It is aggravated by obesity.

      d. Posterior bulging of the vaginal tissue from a rectocele

          (1) A rectocele is the prolapse of the rectum bulging up against the posterior vaginal wall. It is generally related as described earlier.

  4. It may be useful to document any abnormalities by creating a diagram.

K. Inspect perineum and anus.

  1. Posterior skin of the perineum between the vaginal introitus and the anus should appear smooth.

  2. If woman had an episiotomy, a scar may be visible.

  3. Note any skin tags, lesions, fissures, ulcers, or hemorrhoids in the anal area.

PALPATION OF THE EXTERNAL GENITALIA

A. Some comments

  1. Avoid startling the patient by telling her in advance when she will be touched and where.

  2. Palpation of the external genitalia is conducted using a gentle approach and, if tenderness is elicited, a cotton-tipped applicator/swab may be used to assess more specifically the location and severity.

  3. Placing the finger beneath the urethra along the anterior vaginal wall may help identify the presence of a urethral diverticulum or express any liquid/discharge that might be present in the Skene's glands.

4. During palpation of the introitus, obese and parous patients may also be asked to perform a Kegel contraction followed by a Valsalva maneuver to assess tone and laxity of the pelvic musculature to detect any degree of cystocele or rectocele.

5. Avoid excessive palpation of the genitalia, which might be interpreted as sexual. As mentioned previously, it is recommended to have a chaperone/observer present during the gynecologic examination.

B. Assess Bartholin's glands and Skene's glands.

1. **Technique:** Insert index finger into the vagina with thumb remaining outside on the posterior portion of the labia majora. Press thumb and index finger together at the 5 o'clock and 7 o'clock positions of the lateral labia minora.

2. Note any swelling, masses, discharge, or tenderness.

3. **Normal findings:** Skene's and Bartholin's glands are normally not palpable. The surface should be homogeneous, nontender, and without discharge.

4. **Clinical alteration:** Varying degrees of enlarged gland result from a Bartholin's cyst. Marked swelling, increased warmth, and tenderness may indicate an abscess.

5. If discharge is present, a gonorrheal (GC) and chlamydia culture should be performed because gonorrhea and/or chlamydia may cause a Bartholin's abscess.

C. Assess paraurethral gland and urethra.

1. **The technique:** Insert the gloved hand slowly into the vagina, palm upward. Exerting upward pressure, remove finger, milking the urethra.

2. Note tenderness or discharge from the urethra.

3. **Normal findings:** Negative discharge and nontender.

4. **Clinical alteration:** Purulent discharge may be related to gonococcal or chlamydial urethritis.

D. Evaluate vaginal wall support.

1. **Technique:** Spread the vaginal introitus and ask patient to bear down. You may also ask the woman to cough or bear down (Valsalva maneuver). Assess any degree of prolapse.

2. Note any anterior or posterior bulging of the vaginal wall. Some leakage of urine from the urinary meatus may also be noted during this maneuver.

3. **Normal finding:** No protrusion of vaginal walls through the vaginal introitus.

4. Clinical alterations

a. Anterior bulging of vaginal tissue (in varying degrees) at and/or extending beyond the introitus indicates a cystocele or cystourethrocele.

b. Posterior bulging. A rectocele will balloon upward toward the introitus during the Valsalva maneuver.

c. If the cervix is visible at the vaginal opening, it usually indicates a significant uterine prolapse.

E. Assess pelvic muscle tone (see Chapter 31, "Pelvic Organ Prolapse").

1. The pelvic floor muscles (pubococcygeal muscle [PC]), a sling-like structure, are attached to the pubic bone in front and the coccyx/tail bone in back. The character and strength of these muscles are easily accessed during the vaginal digital examination (Figure 5.2).

a. Place one finger 2 cm inside the woman's vagina. Palpate the pelvic floor muscle at the 5 o'clock position. Ask her to tighten her pelvic floor muscle by contracting her rectal muscles. Repeat maneuver in the 7 o'clock position.

b. Compare strength.

2. Examiner should feel upward pressure on the fingers.

3. **Normal findings:** Tension is maintained for 5 seconds.

4. Clinical alteration. Impaired strength due to:

a. Vaginal deliveries (traumatic or multiple)

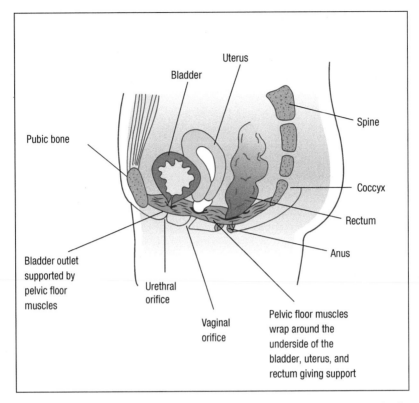

FIGURE 5.2 Side view of a woman's bladder and related structures. Note how the urethral and vaginal orifices and rectum pass through the strap of the pelvic muscles.

    b. Older age, particularly with decreased estrogen levels in women not receiving hormone therapy

    c. Neurologic impairment such as multiple sclerosis

  5. Impaired tone may cause urinary or fecal incontinence.

THE BIMANUAL EXAMINATION

A. Special considerations

  1. Any pelvic mass detected during the bimanual examination should be described in terms of its location, size (in centimeters), tenderness, motility, and consistency (soft, hard, smooth, irregular).

  2. It is important for the patient to relax as much as possible because voluntary guarding of the abdominal muscles will prevent effective palpation of the pelvic structures.

  3. There is a controversy regarding which portion of the pelvic examination should be performed next. Some clinicians believe that the bimanual examination should precede the speculum examination. There are several advantages to this (Box 5.2).

    a. This technique helps facilitate the insertion of the speculum, because the woman's own vaginal secretions can be used as a lubricant, thus eliminating the use of lubricating gels.

    b. If an abnormality is palpated, it can be thoroughly inspected during the speculum examination. Most vaginal lesions are more easily palpated than visually inspected.

> **BOX 5.2 Advantages of Performing the Bimanual Examination Before the Speculum Examination**
>
> - Helps the clinician determine the position of the cervix facilitating insertion of the speculum and visualizing the cervix
> - Able to use woman's own vaginal secretions for lubrication
> - Facilitates insertion of the speculum
> - Eliminates use of lubricating gels
> - Clues the examiner to palpated anomalies that require further inspection
> - Perceived by the patient as less invasive

  c. When the bimanual examination is performed before the speculum examination, the clinician can better determine the position of the cervix, which makes the speculum insertion easier for both the patient and the clinician.

  d. Gentle palpation may be perceived as less invasive to the woman than inserting the speculum first.

  e. A disadvantage of this technique is the possibility of mixing cervical and vaginal flora together, altering the accuracy of any subsequent vaginal microscopic analysis. NOTE: If vaginitis is suspected, a vaginal sample can be obtained with a swab before the bimanual examination is performed.

4. The bimanual examination involves using both hands, inserting one or two fingers vaginally, while with the other hand, palpating the pelvic structures through the abdominal wall.

5. It is important that the patient be relaxed during the bimanual examination because guarding and tightening of the abdominal muscles will impede the examiner's ability to palpate the underlying structures beneath the rigid musculature.

6. A metal speculum can be warmed by keeping it on a heating pad or running it under warm water just before insertion.

7. *While wearing gloves*, some clinicians touch the blades of the speculum to ensure that the temperature is comfortable.

8. An introitus should comfortably accommodate a single examining finger. Should the orifice be too small, a single finger inserted into the rectum can be used to perform a fairly accurate bimanual examination. However, it is important to be sensitive to the invasiveness of this approach.

9. Box 5.3 lists the advantages and disadvantages of using a plastic speculum.

B. Technique
   1. Stand between stirrups.
   2. Insert the index and middle fingers of your gloved hand and exert firm pressure, primarily downward. (The thumb should be abducted, with the ring and little finger flexed into the palm.)

C. Palpation of the cervix: The cervix should be palpated by sweeping the fingers around the protruding cervical knob in the area of the fornices; gently move the cervix side to side.
   1. The cervix should normally be palpable, mobile, and non-tender.
   2. Note the depth and angle of the cervix.
      a. Should the cervix be markedly tilted to the right or left, or fixed, endometriosis and pelvic/uterine/adnexal mass adhesions should be suspected.
   3. Note the size, shape, and consistency (like the tip of the nose).
   4. Note any palpable lumps.
   5. Clinical alterations

> **BOX 5.3 Advantages and Disadvantages of the Plastic (Disposable) Speculum**
>
> **Advantages of the Plastic Speculum**
> - Provides an unobstructed view of the vaginal walls through its clear blades
> - Eliminates the need to warm the speculum
> - Reduces patient anxiety because clear plastic is generally less "threatening" to patients than metal
> - More comfortable due to the rounded edges of the speculum blades
> - Can attach to a light source
> - If attached: Enhances illumination of the cervix and vaginal walls; reduces risk of contamination of lamp from adjusting an external light source
>
> **Disadvantages of the Plastic Speculum**
> - Adds to the accumulation of medical waste
> - The speculum can break or lock in place, making removal challenging—it should not be used with obese or restless patients
> - A click may occur during the opening and closing of the blades, which may startle the patient (be sure to warn the patient)

  a. Presence of cervical motion tenderness (CMT) indicates possible PID
  b. A fixed cervix due to endometriosis or a tumor displacing it
  c. Small smooth, nontender/bumps indicating probable benign nabothian cysts
  d. Prominent anterior cervical lip from maternal use of diethylstilbestrol (DES)
  e. An anterior-pointing (angled toward the introitus) cervix suggests a retroverted uterus
  f. A posterior-pointing (angled downward) cervix suggests anteverted uterus
  g. If the cervix protrudes into the vagina more than 3 cm (1.2 in.) or is located proximal to the introitus, this may indicate a pelvic or ovarian mass or uterine prolapse

D. The vagina should be carefully palpated for tenderness, lesions, masses, or foreign bodies (e.g., forgotten tampons)

E. Palpation of the uterus
  1. Some key points
      a. The uterus is sometimes difficult to palpate effectively.
      b. The uterus may not be palpable in an obese woman or in one whose abdominal muscles are tense and rigid.
      c. If the uterus is not palpable in a thin, relaxed woman, it may be absent, or tipped posteriorly (retroverted).
  2. The technique
      a. Place the dominant hand on the abdomen, midway between the umbilicus and the symphysis pubis.
      b. Insert the index and middle fingers (one finger is acceptable if unable to insert two) of the other hand into the vagina, with the palmar surface facing anteriorly.
      c. Position the two fingers in the vagina under the cervix, then lift the cervix by applying upward pressure. At the same time, press downward, in the suprapubic area, with the abdominal hand using a gentle sweeping technique. Then, palpate the uterus between the two hands. Assess the uterus with the abdominal hand (Figure 5.3).
  3. Note anteflexed, retroflexed, anteverted, or retroverted position
      a. The uterus is normally anteverted and slightly anteflexed.
      b. If it is retroverted and immobile, suspect endometriosis.
      c. A retroverted uterus is not palpable during a bimanual examination (Figure 5.4).

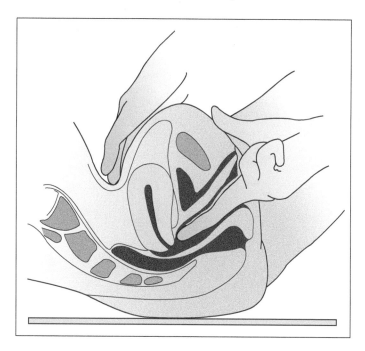

FIGURE 5.3 Bimanual palpation of an anteverted uterus. The examiner is able to palpate the body or fundus of the uterus between the vaginal and abdominal examining fingers.

Source: Gray, R. H. (1980). *Manual for the provision of intrauterine devices (IUDs)*. Geneva, Switzerland: World Health Organization.

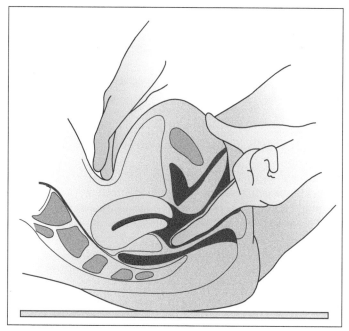

FIGURE 5.4 Bimanual palpation of a retroverted uterus. The examiner is unable to palpate the fundus of the uterus between the vaginal and abdominal examining fingers.

Source: Gray, R. H. (1980). *Manual for the provision of intrauterine devices (IUDs)*. Geneva, Switzerland: World Health Organization.

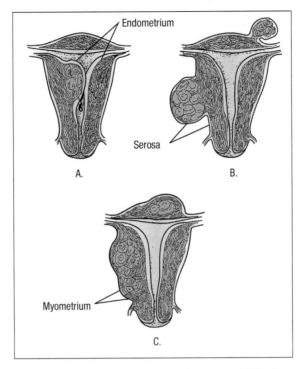

FIGURE 5.5 Appearance of uterine fibroids: (A) submucous leiomyoma, (B) subserous leiomyoma, and (C) intramural leiomyoma.

4. Consistency, size, and shape
   a. Mobility
      (1) It should be normally mobile in the anteroposterior plane.
      (2) It has limited mobility in the transverse plane because it is supported by the cardinal ligaments.
      (3) Immobility in the anteroposterior plane suggests scar tissue due to previous PID, endometriosis, scarring.
   b. Tenderness
   c. Palpable masses
   d. **Normal findings:** Smooth, firm surface; mobile; without tenderness or masses
   e. Clinical alterations
      (1) Soft enlargement caused by an intrauterine pregnancy
      (2) Tenderness of the uterus suggesting possible infection, endometriosis, or pregnancy
      (3) An irregular, firm uterus is related to the various shapes and positions of fibroids (Figure 5.5). In women over 50, an irregular and/or enlarged uterus may be associated with malignancy.
      (4) An immobile, tilted uterus is associated with endometriosis, scarring, or an abdominal mass.

PALPATION OF THE OVARIES AND FALLOPIAN TUBES

A. Some comments
   1. The ovaries are small (the size of an almond) and difficult to assess, particularly in the presence of abdominal obesity or muscle rigidity. In endometriosis, the ovaries may be located behind the uterus (referred to as *holding hands*), making them difficult to assess.

2. The ovaries should NOT be palpable in postmenopausal women; if they are palpated, this should be considered abnormal and be promptly investigated (referral to Ob/Gyn).
3. Advise the patient that there may be a brief sensation of discomfort when the ovaries are palpated.
4. The fallopian tubes are normally not palpable. If they are enlarged, the examiner should suspect salpingitis, an ectopic pregnancy, or cancer—especially if 50 years or older.

B. The technique
1. The ovaries are evaluated by first locating the vaginal fingers to either the right or left side of the lateral fornix (posterior vaginal area).
2. Move the abdominal hand to the lower abdominal quadrant on the same side as the internal hand.
3. Apply firm and steady pressure, beginning medially to the anterior iliac crest. Sweep your abdominal hand inward toward the vaginal hand and down to the mons pubis. This should be a smooth process, not involving a jerky, punching-like action.
4. Repeat the procedure on the opposite side.

C. Note
1. Size, tenderness, and masses
2. Location
3. Thickening or enlargement

D. Normal findings
1. Ovaries may normally be slightly tender when palpated.
2. The fallopian tubes should be nonpalpable, nontender, and not thickened.

E. Abnormal findings
1. Enlarged, cystic ovaries are often associated with polycystic ovarian syndrome.
2. An enlarged ovary may be secondary to an ovarian cyst or ovarian cancer. If either condition is suspected, a pelvic ultrasound should be ordered to confirm the diagnosis.
3. Palpable tubes may feel like fibrous bands, suggesting previous salpingitis or endometriosis, or possible rare fallopian tube cancer in a woman older than 50 years. Prompt referral to Ob/Gyn is essential if cancer is suspected.

RECTOVAGINAL EXAMINATION

A. This examination is not always necessary, but if infection is suspected and/or the uterus is thought to be retroverted, or if abnormalities are suspected, this examination should be considered.
B. As you insert your finger into the rectum, instruct the client to bear down, then to relax and continue to inhale and exhale slowly. The examination is often slightly uncomfortable and is considered invasive. Be sure to screen your patient for sexual abuse.
C. Technique
1. After applying a new glove, insert one lubricated, gloved finger rectally and one gloved finger vaginally, palpating the rectovaginal septum.
2. Insert your fingers as far in as possible.
3. With the other hand on the abdomen, push the uterus as posteriorly as possible.
4. Palpate the posterior aspect of the uterus and the rectal wall with your internal fingers.
5. Note any masses, tenderness, hemorrhoids, or the presence of a retroverted uterus (size, shape, angle, contour [smooth, irregular, etc.], mobility, tenderness).
D. Guaiac assessment for occult blood (not very accurate according to recent research)
1. Take stool adhered to the examining glove and wipe on the appropriate section of the test paper.

2. Place one to two drops of developing solution over sample.
3. Wait for 30 seconds.
4. A positive result is indicated by the appearance of a blue or dark green color.

E. Colonoscopy screening
1. Colon cancer is the third most common cancer diagnosed in both men and women in the United States. It is also the third most common cause of cancer-related death among men and women in the United States. The death rate (number of deaths per 100,000 people per year) from colorectal cancer has been dropping in both men and women for several decades. This is thought to be due to increased screening and early management (such as removal of pre-cancerous polyps).
2. Early screening for asymptomatic colorectal cancer is lifesaving.
3. Suggest screening of average-risk women from 45 years of age every 10 years.
4. High-risk women include those with advancing age, a diet high in fat, or a family history of colon cancer.
5. Colorectal cancer risk factors include:
   a. Older age
   b. Inflammatory bowel disease (Crohn's disease or ulcerative colitis)
   c. Personal or family history of colorectal cancer or colorectal polyps.
   d. Genetic syndrome such as familial adenomatous polyposis (FAP) or hereditary non-polyposis colorectal cancer (Lynch syndrome).
6. Lifestyle factors that may increase risk of colorectal cancer
   a. Lack of regular exercise
   b. Diet low in fruit and vegetables
   c. Low-fiber and high-fat diet, or a diet high in processed meats.
   d. Overweight and obesity
   e. Alcohol consumption
   f. Tobacco use
7. Recommendations for screening of high-risk women depends on their specific risks as described and recommended in the 2019 American Cancer Society screening guidelines.
8. Education is critical.

SPECULUM EXAMINATION

A. Some comments
1. The size (diameter) and tone of the introitus (vaginal opening) influence the size and type of the speculum that is selected. If the cervix is palpated prior to speculum insertion, the examiner will have a better idea of what size speculum might be most appropriate.
2. Select a speculum size that will be comfortable for the patient while allowing optimal viewing of the cervix (the largest comfortable size).
3. If a metal speculum is used, it should be warmed or lubricated with tap water. Another strategy to ease insertion is to apply a small amount of lubricant to the tips of the speculum blades.
4. Utilizing liquid-based cytology reduces the likelihood that lubricant will interfere with the test; nonetheless, to minimize the risk, only a small amount of lubricant should be used if it is needed.
5. The patient should be informed when the speculum will be inserted. Showing the patient the speculum before it is inserted may lessen anxiety during the procedure. (However, it may increase anxiety in others.)

B. **Choice of speculum:** Either a plastic or metal speculum may be used.
1. Plastic speculums can be purchased with an attached light (corded or cordless). This feature enhances visualization because it allows direct illumination of the vaginal vault.

C. Technique
  1. Palpating the cervix before inserting the speculum will help the clinician locate the cervix. This in turn will help the clinician insert the speculum in the appropriate direction and angle (slightly up, down, left, right, front, or back of the vagina).
  2. Using your nondominant hand, separate the labia with your index and middle fingers. At the same time, holding the speculum between your index (over top blade) and middle finger (under bottom blade), insert the speculum while applying gentle downward pressure. This helps avoid injuring the clitoral area as the speculum is inserted.
  3. Hold the speculum at a slight side angle during insertion.
  4. Next, gently direct the speculum downward toward the sacrum, while applying downward pressure against the peritoneum until the speculum is fully inserted.
  5. Gradually open the blades as the cervix comes into view (shiny and smooth).
  6. When inserting the speculum, be careful not to pinch pubic hair.
  7. Sometimes, a slight side-to-side movement (shimmy) of the blades will help you visualize the cervix (as you open the speculum blades).
  8. Small adjustments in speculum angle may also be helpful.
  9. The blades may be held open with one hand, or by either tightening the screw of a metal speculum (be careful not to catch any pubic hair) or by clicking the plastic blades into an open position.
      a. There is no need to secure the blades wide open. It is sometimes more comfortable for the patient if the blades are held partially open for the short time during which the vagina and cervix are inspected.
  10. The vaginal canal is inspected as the speculum is removed. This is enhanced with a lighted plastic speculum.

D. Inspection of the vagina
  1. The vaginal mucosa should be examined while the speculum is in place and also as the speculum is slowly rotated and withdrawn from the vagina. This is facilitated by the use of a clear plastic speculum. Special attention should be given to any lesions that were palpated earlier.
  2. Note any abnormal alterations.
      a. **Presence of rugae (mucosal folds):** Rugae indicate a good estrogen effect. In a woman with low estrogen levels, the mucosa will be thin, atrophic, and lack rugation.
      b. A spatula or cotton-tipped applicator may be used to collect a lateral vaginal wall sample to assess pH, perform a whiff test, and prepare the wet mount.
      c. Cervical mucus may alter the pH and wet mount reading, so it should be avoided, if possible.
  3. Note the quantity, quality, color, and odor of any vaginal discharge.
      a. A vaginal pH, whiff test, and a wet mount may be considered (based on history and risk) to assess for vaginal infections and to confirm the presence of normal vaginal flora (pH only) or estrogen deficiency (see Chapter 6, "Vaginal Microscopy and Vaginal Infections").
      b. Research suggests that bacterial vaginosis (BV) may be linked to preterm labor and many gynecologic problems.
      c. It is now recognized that lactobacilli-dominant flora is important for all women of reproductive age, including those who are attempting pregnancy. A culture for gonorrhea or chlamydia and possibly other STIs, like trichomoniasis and/or genital herpes, may be indicated especially if the vaginal pH or whiff test are abnormal and/or if the wet mount shows excessive polymorphonuclear white blood cells (greater than 5 per high power field).

E. **Visualization of the cervix:** If discharge obscures the view, collect the cervical cancer screening sample first, then gently remove the discharge with a Dacron swab; evaluate/test any unusual discharge; pay special attention to any anomalies previously palpated; note the following:

TABLE 5.3 Conditions Affecting the Cervix

CONDITION	SYMPTOMS IDENTIFIED DURING ASSESSMENT
Nulliparous cervix	Os is small and either round or oval Covered by smooth epithelium
Parous cervix	Slit-like appearance
Cervical polyp	Small, often friable, bright-red, berry-like protrusion(s) Usually arises from the endocervical canal and becomes visible when it protrudes through the cervical os
Nabothian cyst	Vary in size, can be single or multiple Appear as translucent, smooth, nontender nodules on the cervical surface May be caused by chronic cervicitis
Ectropion	An extension of the endocervical columnar epithelium onto the ectocervix Often seen with increased estrogen production, such as pregnancy or use of birth-control pills
Erosion	Friable tissue surrounding os from an infected ectropion Might be first evidenced by bleeding with a Pap test

1. Size and shape of the cervical os
   a. Normal findings and clinical alterations
      (1) Slit associated with vaginal delivery
      (2) Lacerations from a tear during a precipitous delivery
      (3) An oval or round os is noted in nulliparous women
      (4) A tiny os may be noted in post-menopausal women who are not taking hormone replacement therapy
2. Characteristics of the cervix, such as friability or lesions
   a. A friable cervix may be related to a cervical infection, such as chlamydia or vaginitis.
   b. Nabothian cysts appear smooth, round, small, yellow, raised and are nontender.
   c. A wartlike friable growth may be associated with cervical cancer or noncancerous genital warts (from low-risk human papillomavirus [HPV] subtypes 6 or 11; cervical cancer is usually not visible in the early stages).
3. Cervical surface
   a. A cervical erosion is a denuded area of squamous epithelium with a clearly defined but slightly irregular border.
   b. Varying amounts of squamous epithelium (pink tissue) are visible on the ectocervix, depending on the patient's age and hormonal status.
   c. Conditions affecting the cervix are listed in Table 5.3.
4. **Cervical mucus:** Evaluate for quality and quantity, including clarity, opacity, and mucus; perform a wet mount if indicated (see Chapter 6, "Vaginal Microscopy and Vaginal Infections").
   a. Clear mucus indicates a healthy cervix without infection.
   b. Yellow, thick mucus suggests infection such as cervicitis, STIs, or PID.
5. Signs of DES exposure (Box 5.4)
6. **Color of the cervix:** It is normally pink but may have a bluish hue in early pregnancy or increased vascularity
   a. A red, friable cervix suggests infection (especially if yellow cervical mucus).
7. Any cervical lesion, regardless of the cervical cancer screening test results (even if negative) should be referred for colposcopy.

BOX 5.4 Signs of Diethylstilbestrol Exposure

Cockscomb: Prominent anterior portion of the cervix
Collar: Flat rim or hood surrounding the posterior cervix, covered with columnar epithelium
Pseudopolyp: Lypoid appearance of cervix resulting from circumferential groove, thickening of stroma of anterior or posterior endocervical canal
Hypoplastic cervix: Cervix less than 1.5 cm in diameter
Other: Columnar epithelium that covers most of the cervix; may extend to the vaginal wall

---

UPON COMPLETION OF THE PELVIC EXAMINATION

A. The woman should be provided with verbal reassurance, be advised to get dressed, and offered tissue to wipe off any excessive lubricant. A sanitary pad should be provided if any bleeding is present.

B. Provide the woman privacy to dress, then return to complete the visit. Allow time to address any questions arising from the examination or overall visit.

C. At this point, information obtained from the comprehensive health history is combined with findings from the physical examination to determine the assessment and/or diagnosis/diagnoses.

D. The plan of care based on the workup, probable diagnoses should be thoroughly reviewed and negotiated with the patient.

E. Provide education, counseling, and support as appropriate.

F. Review timeline for test results (if any were performed).

G. Document findings accurately (Box 5.5).

H. Arrange for any follow-up or additional testing.

RESOURCE

Nurse Practitioners in Women's Health (NPWH). 2021. Well Women Visit App.

BOX 5.5 Charting a Normal Pelvic Examination (Sample)

External genitalia: Normal distribution of pubic hair; no lesions, masses, or lymphadenopathy; non-tender; no discharge from the Bartholin's glands or urethra
Vagina: Pink, rugated without bulging or lesions; scant opaque, white discharge without odor; good muscle tone
Cervix: Pink, non-tender, without lesions. Cervical mucus scant and clear, no cervical motion tenderness (CMT).
Uterus: Anterior; normal size, firm without enlargement, tenderness, or masses; mobile
Adenexae: Ovaries palpated without enlargement, tenderness, or masses
Rectovaginal: Non-tender, without fissures, masses, or lesions

BIBLIOGRAPHY

American Cancer Society. (2018). *2018 colorectal cancer screening guideline for men and women at average risk*. Retrieved from https://www.cancer.org/content/dam/cancer -org/online-documents/en/pdf/infographics/colorectal-cancer-screening-guideline-for-men-and-women-at-average-risk.pdf

Bates, C. K., Carroll, N., & Potter, J. (2011). The challenging pelvic examination. *Journal of General Internal Medicine, 26*(6), 651–657. https://doi.org/[0-9A-z]0.1007/s11606-010-1610-8

Bickley, L. S., Szilagyi, P. G., Hoffman, R. M., Soriano, R. P. (2020). *Bates' guide to physical examination and history taking* (13th ed.). Wolters Kluwer.

Committee on Gynecologic Practice. (2016). Committee opinion no. 534: Well-woman visit. *Obstetrics and Gynecology, 120*(2 Pt. 1), 421–424. https://doi.org/[0-9A-z]0.1097/AOG.0b013e3182680517

Hamza, A., Warczok, C., Meyberg-Solomayer, G., Takacs, Z., Juhasz-Boess, I., Solomayer, E. F., Radosa, M. P., Radosa, C. G., Stotz, L., Findeklee, S., & Radosa, J. C. (2020). Teaching undergraduate students gynecological and obstetrical examination skills: The patient's opinion. *Archives of Gynecology and Obstetrics, 302*(2), 431–438. https://doi.org/10.1007/s00404-020-05615-1

Harmanli, O., & Jones, K. A. (2010). Using lubricant for speculum insertion. *Obstetrics and Gynecology, 116*(2 Pt. 1), 415–417. https://doi.org/[0-9A-z]0.1097/AOG.0b013e3181e750f1

Kirubarajan, A., Li, X., Got, T., Yau, M., & Sobel, M. (2021). Improving medical student comfort and competence in performing gynecological exams: A systematic review. *Academic Medicine: Journal of the Association of American Medical Colleges, 96*(9), 1353–1365. https://doi.org/10.1097/ACM.0000000000004128

Richman, S. M., & Drickamer, M. A. (2007). Gynecologic care of elderly women. *Journal of the American Medical Directors Association, 8*(4), 219–223. https://doi.org/[0-9A-z]0.1016/j.jamda.2006.12.019

Secor, M., & Fantasia, H. (2018). *Fast facts about the gynecologic exam: A professional guide for NPs, PAs, and midwives* (2nd ed.). Springer Publishing.

6
VAGINAL MICROSCOPY AND VAGINAL INFECTIONS

HANNE S. HARBISON AND R. MIMI SECOR

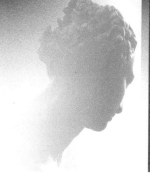

VAGINAL MICROSCOPY SUMMARY

A. Overview
1. Five conditions cause most abnormal vaginal discharge and infections (Box 6.1).
2. Vaginal microscopy is an important point of care laboratory tool for the differential diagnosis of vaginitis.
3. The two components of a wet mount are: (a) normal saline and (b) 10% potassium hydroxide (KOH).
4. The sensitivity depends on the expertise of the clinician and the adequacy of the sample, and ranges between 60% and 90%.

B. Indications
1. On every patient presenting with vaginal symptoms or with clinical features suggestive of a cervical or vaginal condition
2. With high clinical suspicion for a specific diagnosis because many conditions can mimic each other and mixed infections are common
3. In a patient with urine sediment that contains white cells and many squamous epithelial cells to determine the source of infection (vagina or urinary tract)
4. To determine treatment success or to evaluate continued symptoms (Table 6.1)

VAGINAL ECOLOGY

A. The vaginal pH is normally acidic, ranging from 4.5 to 4.6.
1. Factors that increase the glycogen content (high levels of estrogen or uncontrolled diabetes) increase the acidity of the vaginal secretions.
2. Glycogen present in the epithelial cells is used by the peroxide-producing lactobacilli to produce lactic acid, which maintains an acid environment.
3. *Candida* species thrive in a mildly acidic environment.

BOX 6.1 The Five Conditions Causing the Majority of Vaginal Discharge or Infection (In Order of Prevalence)

1. Bacterial vaginosis (BV)
2. *Candida*
3. *Trichomonas vaginalis* (TV)
4. Genito-urinary syndrome of menopause (GSM)
5. Desquamative inflammatory vaginitis (DIV) (diagnosis of exclusion, often confirmed by specialist)

TABLE 6.1 Pharmacological Management of Vaginitis

BACTERIAL VAGINOSIS

GENERIC (BRAND) AVAILABILITY	DOSAGE: ADULT	SIDE EFFECTS/MONITORING	COMMENTS
Metronidazole 250 and 500 mg tablet (Flagyl)	500 mg tablet PO BID for 7 days	Dyspepsia, headache, nausea, vomiting, diarrhea, constipation, anorexia, abdominal cramps, rash, dizziness, metallic taste, urine discoloration WBC with differential at baseline, during and after treatment if prolonged or repeated	
Metronidazole vaginal 0.75% gel (Metro Gel)	1 applicator intravaginally QHS for 5 nights	Vulvovaginal irritation, candidiasis	
Clindamycin cream 2% (Cleocin Vaginal, ClindaMax Vaginal, Clindesse)	1 applicator intravaginally QHS for 7 nights	Vaginal discharge, irritation, candidiasis, abdominal cramps, nausea, vomiting, diarrhea, headache, rash, urticaria	"Clindesse" Single dose, bioadhesive, time-released for 7 days

VAGINAL CANDIDIASIS

GENERIC (BRAND) AVAILABILITY	DOSAGE: ADULT	SIDE EFFECTS/MONITORING	COMMENTS
Clotrimazole 1% cream (generic)	5 g intravaginally QHS for 7–14 days	Vaginal burning, pruritis, soreness, swelling, pelvic pain, abdominal pain, pelvic cramps	
Clotrimazole 2% cream (generic)	5 g intravaginally QHS for 3 days	Vaginal burning, pruritis, soreness, swelling, pelvic pain, abdominal pain, pelvic cramps	
Miconazole 2% cream (Monistat 7)	5 g intravaginally QHS for 7 days	Vaginal burning, pruritis, soreness, swelling, pelvic pain, abdominal pain, pelvic cramps	
Miconazole 4% cream (Monistat 3)	5 g intravaginally QHS for 3 days	Vaginal burning, pruritis, soreness, swelling, pelvic pain, abdominal pain, pelvic cramps	
Miconazole 100 mg suppository (Monistat 7)	1 suppository intravaginally QHS for 7 days	Vaginal burning, pruritis, soreness, swelling, pelvic pain, abdominal pain, pelvic cramps	
Miconazole 200 mg suppository (Monistat 3)	1 suppository intravaginally QHS for 3 days	Vaginal burning, pruritis, soreness, swelling, pelvic pain, abdominal pain, pelvic cramps	
Miconazole 1,200 mg suppository (Monistat 1)	1 suppository intravaginally QHS for 1 day	Vaginal burning, pruritis, soreness, swelling, pelvic pain, abdominal pain, pelvic cramps	

(continued)

TABLE 6.1 Pharmacological Management of Vaginitis (*continued*)

VAGINAL CANDIDIASIS (*CONTINUED*)

GENERIC (BRAND) AVAILABILITY	DOSAGE: ADULT	SIDE EFFECTS/MONITORING	COMMENTS
Tioconazole 6.5 % ointment (Monistat 1-Day)	5 g intravaginally QHS for 1 day	Vaginal burning, pruritis, soreness, swelling, pelvic pain, abdominal pain, pelvic cramps	
Butaconazole 2% cream (Gynazole-1)	5 g intravaginally in single application	Vaginal burning, pruritis, soreness, swelling, pelvic pain, abdominal pain, pelvic cramps	More broad spectrum than other "azoles," bioadhesive, extended release for 7 days Avoid in pregnancy (Category C)
Terconazole 0.4% cream (Terazol 7)	5 g intravaginally QHS for 7 days	Headache, vaginal burning, dysmenorrhea, pelvic pain, abdominal pain	
Terconazole 0.8% cream (Terazol 3)	5 g intravaginally QHS for 3 days	Headache, vaginal burning, dysmenorrhea, pelvic pain, abdominal pain	
Terconazole 80 mg suppository (Terazol)	1 suppository intravaginally QHS for 3 days	Headache, vaginal burning, dysmenorrhea, pelvic pain, abdominal pain	
Fluconazole 150 mg tablet (Diflucan)	1 tablet PO single dose		Avoid in pregnancy Narrow spectrum
NEW: Ibrexafungerp (Brexafemme) 150 mg tab	300 mg PO q12 hr for 1 day	Diarrhea, nausea, vomiting, abdominal pain, dizziness	Avoid in pregnancy, expensive, first in class, fungicidal – triterpenoid; consider referring to specialist for this medication; diagnosis should be confirmed with culture.

TRICHOMONAS

GENERIC (BRAND) AVAILABILITY	DOSAGE: ADULT	SIDE EFFECTS/MONITORING	COMMENTS
Metronidazole 250 and 500 mg tablet (Flagyl)	500 mg tablet PO BID for 7 days	Dyspepsia, headache, nausea, vomiting, diarrhea, constipation, anorexia, abdominal cramps, rash, dizziness, metallic taste, urine discoloration WBC with differential at baseline, during and after treatment if prolonged or repeated	
Tinidazole 250 mg and 500 mg tablet (Tindamax)	2 g PO once	Nausea, vomiting, anorexia, fatigue, weakness, flatulence, urinary tract infection, pelvic pain, vulvovaginal discomfort, vaginal odor, candidiasis, metallic taste, menorrhagia, upper respiratory infection Creatinine at baseline; WBC with differential if retreatment	Avoid in pregnancy

(*continued*)

TABLE 6.1 Pharmacological Management of Vaginitis (*continued*)

DESQUAMATIVE INFLAMMATORY VAGINITIS

GENERIC (BRAND) AVAILABILITY	DOSAGE: ADULT	SIDE EFFECTS/MONITORING	COMMENTS
Clindamycin 2% cream (Cleocin Vaginal, ClindaMax Vaginal, Clindesse)	1 applicator intravaginally QHS for 7–21 nights	Vaginal discharge, irritation, candidiasis, abdominal cramps, nausea, vomiting, diarrhea, headache, rash, urticaria	No standardized, approved treatment
Hydrocortisone 10% cream (Cortisone 10)	300–500 mg intravaginally QHS for 21 days	Burning, pruritis, irritation, dryness, hypopigmentation, allergic contact dermatitis, secondary infection, atrophy	

Source: https://www.cdc.gov/std/treatment-guidelines/default.htm

4. Lactobacilli (LB) usually dominate the flora of the normal estrogenized vagina (96%). LB help maintain a low pH of vaginal discharge by producing lactic acid, which inhibits adherence of bacteria to epithelial cells.
   a. Inhibit growth of organisms that may normally be found in the vagina, such as *Gardnerella vaginalis* and *Mycoplasma hominis.*
   b. LB are estrogen dependent so increase after menarche and markedly decrease after menopause (Table 6.2).
B. Factors that affect normal vaginal flora:
   1. Hormones
      a. Estrogen causes glycogen to be deposited in the vagina, mainly in the intermediate cells. Glycogen is then metabolized into lactic acid, lowering vaginal pH by increasing vaginal acidity.
   2. Medications
      a. Antibiotics may increase the incidence of *Candida* infection. Possible mechanisms include less competition, direct stimulation, and decrease in antifungal secretions by other bacteria.
      b. Corticosteroids act as an immune suppressant.
   3. **Douching:** Disrupts normal flora and may increase the risk for BV, sexually transmitted infections (STIs), and possibly ovarian cancer.

TABLE 6.2 pH in Relation to Life Cycle Changes Affected by the Presence or Absence of Lactobacilli

PHASE OF REPRODUCTIVE LIFE CYCLE	pH
Preadolescence	7.0
Reproductive years	3.8–4.6
Postmenopausal years	4.7–7.0

HISTORY AND EXAMINATION

A. Obtain a thorough focused history. Questions to ask are included in Box 6.2. It is important to inform the patient that certain substances in the vagina can affect the accuracy of the examination and wet mount (e.g., medications, semen, blood), and if possible, the patient should avoid these for 48 to 72 hours prior to the examination (Vieira-Baptista, 2021).

B. Obtain consent for examination using trauma-informed care principles. Perform clinical evaluation. Box 6.3 shows the sequence of the examination.

C. Observe and document characteristics of any vaginal discharge (Table 6.3).

D. Equipment needed:
   1. Gloves
   2. Speculum (metal or plastic)
   3. Dacron-tipped swabs or plastic spatula
   4. Frosted-glass slide (one or two)
   5. Coverslips (one or two)
   6. Bottle of normal saline (slightly warmed if possible)
   7. Bottle of 10% potassium hydrochloride (KOH) or single-use units
   8. Vaginal pH test paper or pH swab
   9. Microscope with 10× and 40× objectives
   10. Small test tubes (3 to 4 in. long)

BOX 6.2 Key History-Taking Questions and Considerations

History and Chronology
- Onset of symptoms
- Duration of current episode
- Self-diagnosis and use of OTC treatments

Symptoms
- Description
- Location
- Severity
- Associated symptoms: urinary, dermatologic, menstruation

Aggravating Factors
- Allergies
- Prescription and OTC medications
- Sexual activities including oral sex
- Sex toys
- Douching
- Soaps/hygiene sprays
- Shaving

Sexual History
- Date of last sexual/genital contact
- Gender of partner(s)
- STI history
- Partner symptoms
- Sexual practices (i.e., vaginal, anal, oral exposure)
- Condom use
- Sexual devices or toys
- Lubricants (specify type)
- Dyspareunia (superficial vs. deep)

Obstetric and Gynecologic Factors
- Last menstrual period
- Duration of menses
- Use of menstrual products
- Pelvic or genital surgeries
- Cervical cancer screening history

Relieving Factors
- Vulvar care measures
- Prescription and OTC medications
- Alternative treatments

OTC, over-the-counter; STI, sexually transmitted infections.

BOX 6.3 Sequence of Examination During a Vaginitis Office Visit

- Obtain a thorough, focused history
- Using principles of "trauma-informed care,*" explain the procedure to the patient and obtain consent to perform examination
- Offer the patient a hand mirror to observe during the exam (telescoping type works best)
- Inspect external genitalia
- May palpate cervix in advance of speculum insertion (helps clinician locate cervix)
- Insert speculum
- Determine vaginal pH (pH swab or vaginal pH paper)
- Collect sample of discharge from the posterior lateral vaginal walls
- Collect STI cultures from vaginal, or cervical samples, if indicated
- Remove speculum
- Perform bimanual exam if indicated
- Remove examination gloves and put on new gloves
- Label any specimens
- Perform wet mount evaluation
- Document results
- Review results with the patient
- Treat infection as appropriate

*Trauma-informed care (TIC) is an approach that assumes an individual is more likely than not to have a history of trauma.

pH ASSESSMENT

A. pH measurement can be done with individual strips or rolls of pH paper or pH swab (nonnumerical). If using a roll, tear off a 0.5- to 1-inch strip before inserting the speculum.

B. Measurement can be done by applying the pH paper to vaginal wall or to the discharge from the collecting spatula. Alternately you can dip the pH strip into the discharge pooled on the upper blade of the vaginal speculum. A sample from a swab may also be applied to the pH paper.

C. Common diagnoses associated with pH measurements are included in Table 6.4.

TABLE 6.3 Analysis of Vaginal Discharge

CHARACTERISTIC	POSSIBLE FINDINGS
pH	3.8–7.0
Amount (quantify)	Small/scant, moderate, large, copious
Color	Off-white Creamy Whitish-gray Yellow Green Pink-red
Character	Watery, thick, thin, curd-like/clumpy, homogeneous, flocculent, frothy, bubbly
Odor	Fishy, foul, no odor
Blood	Present (amount), thin, thick, clots, absent

TABLE 6.4 Measurement of Vaginal pH		
pH	**CONDITION**	**COLOR CHANGE**
3.8–4.6	Normal flora	Light yellow
4.0–4.6	Vulvovaginal candidiasis (not as diagnostic)	Medium to dark yellow
4.7–6.0	Bacterial vaginosis or Trichomoniasis	Light to dark olive green or bluish
7.0	Trichomonas, cervical secretions, blood, semen	Bluish

SALINE WET MOUNT

A. Obtain the sample from the mid lateral fornix and lower third of vagina using a Dacron-tipped swab or plastic spatula (Vieira-Baptista, 2021). Avoid cervical mucus (high pH).

B. Slide method
 1. Place two separate samples of vaginal discharge on the same frosted-glass slide or use two slides (one for each sample). Using two slides works best with frosted-tipped slides.
 2. Add one to two drops of normal saline to the sample on the left. Add one to two drops of KOH to the sample on the right.
    a. Be careful not to mix the solutions or the sample must be collected again because the KOH will dissolve the cellular material of both samples. This is why two slides may be preferred.
 3. Mix each specimen thoroughly, stirring until smooth, to create a turbid suspension. May use same device if saline is mixed first. May also mix as the coverslip is applied.

C. Saline immersion/test tube method
 1. Place 7 to 10 drops (1–2 mL) of normal saline in a small test tube. (Saline must be at room temperature or warmer.)
 2. Collect sample and immerse into the saline-filled tube (approximately 1–2 mL).
 3. Place several drops of the suspension on the slide forming a puddle approximately 0.5 in. in diameter.
 4. Gently place separate coverslips over the specimen just before viewing to prevent drying. Hold one edge of the coverslip against the slide (like a hinged door) and slowly drop the coverslip over the liquid specimen to reduce the number of air bubbles.
 5. If necessary, take a paper towel and gently dab the side of the slide to absorb any excess fluid leaking from the slide.
 6. Interpret findings immediately, viewing saline slide first.
 7. A minimum of 10 to 12 fields should be analyzed for a total of 2 to 3 minutes.

KOH PREP

A. Purpose
 1. Dissolves leukocytes, *Trichomonas,* and background debris, making identification of fungal structures easier.
 2. Effects on epithelial cells
    a. KOH dissolves intracellular structures and breaks down the cell wall, changing the wall from cuboid and translucent to ovoid and transparent.
    b. Epithelial cells become enlarged and faint; called *ghost* cells.
 3. Branching hyphae (long non-segmented), pseudohyphae (segmented branches like sausage links), and buds are alkali resistant and stand out in sharp contrast.

B. Obtaining and preparing the sample
  1. Use a Dacron swab or plastic spatula to collect the specimen.
  2. Either mix the sample into two to three drops of KOH (10%) placed on a slide or add two to three drops of KOH to saline immersion tube. NOTE: Due to the dilution of a test tube sample, adding KOH to that sample may produce a false-negative test.
    a. Material should be fairly thick with epithelial cells clustered to concentrate the yeast forms.
  3. Perform the whiff test.
    a. Volatile amines are released into the air when anaerobic bacteria come in contact with an alkaline solution such as KOH.
    b. Amines are produced by converting lysine to cadaverine, arginine to putrescine, and trimethylamine oxide to trimethylamine.
    c. Immediately after mixing the sample with KOH, pass the swab, slide, or test tube under your nose.
    d. Note the presence of a fishy odor. If odor is present, it is recorded as a positive result.
  4. Blot the side of the slide with a paper towel if there is excess fluid because KOH can damage the microscope objective.
C. Observe the sample.
D. Wait for 1 to 2 minutes to allow KOH to lyse the cellular material.
  1. Scan the slide.
    a. **Low power (10×):** Locate sections of yeast forms, which may appear as thin sticks (hyphae), elongated balloons (pseudohyphae), or sausage links (pseudophyphae).
    b. **High power (40×):** Focus on identifying buds and examining the morphology of the hyphae/pseudohyphae.

THE MICROSCOPE

A. Wet mount microscopy should be performed on a phase contrast microscope (Vieire-Baptista, 2021).
  1. **Magnification:** There are two magnifications used to examine wet mounts:
    a. Low-power objective (eye piece 10× = 100× magnification)
    b. High-power objective (eye piece 40× = 400× magnification)
  2. **Light source:** Helps increase the examiner's ability to visualize details by controlling the illumination. The light source is controlled by the following features:
    a. Brightness setting of the light source
    b. The field diaphragm ring
    c. The position of the condenser
  3. Mechanics of observing the saline smear
    a. Position the slide on the stage of the microscope with the saline preparation under the objective and secure with stage clips.
    b. Turn the light on and adjust shutter as needed.
    c. Click low objective (10X) into place over the specimen.
    d. Turn the condenser to the lowest position; dispersed light is best to accentuate fine details.
    e. Adjust the eyepiece until a single round field is seen (interpupillary diameter).
    f. While looking through the eyepiece, turn the coarse adjustment knob until the microscopic field comes into focus.
    g. Turn the fine-adjust knob slowly back and forth to adjust to the different planes and bring the image into sharper focus.
    h. Move the saline specimen under the objective and scan the slide to locate representative sections.
      (1) Scan fields in a zig-zag pattern.

(2) It is important to avoid contact between the objective and the KOH that might be leaking along the edges of the coverslip. This can cause scratching of the glass surface and require replacement of the microscope objective.

    i. Switch to high-power objective (40X) magnification.

      (1) It may be necessary to increase the light source slightly.

      (2) Raise the condenser to focus the light.

    j. Use the fine-adjustment knob to focus; coarse adjustment should not require readjustment.

    k. Using the stage adjustment knobs, move the slide in a zig-zag pattern.

4. Mechanics of observing the KOH preparation:

    a. Move the KOH slide into position on the stage.

    b. Switch back to low-power objective to scan fields for yeast forms. Hyphae and pseudohyphae are easiest to identify on low power.

    c. If yeast forms are noted, switch to high power to confirm their presence and type. Observing only buds suggests a possible *Candida glabrata* infection, but this should be confirmed by culture, preferably with polymerase chain reaction (PCR) testing.

5. Completion

    a. Turn off the microscope light source and dispose of the slide(s) in a biohazard container.

    b. Clean the microscope stage if it is soiled and clean the lenses with special paper or a cotton swab with lens cleaner.

    c. Record findings and review the findings with the patient.

6. Common findings on saline wet mount

    a. Vaginal epithelial cells

      (1) Slightly grainy cytoplasm-containing vacuoles

      (2) Distinct cell walls

      (3) Evaluate cells for the following features:

        • Quantity of mature cells present

        • Presence of immature cells and their relative frequency may indicate decreased estrogen or inflammatory reaction.

    b. Clue cells

      (1) Significant bacterial adherence to cell surfaces (epithelial cell mucin gel barrier is stripped away by succinic acid produced by BV-associated bacteria, allowing adherence of bacteria to cell surfaces)

      (2) Have a "lacy" or obscured border and nucleus is often obscured

    c. Lactobacilli (Figure 6.1)

      (1) Pleomorphic, gram-positive, aerobic, or facultative anaerobic, non-spore-forming organism

      (2) Elongated, rod-shaped bacilli that appear as straight rods of varying lengths, which may be motile depending on amount of fluid in specimen

    d. White blood cells (WBCs) (or polymorphonuclear leukocytes [PMNs])

      (1) Present as dark and granular cells with clearly segmented nuclei

      (2) May also appear as cytoplasmic granules with an indistinct nucleus (often with chronic infection)

      (3) Slightly larger than the nucleus of a mature epithelial cell

      (4) The number of WBCs helps determine the extent of inflammation (Table 6.5)

      (5) Increased in many conditions (Box 6.4)

    e. Motile trichomonads

    f. Immature squamous epithelial cells (see Chapter 24, "Genitourinary Syndrome of Menopause and Vulvovaginal Atrophy")

    g. Red blood cells (RBCs) as small concave spheres, approximately half the size of a WBC

    h. Artifact may interfere with interpretation of the wet mount (Box 6.5)

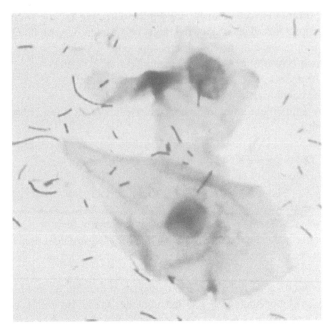

FIGURE 6.1 Lactobacilli.

TABLE 6.5 Significance of White Blood Cells (WBCs)

	NUMBER IN HPF	RATIO OF WBCS TO EPITHELIAL CELLS
Normal	0–4	<5:1
Moderate	5–10	>5:1
Severe	10 or more	>10:1

Note: May be influenced by the concentration of the smear. If inflammation is present, observe for the presence or absence of parabasal cells.

HPF, high-power field.

BOX 6.4 Causes of the Presence of Leukocytes (White Blood Cells) on Wet Mount

Moderate increase of leukocytes found with:
- Intrauterine contraception use
- Postpartum reparative process
- Genitourinary syndrome of menopause (GSM)
- Allergic reaction to spermicides, douches, and other substances
- Medroxyprogesterone acetate (MPA; Depo-Provera) users with low estrogen levels (indicated by elevated pH >4.6)

Possible marked increase of leukocytes found with:
- Trichomoniasis
- Candidiasis
- Chlamydia or gonorrhea
- Desquamative inflammatory vaginitis (DIV)

Note: If many leukocytes are seen but neither *Candida* nor *Trichomonas* are present, consider an STI culture. Also consider dysplasia or metaplasia as a possible cause.

> **BOX 6.5 Artifacts That May Interfere With the Interpretation of a Wet Mount**
>
> - Powder granules from gloves (resemble umbilicated marshmallows)
> - Tiny bubbles of emulsified vaginal creams or lubricants
> - Dust on microscope lenses or coverslips
> - Cotton fiber from cotton-tipped swab, undergarments, or tampons

7. Normal findings include:
   a. Absence of or less than 5 WBCs/high-power field (hpf)
   b. pH less than 4.7
   c. Presence of moderate amounts of Lactobacilli
   d. Absence of demonstrable pathogens, such as *Trichomonads* or clue cells
   e. Figure 6.2 shows the characteristics of a normal smear.
8. Interpretation of results
   a. Acidic finding (pH less than 4.7) indicates the presence of vaginal lactobacilli in the vaginal flora.
   b. Factors that interfere with the determination of pH, which, if present, eliminate use of pH as a diagnostic tool:
      (1) **Menses:** Greater than 7
      (2) **Semen:** Greater than 7
      (3) **Cervical mucus:** Greater than 7
      (4) Lubricating jelly
      (5) Intravaginal medications

VAGINAL CANDIDIASIS

A. Pathogenesis
   1. It is hypothesized that infection occurs when there is dysbiosis (i.e., an altered vaginal microbiome) in combination with an abnormal host response to the normal presence of *Candida* in the vagina (Swidsinski, 2019).
   2. Candidiasis is not a sexually transmitted infection.

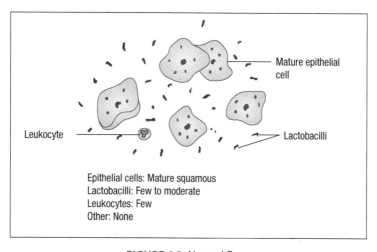

FIGURE 6.2 Normal flora.

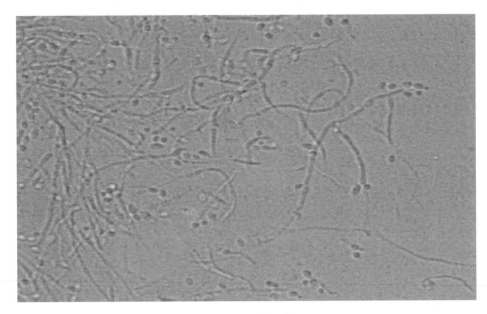

FIGURE 6.3 *Candida albicans.*

B. Six genera typically inhabit the vagina (in order of occurrence) (Pappas, 2016).
1. *Candida albicans* (cause of vulvovaginal candidiasis in 90% to 95% of cases)
    a. Dimorphic, forming both blastospores (buds) and mycelia (filaments, hyphae, and pseudohyphae; Figure 6.3)
2. *Candida tropicalis* (23%): Dimorphic
3. *Candida glabrata* (5%–10%): Monomorphic; forms only spores (buds)
4. *Candida krusei*
5. *Candida parapsilosis*
6. *Candida pseudotropicalis*

C. Relationship to estrogen
1. There is some evidence that there are estrogen receptors on *C. albicans* and that any condition that increases estrogen may increase risk for the development of candidiasis, such as:
    a. Pregnancy
    b. Local estrogen treatment with vaginal medication
    c. Estrogen-containing contraception

D. Relationship to pH
1. Presence of yeast does not usually change the acidity of the vaginal secretions.

E. Predisposing risk factors for the development of candidiasis
1. Immune suppression
    a. HIV
    b. Pregnancy
    c. Corticosteroids
2. Increased vaginal glycogen associated with poorly controlled diabetes

F. Clinical features of *C. albicans* (see Table 6.6)
1. Subjective findings
    a. Vulvovaginal erythema, edema, intense pruritus, pain, dyspareunia
    b. Increased, cottage cheese–like, clumpy discharge.
    c. External dysuria (burning when the urine touches the vulva)

TABLE 6.6 Differential Diagnosis of Vaginal Conditions

CONDITION	VULVOVAGINAL SYMPTOMS	VAGINAL DISCHARGE	LACTOBACILLI	pH	MICROSCOPY
Candida albicans	Mild to severe itching Cyclic Marked vulvovaginal erythema	Increased amount White, curdy, cottage cheese–like	Moderate	<4.7	KOH Hyphae, pseudohyphae, and spores
C. glabrata and other non-*C. albicans* infections	Mild to moderate burning/itching Chronic, cyclic Mild vulvovaginal erythema	Increased White, green Less commonly yellow/green	Moderate	<4.7	KOH Spores only Vary in size and shape Need culture to confirm
BV	Mild to moderate itching Absent to mild inflammation Mild vulvovaginal erythema No itching or mild-to-moderate itching and/or irritation	Adherent, malodorous, homogeneous discharge White/grey Fishy odor, particularly after intercourse	Rare	>4.6	Saline Clue cells, few to many WBCs KOH + whiff test Usually negative KOH
Trichomonas	Mild to severe vulvar itching Petechiae of cervix and vagina Vulvar Erythema May be asymptomatic	Copious Yellow-green May be frothy Malodorous	Varies	>4.6	Saline trichomonads Many WBCs Usually negative KOH
GSM/VVA	Pruritus, irritation Vaginal dryness and dyspareunia Smooth vaginal walls	Pale or red, tender vestibule and vagina Scant discharge Lack of rugae	Rare	>4.6	Saline Parabasal cells Few to many WBCs Negative KOH
DIV	Erythema of vulva, vagina, and cervix Dyspareunia, pruritus, or irritation	Often yellow, thick profuse No odor	Rare	>4.6	Saline Basal/parabasal cells Many WBCs Negative KOH

BV, bacterial vaginosis; DIV, desquamative inflammatory vaginitis; GSM, genitourinary syndrome of menopause; KOH, potassium hydroxide; WBC, white blood cell.

TABLE 6.7 *Candida* Species and Morphology		
YEAST FORM	**DESCRIPTION**	**SPECIES NAME***
Pseudohyphae	Long, segmented "sausage links" with minimal tapering points along the length. Similar diameter from proximal to distal. Larger than lactobacilli	*Candida albicans*
Hyphae	Long, continuous filaments appearing as if blown out of glass; smooth, tube-like elongated circus balloons tied together, end to end	*C. tropicalis*
Chlamydiaspores	Look like clusters of glass beads at terminal ends of the hyphae Uniform in size, associated with hyphae forms	*C. albicans*
Blastospores	Budding ovoid spores of variable size (2–10 microns) Round to ovoid; no filaments	*C. glabrata*
	May be budding or grouped in clusters interspersed with filaments Smaller than red blood cells Located at the proximal branches, appearing much like a fern	*C. tropicalis*

*recommend culture and speciation to confirm type of fungal species.

2. Objective findings
    a. Vulvovaginal erythema, swelling, excoriations, fissures
    b. Thick, curd-like discharge that may be white, yellow, or green tinged
        (1) Classic, clumpy, curd-like discharge noted 20% to 50% of the time
        (2) Loosely adherent to the vaginal mucosa or vestibule
        (3) May coat entire vagina or appear in patches
G. Diagnosis
    1. Use of vaginal microscopy in the diagnosis of candidiasis is about 60% sensitive and 90% specific (Schwebke, 2018).
    2. Yeast forms are viewed more easily with KOH preparation than with saline.
    3. pH less than 4.7
    4. Observations using saline
        a. Presence of varying numbers of leukocytes (PMN)
        b. Lactobacilli are present in moderate numbers
        c. Presence of yeast forms
        d. Abundance of epithelial cells (increase in exfoliation)
    5. Observations using KOH
        a. Negative whiff test
        b. Note the presence of yeast forms (described in Table 6.7).
H. Other testing modalities
    1. Molecular tests (BD MAX, BD Affirm VPIII):
        a. May have higher sensitivity and specificity than wet mount (Schwebke, 2018, 2020)
        b. Can test for multiple infections simultaneously (TV, VVC, BV)
        c. PCR tests are available through certain commercial labs and can speciate yeast and also report various specific BV-associated bacteria.
        d. The Centers for Disease Control and Prevention (CDC) recommends BV diagnosis be based on Amsel's criteria not lab testing for specific organisms.
    2. Fungal culture (Fungal cultures are not always available through commercial labs and when they are available, results may take 72 hours and sometimes even a week or longer.)

   a. Indications
      (1) Signs and symptoms of candida infection, but no yeast forms seen on microscopy
      (2) Recurrent or persistent symptoms
3. Cervical cancer screening test
   a. Sensitivity is very low.
   b. Not indicated as a diagnostic tool for vulvovaginitis.

BACTERIAL VAGINOSIS

A. Overview
   1. BV is the most common cause of vaginitis (Peebles, 2019).
   2. BV is associated with an increased risk of STIs, including HIV, postsurgical gynecologic infections, PID, infertility, complications of pregnancy and recurrence of BV (Workowski, 2021; Ravel 2021).
   3. An estimated 84% of people with BV do not have symptoms. This may be because some people are not aware of the differences between normal and abnormal vaginal discharge. This emphasizes the need to provide education about the symptoms of vaginal infections versus the nature of normal vaginal discharge.
   4. BV is a sexually *associated* infection—the same causative bacteria have been cultured from the prepuce of cis-male sexual partners of cis-females with BV. However, treating male partners has not increased the cure rate nor reduced recurrent infections (Schwebke, 2021). There is evidence that BV is sexually transmitted between cis-female partners (Muzny, 2019).

B. Predisposing factors
   1. Douching (RR 2.1)
   2. Not using condoms for vaginal intercourse
   3. New sexual partner, multiple partners, partner with BV
   4. Copper-containing intrauterine contraceptive (IUC)
   5. Menstruation

C. Pathogenesis
   1. Dysbiosis of vaginal microbiome and formation of a poly-microbial biofilm (Muzny, 2019).
   2. Decrease in hydrogen peroxide–producing lactobacilli
   3. Increase in various anaerobic bacterial pathogens including *Gardnerella vaginalis*, *Prevotella* species, *Mobiluncus* species, *Atopobium vaginae*, and other BV-associated bacteria.

D. Clinical features (see Table 6.6)
   1. Subjective findings
      a. Increase in vaginal discharge: thin, watery, white/grey in color
      b. Fishy odor, particularly notable after intercourse
   2. Objective findings
      a. Homogeneous white/grey discharge that adheres to the vulva and vaginal walls.
      b. Mild erythema or absence of inflammation of vulvar or vaginal tissues

E. Diagnosis (Muzny, 2020)
   1. Wet mount Amsel's criteria; must have three out of four for diagnosis
      a. pH greater than 4.6
      b. KOH: Positive whiff test
      c. Homogeneous vaginal discharge
      d. Greater than 20% "clue cells" in saline preparation (Figure 6.4)
   2. Additional findings
      a. Absence or relative scarcity of lactobacilli
      b. Possible presence of *Mobiluncus* species, such as *M. curtisii* or *M. mulieris*

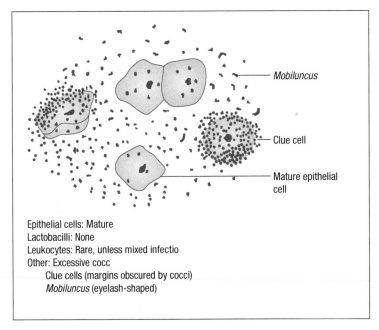

Epithelial cells: Mature
Lactobacilli: None
Leukocytes: Rare, unless mixed infectio
Other: Excessive cocc
    Clue cells (margins obscured by cocci)
    Mobiluncus (eyelash-shaped)

FIGURE 6.4 Bacterial vaginosis.

    (1) Highly motile, anaerobic, Gram negative
    (2) Tiny, short-curved, "comma"-shaped bacteria
  c. Few leukocytes (unless a concomitant infection is present)
  d. Floating background bacteria
 3. Gram stain – Nugent criteria
  a. Not a point-of-care test; used in research studies primarily
  b. The diagnosis is based on the stippled appearance of epithelial cells due to uniformly spaced coccobacilli, a reduction of *Lactobacillus* morphotypes, and an increase in small gram-negative rods and gram-positive cocci.
 4. **Point-of care tests:** Osom BV Blue, BD Affirm VPIII
  a. High sensitivity and specificity
  b. Cost and availability limit use
 5. **NAAT tests:** BD Max Vaginal Panel, Aptima BV (Gaydos, 2017)
  a. High sensitivity and specificity
  b. Results take 1 to 5 days depending on processing lab

TRICHOMONIASIS

A. Overview
 1. Most common curable STI; incidence estimated as 6.9 million in 2018 (CDC, 2021)
 2. Is a sexually transmitted parasite
 3. Is a cause of nongonococcal urethritis (NGU) in people with penises.
 4. Chronic trichomoniasis can reduce the glycogen content of the cells, causing the vaginal lining to become thinner and more prone to ulceration.
 5. Primarily affects the vagina but can affect the cervix, Bartholin's and Skene's glands, and urethra.
 6. Many infections are asymptomatic and may be for decades.

B. Identification of trichomoniasis
   1. Trichomonads are unicellular, anaerobic protozoans.
   2. Actively motile by virtue of four filaments of equal length
      a. One to two times the length of the organism itself
      b. Protrude from the forward end of the trichomonad
   3. Teardrop shape of various sizes
      a. A little larger than PMN leukocytes
      b. Smaller than a mature epithelial cell but larger than its nucleus
C. Replication
   1. Binary division
   2. Transfer from one host to another only in the presence of moisture
D. Effects of pH
   1. If less than 4.7, the organism is rounded. It is difficult to distinguish from a WBC.
   2. Usually pH is greater than 4.6.
E. Predisposing factors (CDC, 2021)
   1. Incarceration
   2. Two or more sexual partners in the past year
   3. Less than high school education, living below the poverty level
F. Clinical features (see Table 6.6)
   1. Subjective findings
      a. Profuse, often malodorous discharge
         (1) **Classic appearance:** Frothy, yellow to green
      b. Pruritus, vaginal burning
   2. Objective findings
      a. Vulvar and vaginal edema and erythema
      b. Strawberry cervix (ecchymotic petechiae)
G. Diagnosis
   1. **Wet mount (sensitivity 36%–70%):** Timing is critical; should be examined within 10 minutes of collection. If wet mount cannot be performed immediately, place cotton-tipped applicator with vaginal secretions in a test tube with 0.5 inch (1–2 mL) normal saline.
      a. Trichomonads are visible only in saline; lysed in KOH.
      b. Squamous epithelial cells are present.
      c. PMN leukocytes are increased due to the inflammation.
      d. Lactobacilli may be present.
      e. KOH whiff likely positive
   2. Characteristics of trichomonads in saline
      a. Flagella are not visible under low power and sometimes visible under high power.
      b. Healthy trichomonads undulate, jerk, twitch, or actively move in the direction of the flagella.
      c. Trichomonads assume a rounder shape when they are dry or drying and thus can look like WBCs.
      d. Figure 6.5 demonstrates the characteristics of trichomoniasis.
   3. **NAAT tests:** Amplivue, Aptima, TV Q, Cepheid Xpert, Solana (Muzny, 2014)
      a. Sensitivity 94%-100%
      b. Some NAATs can run CT/GC and TV simultaneously
      c. Only option for people with penises
      d. Processing takes 3 to 5 days depending on lab
   4. **Point-of-care test:** Osom Trich
      a. Sensitivity 83% to 92%
      b. Takes 10 to 15 minutes to process

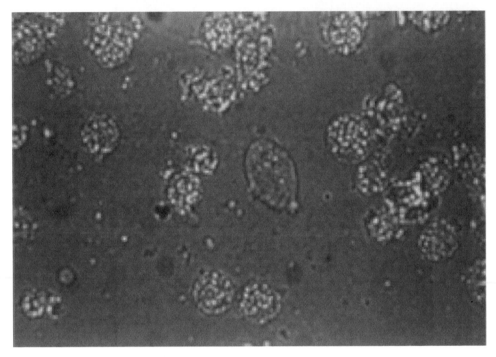

FIGURE 6.5 Characteristics of trichomoniasis.

5. Culture
   a. Sensitivity 70% to 85%
   b. Not readily available; used primarily in research.
6. Cervical cancer screening test
   a. Not a diagnostic tool for Trichomonas.
   b. If seen on cervical cancer screening, treat and retest with a NAAT

DESQUAMATIVE INFLAMMATORY VAGINITIS

A. Inflammatory vaginitis of unknown etiology is characterized by minimal to no lactobacilli
   (Paavonen, 2018). May be an infection (*Streptococcus* spp., *S. aureus, Group B streptococci,
   Escherichia coli* or *E. faecalis*) or a dysbiosis (Paavonen, 2018; Qi, 2021).
   1. Clinical features (Table 6.6)
      a. Subjective findings
         (1) Dyspareunia
         (2) Stinging and burning
         (3) Sticky, yellow vaginal discharge
      b. Objective findings
         (1) Homogeneous yellow/green purulent discharge
         (2) Vaginal and vulvar erythema
         (3) Vulvar edema
         (4) Thinning of vaginal mucosa
         (5) Cervico-vaginal petechiae
   2. Diagnosis
      a. Wet mount (Paavonen, 2018)
         (1) Many PMN cells
         (2) Increased parabasal cells

(3) Few mature epithelial cells

(4) Negative clue cells, yeast forms, or trichomoniasis

(5) Few to no lactobacilli

(6) Red blood cells may be present

b. KOH

(1) Negative whiff test

c. pH greater than 4.6

GENITOURINARY SYNDROME OF MENOPAUSE FORMERLY VULVOVAGINAL ATROPHY (VVA) (See Chapter 24, "Genitourinary Syndrome of Menopause and Vulvovaginal Atrophy")

A. Overview

1. Inflammation and thinning of the vaginal epithelium due to a lack of estrogen.

2. Found in lactating people, those who underwent natural or surgical menopause, or in patients taking anti-estrogen medications.

B. Clinical features (see Table 6.6)

1. Subjective findings

a. Vaginal dryness

b. Dyspareunia

c. Vulvar and vaginal irritation and burning

d. Possible spotting

e. Urinary symptoms

2. Objective findings

a. Pale, dry vulvar tissues, possible erythema (focal or generalized), excoriations

b. Thin and smooth vaginal walls; lack of rugae

c. Inflammation or exudate may be present

d. Smooth, shiny vulva with adherence of labia

e. Urethral caruncle or prolapse

f. Presence of parabasal cells and increased PMNs (Figure 6.6)

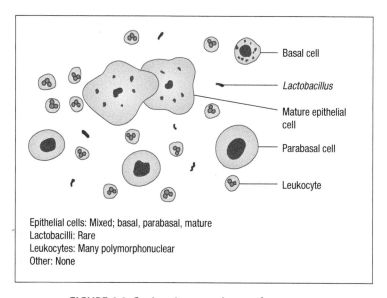

Epithelial cells: Mixed; basal, parabasal, mature
Lactobacilli: Rare
Leukocytes: Many polymorphonuclear
Other: None

FIGURE 6.6 Genitourinary syndrome of menopause.

C. Assessment of the maturation index in the diagnosis of atrophic vaginitis (see Chapter 22, "Assessment of Menopausal Status")

CHEMICAL VAGINITIS

A. Irritation and inflammation of the vulva and vagina can occur from contact with several potential chemical irritants. The history should include questions about a history of contact dermatitis and exposure to any new products. Some potential irritants are listed in Box 6.6.

VAGINAL GRAM STAIN

A. The procedure
   1. Briefly heat-fix the slide that contains the smear of vaginal secretions.
   2. Flood the slide with gentian violet stain solution for 60 seconds.
   3. Wash the slide in water.
   4. Flood it with Gram's iodine solution for 60 seconds.
   5. Rinse it again with water.
   6. Decolorize it with acetone and alcohol solution until it runs clear.
   7. Flood it with safranin stain for 60 seconds.
   8. Wash it in water a third time.
   9. Add a drop of oil to use the oil immersion lens (100x).

BOX 6.6 Substances That May Cause Chemical Vulvovaginitis

Substances Associated With Laundering
- Chlorine bleach
- Laundry detergent
- Fabric softeners

Intravaginal Preparations
- Propylene glycol found in spermicides, lubricants, and vaginal medications, including the base that vaginal medications are prepared in, such as petrolatum or a cream base.

Feminine Hygiene Products
- Deodorant tampons, liners, and sanitary napkins
- Douches and vaginal sprays

Body Secretions
- Semen
- Saliva

Vulvar or Vaginal Medications
- Antifungals
- Lidocaine
- Crotamiton
- Estrogen creams and suppositories
- Antibiotic preparations

Clothing
- Synthetic fibers
- Fabric dyes
- Nylon (can give off formaldehyde vapors)
- Fiberglass particles on underwear

B. Stain of various organisms
  1. **Gonorrhea:** Intracellular gram-negative diplococci
  2. **Gardnerella vaginalis associated with BV:** Gram-positive

BIBLIOGRAPHY

Centers for Disease Control and Prevention. (2021). *Sexually Transmitted Infections Prevalence, Incidence, and Cost Estimates in the United States.* https://www.cdc.gov/std/statistics/prevalence-2020-at-a-glance.htm. Accessed 11/28/2021

Gaydos, C. A., Beqaj, S., Schwebke, J. R., Lebed, J., Smith, B., Davis, T. E., Fife, K. H., Nyirjesy, P., Spurrell, T., Furgerson, D., Coleman, J., Paradis, S., & Cooper, C. K. (2017). Clinical validation of a test for the diagnosis of vaginitis. *Obstetrics and Gynecology, 130*(1), 181–189. https://doi-org.proxy.library.upenn.edu/10.1097/AOG.0000000000002090

Muzny C. A., Blackburn R. J., Sinsky R. J., Austin E. L., & Schwebke J. R. (2014). Added benefit of nucleic acid amplification testing for the diagnosis of *Trichomonas vaginalis* among men and women attending a sexually transmitted diseases clinic. *Clinical Infectious Diseases, 59*, 834–41. https://doi.org/10.1093/cid/ciu446 1061.

Muzny, C. A., & Kardas, P. (2020) A narrative review of current challenges in the diagnosis and management of bacterial vaginosis. *Sexually Transmitted Diseases, 47*(7), 441–445. https://doi.org/10.1097/OLQ.0000000000001178.

Muzny, C. A., Lensing, S. Y., Aaron, K. J., & Schwebke, J. R. (2019). Incubation period and risk factors support sexual transmission of bacterial vaginosis in women who have sex with women. *Sexually Transmitted Infections, 95*(7), 511–515. https://doi-org.proxy.library.upenn.edu/10.1136/sextrans-2018-053824

Muzny, C. A., Taylor, C. M., Swords, W. E., Tamhane, A., Chattopadhyay, D., Cerca, N., & Schwebke, J. R. (2019). An updated conceptual model on the pathogenesis of bacterial vaginosis. *The Journal of Infectious Diseases, 220*(9), 1399–1405. https://doi-org.proxy.library.upenn.edu/10.1093/infdis/jiz342

Paavonen, J., & Brunham, R. C. (2018). Bacterial vaginosis and desquamative inflammatory vaginitis. *The New England Journal of Medicine, 379*(23), 2246–2254. https://doi-org.proxy.library.upenn.edu/10.1056/NEJMra1808418

Pappas, P. G., Kauffman, C. A., Andes, D. R., Clancy, C. J., Marr, K. A., Ostrosky-Zeichner, L., Reboli, A. C., Schuster, M. G., Vazquez, J. A., Walsh, T. J., Zaoutis, T. E., & Sobel, J. D. (2016). Clinical practice guideline for the management of candidiasis: 2016 update by the infectious diseases society of america. *Clinical Infectious Diseases: An Official Publication of the Infectious Diseases Society of America, 62*(4), e1–e50. https://doi.org/10.1093/cid/civ933

Peebles K., Velloza J., Balkus J.E., McClelland R.S., & Barnabas R.V. (2019). High global burden and costs of bacterial vaginosis: A systematic review and meta-analysis. *Sex Transm Dis, 46*, 304–11. https://doi.org/10.1097/OLQ.0000000000000972 973.

Qi, W., Li, H., Wang, C., Li, H., Zhang, B., Dong, M., Fan, A., Han, C., & Xue, F. (2021). Recent advances in presentation, diagnosis and treatment for mixed vaginitis. *Frontiers in Cellular and Infection Microbiology, 11*, 759–795. https://doi-org.proxy.library.upenn.edu/10.3389/fcimb.2021.759795

Ravel, J., Moreno, I., & Simón, C. (2021). Bacterial vaginosis and its association with infertility, endometritis, and pelvic inflammatory disease. *American Journal of Obstetrics and Gynecology, 224*(3), 251–257. https://doi-org.proxy.library.upenn.edu/10.1016/j.ajog.2020.10.019

Schwebke, J. R., Gaydos, C. A., Nyirjesy, P., Paradis, S., Kodsi, S., & Cooper, C. K. (2018). Diagnostic performance of a molecular test versus clinician assessment of vaginitis. *Journal of Clinical Microbiology, 56*(6), e00252–18. https://doi-org.proxy.library.upenn.edu/10.1128/JCM.00252-18

Schwebke, J. R., Lensing, S. Y., Lee, J., Muzny, C. A., Pontius, A., Woznicki, N., Aguin, T., & Sobel, J. D. (2021). Treatment of male sexual partners of women with bacterial vaginosis: A randomized, double-blind, placebo-controlled trial. *Clinical Infectious Diseases: An Official Publication of the Infectious Diseases Society of America, 73*(3), e672–e679. https://doi-org.proxy.library.upenn.edu/10.1093/cid/ciaa1903

Schwebke, J. R., Taylor, S. N., Ackerman, R., Schlaberg, R., Quigley, N. B., Gaydos, C. A., Chavoustie, S. E., Nyirjesy, P., Remillard, C. V., Estes, P., McKinney, B., Getman, D. K., & Clark, C. (2020). Clinical validation of the aptima bacterial vaginosis and aptima *candida/trichomonas* vaginitis assays: Results from a prospective multicenter clinical study. *Journal of Clinical Microbiology, 58*(2), e01643–19. https://doi-org.proxy.library.upenn.edu/10.1128/JCM.01643-19

Swidsinski A., Guschin A., Tang, Q. et al. (2019) Vulvovaginal candidiasis: Histologic lesions are primarily polymicrobial and invasive and do not contain biofilms. *American Journal of Obstetrics and Gynecology, 220*(91), e1–8. https://doi.org/10.1016/j.ajog.2018.10.023.

Vieira-Baptista P., Grinceviciene S., Oliveira C., Fonseca-Moutinho J., Cherey F., Stockdale C. K. (2021). The international society for the study of vulvovaginal disease vaginal wet mount microscopy guidelines: How to perform, applications, and interpretation. *Journal of Lower Genital Tract Disease, 25*(2), 172–180. https://doi.org/10.1097/LGT.0000000000000595

Workowski, K. A., Bachmann, L. H, Chan, P. A., et al. (2021). Sexually transmitted infections treatment guidelines, 2021. *MMWR Recomm Rep 2021;70*(No. RR-4):1–187. https://doi.org/10.15585/mmwr.rr7004a1external icon.

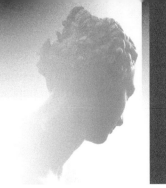

7

SEXUALLY TRANSMITTED INFECTIONS

DEBRA ILCHAK, R. MIMI SECOR, AND IRIS STENDIG-RASKIN

EXPERT REVIEWER: HANNE S. HARBISON

SEXUALLY TRANSMITTED INFECTIONS EXPLAINED

A. Statistics and trends
   1. Previously known as *sexually transmitted diseases*, now referred to as sexually transmitted infections (STIs). This chapter includes all STIs except HIV.
   2. Approximately 26 million new infections occur each year (incidence) in the United States per the Centers for Disease Control and Prevention (CDC). The CDC also estimated 67.6 million prevalent and 26.2 million incident STIs in the United States.
   3. Almost half of new STIs is among 15- to 24-year-olds.
   4. One in five individuals in the United States have been diagnosed with either a viral or bacterial STI.
   5. Non-Hispanic African Americans and Hispanic individuals have disproportionately higher rates of STIs.
   6. Significant physical and psychological consequences result from STIs, such as infertility, stigma, pain, and death, to name a few.
   7. The total direct medical costs of managing STIs are estimated to be $16 billion (in 2020 dollars); these estimates are based on CDC's analyses of eight common STIs: chlamydia, gonorrhea, hepatitis B virus (HBV), herpes simplex virus type 2 (HSV-2), HIV, human papillomavirus (HPV), syphilis, and trichomoniasis.
   8. Reportable STIs include gonorrhea, chlamydia, syphilis, and HIV.
   9. STIs that are not reportable include HPV, HSV, and trichomoniasis.
   10. Biological factors place people with vaginas at greater risk than people with penises for acquiring STIs and suffering from more severe health consequences associated with STIs.
B. Epidemiology; see Table 7.1 for a summary of STI assessment of people with vaginas.
   1. Chlamydia is the most common reportable STI.
      a. An estimated 1.6 million (in 2020) new cases each year
      b. More than half of new cases are undiagnosed and therefore unreported.
      c. Leading cause of pelvic inflammatory disease (PID) and infertility in the United States
   2. Gonorrhea is the second most common reportable STI.
      a. An estimated 677,769 cases were reported in 2020—an increase of 111% since 2009; gonorrhea is also underdiagnosed and underreported.
      b. More common in men having sex with men (MSM)
      c. Increases susceptibility to HIV three- to fivefold
      d. Widespread fluoroquinolone-resistance. In suspected cephalosporin treatment failure, contact an infectious disease specialist.

TABLE 7.1 STI Assessment

INFECTION	CAUSE	PREVALENCE	SYMPTOMS	DIAGNOSIS
Chlamydia	Obligate intracellular parasite susceptible to antibiotics	Most common reported STI; leading cause of preventable infertility	Often asymptomatic, so need for widespread screening in <25 years old	Annual screening in individuals with a vagina if <25 years old is recommended by the CDC; diagnosis screening: urine, cervico-vaginal swab, cervical, or urethral NAAT/PCR testing
Genital herpes	Type 1 or 2 herpes virus; both can infect genitals	Estimated 18.6 million Americans infected with HSV-2	Most asymptomatic, most transmission when asymptomatic; symptoms may include painful genital lesions; first infection most severe; recurrences most common with HSV-2; widely variable symptoms	Classic symptoms suspect HSV; culture if lesions. PCR culture more sensitive, expensive; type-specific serology IgG/herpes select; 98% seroconversion 4 months post-HSV acquisition
Genital warts	Nononcogenic HPV 6, 11	Nearly all sexually active individuals will get HPV	Single or multiple, soft, fleshy, nontender, cauliflower-like lesions in genital area including vulvovaginal, anal, or cervix	By examination, HPV DNA testing not recommended; RPR to rule out condylomata lata of syphilis; colposcopy and/or biopsy of atypical lesions
Gonorrhea	*Neisseria gonorrhoeae*, gram-negative diplococcus bacteria	Second most common STI in the United States, especially among MSM	Commonly asymptomatic, or abnormal vaginal discharge, dysuria, abnormal bleeding	Gram stain, (50% sensitivity) culture, NAAT of cervical or vaginal secretions; urine NAAT an option too
PID	Polymicrobial, various combinations, *N. gonorrhoeae, Chlamydia trachomatis,* anaerobes, and others	Leading cause of female infertility	Many have no symptoms or atypical symptoms; symptoms include pain/tenderness in lower abdomen, uterus, ovaries; fever, chills, elevated WBCs/ESR, associated with menses	High index of suspicion, low threshold for diagnosis, + cultures, CDC criteria, pelvic exam tenderness, mucopus, WBCs on vaginal microscopy
Syphilis	*Treponema pallidum* spirochete	Increasing among heterosexual women, high rates in MSM	Primary: Classic chancre is painless indurated ulcer in genital area at site of exposure, may evade diagnosis if vaginal Secondary: Variable skin rash, may involve palms, and/or soles Latent: No signs or symptoms, positive serology, negative spinal tap, except in the case of neurosyphilis	Primary: Darkfield examination of chancre, with non-treponeal and treponemal serology Secondary and latent: Non-treponemal and treponemal serology

(continued)

TABLE 7.1 STI Assessment (*continued*)				
INFECTION	**CAUSE**	**PREVALENCE**	**SYMPTOMS**	**DIAGNOSIS**
Trichomoniasis	Motile protozoan	Most common curable STI in the United States and worldwide; 2.6 million U.S. women infected yearly; may be asymptomatic for years	Excessive, frothy, yellow-green vaginal discharge; examination findings variable, sometimes with genital erythema, swelling, and pruritus	Vaginal microscopy for typical motile trichomonads and WBCs; Pap should be verified with culture or microscopy; various vaginal cultures may also be used, including PCR

CDC, Centers for Disease Control and Prevention; ESR, erythrocyte sedimentation rate; HPV, human papillomavirus; HSV, herpes simplex virus; IgG, immunoglobulin G; MSM, men having sex with men; NAAT, nucleic acid amplification test; PCR, polymerase chain reaction; PID, pelvic inflammatory disease; RPR, rapid plasma regain; STI, sexually transmitted infection; WBC, white blood cell.

3. Genital herpes (HSV 2) is a common STI.
    a. **Prevalence:** One in five Americans; 25% of people with vaginas, one out of three older than 30, and more than 50% of non-Hispanic Blacks are seropositive for HSV-2.
    b. Most transmission occurs when people are asymptomatic.
    c. Most symptoms are atypical.
    d. When symptoms occur, they typically appear as one or more painful blisters in the urogenital area or rectum. The fluid-filled blisters soon break, leaving tender ulcers (sores) that may take 2 to 4 weeks to heal if it is the primary outbreak. Recurrent infections typically are unilateral, less severe than the primary outbreak, with a duration of about 3 to 7 days without treatment
    e. HSV 1 accounts for up to 50% of primary genital infections and rarely causes recurrences after the first year of infection.
    f. HSV 2 is associated with the highest shedding and recurrence rate the first year with up to 1 to 3 days associated with asymptomatic or symptomatic shedding. Recurrences and/ or asymptomatic shedding may continue over a lifetime, waxing and waning in variable ways per individual.
4. HPV is the most common STI with the highest incidence among young populations in their late teens and early 20s.
    a. Approximately 85% of sexually active people will contract HPV.
    b. Infection is usually transient, clearing within 2 years.
    c. HPV is the cause of cervical cancer. Development of cancer is associated with persistent HPV infection with high-risk subtypes, including 16, 18, 31, and others. HPV can also cause anogenital warts and other HPV-associated cancers.
    d. More than 100 different strains or subtypes exist, 30 of which are sexually transmitted.
    e. HPV can infect the genital area, including the skin of the penis, vulva, anus, and the vagina, cervix, and rectal mucosa.
    f. HPV vaccination is recommended for all adolescents at age 11 or 12 years.
5. Primary and secondary syphilis rates in women have increased 147.4% over the last 5 years. The reason is unclear.
    a. Rates are higher in MSM than among heterosexual women.
    b. Syphilis is known as *the great imitator* because the signs and symptoms can mimic those associated with other STIs and nonvenereal skin problems.
6. *Mycoplasma genitalium*
    a. Associated with cervicitis, PID, preterm delivery, spontaneous abortion, and infertility in women.
    b. Frequently asymptomatic
    c. NAAT available for testing with urine and vaginal and cervical samples

C. Complications associated with STIs
1. Chlamydia and gonorrhea, if untreated, may lead to PID, ectopic pregnancy, chronic pelvic pain, and infertility.
2. Long-term complications of chlamydia are much more serious in people with uteruses.
3. Many STIs, including gonorrhea, herpes, bacterial vaginosis, and syphilis, increase the risk of acquiring HIV.
4. Several infections are associated with preterm labor, including trichomoniasis and bacterial vaginosis.
5. Cervical cancer is a rare complication from persistent HPV infection.
D. Considerations for people with vaginas and uteruses
1. Females are more susceptible to STIs due to the extensive mucous membrane tissue lining the genital tract.
2. Many STIs are asymptomatic and can go undiagnosed and untreated.
3. Rates of syphilis have increased in reproductive-aged people along with rates of congenital syphilis. Reinfection can happen if their partners are not diagnosed and appropriately treated.
4. STIs can complicate a pregnancy and contribute to negative health outcomes for parents and their babies. For CDC STI screening recommendations during pregnancy, visit https://www.cdc.gov/std/pregnancy/stdfact-pregnancy-detailed.htm#table1

CLINICAL EVALUATION OF PEOPLE WITH VAGINAS AND UTERUSES

A. History
1. Symptoms
   a. Onset, duration, location, severity, course, precipitating factors
   b. Past history of STIs, symptoms, diagnosis, management
   c. Self-care to present
   d. Associated symptoms with review of symptoms (ROS)
      (1) Constitutional
         • Malaise, fatigue, myalgia, chills, fever, weight loss, anorexia
      (2) Head, eye, ear, nose, and throat (HEENT; HSV 1, HSV 2, gonorrhea, syphilis)
         • Sores, lesions, oropharnygeal erythema, exudate, tenderness
      (3) Cardiac (syphilis, gonorrhea-associated endocarditis)
         • Murmurs, irregularity, other abnormal findings
      (4) Gastrointestinal (hepatitis, PID, HIV)
         • Abdominal pain, PID, back pain (pyelonephritis), upper right quadrant pain (liver), bloating, indigestion, nausea, vomiting, diarrhea, anorexia, weight loss
      (5) Genital/urinary (HSV 1, HSV 2, gonorrhea, chlamydia, trichomoniasis, bacterial vaginosis, candidiasis)
         • Urinary symptoms of frequency, urgency, dysuria, hematuria, odor, abnormal color to urine, back pain
         • Genital or anal itching, sores, tears, lesions, burning, pain, discharge, bleeding, odor, dyspareunia
      (6) Neurological (syphilis, HSV)
         • Mental status changes, headache
      (7) Skin (syphilis, gonorrhea, HSV, HPV)
         • Sores, lesions, blisters, rashes, warts, tattoos, branding, body piercings, icterus (hepatitis)
      (8) Extremities (gonorrhea, syphilis, lymphogranuloma venereum [LGV])
         • Arthralgias, joint stiffness, pain, swelling
2. Gynecologic history
   a. Pregnancy history, including gravida, parous, pregnancy intention

        (1) Abortions
- Spontaneous, medical, surgical, miscarriage

  b. Menstrual history

      (1) Last menstrual period, characteristics, timing

      (2) Age of first period or menarche; cycle length and duration; dysmenorrhea (new onset or worsening of dysmenorrhea); abnormal bleeding; bleeding between periods or after intercourse; type of products used (tampons, pads, menstrual cup)

  c. STI history

      (1) Record all STIs, including vaginal infections; dates of infections, how previously diagnosed and treated, inquire about any incomplete treatments; record follow-ups, partner notification, and subsequent treatments

      (2) Date last tested, what tests done, and results

  d. Sexual history

      (1) Sexual partner(s), date of most recent sexual encounter; total number of sex partners in a specific time frame (1 month, 3 months, 6 months), last sexual encounter, sexual orientation

      (2) Behaviors
- Unprotected vaginal, anal, oral (receptive, expressive); use of condoms (percentage); sex with money or drug exchange; injection drug use; tattooing; body piercing; branding; violence; rape; abuse, including violent sex play; using dirty sex toys
- High-risk partner(s)
  - Exposure to HIV, hepatitis B, hepatitis C, chlamydia, gonorrhea, IV drug use, sex worker, MSM, bisexual, group sex, abusive controlling partner with unknown history or suspected high-risk history

      (3) Contraceptive history
- History of unprotected intercourse, consenting, rape, reluctant consent, reproductive coercion, access to emergency contraception (Plan B, ulipristal [Ella], or intrauterine contraception [IUC])
- Current contraceptive method, methods used in past, dates, problems, satisfaction with current method, complaints, and compliance with method of choice

      (4) Infertility

  e. Gynecologic surgery, procedures, problems

  f. Personal hygiene

      (1) Douching may increase risk of recurrent vaginal infections (e.g., bacterial vaginosis [BV]) and PID

      (2) Tampon, pad, or menstrual cup use; deodorant tampons, synthetic or cotton, note brand; use of panty liners; frequency of wear (daily vs. with menses only)

      (3) Type of underwear (e.g., thong underwear associated with vaginal infections)

      (4) Hygiene practices
- Including poor hygiene, not wiping front to back, not washing after anal intercourse, not washing sex toys, poor oral hygiene, not washing hands or genitals before sex
- Use of soap, type, amount used, bubble baths, feminine-hygiene sprays, other chemicals
- Baths versus showers; source of water in bath or shower

      (5) Tight clothing, workout clothing, pantyhose, bathing suit, duration of wear particularly extended hours

      (6) Genital and oral piercings

3. Social history

  a. History of sexual, physical, and verbal abuse or trauma

  b. Lifestyle history: diet, exercise, sleep, stressors, occupation, recreation

  c. **Substance use:** Alcohol, nicotine, marijuana

4. Medical history
   a. **Medical conditions:** Past and present, stable or unstable
   b. Immunization status, including HPV, hepatitis A, hepatitis B
5. Current medications
   a. Prescription medications; over-the-counter medications
   b. Medication allergies
6. Family history

B. Examination
   1. Vital signs (if fever, consider PID)
   2. Skin
      a. Lesions, rashes, warts, ulcers, palmar or foot sole rash (syphilis), tattoos, piercings, brandings, pallor, jaundice
   3. Oral
      a. Erythema, tenderness, sores, lesions; warts, exudate, plaques, thrush, Kaposi's sarcoma (KS)
      b. Foul odor, gum disease, plaque, dental caries, poor hygiene
   4. Cardiac
      a. Tertiary syphilis
   5. Abdominal
      a. Absence of bowel sounds or increased bowel sounds
      b. Masses, enlargement
         (1) Lower abdominal mass, consider PID with tubo-ovarian abscess (TOA)
         (2) Right upper abdominal mass, consider hepatitis
         (3) Inguinal nodes swelling and/or tenderness, consider HIV, pelvic, genital infection
      c. Tenderness
         (1) Costovertebral angle (CVA) tenderness with pyelonephritis
         (2) Right upper quadrant, consider hepatitis
         (3) Lower abdomen, consider PID, cystitis
   6. Pelvic examination
      a. External genitalia
         (1) Inguinal node tenderness or enlargement
         (2) Erythema, lesions, urethral discharge, fissures, tears, tenderness
         (3) Bartholin gland areas are located at 5 o'clock and 7 o'clock at the vaginal introitus
         (4) Skene's glands at 3 o'clock and 9 o'clock positions of urethral meatus
         (5) Urethral caruncle, discharge
      b. Vagina
         (1) Introital erythema (focal or diffuse), lesions, tenderness, particularly between labial folds (displace tissue to fully visualize tissues)
         (2) Discharge
            • Color, quality; flocular, creamy, homogeneous, clumpy, frothy; amount
         (3) Vaginal pH, amine potassium hydroxide (KOH) test; foul-fishy odor is positive
         (4) Vaginal microscopy/wet mount (see Chapter 6, "Vaginal Microscopy and Vaginal Infections")
      c. Cervix
         (1) Redness, cervical erosion, ectropion, mucopus, friability, bleeding
         (2) Cervical os, size, shape, mucopus from os, quantity
         (3) Cervical motion tenderness; mild, moderate, severe, or positive chandelier test suggestive of PID
      d. Bimanual examination of uterus and adnexa
         (1) Tenderness; mild, moderate, severe, rebound, localized, masses, mobility
         (2) Uterus size, shape, mobility, firmness, tenderness
         (3) Ovaries

- Palpable or nonpalpable
- Tenderness; mild, moderate, severe
- Fullness or masses

 e. Rectal

  (1) Lesions; sores, blisters, warts, tags, fissures, tears, hemorrhoids

  (2) Erythema, hemorrhoids, lesions, tenderness, discharge, itching, bleeding

 7. Extremities

  a. Joint swelling, tenderness, increased heat, reduced range of motion

 8. Neurological

  a. Visual changes, mental status, altered behavior

C. Diagnostic testing per the CDC STI Guidelines

 1. Chlamydia testing

  a. Yearly screening of all sexually active people with vaginas younger than 25 years

  b. Screen people with vaginas 25 years old and older if new or multiple sexual partners or history of high-risk behaviors

  c. Retest 3 months after treatment to detect reinfection

  d. If retesting in 3 months does not occur, then retesting within 12 months following initial treatment is recommended

 2. Gonorrhea testing

  a. Yearly screening of all sexually active people with vaginas younger than 25 years

  b. Screen people with vaginas 25 years old and older if new or multiple sexual partners, history of high-risk behaviors, MSM, bisexual, heterosexual females with sex partners of unknown risk, or who have high-risk partners, or females not using condoms

  c. Women with previous or current STI, those who engage in commercial sex work and drug use, women in certain demographic groups, and those living in communities with a high prevalence of disease

  d. Screening is not recommended for heterosexual men and women 25 years and older who are at low risk

 3. Genital herpes

  a. The U.S. Preventive Services Task Force (USPSTF) does not recommend routine serologic screening for genital herpes for asymptomatic individuals.

  b. Culture needed if fluid-filled blisters or very moist lesions.

  c. Polymerase chain reaction (PCR) is four times more accurate than non-PCR; therefore, non-blistering lesions may be tested with greater accuracy.

  d. Culture and PCR results should be typed to determine if HSV 1 or 2

  e. HSV 1- and 2-specific immunoglobulin G (IgG) antibody testing are the gold standard diagnostic tests for non-primary HSV testing.

   (1) Nearly 100% seroconversion within 4 months of infection

   (2) Initial negative test indicates probable primary infection with recent acquisition of infection

   (3) There is no type-specific immunoglobulin M (IgM) antibody test and therefore IgM should not be ordered

 4. Syphilis

  a. CDC recommends screening asymptomatic adults at increased risk and all pregnant women at first prenatal visit and if high risk again at 28 weeks of gestation and delivery.

  b. Risk populations: MSM, bisexual, injection drug use, HIV infection, high-risk partner.

  c. Rate of infection is increasing among heterosexual women contributing to an increase in congenital syphilis.

 5. Trichomoniasis

  a. CDC recommends screening with the presence of vaginal discharge.

b. The preferred diagnostic test is a microscopy wet mount because it is inexpensive; however, microscopy has a lower sensitivity (44%–68%) rate as compared to a culture (44%–75% sensitivity).

c. NAATs are more sensitive than performing a wet mount.

d. Trichomoniasis is considered an incidental finding on a Pap test and is not considered a diagnostic test if present; the CDC recommends treatment after testing with a sensitive diagnostic test.

D. Pharmacological management of sexually transmitted infections (STIs): see Table 7.2.

TABLE 7.2 Pharmacological Management of Sexually Transmitted Infections

INFECTION	REGIMEN TYPE	MEDICATION	DOSAGE	COMMENTS
Chlamydia[a]	Recommended regimen in adults and adolescents	Doxycycline	100 mg orally 2x/day for 7 days	• Contraindicated during second and third trimesters of pregnancy due to risk of tooth discoloration • Take with food to decrease GI irritation • More efficacious for rectal chlamydia infection than azithromycin
	Recommended regimen in pregnancy	Azithromycin	1 g orally in a single dose	• Alternative regimen for non-pregnant adults and adolescents
Genital herpes (HSV 2)	First clinical episode	Acyclovir	400 mg orally 3x/day for 7–10 days	• If healing is incomplete after 10 days of therapy, treatment can be extended
		Famciclovir	250 mg orally 3x/day for 7–10 days	
		Valacyclovir	1 g orally 2 x/day for 7–10 days	
	Episodic therapy	Acyclovir	800 mg orally 2x/day for 5 days OR 800 mg orally 3x/day for 2 days	• Initiate as soon as possible after onset of symptoms
		Famciclovir	1 g orally 2x/day for 1 day OR 500 mg orally once, followed by 250 mg 2x/day for 2 days OR 125 mg orally 2x/day for 5 days	

(continued)

TABLE 7.2 Pharmacological Management of Sexually Transmitted Infections (*continued*)

INFECTION	REGIMEN TYPE	MEDICATION	DOSAGE	COMMENTS
Genital herpes (HSV 2) (*cont.*)		Valacyclovir	500 mg orally 2x/day for 3 days OR 1 g orally once daily for 5 days	
	Suppressive therapy	Acyclovir	400 mg orally 2x/day	• In persons with ≥10 episodes/year, valacyclovir 500 mg once a day might be less effective than other dosing regimens • Suppressive therapy in pregnant women starts at 36 weeks of gestation
		Valacyclovir	500 mg orally once a day OR 1 g orally once a day	
		Famciclovir	250 mg orally 2 times/day	
	Suppressive therapy in pregnant women	Acyclovir	400 mg orally 3x/day	• Starting at 36 weeks of gestation
		Valacyclovir	500 mg orally 2x/day	
Gonorrhea[a]	Recommended regimen for uncomplicated infections of the cervix, urethra, and rectum	Ceftriaxone PLUS If chlamydia infection not excluded, doxycycline	500 mg IM in a single dose 100 mg orally 2x/day for 7 days	• Safe in pregnancy • In persons weighing ≥150kg, 1 g ceftriaxone should be administered • Can dilute with 1% lidocaine to reduce injection pain
Mycoplasma genitalium	Recommended regimen if detected by FDA-cleared NAAT and resistance testing is not available	Doxycycline 100 mg orally 2x/day for 7 days FOLLOWED BY Moxifloxacin 400 mg orally 1x/day for 7 days		• Doxycycline contraindicated during second and third trimesters of pregnancy • See guidelines for recommended regimen if resistance testing done • Test of cure not needed if treated with recommended regimen
Pelvic inflammatory disease	Intramuscular/oral treatment	Ceftriaxone 500 mg IM in a single dose PLUS Doxycycline 100 mg orally 2x/day for 14 days WITH Metronidazole 500 mg orally 2x/day for 14 days		• See guidelines for all treatment options including parenteral • Selection based on severity of symptoms, adherence, pregnancy

(*continued*)

TABLE 7.2 Pharmacological Management of Sexually Transmitted Infections (*continued*)

INFECTION	REGIMEN TYPE	MEDICATION	DOSAGE	COMMENTS
Syphilis	Primary and secondary	Benzathine penicillin G	2.4 million units IM in a single dose	• Safe in pregnancy • Jarisch-Herxheimer reaction (fever with headache and myalgia) can occur within first 24 hours after treatment. Considered an adverse side effect of treatment, not an allergy to penicillin • In pregnancy, a second dose of benzathine penicillin G 2.4 million units IM can be administered 1 week after initial dose to help prevent congenital syphilis
	Early latent	Benzathine penicillin G	2.4 million units IM in a single dose	
	Late latent	Benzathine penicillin G	7.2 million units total, administered as 3 doses of 2.4 million units IM each at 1-week intervals	
Trichomoniasis	Recommended regimen for women	Metronidazole	500 mg orally 2x/day for 7 days	• Safe in pregnancy • Refraining from alcohol use while taking metronidazole or tinidazole is unnecessary • Take with food to decrease GI irritation
	Alternative regimen for women	Tinidazole	2 g orally in a single dose	• Avoid use in pregnancy
Warts— external anogenital	Patient-applied	Imiquimod	3.75% or 5% cream	• Imiquimod and sinecatechins may weaken condoms and vaginal diaphragms • Do not use podofilox or sinecatechins in pregnancy • Imiquimod poses low risk in pregnancy, but data are limited
		Podofilox	0.5% solution or gel	
		Sinecatechins	15% ointment	
	Provider-administered	Cryotherapy with liquid nitrogen or cryoprobe		
		Surgical removal by tangential scissor excision, tangential shave excision, curettage, laser, or electrosurgery		
		Trichloroacetic acid (TCA) or bichloroacetic acid (BCA) 80%–90% solution		

Note: Additional recommended and alternative regimens can be found in the CDC's Sexually Transmitted Infections Treatment Guidelines, 2021: https://www.cdc.gov/std/treatment-guidelines/default.htm

[a]Offer expedited partner therapy (EPT) for chlamydia and gonorrhea, if permitted by state laws or regulations. For more information, visit https://www.cdc.gov/std/ept

Source: Centers for Disease Control and Prevention. (2021). Sexually transmitted infections treatment guidelines, 2021. Retrieved from https://www.cdc.gov/std/treatment-guidelines/default.htm

CASE STUDY

Patient Situation

A 23-year-old female presents to the office complaining of "yellow discharge" with odor and vaginal irritation.

Subjective Data

- *Symptoms:* Began 2 weeks ago, treated with over-the-counter fungal cream × 3 days with no improvement. Denies dysuria, pelvic pain, or vaginal sores.
- *Sexual History*: Reports new male partner × 4 months and two sexual partners in the past year, vaginal sex with no condom use, treated for chlamydia 2 years ago.
- *Medications*: levonorgestrel IUD × 2 years, occasional use of marijuana for feelings of anxiety, denies allergies to medications.

Objective Data

- *Pelvic Exam*: No inguinal adenopathy, external genitalia with erythema and no lesions or swelling, vagina with frothy yellow vaginal discharge with fishy odor noted, cervix erythematous with no bleeding noted.
- *Bimanual Exam:* No cervical motion or adnexal tenderness.
- *Vital signs:* Blood pressure 112/78, pulse 68/min, temperature 98.6°F
- Height: 5'6" Weight 180 lbs.

Clinical Analysis

Based on the history and physical exam, you suspect the patient has trichomoniasis.

What diagnostics should be ordered, and why?

- NAAT for T. vaginalis (endocervical or vaginal swab, urine specimen)
- Wet mount if microscopy available in the office (has low sensitivity)
- Offer testing for other STIs (chlamydia, gonorrhea, HIV, syphilis)

The diagnostic test is positive for trichomoniasis. What are the treatment options?

- Metronidazole 500 mg orally 2 ×/daily for 7 days
- Alternative Regimen: Tinidazole 2 g orally in single dose
- Refraining from alcohol use while taking these medications is unnecessary

What patient education and counseling should be provided?

- Trichomoniasis is a sexually transmitted infection that is curable with medication.
- Sex partner(s) needs presumptive treatment. Refer or offer expedited partner therapy (EPT) if permissible by state law.
- Abstain from sex until treatment completed, and sex partner(s) treated (completion of medication, symptoms resolve).
- If not already completed, offer testing for other STIs (chlamydia, gonorrhea, HIV, syphilis).
- Encourage use of condoms to decrease STI transmission.

What follow-up is recommended?

- Retesting for *T. vaginalis* is recommended in 3 months due to high rates of reinfection.
- If not completed at 3 months, retest whenever patient presents for medical care in the 12 months after initial treatment.

ACKNOWLEDGMENT

Thanks to Hanne S. Harbison, MHSPH, MSN, WHNP-BC for reviewing this chapter.

ADDITIONAL RESOURCE

CDC STI Tx Quick Guide: https://www.cdc.gov/STIapp

BIBLIOGRAPHY

American Cancer Society. (2020). *HPV and HPV testing.* https://www .cancer.org/cancer/cancer-causes/infectious-agents/ hpv/hpv-and-hpv-testing.html

Centers for Disease Control and Prevention. (2021a). *Sexually transmitted infections treatment guidelines, 2021.* https:// www.cdc.gov/std/treatment-guidelines/STI-Guidelines-2021.pdf

Centers for Disease Control and Prevention. (2021b). *HIV basics.* https://www.cdc.gov/hiv/basics/index.html

Centers for Disease Control and Prevention. (2022a). *CDC fact sheet: Incidence, prevalence, and cost of sexual transmitted infections in the United States.* https://www.cdc.gov/nchhstp/newsroom/docs/factsheets/2018-STI-incidence-prevalence -factsheet.pdf

Centers for Disease Control and Prevention. (2022b). *Sexually transmitted diseases surveillance 2020.* https://www.cdc.gov /std/statistics/2020/default.htm

Kreisel, K. M., Spicknall, I. H. Gargano, J. W., Lewis, F. M. T., Lewis, R. M., Markowitz, L. E., Robers, H., Johnson, A. S., Song, R., St. Cyr, S. B., Weston, E. J., Torrone, E. A., & Weinstock, H. S. (2022). Sexually transmitted infections among US women and men: Prevalence and incidence estimates, 2018. *Sexually Transmitted Diseases, 48*(4), 208–214. https:// doi.org/10.1097/OLQ.0000000000001355

Planned Parenthood. (2022). *Sexually transmitted diseases.* http://www.plannedparenthood.org/health-topics/stds-hiv-safer -sex-101.htm

U.S. Preventive Services Task Force. (2022). *Recommendation topics.* https://www.uspreventiveservicestaskforce.org/uspstf /recommendation-topics

8

ASSESSMENT OF THE SKIN/AESTHETICS

KATHLEEN HAYCRAFT

DERMATOLOGIC ASSESSMENT: REVIEW OF BASIC CUTANEOUS ANATOMY (FIGURE 8.1)

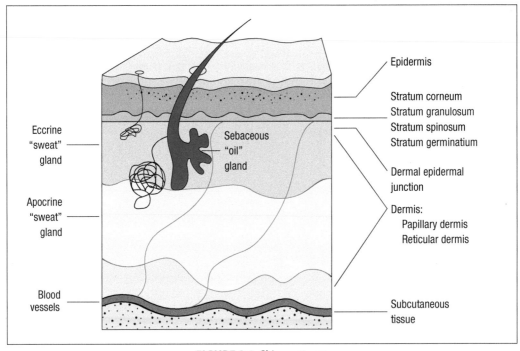

FIGURE 8.1 Skin anatomy.

A. The epidermis and the dermis rest on the subcutaneous layer. These layers form the integumentary system. The skin is the largest organ of the body. It is also the most expressive organ.

B. The epidermis is the outer layer of the skin.
   1. It is composed of the following layers:
      a. Stratum germinatum (above the dermis)
      b. Stratum spinosum
      c. Stratum granulosum
      d. Stratum corneum (top layer of the skin)
   2. The epidermis has four types of cells.
      a. Keratinocytes (produce keratin) create the hornified outer layer of the skin.
      b. Melanocytes (have dendritic connections to keratinocytes) are responsible for the production of melanin (protection from ultraviolet [UV] rays).

    c. Langerhans cells are derived from the bone marrow and are present in the first three layers of the epidermis. They play an important role in the immune system of the skin.

    d. Merkel cells are neuroendocrine cells.

C. Dermis

  1. The papillary dermis is directly below the epidermis. It consists of capillaries, fibers, and collagen.

  2. The thicker reticular dermis consists of dense connective tissue, larger blood vessels, and elastic and collagen bundles.

  3. Fibroblasts are the predominant cell type of the dermis. The cells produce collagen and elastic fibers.

  4. Collagen represents most of the dermis. Elastic fibers represent approximately 1% of the dermis but have a significant role in countering deforming forces.

D. The dermal/epidermal junction is an undulating membrane that connects the dermis to the epidermis. This layer flattens with aging. This is a focal point of attack in diseases like bullous pemphigus.

E. Epidermal appendages include hair follicles, nails, sweat (eccrine) glands, sebaceous glands, apocrine glands, and mammary glands.

F. Vascular supply

  1. The cutaneous vessels play a critical role in thermal regulation.

CUTANEOUS ASSESSMENT

A. The color of the skin can provide valuable information regarding the patient's state of health; it is the largest organ of the body and as such it may give valuable clues regarding systemic disease. To examine the skin, you must *listen* to the patient's history and current concerns; *look* at all of the skin (including soles of the feet, between the toes, scalp, vulva, fingernails, eyes, and ears); *touch* the skin as you examine it; and *smell* for any unusual odors.

B. Pigment changes (Table 8.1)

C. Temperature and turgor

  1. Very cool skin can be seen with exposure to cold or shock.

  2. Skin that is excessively warm may be associated with high fever and/or infection.

TABLE 8.1 Dermatologic Assessment

COLOR	ASSOCIATED WITH
Yellow to orange	Liver, renal, or hypercarotenemia
Blue	Cyanosis (low oxygen) or argyria (excess silver)
Red or erythema	Red-man syndrome (allopurinol, rapid IV fluoroquinolone) or erythroderma (exfoliative dermatitis, which can be fatal and may require hospitalization) Excess flushing from embarrassment, fever, or infection
Absence of pigment	Vitiligo, Addison's disease, uremia, anemia. In a lesion it may represent a morpheaform basal cell cancer
Hyperpigmentation	Medications (minocycline, amiodarone, and many others), post-inflammation: In a lesion it may represent melanoma or a pigmented basal cell cancer.

3. Good skin turgor refers to the ability of the skin to resume its normal shape after being tented with the thumb and forefinger for about 10 seconds. If the skin does not rapidly resume its shape, poor skin turgor is present, and dehydration may exist (this may normally occur with aging skin).

D. Scars
   1. Location
   2. Tenderness
   3. Cause
   4. Hypertrophic (large scar at site) or keloid (large scar that extends beyond the original scar site)

E. Presence of dryness (frequently associated with aging) or oiliness (seen with acne and sometimes Parkinson's disease)

F. Odor may be associated with infection, renal failure, liver failure, intestinal obstruction, diabetic fruitiness, and a wide range of smells specific to the individual

G. Oral assessment
   1. Teeth and gum assessment are important to the complete assessment.
   2. Assess the gums for signs of gingivitis, which include bleeding and inflammation of the gums. Patients with symptoms of gingivitis should be referred to a dentist. Gingival hypertrophy is a side effect of many medications, and either gum disorder requires a dental referral.
   3. Cavities and excessive plaque should be referred to a dentist.
   4. Lesions of the gums, tongue, palate, or buccal mucosa should be referred to a dentist or an ear, nose, and throat (ENT) specialist for prompt evaluation.
   5. A thick-ridged hard palate is a normal finding and is referred to as a *torus palatine*.
   6. Oral health is correlated with overall health. Every opportunity should be taken to stress the health benefits of tooth brushing and regular flossing.

H. Fingernails/toenails may add to the assessment of systemic and localized illness (Table 8.2).

I. Hair
   1. Loss of hair is referred to as *alopecia*.
   2. Examination of the scalp is an important part of hair assessment.
      a. Any unusual scalp lesions should be referred for possible biopsy to rule out cutaneous carcinoma including basal cell carcinoma (BCC), squamous cell carcinoma, and melanoma.
      b. Note whether the scalp is erythematous, boggy, or tender.
      c. Question the patient whether the scalp is itchy.
      d. Erythema and scalp edema are associated with infectious and inflammatory disorders and require referral to dermatology.
      e. The alopecia disorders are numerous.
      f. Scalp pruritus is frequently associated with contact dermatitis and/or excessive hair washing. Sulfite-/sulfate-free shampoos can be helpful.
      g. Persistent pruritus should be referred to dermatology for evaluation.
   3. Loss of hair due to the prolonged resting phase of the hair follicle is referred to as *telogen effluvium* and is common in the postpartum period, with low iron levels, and with the use of some medications. Oral retinoids, antibiotics, contraceptive pills and injections, statins, neuroleptics, hormone replacement therapy, antihypertensives, diuretics, NSAIDs, and steroids are examples, but many medications can be involved, so a thorough history is necessary. It involves less than 15% of the hair follicles and thus alopecia is limited in scope.
   4. Loss of hair due to *anagen effluvium* is rapid and is frequently due to medications, such as chemotherapeutic agents. Anagen effluvium may involve up to 85% of the hair follicles and is much more catastrophic in appearance.

TABLE 8.2 Nail Changes Associated With Systemic Diseases

NAIL CHARACTERISTIC	ASSOCIATED CONDITION
Clubbing of fingernails	Chronic lung/heart conditions
Spoon nails (koilonychia)	Anemia and kidney disease
Melanoma of the nails	Seen as a dark spot or line usually at the proximal nail
Rippled nails	Thyroid, diabetes, and circulation disorders
Nail pitting	Psoriasis, lichen planar pilaris, alopecia areata, and other cutaneous disorders
Yellow nail syndrome	Lymphedema and respiratory conditions
Terry's nails (opaque nails with dark tips)	Diabetes, congestive heart failure, liver disease, and malnutrition
Beau's lines (indentations that run across the nails)	Injury or illnesses where the cuticle growth has been interrupted (e.g., fever, severe illness, malnutrition, other serious illnesses)
Onycholysis (splitting and brittle nails)	Psoriasis, lichen planar pilaris, psoriasis, thyroid disease, drug reactions, and a wide range of other illnesses
Lyndsay's nails (half and half nails)	Renal disease
Leukonychia (white lines or dots on the nails)	Trauma
Thickened white, brown, or yellow nails	Fungal/mold infections of the nails

Note: The interdigital areas of the toes and soles of the feet need to be examined for erythema, scale, and/or maceration associated with yeast, fungal, mold, or mixed-web infections.

5. *Androgenic effluvium* is due to changes in hormonal balance. The hair follicle itself thins and the hair pattern loss is greater at the front than at the back.
6. *Alopecia areata* is hair loss due to immune activity in which the hair follicle is destroyed by the immune system.
   a. It is seen with other autoimmune system disorders.
   b. When promptly treated, alopecia areata may be halted.
   c. It is usually first noted as "spot baldness."
   d. When it occurs all over the body (axilla, genitalia, eyebrows, eyelashes, etc.), it is known as *alopecia universalis*. Alopecia that involves the entire scalp is known as *alopecia totalis.* This type of alopecia is catastrophic and must be referred to dermatology immediately.
7. Scarring alopecias occur with lupus, dissecting cellulitis, lichen planopilaris, and folliculitis decalvans, to name a few conditions.
   a. Most scarring alopecias are associated with an erythematous tender scalp.
   b. They must be promptly identified and referred immediately to prevent permanent hair loss.
8. Tinea capitis is a fungal infection of the scalp. It appears as an annular lesion with peripheral scale, central clearing, and random broken hair follicles. It requires oral antifungal treatment, not topicals. Referral to dermatology may be needed.
J. Rashes or pruritus
   1. How long has it been present? How did it look originally, and how has it changed?
   2. Is it associated with pain? Is it associated with pruritus?
   3. Is it associated with any recent activities or changes in environment?
   4. What has been used or provides relief or worsening of symptoms?

TABLE 8.3 Fitzpatrick Scale

SKIN TYPE	COLOR	FEATURES
I	White/freckled	Always burns, never tans
II	White	Burns easily, tans poorly
III	Olive	Mild burn, gradually tans
IV	Light brown	Burns minimally, tans easily
V	Dark brown	Rarely burns, tans easily
VI	Black	Never burns, always tans

K. Petechiae or ecchymosis should prompt questioning of any trauma, recent or current symptoms of infection, and any other associated bleeding. Bleeding skin lesions should prompt evaluation for immediate biopsy.

L. Hyperhidrosis or hypohidrosis
  1. Excessive sweating can be associated with carcinoma, thyroid disorders, hormonal changes, and infectious disease.
  2. Hyperhidrosis is generally a benign condition but is associated with significant social embarrassment. Treatments are effective.
  3. Hypohidrosis is associated with increased risk of heat stroke/exhaustion.

M. Fitzpatrick scale is used to assess skin color (Table 8.3)

N. Vulvar assessment (Figure 8.2): Melanoma, human papillomavirus (HPV)-related vulvar intraepithelial neoplasia (VIN), lichen sclerosis, and other dermatologic conditions and precancers may be noted during the genital examination.

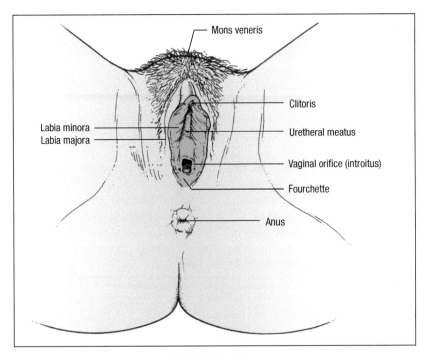

FIGURE 8.2 Vulva.

1. The mons pubis is the rounded mass of skin with underlying fatty tissue over the pubic bone.
   a. Note the hair growth, as sparse hair may be associated with hypoactive endocrine gland activity and heavy hair growth may be associated with hyperactive endocrine gland activity.
   b. Examine for the presence of unusual-looking lesions on the mons pubis. This is of particular importance in those who use sun-tanning beds or who tan without wearing a bathing suit.
2. Labia majora are the two prominent cutaneous folds that extend from the mons pubis to the perineum. Elongated labia majora are called *labia majora elongata* and are a normal variant.
3. Labia minora are the two inner mucosal/cutaneous folds that form the vaginal orifice. The labia minora may also be enlarged and is a normal variant. It is also referred to as *labia minora elongata.*
4. The introitus is the vaginal orifice. The introitus is examined for the presence of prolapse of the uterus.
5. The clitoris is a small mound of erectile tissue found above the urethral meatus and under the clitoral hood near the anterior junction of the labia minora.
   a. It is involved in sexual arousal and orgasm.
   b. Persistent genital arousal disorder is occasionally associated with clitoral priapism. This may be an adverse effect of some antidepressants.
   c. Enlargement of the clitoris may be an effect of excessive androgen production. Also, ask about exogenous ester or testosterone use (prescription and illicit use)
6. The fourchette is the area where the labia minora meet posteriorly. It is an area that is involved if episiotomy is needed during delivery.
7. For more information on the vulvar examination, see Chapter 5, "The Physical Examination."

DERMATOLOGIC ISSUES RELATED TO PREGNANCY

A. **Changes in the skin:** Three factors involved in the development of changes in the skin during pregnancy are increased hormones, compression from the expanding uterus, and intravascular volume expansion.
   1. Estrogen increases melanocytic activity, resulting in increased pigmentation, cutaneous vasodilatation, keratin growth, increased permeability, and increased angiogenesis.
   2. Progesterone also enhances melanocytic activity and reduces the lysis of collagen.
   3. Hormones produced by the pituitary gland (gonadotropins, adrenocorticotrophic hormones, and melanocytic hormones) all have effects on the skin.
   4. The sources of these hormones are the endocrine glands as well as the placenta.
B. Pigment changes
   1. Melasma and chloasma ("mask of pregnancy") occur in 70% of pregnant persons, usually in the third month of pregnancy, and frequently regresses postpartum.
   2. Melasma is worsened by sunlight and is more pronounced in patients with higher Fitzpatrick skin types (types I–VI; see Table 8.3).
   3. Avoid the standard treatments during pregnancy (hydroquinone, retinoic acid, and fluocinolone).
   4. Broad-spectrum sunscreens and sun avoidance are the mainstays of prevention and treatment.
   5. Additional areas of increased pigment changes include the areola, anogenital, axilla, and inner thighs.
   6. Linea nigra is found in 75% of pregnant persons. This is a darkened line from the umbilicus (occasionally substernal) to the symphysis pubis.

7. Freckles, nevi, and scars may become more pigmented during pregnancy. They may expand as the patient expands; however, rapidly expanding lesions are a hallmark of malignancy and need to be carefully evaluated.

C. Vascular changes

1. Vasomotor instability may result in excessive facial flushing. The majority resolve in the postpartum period.

2. Spider telangiectasias occur in 60% of pregnant persons.

   a. These are erythematous macules or papules with central redness that are surrounded by radiating capillaries.

   b. They frequently develop in the first trimester and often resolve after delivery. They occur on the upper part of the body (drained by the superior vena cava). They do not require treatment. If numerous lesions appear suddenly, concern for hepatic disease is raised.

3. Acral (hands/feet) erythema is common in the first trimester and usually resolves in the postpartum phase.

4. Vascular proliferation is evidenced by hyperplasia and erythema of the gingiva.

   a. Pyogenic granulomas (pregnancy epulis/epulis gravidarum) appear as fleshy erythematous growths.

   b. They can occur anywhere but are often found in the oral cavity.

   c. They are fragile and tend to bleed.

   d. Spontaneous regression is observed in the postpartum period.

D. Structural changes

1. Striae gravidarum are of great concern and occur in 60% to 90% of pregnant White people.

   a. They are less common in other ethnic groups.

   b. Risk factors include maternal weight gain, high neonatal birth weight, and younger age.

   c. No proven preventive measures exist.

   d. Laser, focused ultrasound, and retinoid creams may be of some help but should be limited to post partum.

2. Acrochordons (skin tags) are common during the second half of pregnancy and frequently shrink after delivery. If they persist, they may be treated after delivery by electrocautery or snip removal.

E. Adnexal changes

1. Hirsutism

   a. Increased hair can also occur in undesirable hirsutism of the face, trunk, and extremities.

   b. Hirsutism usually reverses postpartum.

   c. Excessive hair loss (shedding) can occur in the postpartum phase.

   d. This generally resolves in 6 to 15 months.

2. Nails grow faster during pregnancy and may become more brittle.

3. Hormonal influence on sebaceous glands may result in acne.

   a. Acne is more common in the last trimester.

   b. All "cyclin" antibiotics should be avoided during pregnancy as well as many retinoids.

   c. Topical benzoyl peroxide and macrolide antibiotics may be used.

4. After the sixth week of pregnancy, the sebaceous glands (Montgomery) of the areola enlarge.

   a. Appear as elevated dark tan papules that regress after delivery.

   b. Occurs in approximately 50% of pregnant people.

5. Eccrine (sweat) glands increase progressively during pregnancy. Milia appear as small papules that appear clear.

6. Angiokeratomas of Fordyce (purplish macules/papules in the labia) usually reduce during pregnancy, as does hidradenitis suppurativa (chronic marble- or pea-sized lumps in the axilla and groin that are painful and drain).

F. Specific dermatologic issues related to pregnancy
  1. Atopic eczema of pregnancy (AEP) is the most frequent dermatosis of pregnancy.
     a. It develops as an itchy rash on the flexural surfaces.
     b. Prurigo features (nodules formation) may occur with eczema of pregnancy.
     c. Soap and water may aggravate the disorder, and mild soaps and limited bathing followed by emollients (not lotions) are the mainstays of treatment.
  2. Polymorphic eruption of pregnancy (PEP) is nonspecific eczema-like patches and papules.
     a. PEP is not associated with elevated immune globulin (AEP has increased immune globulin).
     b. Usually presents in the last trimester of pregnancy. The incidence is less than 1% and is more frequent in the first pregnancy.
     c. Spontaneous remission usually occurs after delivery.
     d. If the pruritus is severe, antihistamines and topical/oral steroids may be needed. The risk/benefit of treatment needs to be evaluated.
  3. Pemphigoid gestation (previously known as *herpes gestationis*) is associated with the development of tense bulla (blisters), usually in the second or third trimester in multiparous patients.
     a. Pruritus usually precedes the development of the blisters.
     b. Pruritus usually develops in the periumbilical area and extends to the abdomen.
     c. Tense bullae develop on the trunk and limbs and usually spare the face.
     d. Treatment with oral or ultra-potent topical steroids may be indicated. The risk/benefit of treatment needs to be evaluated.
  4. Intrahepatic cholestasis of pregnancy usually presents in the third trimester as intense nocturnal pruritus.
     a. If skin lesions are present, they occur due to scratching. The symptoms resolve postpartum, and the disorder is likely to recur in future pregnancies.
     b. This disorder is significant as it is associated with higher incidence of neonatal mortality and morbidity.
     c. Liver enzymes and bile salt levels need to be monitored and the disorder is treated with cholestyramine and/or ursodeoxycholic acid.

DERMATOLOGIC ISSUES RELATED TO CONTRACEPTION

A. Acne is a chronic inflammation of the sebaceous glands of the face, chest, and/or back. Stress the need for chronic treatment and gentle cleansing of the acne areas as the skin is inflamed. Despite popular tradition, the skin should not be inflamed or irritated by rough abrasives or harsh astringents. The lesions of acne include papules, pustules, comedones, cysts, and nodules. The types of lesions as well as the number of lesions determine the severity of acne.

B. Pathology of acne is described in Table 8.4.

C. Treatment focuses on reduction of sebum (benzoyl peroxide, salicylic acid, and retinoids), administration of short-term antibiotics (topical or oral) to reduce *Propionibacterium acnes,* and opening of the pores with retinoids (the mainstay of acne treatment). Birth-control pills are an effective acne treatment.
  1. Acne is generally improved by estrogen and may be affected by progesterone.
  2. Avoid birth-control pills that contain androgenic progestin. Generally, a higher estrogen dose improves acne (30–35 mcg).
  3. Acne is affected by contraception choices.
     a. Combination hormonal contraceptives (birth control pills) are an effective treatment for acne; they raise SHBG levels, which subsequently lower testosterone levels.
     b. Implanted cutaneous hormonal rods, or progestin-containing contraceptives such as medroxyprogesterone acetate (Depo Provera) injections, may precipitate or worsen acne.
     c. Assessing the patient for acne history is a vital component of contraception counseling and selection of contraceptive methods.

TABLE 8.4 The Two Paths of Acne Pathology

PATH 1: HORMONE DRIVEN	PATH 2: INCREASED CELL PRODUCTION
Many hormones (DHEA-S, progesterone, testosterone, insulin-like growth factor) influence the sebaceous gland to increase sebum production	Hyperkeratinization. The cells that are in the duct will join with increased sebum to plug the duct, creating a comedone (open pores are blackheads)
The sebum is rich in triglycerides	Causes plugging of the sebaceous gland
Triglycerides provide abundant food that promotes the proliferation of *Propionibacterium acnes*	Causes inflammation
P. acnes stimulates the TLRs along the sebaceous unit, resulting in inflammation	Results in the development of comedones; when the pore is closed, they become papules or pustules, and when the pore is open, they are commonly known as *blackheads* (oxidized sebum/cells)

DHEA-S, dehydroepiandrosterone sulfate; TLRs, toll-like receptors.

D. Erythema nodosum is an inflammatory condition of the fat cells under the dermis.
 1. It presents as erythematous, tender nodules or lumps over the shins.
 2. May be preceded by a mild fever, fatigue, and arthralgias.
 3. Condition usually resolves within 6 weeks.
 4. May be triggered by a wide variety of infectious processes; autoimmune disorders; carcinoma; pregnancy; and medications, including birth control pills.
 5. Treatment is focused at removing the etiologic agent. Elevation of the legs and compression stockings may provide symptomatic relief.

GENERAL DERMATOLOGY

A. Rosacea is a common dermatologic condition in women's health.
 1. Rosacea is an inflammatory cutaneous condition of the face.
 2. Its pathology involves the presence of a demodex mite with associated inflammation and increased vascularity.
 3. It presents as a central erythema of the face with associated papules and thickening of the skin.
 4. Associated with increased comorbidities.
 5. There are four types of rosacea (Table 8.5).
B. Skin cancers/carcinoma
 1. Cutaneous carcinoma is the most common cancer.
 2. During the well-patient examination, the provider should thoroughly examine the skin and identify skin cancer in the early stages, leading to appropriate treatment and reduction in mortality and morbidity.
 3. Types of skin cancer are listed in Table 8.6.
 4. Risk factors for cutaneous carcinoma are listed in Table 8.7.
 5. See Box 8.1 for clinical warnings of skin cancer.

COSMESIS AND PHOTOAGING

A. Cutaneous aging
 1. Aging is associated with several changes in the skin, including:

TABLE 8.5 Rosacea Types	
Erythrotelangiectatic	Erythema of the central face Treatment includes intense pulsed-light therapy or bromocriptine
Ocular	Onsets frequently with ETR Best treated with oral minocycline or doxycycline (cylins) and/or sulfa ophthalmic drops
Papular/pustular	Erythema associated with these lesions Treatment includes metronidazole, azelaic acid, and oral "cyclins"
Granulomatous	Thickening of the skin Best treated with oral "cyclins," laser, and/or isotretinoin

ETR, erythematotelangiectatic rosacea.

TABLE 8.6 Common Skin Cancer Types	
TYPE OF CANCER	**ID FEATURES/ TREATMENT**
Basal cell carcinoma (BCC) 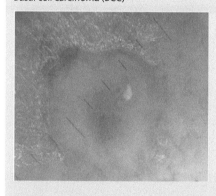	*Most common* skin cancer Rarely occurs in Black persons 85% occur on the head and neck Usually presents as bleeding or scabbed lesions or a pimple that does not heal or recurs *Rarely deadly* If untreated, it can penetrate and infiltrate the surrounding tissues Nodular BCC usually presents as a pearly white or pink, dome-shaped papule Superficial BCC presents as a patch or erythematous skin that extends peripherally and develops telangiectatic vessels Morpheaform BCC presents as a white patch of sclerotic skin and is frequently missed until advanced There are patients who have multiple BCCs that are genetically linked; this is Gorlin syndrome
Squamous cell carcinoma (SCC) 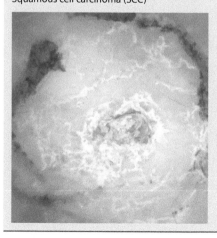	*Second most common* form of skin cancer *Presents on sun-exposed skin* Most common sites are face and back of the hands SCC usually present as an erythematous, scaly papule They may grow rapidly or slowly Although it rarely causes death, the immune-suppressed patient is at much greater risk of death from metastasis and death from SCC If the SCC is found on the mucosa or tongue, it has a much higher risk for metastasis It may occur in burns (Marjorin's ulcer) HPV has been associated with SCC in the anogenital area

(*continued*)

TABLE 8.6 Common Skin Cancer Types (*continued*)

TYPE OF CANCER	ID FEATURES/ TREATMENT
Melanoma 	*Third most common* type of skin cancer Previously referred to as the deadliest skin cancer; however, Merkel cell cancer is much rarer and much more deadly Early detection is important Treatment, prognosis, and 5-year survival is determined by tumor thickness and lymph node involvement Lesions may appear anywhere on the body It does not have to be in a sun-exposed area Lesions may be noted in the scalp; mouth; vulvar area; under nails; and on the feet, including between the toes Although not totally precise, the *ABCDEs of melanoma* detection have helped increase melanoma detection by lay/nonmedical individuals. These are danger signs that may indicate the need for biopsy and/or referral. A—Asymmetry. When viewing the lesion in half, both vertically and horizontally, the two halves do not match. B—Border irregularity. The borders of the lesion may be uneven, scalloped, or notched. C—Color variation. The lesion may have two or more colors. D—Diameter enlargement. The lesion may be larger than 6 mm or ¼ in. This is roughly the size of a pencil eraser. E—Evolving. The lesion may be evolving or changing from its original presentation. Only an experienced provider should excise melanoma. Suspicious lesions should not be monitored but referred promptly to an experienced dermatology provider. Slides of melanoma tissue can be sent for genetic assay to determine the melanoma's risk of metastasis. This adds to traditional methods of assessing risk.

HPV, human papilloma virus.

TABLE 8.7 Risk Factors for Cutaneous Carcinoma

Family history

Sun exposure

Fair skin

Use of tanning beds

History of actinic keratosis

History of sunburns. Sunburns in childhood are problematic but recent research indicates sunburns at any age are a risk factor.

Immune suppression
Genetic mutation at multiple genomes

Melanoma-specific risk factors:
All the preceding risk factors
Multiple melanocytic nevi, especially dysplastic nevi
Past history of melanoma
Family history of melanoma
Living at higher altitude or closer to the Equator. Increased risk of melanoma has been found among airline pilots and flight attendants.

BOX 8.1 Clinical Warnings of Skin Cancer

- Cutaneous carcinoma is the most common cancer.
- A pimple that comes and goes (or persists in the same spot) is frequently a basal cell cancer.
- A lesion that bleeds easily, regardless of size, is suspicious for skin cancer.
- A patch of skin that comes and goes or persists in the same area may be a superficial basal cell cancer or squamous cell cancer in situ.
- A rapidly growing lesion or one that is changing in color should be referred for biopsy.
- When examining the skin for abnormal lesions, look for the "ugly duckling," the "pretty duckling," or "what doesn't belong with the others." In other words, look for the lesion that does not appear like the others.
- Melanoma skin cancer can occur in areas of the body that have never been exposed to the sun (e.g., vulva).
- A Bartholin's cyst that persists despite treatment should be biopsied for carcinoma.
- Persistent genital warts that are not responsive to treatment should be biopsied for squamous cell carcinoma.
- Persistent lichen sclerosis that has not been responsive to treatment should be biopsied for vulvar carcinoma.
- Cellulitis that does not respond to standard evidence-based antibiotic treatment.

---

    a. A reduction in sebaceous glands results in xerosis (dry skin) and a tendency to experience more easily irritated skin and resulting pruritus.

    b. Collagen fibers thicken and dominate over elastin fibers, resulting in rhytids (wrinkles).

    c. Skin thins and paper-like skin that is prone to injury occurs, and angiomas develop.

    d. Blood vessels become more fragile, resulting in easy bruising.

    e. Collagen production is reduced.

    f. Subcutaneous fat is reduced, resulting in hollowing.

    g. Pigment formation is dysfunctional, resulting in "blotchiness."

    h. Keratinocyte repressor genes fail in areas, resulting in seborrheic keratosis.

2. The aforementioned are intrinsic factors associated with aging (genetic and chronologic).

3. Extrinsic factors associated with aging (smoking and UV rays) may result in increased rhytids (wrinkles), lentigo (pigmentation), and telangiectasias (spider veins).

4. Ultraviolet (UV) rays are very harmful to the skin.

    a. UVA waves penetrate deep in the dermis. They are associated with premature aging, skin cancer, and autoimmune disease. UVA waves can penetrate glass and clothing.

    b. UVB waves penetrate the epidermis and result in tanning and sunburns. They are strongly associated with skin cancer.

    c. UVC waves are reflected by the ozone layer and have an oncogenic effect where ozone layers are depleted.

B. Cosmetic approach to reducing/preventing photoaging

    1. To reduce photoaging, use broad-spectrum sunscreen daily, avoid the midday sun, and wear broad-brimmed hats and sunglasses. A recent study in Australia showed that daily application of sunscreen from head to toe reduced cutaneous aging.

    2. Antioxidants reverse the daily damage from UV exposure. Many antioxidants are available and include green tea, vitamin E, vitamin C, coffee berry, blueberry, caffeine, alpha-lipoic acid, hydroquinone, kojic acid, tocopherol, polyphenols, and a wide variety of others.

3. Retinoids will reduce small rhytids (wrinkles) and correct pigmentation and inflammation; they reduce aging.
   a. Retinols are available over the counter, whereas the more powerful retinoids are available by prescription.
   b. Retinoids are much more potent than retinols.
   c. Retinols do convert to retinoids but at a much lower concentration.
4. DNA and stem cell serums are available on the market and promote claims to reverse DNA damage to the skin. The data are inconclusive currently.
5. Dermabrasion is an ablative technique that uses a wire brush or diamond wheel, causing the upper layer of the skin to be injured, resulting in enhanced *collagen formation.*
   a. It is used with acne scarring, for uneven skin tones, and removal of tattoos and striae. This is not to be confused with microdermabrasion, which is performed with brushes and is not done in the office setting.
6. Laser and light therapy can reduce skin laxity, increase collagen, and improve pigment issues. By reducing the appearance of wrinkles, age spots, and pigment changes, these therapies are powerful tools in the armament of cosmetic therapy.
7. There is a wide variety of chemical peels that add to the arsenal of treatment for acne scarring, melasma, hyperpigmentation, acne, and rhytids. Adverse effects from peels include scarring, changes in pigmentation, and infection. Only experienced providers should use them.

C. Fillers and neuromodulators
   1. Botulinum toxin type A (Botox, Dysport, and Xeomin) is a neuromodulator that modulates the neuromuscular synapse by binding to the receptor site on the motor nerve terminal. This inhibits acetylcholine from activating the motor neuron.
      a. These products are very safe.
      b. Side effects are dependent on the site injected and the injector's expertise.
      c. A new topical gel administered in the provider's office is available.
      d. Areas for injection include the glabella (i.e., between the eyebrows), forehead, periocular rims, brow lift, gummy smile reduction, depressor angularis orbicularis (DAO), mentalis (chin), and nasal sidewall. The only U.S. Food and Drug Administration (FDA)–approved sites are the periocular rims (crow's feet) and the glabella.
   2. Fillers
      a. Hyaluronic acid fillers are used around the lips, nasolabial folds, around the mouth, and cheeks.
      b. Calcium hydroxyl apatite is used on the cheeks, nasolabial folds, and temples, but *not on the lips.*
      c. Polylactic acid fillers are used for general volume and *not on the lips.*
      d. Warning: Fillers should never be injected into the glabella, as that may be associated with blindness.

D. **Fat reduction:** Careful patient selection is critical to patient satisfaction with the procedures. Patients may have areas of fat that have been shown to be resistant to diet and exercise. This is not an effective treatment for obesity.
   1. **Cryolipolysis:** This technique is a form of "controlled frostbite." It is useful for the abdomen, flanks, back, chin, and thighs. It is uncomfortable but not painful. One to two procedures per desired site will be needed. Minimal complications occur. The most common are bruising, paresthesias, and rarely, post-procedure neuropathic pain.
   2. **Laser:** The laser is used three times every 3- to 4-week period to achieve its effects. It has few side effects after the procedure but is somewhat painful during the procedure. Side

TABLE 8.8 Aesthetics			
PROCEDURE	**INDICATIONS**	**ADVERSE EFFECTS**	**COST**[a]
Neurotoxin	Reduction of dynamic wrinkles	Headache, bruising, paralysis of undesired areas, asymmetry	$200–$700 depending on the site and the type of agent used
Filler	To restore volume in the temples, chin, cheeks, nasolabial folds, and lips	Blindness, necrosis Injection into areas for which drug is not intended causes undesirable consequences Due to its high side-effect profile, collagen is rarely used Fat transfer is a viable filler option	$500–$3,000 depending on the type of filler used and the number of syringes
Fat-reduction techniques	To reduce focal fat areas Not as effective in older people or others who lack skin elasticity	Laser bruising, burning with scarring Ultrasound postprocedure neuropathy	$650–$1,200 depending on procedure type and location
Nonsurgical facelift	Better results if younger, less sun exposure, and not a smoker	Bruising, swelling, paresthesia Pain may require medication	$1,500–$3,000
Facelift	To reduce rhytids and promote a smoother face	All those associated with a surgical procedure	$10,000–$12,000

Note: The most important accomplishment after skill excellence is the ability to set realistic expectations. Costs were obtained from www.realself.com. This site is excellent for determining costs and expectations and making referrals.

effects include bruising and the risk of burning with scarring. It can be used in the same places as cryolipolysis. Ablative lasers carry higher risks.

E. **Nonsurgical facelift:** Ultrasound is administered with a convex system that allows the energy to be focused and creates thermal coagulation points. When the energy is focused on the superficial musculo-aponeurotic system (SMAS; thin muscles below the skin), it creates increased collagen formation and reduction in laxity and tightens the skin. It is used on the forehead, lower face, and neck. Bruising, burns, and numbness may be side effects (Table 8.8).

F. Varicose veins
 1. Varicose veins occur due to prolonged standing (occupational hazard), pregnancy, trauma, genetic factors, and obesity.
 2. They are veins that are close to the surface of the skin and appear most frequently on the legs.
 3. Nonsurgical treatments include weight loss, dietary sodium reduction, exercise, compression stockings, and avoiding long periods of standing and/or sitting.
 4. Small veins may be injected with sclerotherapy or treated with laser (by an experienced clinician). Larger veins may be treated by laser-guided sclerotherapy, radiofrequency, or surgery.
 5. Sclerotherapy may be performed by hypertonic sclerotherapy or foam sclerotherapy. Both require compression stockings and avoidance of prolonged standing or sitting for up to 2 weeks (some providers may limit this to a few days) after the procedure. Complications include skin ulceration, thromboembolism, and allergic reactions.

BIBLIOGRAPHY

Bickley, L. S. (2017). *Bates' guide to physical examination and history taking* (12th ed.). Wolters Kluwer.

Bobonich, M., & Nolen, M. (2021). *Dermatology for advanced practice clinicians* (2nd ed.). Wolters Kluwer.

Bolognia, J. L., Jorizzo J. L., & Schaffer, J. V. (2018). *Dermatology* (4th ed.). Elsevier.

Habif, T. P. (2020). *Clinical dermatology: A color guide to diagnosis and therapy* (7th ed.). Elsevier.

Hughes, M. C. B., Williams, G. M., Baker, P., & Green, A. (2013). Sunscreen and prevention of aging: A randomized trial. *Annals of Internal Medicine, 158*(11), 781–790. https://doi.org/10.7326/0003-4819-158-11-201306040-00002

James, W. D., Elston, D. M., Berger, T. G., & Andrews, G. C. (2019). *Andrews' diseases of the skin: Clinical dermatology* (13th ed.). Elsevier.

Soutou, B., Régnier, S., Nassar, D., Parant, O., Khosrotehrani, K., & Aractingi, S. (2013). Dermatological manifestations associated with pregnancy. In E. Manzotti (Ed.), *Medscape.* https://www.medscape.org/viewarticle/706-769

9

ASSESSMENT OF THE FEMALE BREAST

KATHRYN TROTTER, LISA ASTALOS CHISM, ALIT YOUSIF, AND HELEN A. CARCIO

BASICS RELATED TO EXAMINATION OF THE FEMALE BREAST

A. The examiner must possess a thorough understanding of the normal anatomy and physiology of breast structure to identify any anomalies.
B. Physical examination of the breast by providers and breast self-awareness may be important for breast cancer detection. Breast cancer is not preventable; it is the early detection of breast cancer that is key to the patient's survival.
C. The examination of the breast includes inspection and palpation of the breasts and palpation of the lymph nodes that drain the breast.
D. Proper positioning of the patient and good lighting are key factors to inspection and palpation of the breast.
E. It is important for the examiner to acknowledge the societal association of the breast with gender and sexuality; this may make the assessment of the breast an emotionally uncomfortable examination for some patients.
F. Assessment of breast symmetry is essential; the patient must have both breasts uncovered for comparison.
G. Ideally, the breast examination should not take place immediately before the patient's menstrual period, when the breast may be normally tender and engorged.
H. The breast examination provides the examiner with an excellent opportunity to demonstrate breast awareness and to reinforce teaching.
I. Approximately 5% of women in the United States have breast implants.
   1. There are limitations in detecting breast cancer in patients with implants.
   2. The breast exam is conducted in the same way as without an implant, including if it is postmastectomy.

IMPORTANT STATISTICS

A. Based on 2020 American Cancer Society (ACS) current incidence rates, 12.8% of women born in the United States will develop breast cancer at some time in their lives. This translates to one woman in eight being affected, with most of the risk occurring after age 50 years.
B. The strongest risk factor (Box 9.1) for breast cancer in women is age.
C. In the United States, breast cancer is the most common cancer among women, and is second to lung cancer for cancer-related deaths.
D. In the United States, approximately 5% of all breast cancer occurs in women younger than 40 years, and current evidence shows it is the leading cause of cancer-related deaths in this age group, likely due to more complex biological features of their cancers.
E. The median age at diagnosis is 62 years, which means that half of the women diagnosed with breast cancer were 62 years or younger; in Black women the median age is 60. Because a

BOX 9.1 Risk Factors Associated With Breast Cancer

Advancing age
  Older than 40 years

Family history
  First-degree relative: Mother, sister, daughter; mother or sister has disease; relative was premenopausal at time of diagnosis; personal history of breast cancer or ovarian cancer

Mantle radiation exposure during teen years (non-Hodgkin lymphoma)

Previous breast biopsy or benign breast disease
  Atypical hyperplasia; lobular neoplasia; reproductive issues

Estrogen exposure
  First pregnancy at age 30 years or older. Early menarche (before age 12). Late menopause (after age 55). Infertility or nulliparity. Never breastfed.

Hormonal treatments
  Estrogen replacement therapy (controversial)
  Recent use (within 5 years)
  Long-term use
  Oral contraceptive use (probably does not increase risk)

Dietary factors
  Obesity (older than 50 years)
  High-fat diet
  Alcohol use (more than two glasses per day)

Lifestyle factors
  Pesticide exposure; smoking; lack of moderate exercise

majority of breast cancer is diagnosed between 60 and 69, it is an important time to maintain screening mammograms.

F. The 5-year relative survival rate in the United States is slightly lower among women diagnosed with breast cancer younger than 40 years (86%) compared with women diagnosed at ages 40 years and older (92%). Although numbers have improved for all races in the last few decades, the survival rate is 10% lower for non-Black women. While the racial gap has narrowed, the disparity is notable for late-stage breast cancer diagnosis. Of note, socioeconomic status affects relative survival rate, with less education and lack of health insurance associated with lower breast cancer survival.

G. Breast cancer is far more curable when the tumor is detected early.

1. The goal of screening examinations for early breast cancer detection is to find cancers before they start to cause symptoms. *Screening* refers to tests and examinations used to find a disease, such as cancer, in people who do not have symptoms.

2. Breast cancers that are found because they are causing symptoms tend to be larger and are more likely to have already spread beyond the breast. In contrast, breast cancers found during screening examinations are more likely to be smaller and still confined to the breast. The size of a breast cancer and how far it has spread are some of the most important factors in predicting the prognosis of a patient with this disease.

3. Table 9.1 comes from the National Cancer Institute's Surveillance, Epidemiology and End Results (SEER) database. It shows survival rates and emphasizes the importance of early detection.

TABLE 9.1 Breast Cancer Survival Rates	
STAGE	**5-YEAR SURVIVAL RATE (%)**
0	100
I	99
II	95
III	86
IV	27

ANATOMY AND PHYSIOLOGY OF THE BREAST

A. Breast tissue

1. Each breast contains 12 to 20 major ducts that intertwine, with each duct opening at the nipple. Most breast cancers originate in these ducts.
2. The breasts extend from the second or third rib to the sixth or seventh rib, and from the sternal edge to the anterior axillary line.
3. Breasts consist of glandular tissue, fibrous tissue, ducts, fat, blood vessels, nerves, and lymph nodes (Figure 9.1).

    a. Glandular tissue is contained in the lobes.
    b. Fibrous tissue is the supporting tissue that lies between the glandular tissue.

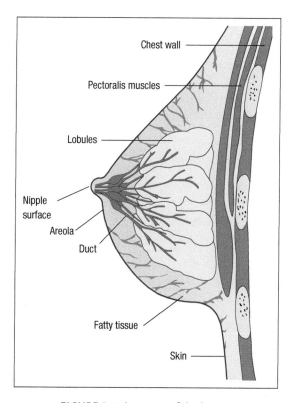

FIGURE 9.1 Anatomy of the breast.

4. Each lobe is subdivided into 50 to 75 lobules, which drain into separate excretory ducts, which in turn drain into the nipple.
5. These lobules in the peripheral breast tissue emerge at the nipple (the hub) like the spokes of a wheel.
6. The lobules produce milk, and the ducts carry the milk to the areola.
7. Each duct dilates as it enters the base of the areola to form a milk sinus, which serves as a reservoir for milk during lactation.
8. Inframammary ridge: The ridge of fat on the lower portion of the breast is called the *inframammary ridge*. The breast tissue here is often more dense than the surrounding tissue and is occasionally palpable in a transverse fashion, usually in more pendulous breasts. Muscle: There is very little muscle in the breast except for a small amount in the areola and the nipple, which causes the nipple to contract, facilitating the emptying of the milk sinuses.
9. The areola and nipple
   a. Dermal papillae contain sebaceous glands. The skin of the areola contains occasional hair follicles.
   b. Sebaceous glands on the areolar surface are the Montgomery tubercles.
10. **Tail of Spence:** More than half the ducts are present in the upper, outer breast quadrant (divide the breast into four parts, with the nipple at the center).
    a. Breast tissue may feel more firm or fibroglandular in those areas.
    b. Breast cancer is more common here in the upper outer quandrant (many cancers arise from ductal tissue).
11. Lymph nodes drain the area in and around the breast (Figure 9.2).
12. The breast undergoes changes during pregnancy and lactation, including enlargement with glandular development.

BREAST SELF-AWARENESS

In recent years, there has been a shift toward breast self-awareness versus the traditional breast self-examination. Breast self-awareness focuses on empowering patients to know what is normal for

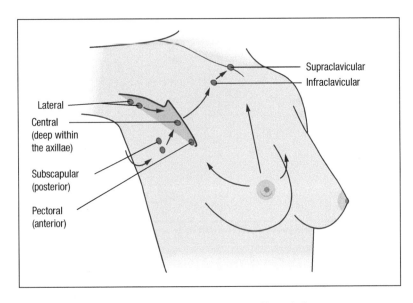

FIGURE 9.2 Arrows indicate direction of lymph flow.

their own breasts and paying attention to any changes that they might feel. Patients should report any breast changes to their health professional, who may do a clinical breast examination (CBE) and/or recommend breast imaging.

A. Breast awareness explained
1. Recent research suggests that breast awareness/self-exam alone has no benefit to breast cancer mortality but does have the effect of reductions in morbidity.
2. Patients are more likely to practice breast awareness if they know what to look for. Health education is vital.
3. Patients should report:
   a. New lumps or thickness of breast or underarm (axilla)
   b. Nipple tenderness or discharge, especially bloody discharge
   c. Skin change such as a pucker, dimple, new crease, or fold
   d. Warm, red, swollen breasts with or without skin resembling the skin of an orange (peau d'orange)
4. Inform the patient that any firm lump that remains unchanged with cyclic variations is suspect and warrants a visit to the healthcare provider.
5. In patients who are disabled, primary caregivers or chaperones should be trained to observe for breast changes.
6. Performing breast awareness provides the patient with a great opportunity to assume an active role in their own healthcare.
7. Point out that breast awareness should not act as a substitute for either CBE or mammography.
B. The technique on a monthly basis (preferably post menses if menstruating)
1. With a mirror, view both breasts without clothes or bra. Look for changes.
2. With the hand from the opposite side of the breast, do a gentle palpation of the breast, moving over the breast to check for new lumps. Often, this is ideal when bathing, and the hand is slightly slippery with soapy water. Checking for nipple discharge is not necessary (it will present itself spontaneously).
3. Educate the patient in the following:
   a. Do not use the tips of your fingers, but use the pads because they have more sensitive pressure receptors.
   b. Be sure to cover the entire breast, beginning in the middle of the armpit, where there are many ducts.
   c. The examination can be performed in the shower, in the bathtub, lying in bed, or standing upright in front of the mirror.
C. If there were breast reduction mammoplasty or implants, inquire about
1. Year surgery was performed; if implant, type (saline/silicone)
2. Presence of any tenderness in area of the implant
3. Acute or gradual onset of pain that may be related to a ruptured implant
4. Occurrence of any trauma in the area of the implant (especially seat belt injury)
5. Reduction mammoplasty often precludes successful breastfeeding
D. Personal history
1. Personal history of cancer of the breast or other reproductive cancer
2. Oophorectomy
3. Family history of breast cancer
E. *BRCA* testing/results

INSPECTION OF THE BREASTS

A. Position
1. The patient should be seated, with arms at the sides; patient should be disrobed from the waist up.

    2. Begin inspection 3 feet from the patient, preferably at eye level, to fully inspect both breasts.

B. Compare the breasts visually.

    1. Note the size, symmetry, ptosis, hair pattern, location, and contour.

    2. Normal findings:

        a. Breasts should be fairly equal bilaterally; a slight asymmetry is common in adolescents.

        b. Breasts extend from the third to the sixth ribs, with the nipple and areola over the fourth or fifth rib; convex contour; sparse hair surrounds areola.

        c. Size of breasts varies with overall body weight and genetic and hormonal influences.

    3. Clinical alterations:

        a. Marked asymmetry resulting from cysts, inflammation, or tumor

C. Assess the breast skin.

    1. Note the color, texture, venous pattern, temperature, and the presence of edema, dimpling or retraction, and lesions.

    2. **Normal findings:** Warm, smooth skin; silver striae; lighter color than exposed areas of skin

    3. Clinical alterations

        a. Edema and dimpling are suggestive of breast cancer.

        b. Inflammation is often caused by mastitis, breast abscess, or, less often, by inflammatory breast carcinoma.

        c. Retraction results from a benign or malignant tumor.

        d. Dilated superficial veins may result from a benign or malignant tumor of the areolar area.

        e. The breasts are engorged in pregnancy and lactation, with dilated superficial veins.

D. Inspect the areolae and the nipples.

    1. Note the size, shape, texture, and pigmentation of the breast, and direction and pigmentation of the nipples; also, note the presence of any discharge or supernumerary nipples.

    2. Normal findings

        a. Symmetrically round or oval areolae

        b. Pigmentation should be pink to dark brown, with roughened Montgomery's tubercles; nipples usually everted and the same color as areolae

    3. Clinical alterations

        a. Inversion (new onset) is often associated with breast cancer. Flat or inverted may be usual for the patient, so ask.

        b. Excoriation is associated with Paget's disease.

        c. Areola is darkened during pregnancy.

E. Observe for milk lines.

    1. Origin: Breast tissue arises out of the ectoderm, extending along the lines from the axilla to the groin.

    2. Accessory or supernumerary mammary glands and nipples are sometimes found along these embryotic lines. Patients may have thought that they were moles or fleshy warts (Figure 9.3).

    3. Supernumerary nipples are often found 5 to 6 cm below the normal nipples.

F. Observe breasts when the patient is in the following positions

    1. Sitting with both arms raised over head

    2. Sitting with both arms pressed firmly on hips, flexing pectoral muscles

    3. Sitting, leaning forward with arms outstretched, allowing breasts to hang freely

    4. Supine with arm above head, on the side being examined. This stretching of the pectoral muscles pulls on breast tissue and exaggerates any dimpling or pucker or retraction.

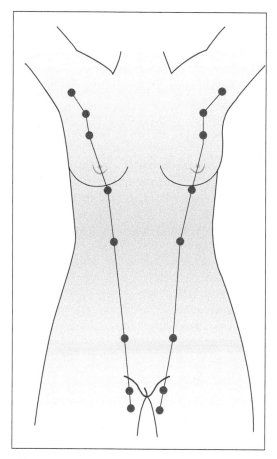

FIGURE 9.3 Milk lines. Possible sites of accessory breast tissue or supernumerary nipples, both of which may become more prominent during pregnancy and the puerperium.

PALPATION OF THE BREAST

A. Basics

1. In a very large breast, it is unlikely that anything but the most obvious lesions will be discovered.
2. The presence of adipose tissue affects the nodularity, density, and fullness of the breast.
   a. In a patient who has recently lost a considerable amount of weight, the breasts are lumpy because some of the cushion of fatty tissue is absent.
   b. Patients who are overweight have fuller breasts.
3. Three to 5 days before menstruation, the breasts may become engorged, increasing slightly in size.
4. Wash hands with warm water before examination.
5. Tilt the exam table back to about 30 degrees, then ask the patient to reach overhead with both arms. This flattens the breast tissue and distributes it evenly across the chest wall to facilitate the detection of masses or accessory breast tissue or supernumerary nipples, both of which may become more prominent during pregnancy and the puerperium.
6. If a patient reports a problem with one of the breasts, examine the unaffected side first to provide a baseline for comparison.
7. Palpation may be performed with one or two hands, but usually one.

8. Lower the patient's arm to relax the pectoral muscles to best examine deep in the muscles in the area of the tail of Spence.
9. Sensory component of fingertips:
   a. Uses sensitive pressure receptors in the fingertips.
   b. The mass will feel more dense than the surrounding tissue.

B. Palpate the four quadrants of the breast.
   1. **Instructions to patient:** Observe how your breast is being examined so that you can be aware. Describe any tenderness.
   2. Technique
      a. While sitting first, gently palpate the breast with the pads of the three to four fingers.
      b. Starting at the 12 o'clock position on the upper aspect of the breast, rotate fingerpads in imaginary concentric circles or lines, toward the center of the breast, the areola, and the nipple.
      c. Do not lift fingers from the breast when moving from one section to another.
      d. In large-breasted patients, use bimanual palpation, compressing the breast between hands.
      e. Next, palpate the breast with the patient supine, with the arm above the head on the side being examined and at 30 degrees elevation. If large breasted, you may also ask the patient to turn to one side and the other.
      f. Repeat for the other breast.
      g. Chart any anomalies. A diagram works best.
   3. Note temperature; size (in centimeters), location, delimitation (borders of the mass), mobility, degree of fixation, and consistency (hardness) of any masses; and breast tenderness. Location is ideally noted with a clock position and number of centimeters from the nipple. (Notation example: *In the left breast, at 2 o'clock, and 8 cm from the nipple, is a 1 cm superficial round, mobile, slightly tender mass. There is no skin color change, dimpling, or nipple retraction or discharge.*)
   4. If a mass is present, assess for retraction.
   5. Normal findings
      a. The breast should be warm, smooth, and elastic.
      b. No masses or discharge should be present; the breast may be more nodular in a geriatric patient.
      c. Generalized, uniform nodularity (may be increased in second half of cycle in a patient taking progesterone supplements)
      d. Increased density and nodularity in the area of the inframammary ridge (firm, crescent-shaped ridge of compressed tissue along the lower edge of the breast)
   6. Clinical alterations (see Table 9.2, which compares different types of lumps):
      a. Nontender, mobile, smooth, well-delineated nodules associated with fibroadenoma
      b. Nontender, immobile, or fixed nodule suggestive of breast cancer
      c. Tender, multiple smooth spongy masses in one or both breasts associated with cysts

PALPATE THE NIPPLE AND THE AREOLA

A. Technique
   1. Gently compress nipple between index finger and thumb.
   2. Repeat for other nipple.
   3. Advise the patient that they do not need to compress the nipple for discharge.

B. Note
   1. The amount, color, and odor of any fluid that is ejected from the nipple. Note location on nipple, similar to clock face if possible. May identify duct location.
   2. Shape and consistency of nipple, including any skin changes.

TABLE 9.2 Comparison of Different Types of Breast Lumps

CHARACTERISTIC	FIBROCYSTIC	FIBROADENOMA	CANCER
Age	25–55 years (rare after menopause)	Puberty to menopause (peak 20–29 years)	Older than 30 years Incidence increases with age
Number	Usually multiple, may be single	Usually single	Usually single; two primary lesions may occur in the same breast
Shape	Smooth, round, may be multilobular	Smooth, lobular, round	Irregular
Delimitation	Well circumscribed	Well circumscribed	Poorly delineated from surrounding tissues
Mobility	Mobile	Mobile	Limited mobility; fixed to surrounding skin or underlying tissue
Pain	Present, cyclic (second half of menstrual cycle)	Usually not painful	Usually nontender
Axillary involvement	None	None	May be present with regional metastasis to axillary lymph nodes
Nipple discharge	Absent	Absent	Often present

C. Evaluation of the discharge (Table 9.3)
   1. Using a white napkin to dab the nipple may help see the color of the discharge.
   2. If bilateral nipple discharge is present, suspect galactorrhea. Measure prolactin levels to check for a pituitary tumor/adenoma.
D. **Normal findings:** No discharge, except during lactation; nipple is erect.
E. Clinical alterations (see Table 9.3):
   1. Unilateral, serous, clear, or serosanguineous discharge is suggestive of physiologic discharge or intraductal papillomas.
   2. Sanguineous or dark-red discharge is associated with cancer or Paget's disease.
   3. Galactorrhea is associated with the use of tranquilizers, antipsychotics, marijuana, and high estrogen levels.

TABLE 9.3 Comparison of Types of Nipple Discharge

TYPES OF NIPPLE DISCHARGE	DESCRIPTION	COMMENTS
Milky white, thin	White, thin	Lactation
Serous, thin, clear, and yellowish	Thin, clear, or yellowish	Suggests physiologic discharge or intraductal papilloma
Serosanguineous, thin	Thin, clear, and pink	Suggests fibrocystic changes or cancer
Bloody	Thick, opaque, and red	Suggests cancer
Purulent	Thick, opaque, greenish or yellowish	Suggests infection

PALPATION OF LYMPH NODES

A. Technique
   1. Using the same fingertip pads, gently palpate the supraclavicular and infraclavicular areas.
   2. For axilla exam, face the patient, abduct the right arm with your right hand, and place your left hand against the chest wall, high into the axilla.
   3. Rotate your hand, cup the examining fingers, and reach high into the axilla using gentle pressure to palpate the subscapular, central, pectoral, and lateral axillary nodes as the hand slides down the axilla.
   4. Support the patient's arm with the opposite hand. This approach relaxes the pectoralis muscle and permits careful evaluation of the axilla.
   5. Repeat for the opposite axilla. If unable to get a good exam while sitting, repeat with the patient supine with arm over head.
B. Note the location (axilla or which quadrant), size (in centimeters), shape, consistency, mobility, and tenderness of any nodes palpated; a diagram is helpful.
C. Normal findings: None
D. Clinical alterations
   1. Nontender, hard enlarged lymph nodes are indicative of metastatic breast cancer.
   2. **Lymphadenitis:** Freely mobile 3 to 5 mm are usually associated with an infection of the patient's hand or arm. We have seen this in about 10% of patients post COVID vaccine, on the vaccinated arm side, with resolution in 4 to 6 weeks.
E. Refer any abnormal findings for further evaluation.

PHYSICAL EXAMINATION OF AN AUGMENTED BREAST

A. Physical examination is similar to that for a natural breast and includes evaluation of both the natural breast tissue and the implant. The breast must also be examined for possible complications related to the implants.
B. In both the upright and supine positions
   1. Assessment procedure is performed when the patient is upright with arms at the sides.
      a. Instruct the patient to elevate the arms over the head and then to place the hands on the hips and lean forward, flexing the pectoralis muscle when asked.
      b. Palpation of the natural breast tissue with the patient upright is often easier if the patient leans slightly forward.
   2. Assessment procedure is done with the patient in the supine position.
      a. The patient's arm should not be elevated above the head, but rather relaxed at the side to relax the pectoral muscles, making the implants more mobile and compressible.
      b. Contraction of the pectoralis muscle contracts the implant into a ball.
      c. Push the implant away from each wedge of tissue as it is examined.
         (1) Some implants are soft and easily displaced.
      d. Palpate the axillary and supraclavicular area for lymph nodes as described previously.
      e. Evaluate the implant for compressibility and mobility.
C. Note the following elements of the implant
   1. Contour
      a. Flatness
      b. Bulges
      c. Indentations
   2. Abnormal skin changes
      a. Thickening

   b. Lesions

   c. Nipple abnormality

3. Compare the size of the breasts, observing the location of the augmentation scar.
4. Determine whether the implants are visible.
5. Observe for signs of capsular contraction or abnormal shape of implants.
6. Assess the integrity of the implant by evaluating any capsular scarring or contraction.

   a. A ruptured implant may not be evident clinically.

   b. May feel firm or hard from silicone granuloma formation

CHARTING

A. Carefully document physical examination findings.

1. A diagram is helpful because it graphically documents any suspected anomalies.
2. Divide the breast into four quadrants by drawing two imaginary lines through the nipple at right angles to each other. Tail of Spence is an extension of the upper outer quadrant.

B. **Record:** Breasts symmetric; normal contour; no dimpling, retraction, or erythema; nipples erect, no discharge; areola pink/brown; firm, smooth, elastic breasts; no masses or palpable lymph nodes.

MAMMOGRAM

A. Mammography explained

1. Radiographic examination of the breast
2. Standard means of detecting breast cancer before palpation
3. Digital tomosynthesis is a technology that gives a 3D picture of the breast; this testing is ideal for patients with increased density in their breast tissue.

B. Mammography can pick up soft tissue densities not yet palpable, as well as calcifications that are too small to feel; a clinical breast exam is considered complementary to mammography.

C. Indications

1. To obtain a baseline mammogram in patients 40 years, or earlier if clinically indicated
2. To evaluate a lump or mass found during palpation of the breast by either the patient or the clinician
3. To screen a patient for breast cancer, particularly those at risk for development of breast cancer

D. Advantages

1. Easy to perform (assuming the patient can stand; some sites are able to do seated mammograms).
2. The sensitivity of mammography is determined by the percentage of breast cancers detected in a given population when breast cancer is present. According to the National Cancer Institute, overall sensitivity is approximately 80% but is lower in younger patients and in those with dense breast tissue. Digital tomosynthesis mammograms are improving sensitivity. It takes multiple x-ray pictures of each breast from many angles, providing a 3D image.
3. The test is relatively inexpensive.

E. Disadvantages

1. Requires special equipment and trained personnel
2. Lower sensitivity in patients younger than 50 years
3. False positive rate of more than 50% in patients screened annually over a 10-year period. This is more common in younger patients, those with dense breasts or who have had breast biopsies, and those taking estrogen.
4. May be uncomfortable for the patient.

F. Role of ultrasound
  1. Used to distinguish between solid and cystic masses
     a. If the mass is cystic, refer for possible aspiration if tenderness is significant. If complicated cyst, will need biopsy.
     b. If solid, refer for needle localization biopsy.
G. Role of breast MRI
  1. Used to screen high-risk patients.
  2. Acquires more information about areas of suspicion.
H. Screening parameters as recommended by the American Cancer Society (ACS)
  1. Mammography
     a. Using shared decision-making, discuss baseline mammography by age 40 to 44 years.
        (1) May start earlier if there is a strong family history of breast cancer, positive *BRCA* test results, fibrocystic disease (makes palpation more difficult), or breast augmentation.
     b. Mammography should be performed every year between ages 45 and 54 years. Patients can switch to mammogram every 2 years or can continue yearly screening over age 55 years, based on individual risk factors.
        (1) The ACS believes that age alone should not be the reason to stop having regular mammograms.
        (2) Patients with serious health problems or short life expectancies should discuss with their doctors whether to continue to have mammograms or not.
     c. They recommend against clinical breast exams.
I. U.S. Preventive Services Task Force (USPSTF) recommendations are being updated in 2022. To date, the 2016 recommendations remain:
  1. Routine screening of average-risk patients should begin at age 50 years.
     a. Routine screening should end at age 74 years.
     b. Patients should get screening mammograms every 2 years instead of annually.
     c. Breast self-exam have little value, based on findings from several large studies.
     d. Decision to screen patients age 40 to 49 years should be made on an individual basis regarding their value and the potential benefits versus the potential harm, and on individual risk factors.
  2. Digital mammography
     a. Similar to traditional mammograms; system uses a digital receptor and computer
  3. Clinical breast exam
     a. USPSTF concludes that current evidence is insufficient on the additional benefits versus harms of clinical breast exams beyond screening mammogram in those older than 40 years.
J. American College of Obstetricians and Gynecologists (ACOG) recommendations
  1. Shared decision-making: The patient and the provider should share in the decision regarding screening based on health history, individual concerns, and priorities.
  2. Screening mammogram offered starting at age 40 years, begin screening no later than 50 years.
  3. Average-risk patient can have screening every 1 or 2 years based on shared decision-making.
  4. Screening should continue until at least age 75 years. Beyond this age, decision to continue to screen should be made on the basis of shared decision-making.
K. The National Comprehensive Cancer Network (NCCN) recommends screening start at age 40 years with annual interval. No age recommendation for when to stop screening mammography. They recommend doing clinical breast exam.
L. Special findings
  1. Microcalcifications
     a. Tiny specks of calcium in the breast
     b. Often found in areas of rapidly dividing cells

  c. Appear benign
  d. Subsequent mammography in 3 to 6 months
  e. If the microcalcifications are clustered or in small groupings, refer the patient for needle localization biopsy or removal.
2. Macrocalcification
  a. Calcium deposits are frequently associated with degenerative changes in the breast
  b. Due to aging, old injuries, or inflammation
  c. Usually benign
  d. First appearance; subsequent mammography in 6 months
  e. Stable—mammography should be performed every year

CASE STUDY

Patient Situation

A 35-year-old White woman presents to the outpatient clinic with concern of a possible new right breast mass.

Subjective Data

Nickel-sized lump for a few weeks. She has mild premenstrual tenderness in outer quadrants about a week prior to her period for years, but the lump seems new. It is tender only when she presses it, and it has not changed in size since she first noticed it. Denies nipple discharge or axillary swelling, or skin color change. No previous breast biopsy or imaging.

G2P1102, LMP: 2 weeks ago, regular q 30 days × 1–2 d spotting, has progesterone IUD for 2 years. Family hx: unremarkable for cancers, except for MGM who had breast cancer at age 60 years.

Objective Data

HEENT: PERRL, normocephalic, neck is supple, no thyromegaly or cervical LAD
  Breasts: Examined in the seated and supine position. Fairly symmetric with left slightly larger than right, mild ptosis, and without nipple retraction, dimpling, or skin color change. Left: without dominant mass or tenderness. Right: 2-cm round mobile nontender mass at 10 o'clock, 5 cm from nipple. Diffuse fibroglandular tissue bilaterally in outer quadrants.
  LAD: No supra- or infraclavicular or axillary nodes palpable.

Clinical Analysis

What diagnostics do you anticipate will be ordered and why? You reassure her this is likely a breast cyst, or other benign condition. You order a diagnostic mammogram (with tomosynthesis) and right breast ultrasound, preferably in the next 2 weeks because the patient is age 30 or older with palpable mass.

What is the priority intervention based on the patient's clinical presentation? Diagnostic imaging. Bilateral mammogram and right breast ultrasound reported right breast hypoechoic 2-cm round mass at 10 o'clock, consistent with a simple cyst. BIRADS 2, benign, no further treatment recommended. Begin screening mammogram at age 40 years.

What should be included in this patient's plan of care? Discuss benign nature of simple cysts, use of aspiration if it becomes uncomfortable. Perform breast cancer risk assessment. Discuss breast awareness and follow-up with new changes. Offer annual clinical breast exam per shared decision-making. Screening mammogram starting at age 40 to 49 years, depending on risk assessment results.

BIBLIOGRAPHY

American Cancer Society. (2015). *Breast cancer screening guideline.* https://www.cancer.org/health-care-professionals/american-cancer-society-prevention-early-detection-guidelines/breast-cancer-screening-guidelines.html

American Cancer Society. (2021). Breast *cancer facts and figures 2019–2020.* American Cancer Society.

American College of Obstetricians and Gynecologists. (2017). *Breast cancer risk assessment and screening in average risk women.* Practice bulletin 179. Author.

National Cancer Institute. (2020). *Cancer stat facts: Female breast cancer.* https://seer.cancer.gov/statfacts/html/breast.html

National Cancer Institute. (2021). *Breast cancer screening.* https://www.cancer.gov/types/breast/hp/breast-screening-pdq#_51

National Comprehensive Cancer Network. (2021). *NCCN clinical practice guidelines in oncology: Breast cancer screening and diagnosis, Version 1.2021.* https://www.nccn.org/guidelines/guidelines-detail?category=2&id=1421

U.S. Preventive Services Task Force. (2016). *Breast cancer: Screening.* http://www.uspreventiveservicestaskforce.org

10

BREAST IMAGING

ALIT YOUSIF

BREAST IMAGING

A. Routinely performed on an outpatient basis.

B. **Two main uses:** Screening and diagnosis

1. Screening exams refer to scheduled (annual, sometimes biennial) imaging of the breasts in women who have no new breast complaints.

   a. Screening mammogram has approximately 87% sensitivity and 90% specificity (Lehman et al., 2017), meaning mammography correctly identifies about 87% of women who truly have breast cancer and is normal for 90% of women who have no breast cancer.

   b. Numerous randomized control studies have demonstrated a significant reduction in mortality from breast cancer when women are invited to yearly screening mammogram (22% reduction for women aged 50 to 74; 15% reduction for women aged 39 to 49; Duffy et al., 2020).

2. Diagnostic imaging involves interrogation of either a symptomatic breast or an imaging abnormality identified on screening.

C. Goal of screening is early detection of breast cancer, earlier even than when a lump can be felt by the patient, in hopes of decreasing associated morbidity and mortality.

D. A variety of modalities are utilized for screening.

1. Mammogram; most commonly used form of screening
2. Ultrasound
3. Magnetic resonance imaging (MRI)
4. Molecular breast imaging (MBI); less commonly used screening method
5. Each modality has its own advantages and disadvantages; unfortunately, there is no one perfect screening tool.

MAMMOGRAM

A. Screening mammogram (SMG)

1. Officially recommended by the American Cancer Society in 1976, and at the time, comprised of x-ray film which was illuminated by white light in order to detect "dense" tumor among the breast tissue.

2. In 2000, the FDA approved 2D digital mammogram which offered better resolution and higher accuracy (Hambly et al., 2009) over film screen, and in 2011, digital breast tomosynthesis (DBT) "3D" mammograms were introduced, further improving accuracy (Durand et al., 2020).

3. Under the Affordable Care Act in 2010, an annual screening mammogram in the United States is available to all women aged 40 and older, without prescription or out-of-pocket fee.

B. **Screen film mammogram:** The developed film is hung on a white light viewbox.

C. **Digital mammogram:** The digital image is evaluated on high resolution (minimum 5 megapixel) monitors

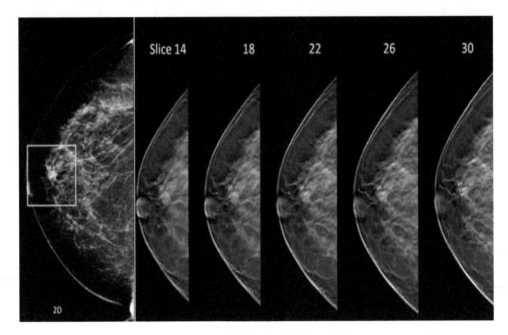

FIGURE 10.1 Multiple "slices" of breast tissue.

D. **DBT:** Multiple "slices" of breast tissue are evaluated on high resolution monitors (Figure 10.1)

E. Regardless of the type of mammogram, all mammography units function similarly and use ionizing radiation to produce an image of the breast tissue.

F. The average radiation dose for a standard mammogram of both breasts (2D or 3D/DBT) is about 0.4 mSv, similar to 2 months of background radiation and well below the annual allowed radiation dose.

G. Mammography facilities are highly regulated by the FDA to ensure lowest dose possible and proper maintenance of equipment.

BI-RADS: BREAST IMAGING REPORTING AND DATA SYSTEM

A. In order to standardize communication of test results and follow up recommendations, the American College of Radiology (ACR) instituted the Breast Imaging Reporting and Data System (BI-RADS) in the 1980s.

B. The interpreting radiologist assigns a BI-RADS number score to each mammogram, whether screening or diagnostic, to convey the results.

C. BI-RADS scores
   1. **BI-RADS 0:** Incomplete; additional images are needed
      a. Most of these are deemed benign after further evaluation and will become BI-RADS 1, or 2; if a suspicious finding is confirmed then a BI-RADS score of 4 or 5 is assigned.
   2. **BI-RADS 1 or 2:** Negative/benign
   3. **BI-RADS 3:** Assigned after diagnostic imaging is performed when there is greater than 98% likelihood of benign finding.
   4. **BI-RADS 4:** Suspicious finding; biopsy is recommended.
   5. **BI-RADS 5:** Highly suspicious for cancer; biopsy strongly recommended.
   6. **BI-RADS 6:** Biopsy-proven breast cancer; appropriate action should be taken.

WHAT DOES THE RADIOLOGIST ASSESS ON MAMMOGRAM?

A. Breast density
1. Although mammography has improved over the years, its most significant limitation is breast density.
2. In this context, breast density refers to how radiopaque the breast tissue is, regardless of how "firm" the tissue may feel on clinical exam.
3. DBT offers improved visualization of dense breast tissue compared to the 2D digital mammogram, with increased sensitivity and specificity (Durand et al., 2020).

B. The BI-RADS system assigns letter classification to breast density (Figure 10.2A–D)
1. **A:** Mostly fatty
2. **B:** Scattered fibroglandular density
3. **C:** Heterogeneously dense breast tissue
4. **D:** Extremely dense breast tissue
5. For many women, breast density decreases with age.
   a. About half of women aged 40 to 44 have dense breast tissue, while only about a third of women aged 70 to 74 have dense breast tissue (Nazari et al., 2018).

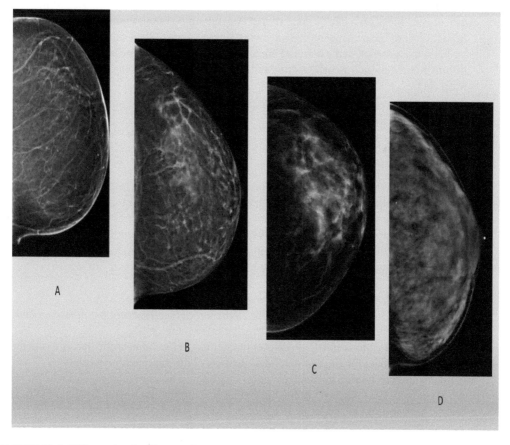

FIGURE 10.2 Different levels of breast density: A. mostly fatty; B. scattered fibroglandular density; C. heterogeneous density; D. extreme density.

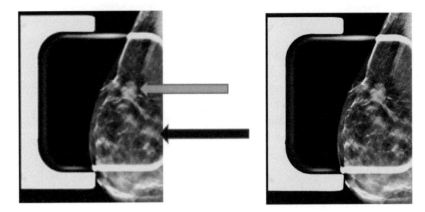

FIGURE 10.3 Case study: 57-year-old BI-RADS 0; called back from SMG. Spot compression demonstrates a mass. Note that the density ("whiteness") of the mass (grey arrow) is similar to dense breast tissue (black arrow). In this case, targeted breast ultrasound demonstrated a suspicious mass, which proved to be carcinoma on biopsy.

    b. Dense breast tissue limits detection of breast cancer because both normal dense tissue and breast cancer can appear dense (white) on mammogram (Figure 10.3), so a small cancer can "hide" on a background of dense tissue. In addition, there is a small increased lifetime risk of breast cancer associated with dense breast tissue (Advani et al., 2021).

    c. In 2019, Congress passed a national breast density notification law, intended to inform women of their density status, and of possible adjunct screening (described in the following).

        (1) The law hopes to allow women to pursue adjunct screening if they choose, which may include ultrasound, MRI, or MBI.

C. Masses

  1. Calcifications

    a. Mammography is an excellent modality to visualize calcifications.

    b. Most calcifications in breast tissue are benign, and usually described as punctate, round, dystrophic, dermal. These benign calcifications often increase with age and are not related to dietary intake of calcium.

    c. Suspicious calcifications demonstrate nonuniform shape (pleomorphic) and can be arranged in linear, grouped, or segmental distribution. Image-guided biopsy of suspicious microcalcifications can be performed to identify ductal carcinoma in situ (DCIS; Figure 10.4).

    d. The majority of DCIS presents with new abnormal calcifications.

    e. DCIS accounts for approximately 20% to 25% of all screen-detected malignancies and is considered a nonobligate precursor to invasive breast carcinoma.

    f. The microcalcifications in DCIS represent malignant cells and necrotic debris in the ducts or the terminal duct lobular unit, without invasion of the basement membrane.

  2. Asymmetry, architectural distortion

    a. An asymmetry is a "density" in one breast that does not have a mirror image in the other breast. Architectural distortion is an abnormal configuration of the tissue.

    b. Asymmetries and regions of architectural distortion are usually called back from SMG and evaluated with spot compression mammogram and targeted ultrasound.

    c. If the abnormality persists on additional views, image-guided biopsy can be performed.

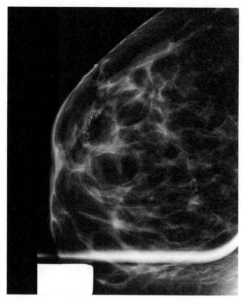

FIGURE 10.4 Pleomorphic calcifications in a 43-year-old patient are suspicious (BI-RADS 4). Image-guided biopsy (stereotactic biopsy) demonstrated ductal carcinoma in situ (DCIS), grade 2.

GUIDELINES FOR SCREENING MAMMOGRAM

A. Most health providers agree on the utility of screening mammogram (SMG)
   1. Easily accessible
   2. Affordable breast cancer screening tool
   3. Acceptable sensitivity and specificity
B. There is great variation in screening guidelines offered by an alphabet soup of societies, often frustrating for patients and providers alike.

SCREENING MAMMOGRAM RECOMMENDATIONS FOR AVERAGE-RISK WOMEN

A. **American College of Radiology (ACR), Society of Breast Imaging (SBI), American Society of Breast Surgeons (ASBrS):** Annual SMG beginning at age 40
B. **American Cancer Society (ACS):** Optional at 40 to 44; annual at 45 to 54; biennial at 55 and older
C. **U.S. Preventive Services Task Force (USPSTF):** Biennial, beginning at age 50 for most
D. These guidelines are based on the SEER data (see the following), and although the guidelines vary by organization, *all* societies agree that annual SMG beginning at age 40 saves lives. The difference of opinion regarding screening schedule is based on practical and economic considerations.
E. SEER (Surveillance, Epidemiology, and End Results Program) data on risk of developing breast cancer in the next 10 years
   1. **At age 30:** 1 in 201 women
   2. **At age 40:** 1 in 65 women
   3. **At age 50:** 1 in 42 women

BREAST ULTRASOUND

A. Sonography of the breast has been traditionally used in diagnostic evaluation where a targeted area of the breast is scanned to visualize masses or cysts (Figures 10.5 and 10.6).

B. High-frequency linear-array transducers are generally used, where fluid appears anechoic (black) and masses are usually hypoechoic (grey).

C. When a mass is identified on mammography, targeted ultrasound in that region of the breast can be performed.

D. Breast ultrasound is usually more comfortable for the patient than mammogram, and ultrasound-guided biopsies are more tolerable for many patients than stereotactic biopsy.

E. Evaluation of axillary lymph nodes is also performed with ultrasound.

F. When a suspicious breast mass is seen, ultrasound can identify smaller satellite lesions which may not be appreciated on mammography.

G. Ultrasound uses sound beams to produce an image of the breast tissue and uses no radiation. Recent studies have shown an increased cancer detection offered by screening ultrasound (Ohuchi et al., 2016), which can be performed as handheld exam or with use of automated breast ultrasound (ABUS; Figure 10.7).

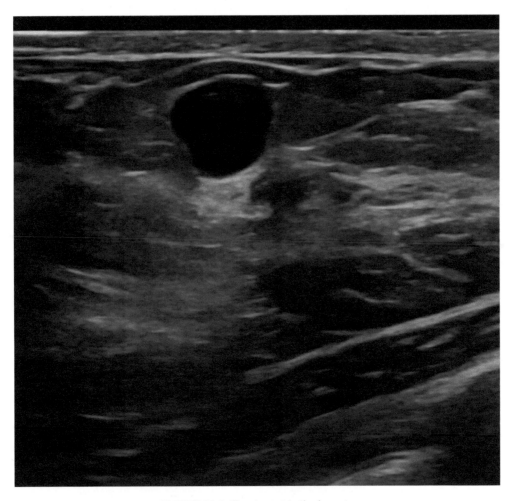

FIGURE 10.5 Simple cyst in the breast.

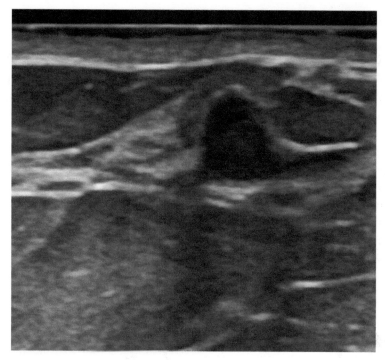

FIGURE 10.6 Solid mass in the breast.

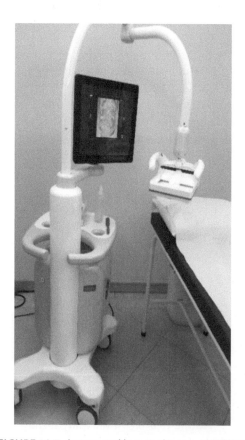

FIGURE 10.7 Automated breast ultrasound (ABUS).

MAGNETIC RESONANCE IMAGING OF THE BREAST (FIGURE 10.8)

A. MRI can be performed as a screening exam, or for surgical planning and treatment monitoring in women diagnosed with breast cancer.

B. The exam uses powerful magnets and radio waves to produce images of the breast.

C. No radiation is utilized in this modality. Intravenous gadolinium contrast is administered, and multiple dynamic images of the breast tissue are obtained (Figure 10.9).

D. Screening breast MRI is recommended for women with greater than 20% lifetime risk of developing breast cancer and can be considered for those at intermediate risk (15%–20%).

E. Because the injected contrast is excreted in urine, adequate renal function should be documented in patients prior to the exam.

F. For patients who suffer from claustrophobia, a mild relaxant prior to the exam may be helpful.

MOLECULAR BREAST IMAGING

A. Molecular breast imaging (MBI) is a nuclear medicine exam that uses intravenous injection of radioisotope (usually Tc-99m sestamibi) to show lesions with increased blood flow and/or increased metabolic activity.

B. MBI images are obtained in the same orientation as mammography, and are interpreted side by side.

C. Small tumors in dense breasts are not well visualized on mammogram but is clearly identified on MBI (Figure 10.10).

THERMOGRAM BREAST IMAGING EXAMS

A. Thermograms are images generated by heat at or near the body surface. To date, no studies have shown efficacy in early cancer detection by thermography.

B. The FDA has classified thermograms as a Class I device, which "present minimal potential for harm to the user" and include items like bandages and enema bags.

C. Thermograms should never replace screening mammograms, but pose no physical harm as an additional tool.

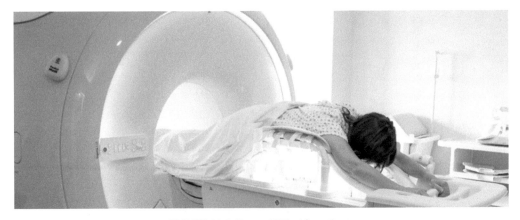

FIGURE 10.8 Breast MRI with patient.

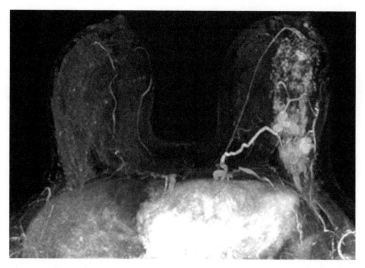

FIGURE 10.9 Extensive enhancing tumor throughout the left breast in a 24-year-old patient with invasive ductal carcinoma.

PROS AND CONS OF BREAST IMAGING MODALITITES

A. Mammogram
   1. **Pros:** Easily accessible, screening is covered by insurance
   2. **Cons:** Limited by breast density, uncomfortable, uses radiation
B. Ultrasound
   1. **Pros:** Comfortable for patient, no radiation, can identify small mass even in dense breast tissue
   2. **Cons:** Cannot always identify DCIS, screening ultrasound is not available universally
C. MRI
   1. **Pros:** High sensitivity for breast cancer
   2. **Cons:** Expensive, difficult for claustrophobic or large patients, contrast cannot be used if patient has severe renal failure or gadolinium allergy
D. MBI
   1. **Pros:** Can be performed on women who cannot have MRI (cannot fit in the magnet gantry; cannot have gadolinium injection)
   2. **Cons:** Radioactive injection, not performed at most breast centers

SCREENING IN SPECIAL CASES: PREGNANCY AND LACTATING

A. Mammography is not contraindicated during pregnancy, and the fetal radiation dose from a screening mammogram is far below the dose related to teratogenic effects (Tremblay et al., 2012). However, the breast tissue can be considerably denser during pregnancy and lactation, which limits evaluation.
B. SMG is not recommended for pregnant and lactating women aged 30 to 39 of average lifetime risk (LTR) but can be appropriate for pregnant women aged 30 to 39 of intermediate or high LTR.
C. For lactating patients, pumping or nursing prior to imaging is recommended to improve the sensitivity of mammography.

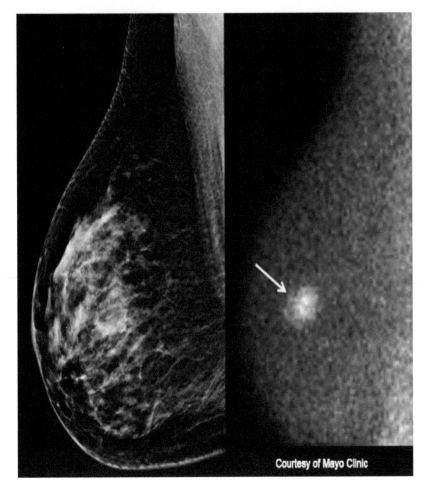

FIGURE 10.10 Small tumor in dense breast, mammogram versus MBI.

Source: Image courtesy of the Mayo Clinic.

D. Any new palpable breast mass in a pregnant patient should be evaluated with imaging, which may or may not include mammography but should include targeted breast ultrasound.

E. Pregnancy-related breast cancer (PRBC) is defined as breast cancer diagnosed during pregnancy, throughout the first postpartum year, or during lactation and represents 3% of all breast cancer diagnoses (Langer et al., 2014).

1. Epidemiologic studies show a slight increased incidence of PRBC with advanced maternal age (Botha et al., 2018; Vashi et al., 2013).

BIBLIOGRAPHY

Advani, S., Zhu, W., Demb, J., Sprague, B. L., Onega, T., Henderson, L. M., Buist, D. S. M, Zhang, D., Schousboe, J. T., Walter, L. C., Kerlikowske, K., Miglioretti, D. L., & Braithwaite, D. (2021). Association of breast density with breast cancer risk among women aged 65 years or older by age group and BMI. *JAMA Network Open. 4*(8), e2122810. https://doi.org/10.1001/jamanetworkopen.2021.22810

Botha, M., Rajaram, S., Karunaratne, K. (2018). Cancer in pregnancy. *International Journal of Gynecology & Obstetrics FIGO Cancer Report 2018, 143*(2), 137–142. https://doi.org/10.1002/ijgo.12621

Duffy, S. W., Vulkan, D., Cuckle, H., Parmar, D., Sheikh, S., Smith, R. A., Evans, A., Blyuss, O., Johns, L., Ellis, I. O., Myles, J., Sasieni, P. D., & Moss, S. M. (2020). Effect of mammographic screening from age 40 years on breast cancer mortality (UK Age trial): Final results of a rondomised, controlled trial. *Lancet Oncology, 21*(9), 1165–1172. https://doi .org/10.1016/S1470-2045(20)30398-3. www.thelancet.com/article/S1470-2045(20)30398-3/fulltext

Durand, M. A., Friedewald, S. M., Plecha, D. M., Copit, D. S., Barke, L. D., Rose, S. L., Hayes, M. K., Greer, L. N., Dabbous, F. M., & Conant, E. F. (2020). False-negative rates of breast cancer screening with and without digital breast tomosynthesis. *Radiology. 298*(2), https://pubs.rsna.org/doi/10.1148/radiol.2020202858

Hambly, N. M., McNicholas, M. M., Phelan, N., Hargaden, G. C., O'Doherty, A., & Flanagan, F. L. (2009). Comparison of digital mammography and screen-film mammography in breast cancer screening. *American Journal of Roentgenology, 218*(2), 1010–1018. https://www.ajronline.org/doi/pdf/10.2214/AJR.08.2157

Langer, A., Mohallem, M., Stevens, D., Rouzier, R., Lerebours, F., & Cherel, P. (2014). A single-institution study of 117 pregnancy-associated breast cancers (PABC): Presentation, imaging, clinicopathological data and outcome. *Diagnostic and Interventional Imaging, 95*(4), 435–41. https://doi.org/10.1016/j.diii.2013.12.021

Lehman, C. D., Arao, R. F., Sprague, B. L., Lee, J. M., Buist, D. S, Kerlikowske, K., Henderson, L. M., Onega, T., Tosteson, A. N., Rauscher, G. H., & Miglioretti, D. L. (2017). National performance benchmarks for modern screening digital mammography: Update from the Breast Cancer Surveillance Consortium. *Radiology, 283*(1), 49–58. https://doi.org/10.1148/radiol.2016161174.

Nazari, S., & Mukherjee, P. (2018). An overview of mammographic density and its association with breast cancer. *Breast Cancer, 25*(3), 259–267. https://www.ncbi.nlm.nih.gov/pmc/articles/PMC5906528/

Ohuchi, N., Suzuki, A., Sobue, T., Kawai, M., Yamamoto, S., Zheng, Y. F., Shiono, Y. N., Saito, H., Kuriyama, S., Tohno, E., & Endo, T. (2016). J-START investigator group. Sensitivity and specificity of mammography and adjunctive ultrasonography to screen for breast cancer in the Japan Strategic Anti-cancer Randomized Trial (J-START): A randomised controlled trial. *Lancet, 387*(10016), 341–348. https://doi.org/10.1016/S0140-6736(15)00774-6

Tremblay, E., Therasse, E., Thomassin-Naggara, I., & Trop I. (2012). Quality initiatives: Guidelines for use of medical imaging during pregnancy and lactation. *Radiographics: A review Publication of the Radiological Society of North America, Inc, 32*(3), 897–911. https://doi.org/10.1148/rg.323115120

Vashi, R., Hooley, R., Butler, R., Geisel, J., & Philpotts, L. (2013). Breast imaging of the pregnant and lactating patient: Physiologic changes and common benign entities. *AJR American Journal of Roentgenology, 200*(2), 329–36. https://doi.org/10.2214/AJR.12.9845

11

MENTAL HEALTH SCREENING:
Anxiety, Depression, Eating Disorders, PTSD, Substance Abuse, Suicide, and Dementia

ELISABETH MAHER AND TIMOTHY LEGG

GENERAL MENTAL HEALTH

A. According to the World Health Organization, mental health is more than the absence of mental illness (2022).

B. Mental health is impacted by multiple factors, including biological, environmental, and socioeconomic factors.

C. Mental illness is one of the most common health problems in the United States, with more than 50% of the population experiencing at least one mental illness episode during their lifetime (Centers for Disease Control and Prevention [CDC], 2018).

D. According to the CDC (2020), women were more likely than men to have taken medication for their mental health (20.6% and 10.7%, respectively) and received counseling or therapy from a mental health professional (11.7% and 7.2%, respectively) in the past 12 months.

E. Disorders such as anxiety and depression are more common among women.

F. Certain mental health issues are unique to women, such as perinatal depression, premenstrual dysphoric disorder, and perimenopause-related depression (National Institutes of Mental Health, 2019).

G. This chapter reviews various mental health conditions commonly seen in primary care and specialty practices like women's health. Screening using appropriate instruments (Box 11.1) will assist in case finding. Evidenced-based management focusing on pharmacotherapeutics are summarized, and referral guidelines reviewed. It should be noted that many patients benefit from various types of therapy with or without medication. Evidence supports the most effective treatment approaches incorporate both therapy and medication.

ANXIETY

A. The annual prevalence of anxiety disorders in United States adults is 19.1% or about 48 million people.

B. Women have twice the risk of developing generalized anxiety disorder (GAD).

C. Although it can occur at any age, the average age of onset is approximately 21 years.

D. Of those diagnosed with GAD, approximately 90% will develop at least one other mental health disorder in their lifetime (College of Psychiatric and Neurologic Pharmacists, 2020–2021, p. 8.).

BOX 11.1 Assessment Instrument Links

GAD-2: https://depts.washington.edu/uwhatc/PDF/TF-%20CBT/pages/3%20Assessment/Standardized%20Measures/GAD%202.pdf

GAD-7: https://adaa.org/sites/default/files/GAD-7_Anxiety-updated_0.pdf

PHQ-9: https://med.stanford.edu/fastlab/research/imapp/msrs/_jcr_content/main/accordion/accordion_content3/download_256324296/file.res/PHQ9%20id%20date%2008.03.pdf

Columbia Suicide Severity Rating Scale: https://www.cms.gov/files/document/cssrs-screen-version-instrument.pdf

SAFE-T: https://store.samhsa.gov/product/SAFE-T-Pocket-Card-Suicide-Assessment-Five-Step-Evaluation-and-Triage-for-Clinicians/sma09-4432

V.A./DoD Clinical Practice Guidelines for the Management of Major Depressive Disorder: https://www.healthquality.va.gov/guidelines/MH/mdd/MDDCPGPocketcardFINAL1.pdf

Canadian Network for Mood and Anxiety Treatments: https://www.canmat.org/resources/#health-professionals

Primary care PTSD-5 scale: https://www.ptsd.va.gov/professional/assessment/documents/pc-ptsd5-screen.pdf

CAGE Questionnaire: https://www.uspreventiveservicestaskforce.org/home/getfilebytoken/QETZFZLBsJbtPmVNVCgA7Z

CAGE-AID Questionnaire: https://www.bhevolution.org/public/document/cage-aid.pdf

Mini Mental State Exam: https://www.ncbi.nlm.nih.gov/projects/gap/cgi-bin/GetPdf.cgi?id=phd001525.1

E. "Anxiety disorders" encompass a wide range of disorders, but share features of excessive fear and anxiety and related behavioral disturbance" (American Psychiatric Association [APA], 2013, p. 189). Those most relevant to adult females of childbearing age include: specific phobia, social anxiety disorder (social phobia), panic disorder, agoraphobia, GAD, substance-/medication-induced anxiety disorder, anxiety disorder due to another medical condition, and other specified anxiety disorder/unspecified anxiety disorder.

F. While the primary care woman's healthcare provider need not be aware of all of the diagnostic criteria for each condition, generalized screening for an anxiety disorder is essential for case finding and treatment/referral to specialty care.

   1. There are several screening tools available to assess anxiety, the most common used in primary care include:

      a. The Generalized Anxiety Disorder scale-2 (GAD-2)

        (1) Fast and easy to use, consisting of two questions

        (2) Positive response to either question should prompt use of GAD-7

      b. Generalized Anxiety Disorder scale-7 (GAD-7)

        (1) Consists of five questions

        (2) Scores range from 0 to 21, with higher scores suggesting higher levels of anxiety

        (3) Positive screening (scores higher than 8, the mid-range of "mild anxiety") should prompt a more in-depth assessment of anxiety using *Diagnostic and Statistical Manual of Mental Disorders, Fifth Edition* (*DSM-5*; APA, 2013) criteria (Sapra et al., 2020).

G. Management of anxiety

   1. Treatment should follow a stepwise approach and should consider both nonpharmacologic and pharmacologic treatments.

a. Non-pharmacologic treatments
  (1) Cognitive behavioral therapy is among the most effective psychological therapies for the treatment of anxiety disorders.
  (2) Efficacy is comparable to medication treatment.
  (3) Other treatments may include relaxation training, mindfulness, and meditation exercises.
b. Pharmacologic treatments
  (1) The College of Psychiatric and Neurologic Pharmacists (2020–2021) has compiled stepwise approaches to medication intervention for the treatment of anxiety and anxiety-related disorders.
  (2) Psychopharmacologic approaches can be used in conjunction with non-pharmacologic treatments.
c. Selective serotonin reuptake inhibitors (SSRIs)
  (1) Recommended initiating one half of starting dose to minimize "activation" or transient increases in anxiety which are often a side effect of SSRI treatment.
  (2) No differences in efficacy and none superior to others. Treatment instead is guided by efficacy and side effects.
  (3) Can take several weeks (up to 12 weeks in some cases) to exert full anti-anxiety effects and may not alleviate all anxiety symptoms.
d. Serotonin norepinephrine reuptake inhibitors (SNRIs)
  (1) Venlafaxine seems to help with the ruminative worry associated with GAD.
  (2) Duloxetine has been associated with decreases in relapse when used at target doses but should be used cautiously in those who struggle with alcohol use disorder.
e. Benzodiazepines
  (1) Some of the most frequently prescribed drugs for treatment of anxiety, however, they are only recommended as second-line agents and should be considered only after intolerance to antidepressants has been established.
  (2) Associated with rapid relief of anxiety symptoms which paradoxically makes it more apt to be abused; rebound anxiety reported with cessation.
  (3) Physical and psychological dependence can develop rather quickly, and up to 44% of patients who have used benzodiazepines for 4 to 6 weeks have reported withdrawal symptoms on cessation.
  (4) Conflicting risks of congenital abnormalities (comparing early to later studies which failed to show risk)
  (5) All benzodiazepines are rapidly absorbed and distributed in breast milk in sufficient quantities to produce pharmacologic effects in newborns.
f. Buspirone
  (1) Second-line therapy
  (2) Can take 2 weeks or longer to begin working; not useful in acute anxiety.
  (3) Animal reproductive studies have shown no birth defects or changes in fertility which suggest low human risk; limited data regarding buspirone excretion breast milk.
g. Hydroxyzine
  (1) Second-line therapy secondary to its side effect profile and lack of efficacy for comorbid disorders
  (2) Little human data exist regarding teratogenic risks of hydroxyzine.

DEPRESSION

A. Annual prevalence for major depressive disorder (MDD) in U.S. adults is 8.4%, or about 21 million people (National Alliance for Mental Illness, n.d.).

B. Multiple disorders fall under the category of depressive disorders in the *DSM-5*. Those of interest to women of childbearing/child-rearing ages include MDD, persistent depressive disorder (also known as dysthymia), premenstrual dysphoric disorder, substance-/medication-induced depressive disorder, depressive disorder due to another medical condition, other specified depressive disorder, and unspecified depressive disorder.

C. According to the *DSM-5*, the common feature of depressive disorders is a sad, empty, or irritable mood, which is accompanied by somatic and cognitive changes significantly affecting the person's functional capacity (APA, 2013).

D. Risk factors associated with depression:
   1. Female gender, low income, and having a first-degree relative with depression.
   2. Average age of onset is the late 20s, but the first episode of major depression can develop at any age.
   3. Fifty percent of individuals who have a single episode of MDD will recover without recurrence; however, those who have had two prior major depressive episodes correlate with approximately 70% future risk of developing another episode of major depression.

E. A variety of screening instruments can be used to screen for depression in women.
   1. The simple mnemonic SIGECAPS is one example:
      a. Sleep disturbance (insomnia or hypersomnia)
      b. Interest (loss of)
      c. Guilt (excessive)
      d. Energy (loss of energy or fatigue)
      e. Concentration (impaired)
      f. Appetite changes (i.e., anorexia or hyperphagia)
      g. Psychomotor agitation or retardation
      h. Suicidal ideations or actions
   2. The patient health questionnaire-9 (PHQ-9) is a series of nine questions based on the *DSM-5*.
      a. It can be self-administered or clinician-administered.
      b. Higher scores are related to more severe depressive symptoms.

F. Management of depression
   1. General treatment considerations
      a. The decision to take medications is highly personal and involves multiple considerations, including but not limited to patient preference, prior response, safety and tolerability of side effects associated with antidepressant medications, and comorbid disorders.
      b. A variety of organizations have developed treatment guidelines for MDD, including the Veterans Administration/Department of Defense and the Canadian Network for Mood and Anxiety Treatments.
   2. Non-pharmacologic approaches
      a. Psychotherapy, which includes a variety of approaches such as: interpersonal therapy, cognitive behavioral therapy, and psychodynamic therapy
      b. Bright light therapy, which is considered first-line treatment for MDD with a seasonal pattern
   3. Pharmacologic approaches
      a. The College of Psychiatric and Neurologic Pharmacists (2020–2021) has compiled stepwise approaches to medication intervention to treat depressive disorders.
      b. Psychopharmacologic approaches can be used in conjunction with nonpharmacologic treatments.
         (1) SSRIs
         (2) SNRIs

        (3) Norepinephrine and dopamine reuptake inhibitors (NDRIs)

        (4) Serotonin, norepinephrine receptor antagonists (SN-RAn) such as mirtazapine

        (5) Tricyclics (may be contraindicated in persons with suicidal ideation)

        (6) Monoamine oxidase inhibitors (MAOIs)

   4. Other treatment approaches

      a. For those who do not respond to pharmacologic treatment, there is a variety of other treatment options available

      b. Transcranial magnetic stimulation

        (1) The use of magnetic fields to stimulate nerve cells in the regions of the brain involved with mood regulation and depression

        (2) Sessions last between 30 to 40 minutes 5 days a week

        (3) Treatment can take 4 to 6 weeks

        (4) Adverse events include headache and transient scalp discomfort

        (5) Maintenance treatment may be required.

      c. Electroconvulsive therapy (ECT)

        (1) Up to 80% to 90% effective for the treatment of MDD

        (2) Can be used during pregnancy

        (3) Treatment of choice for patients with severe suicidal ideation or food refusal

        (4) Ten to 14 treatments are often required before responses seen

        (5) Maintenance treatment may be required

        (6) Adverse events include confusion during the post-ictal phase. Impaired memory following the procedure, headaches, and muscle aches.

   5. NOTE: While bipolar and related disorders are not reviewed in this chapter, before treating depression with an SSRI, ask if there is a personal or family history of mania or hypomania. If there is a positive history of mania or hypomania, do not start medication for depression and refer to psychiatry due to the potential activation from the SSRI that could precipitate a manic episode.

SUICIDE

A. Defined as the act of terminating one's life.

B. Suicidal ideation is a medical emergency and should be treated as such.

C. Suicidal ideation is a symptom found in several mental illnesses (e.g., depression, bipolar, anxiety disorders, psychotic disorders). Unfortunately, there is no single treatment or medication to treat suicide; only the underlying condition resulting in the suicidal ideation can be treated.

D. The annual prevalence of suicidal ideation in U.S. adults is 4.9% or about 12.2 million people (National Alliance of Mental Illness, n.d.).

E. According to the American Foundation for Suicide Prevention (2022), in 2019, there was an average of 13.93 suicides completed per 100,000 individuals—or an average of 130 suicides per day in America.

F. Ahmedani et al. (2014) reported that approximately 45% of people who die by suicide had seen their primary care provider within 1 month before their death. They further reported that only about 20% of persons who died by suicide will have seen a mental health professional in the preceding month.

G. Primary care providers must appreciate the importance of routine screening for suicide.

   1. Not done as providers do not know how to assess for suicide risk

   2. The myth of "introducing the idea to the person" continues to persist, even though the individual with suicidal ideation had been thinking about it before their provider asked them.

H. Assessment should include screening for suicidal ideation, including self-injurious behaviors, and an assessment of the client's risk of imminent harm.

I. Prompt referral to mental health providers and/or emergency psychiatric care is essential.

J. There is a variety of screening tools that can be used to assess suicide.
   1. The mnemonic "IS PATH WARM" is ideal in primary care as it is quick and easy to use:
      a. Ideation (suicidal)
      b. Substance abuse
      c. Purposelessness
      d. Anxiety
      e. Trapped (feelings that the person is trapped in a bad situation or has no way out)
      f. Hopelessness
      g. Withdrawal
      h. Anger
      i. Recklessness
      j. Mood change (dramatic)
   2. Suicide assessment to five-step evaluation and triage (SAFE-T; Substance Abuse and Mental Health Services Administration [SAMHSA], 2009)
      a. Recommended being used at first patient contact, with any subsequent suicidal behavior, increased ideation, or pertinent clinical changes.
      b. Explores risk factors, protective factors, suicide inquiry, risk level/intervention, and documentation.
      c. Available as a pocket card for quick reference for free through SAMHSA.
   3. Columbia Suicide Severity Rating Scale (screen version-recent)
      a. Contains a set of six questions with guided logic (negative answers to questions 1 and 2 prompt the screener to move to question 6; whereas a positive response to question 2 prompts asking questions 3 through 6).
      b. Assists with risk stratification into low-, moderate-, and high-risk groups.

EATING DISORDERS

A. The term *eating disorder* is a broad, general term that encompasses several different disorders.

B. The most familiar eating disorders are anorexia nervosa and bulimia; however, there are numerous conditions regarding food and eating.

C. According to the APA, a persistent disturbance of eating or eating-related behavior characterize an eating disorder and results in altered consumption or absorption of food which impairs physical health or psychosocial functioning to a great degree (APA, 2013).

D. The annual prevalence of eating disorders in U.S. adults is 9%, or about 28.8 million people (National Association of Anorexia Nervosa and Associated Disorders, 2021).

E. Prevalence/clinical course
   1. Some studies suggest peak incidents between ages 19 and 20 years.
   2. Average episode duration is 8 months, with a mean duration of illness between 9.3 and 14.7 years.

F. Screening
   1. Eating disorder screen for primary care (ESP)
      a. A set of five questions that were taken from other normed and validated eating disorder questionnaires
      b. Very useful as a screening instrument
      c. Positive screening should herald the need for additional assessment (Cotton et al., 2003).
   2. SCOFF questionnaire
      a. A short instrument used to screen for anorexia and bulimia

b. Consists of five questions

c. Positive screening should prompt for thorough assessment measures (Morgan et al., 2000)

3. Eating eisorder examination (EDE) and eating disorder examination questionnaire (EDE-Q)

a. The EDE is clinician administered in the form of an assessment.

b. The EDE-Q can be self-administered.

c. Both are considered the "gold standard" for assessing eating disorders as their questions are based on *DSM-5* criteria (Berg et al., 2012).

G. Treatment of eating disorders

1. There is no one treatment for eating disorders through medication support for co-occurring symptoms, such as anxiety, which can be managed with medication.

2. Prioritization is given to determining whether or not inpatient or outpatient treatment is most appropriate for the client.

3. Inpatient hospitalization may be appropriate with decreases in systolic blood pressure, presence of arrhythmias, hyponatremia, hypokalemia, suicidal ideation, and/or act of self-harm and to minimize risk of re-feeding syndrome.

4. Psychopharmacology is often ineffective as many psychopharmacologic treatments result in weight gain, which could be found objectionable by the person with anorexia or bulimia.

5. Nutritional rehabilitation is a comprehensive approach that incorporates individual and family therapy.

6. There is no significant evidence suggesting that the treatment of eating disorders in pregnant patients differs dramatically from those who are not pregnant.

POSTTRAUMATIC STRESS DISORDER

A. Posttraumatic stress disorder (PTSD) is one of the "trauma-and stressor-related disorders" found in the *DSM-5*.

B. Disorders of this category include exposure to traumatic or stressful events (APA, 2013).

C. The annual prevalence for PTSD in U.S. adults is 3.6%, or about 9 million people (National Alliance for Mental Illness, n.d.).

D. It is believed that personal predisposition is needed to develop PTSD symptoms after a traumatic event. The body's failure to return to its pre-traumatic state differentiates PTSD from a simple fear response (College of Psychiatric and Neurologic Pharmacists, 2020–2021, p. 33).

E. Screening for PTSD

1. The gold standard for screening for PTSD in primary care is the primary care-PTSD-5 (PC-PTSD-5) scale.

a. The scale is self-administered, consisting of five questions which attempt to identify those with "probable PTSD."

b. If the client answers "no" to question number 1, the screening is stopped. If they answer "yes," then the screening continues.

2. There are several other rating scales for PTSD, including the clinician-administered PTSD scale (CAPS); however, these are more useful for diagnostic purposes.

F. Pharmacologic management of PTSD

1. First-line treatment of PTSD includes "trauma-focused" psychotherapy (adopting either exposure-based or cognitive behavioral therapy approach), coupled with an SSRI or SNRI.

2. Benzodiazepines should not be used in this population as they have not been shown to have longitudinal efficacy.

a. There is no evidence that benzodiazepines will decrease the course symptoms of PTSD.

b. Benzodiazepine use may potentiate acquisition of fear response and worse in recovery for trauma.

3. Augmentation strategies include the use of mirtazapine.

4. If failure of three trials, including augmentation, consider switching to a tricyclic antidepressant, or the use of phenelzine, a monoamine oxidase inhibitor (MAOI; College of Psychiatric and Neurologic Pharmacists, 2020–2021, p. 35).

SUBSTANCE ABUSE

A. For the purpose of this section, "substance abuse" is used in the broadest possible sense to apply to any psychoactive substance that is used for purposes other than the intended use, for a longer duration than the intended/prescribed use, or despite negative consequences associated with use.

B. A diagnosis of "substance use disorder" (SUD) can be applied to various types of substances (with the exception of caffeine; *DSM-5*).

C. Important characteristics of SUDs include changes in the underlying brain circuitry that persist beyond detoxification and are particularly pronounced in those who have severe disorders (APA, 2013, p. 483).

D. According to the National Center for Drug Abuse Statistics (2022):
   1. SUDs affect over 20 million Americans aged 12 years and over.
   2. Accounting for both alcohol and tobacco, approximately 165 million or 60.2% of the U.S. population aged 12 years or older have used drugs within the last 30 days.
   3. Most common disorders are related to the use of cannabis and prescription pain relievers.
   4. Despite the prevalence, only 20% of individuals in active drug treatment programs in the United States are women.

E. Dual diagnosis is another important consideration in working with women who struggle with SUDs.
   1. "Dual diagnosis" refers to the presence of a SUD and a second disorder, typically a mental health disorder (however, in recent years, the term dual diagnosis has been used to refer to physical health disorders, as well).
   2. The presence of a dual diagnosis requires more intensive treatment and should involve appropriate mental health professionals.

F. Screening tools for substance abuse
   1. Several screening tools can be used to screen for SUDs.
   2. The CAGE questionnaire should be considered in the primary care setting when screening for alcohol use disorder.
   3. The CAGE questionnaire has been adapted to include other drugs and is known as the "CAGE-AID" questionnaire.
      a. Affirmative responses to one or more questions are considered a positive screen and should herald the need for additional assessment.

G. Treatment of SUDs
   1. Treatment of SUDs is complex, often requiring interdisciplinary approaches.
   2. Depending on the substance involved, medically supervised detoxification should be considered (especially in the cases of alcohol and opioid use disorders).
      a. At home detoxification from alcohol is not recommended secondary to the risk of seizure activity.
      b. Detoxification from opioids is associated with considerable discomfort and should be medically managed in an appropriate setting.
   3. The American Society of Addiction Medicine (ASAM) criteria should be used to determine clients' placement along a continuum (community-based care vs. medically managed care on an inpatient basis).
   4. Today there are various psychopharmacologic approaches to help individuals maintain abstinence and control cravings.

      a. Medications such as naltrexone, which blocks the effects of exogenously administered opioids, thus preventing relapse to opioid dependence, have also been shown to improve the symptoms of alcohol dependence.

      b. Medications such as acamprosate and disulfiram are useful in treating alcohol dependence.

5. Many individuals respond well to support groups such as Alcoholics Anonymous (AA) and Narcotics Anonymous (NA).

6. Recent Cochrane reviews have demonstrated some support for the longitudinal efficacy of peer support groups.

7. Many individuals find the religious components associated with AA and NA objectionable. To this end, there are a variety of secular approaches to the treatment of substance use disorder and include:

      a. Self-management and recovery training (SMART) recovery.

      b. Secular organizations for sobriety (SOS)

DEMENTIA

A. An outdated term that refers to one of the multiple neurocognitive disorders found in the *DSM-5*.

B. Although the current term "neurocognitive disorder" is used in *DSM-5*, "dementia" is still quite prevalent in the literature.

C. The *DSM-5* recognizes the categories of "major neurocognitive disorder" and "mild neurocognitive disorder."

D. Although differing in their etiologies, neurocognitive disorders typically represent alterations in one or more of the major neurocognitive domains, which include:

1. Complex attention (including sustained attention, divided attention, selective attention, and cognitive processing speed)

2. Executive function (which includes planning, decision-making, the use of working memory, response inhibition, and mental flexibility)

3. Learning and memory (which includes immediate memory, recent memory/free recall, long-term memory, which includes semantic, and autobiographical, as well as implicit learning)

4. Language (including the use of expressive language and receptive language)

5. Perceptual-motor (which includes abilities to use visual perception, visual constructional abilities, perceptual-motor abilities, praxis, and gnosis)

6. Social cognition (recognition of our emotions)

E. The most common neurocognitive disorder is related to Alzheimer's disease.

1. The annual prevalence of Alzheimer's disease in U.S. adults over 65 years old is about 5.6 million people (Centers for Disease Control and Prevention [CDC], 2019).

F. Screening for dementia

1. One of the most valuable screening tools for the presence of alterations in neurocognitive functioning is the Mini-mental state exam (MMSE).

      a. Consist of 11 questions

      b. Measures five areas of cognitive function (orientation, registration, attention calculation, recall, and language).

      c. The maximum score is 30; scores of 23 or less indicate cognitive impairment.

G. Treatment of dementia

1. The treatment of dementia depends on the etiology.

2. Possible etiologies can include (but are not limited to): Alzheimer's disease, frontotemporal lobar degeneration, Lewy body disease, vascular disease, traumatic brain injury, substance-medication-induced, HIV infection, prion disease, Parkinson's disease, Huntington's disease, due to another medical condition, or due to multiple etiologies.

CASE STUDY

Patient Situation

A 32-year-old Hispanic American female presents to your office for her first prenatal check-up since it was discovered that she was pregnant earlier last week. She is concerned about her current prescription medication Lexapro 10 mg orally daily for treatment of anxiety and depression. She reports that she sees a psychiatric/mental health care provider to treat her "generalized anxiety disorder" and "major depressive disorder" and has been on this medication for the past 3 years. She tells you that it is the "only thing that has ever helped." Further clinical interview reveals that she had a history of a suicide attempt when she was 28 years old. She states, "I know that you shouldn't take medications when you are pregnant, but I am afraid of what will happen if I stop taking my prescription. When I was hospitalized 4 years ago, the doctor told me I nearly died from my suicide attempt." The client also admits that she is afraid to stop taking her medication because her mother was diagnosed with bipolar disorder when she was around the client's age. The client also states that she would like to improve her general health by starting an exercise program to help control her weight as she doesn't want to get "too fat" while she is pregnant.

Subjective Data

- Denies feelings of depression or anxiety at this time.
- Reports good sleep, appetite, and energy levels.
- Current medical history: No chronic conditions
- Home medications: Lexapro (escitalopram) 10 mg orally daily
- Hospitalization 4 years ago for suicide attempt via intentional overdose on acetaminophen, ibuprofen, and other medications found in her at-home medicine cabinet
- Quit smoking about 2 years ago (the client was smoking approximately one-half pack of cigarettes per day x 12 years)

Objective Data

- The client is well dressed/groomed.
- Smiles easily when discussing the prospect of her becoming a mother for the first time.
- Alert and oriented to person, place, time
- Vital signs: blood pressure 116/72, pulse 70, respiration 18/min
- Height: 5'3" Weight 135 lbs.

Clinical Analysis

- What assessments and other diagnostic tests do you anticipate will be ordered, and why?
- Identify this patient's modifiable and non-modifiable risk factors.
- What is the priority intervention based on the patient's clinical presentation?
- What should be included in this patient's plan of care?

BIBLIOGRAPHY

Ahmedani, B. K., Simon, G. E., Stewart, C., Beck, A., Waitzfelder, B. E., Rossom, R., Lynch, F., Owen-Smith, A., Hunkeler, E. M., Whiteside, U., Operskalski, B. H., Coffey, M. J., & Solberg, L. I. (2014). Health care contacts in the year before suicide death. *Journal of General Internal Medicine, 29*(6), 870–877. https://doi.org/10.1007/s11606-014 -2767-3.

American Foundation for Suicide Prevention. (2022). *Additional facts about suicide in the U.S.* https://afsp.org/suicide -statistics

Berg, K. C., Peterson, C. B., Frazier, P., & Crow, S. J. (2012). Psychometric evaluation of the eating disorder examination and eating disorder examination-questionnaire: A systematic review of the literature. *The International Journal of Eating Disorders, 45*(3), 428–438. https://doi.org/10.1002/eat.20931

Centers for Disease Control and Prevention. (2018). *Learn about mental health.* https://www.cdc.gov/mentalhealth/learn/index.htm

Centers for Disease Control and Prevention. (2019, August 20). *The truth about aging and dementia.* https://www.cdc.gov/aging/publications/features/Alz-Greater-Risk.html

Centers for Disease Control and Prevention (2020, September 23). *Mental health treatment among adults: United States, 2019.* https://www.cdc.gov/nchs/products/databriefs/db380.htm

College of Psychiatric & Neurologic Pharmacists. (2020–2021) *Psychiatric psychopharmacology review.* Author.

Cotton, M. A., Ball, C., & Robinson, P. (2003). Four simple questions can help screen for eating disorders. *Journal of General Internal Medicine, 18*(1), 53–56. https://doi.org/10.1046/j.1525-1497.2003.20374.x

Morgan, J. F., Reid, F., & Lacey, J. H. (2000). The SCOFF questionnaire: A new screening tool for eating disorders. *The Western Journal of Medicine, 172*(3), 164–165. https://doi.org/10.1136/ewjm.172.3.164

National Alliance on Mental Illness. (n.d.). *Mental health by the numbers.* https://nami.org/mhstats

National Association of Anorexia Nervosa and Associated Disorders. (2021, November 3). *Eating disorder statistics: General & diversity stats.* https://anad.org/eating-disorders-statistics

National Center for Drug Abuse Statistics. (2022). *Drug abuse statistics.* https://drugabusestatistics.org/#:~:text=9.5%20million%20or%203.8%25%20of,Americans%20aged%2012%20and%20over.

National Institutes of Mental Health. (2019). *Women and mental health.* https://www.nimh.nih.gov/health/topics/women-and-mental-health

Roberts, L. W. (Ed.). (2019). *American Psychiatric Association publishing textbook of psychiatry* (7th ed.). American Psychiatric Association Publishing.

Sapra, A., Bhandari, P., Sharma, S., Chanpura, T., & Lopp, L. (2020). Using generalized anxiety disorder-2 (GAD-2) and GAD-7 in a primary care setting. *Cureus, 12*(5), e8224. https://doi.org/10.7759/cureus.8224

Substance Abuse and Mental Health Services Administration. (2009). *Suicide assessment five-step evaluation in triage (SAFE-T).* https://store.samhsa.gov/sites/default/files/d7/priv/sma09-4432.pdf

World Health Organization. (2022). *Mental health: Strengthening our response.* https://www.who.int/news-room/fact-sheets/detail/mental-health-strengthening-our-response#:~:text=The%20WHO%20constitution%20states%3A%20%22Health,of%20mental%20disorders%20or%20disabilities

12

PRECONCEPTION CARE

KOMKWUAN P. PARUCHABUTR

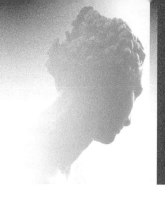

PRECONCEPTION CARE

A. The United States ranks last of all developed nations for maternal mortality (Tikkanen et al., 2020). Patient and provider gaps in knowledge of chronic disease and management were found to be key factors to cardiovascular and coronary conditions that affect maternal health and mortality as well as non-cardiovascular conditions. Approximately 18% of infant mortalities were associated with preterm birth and low birth weight infants, and 20% related to congenital birth defects, which may be associated with maternal health (Matthews et al., 2015).

B. A majority of women reported they did not receive preconception counseling and most providers did not recommend counseling to patients of reproductive age (Wilkes, 2016).

C. Approximately 45% of pregnancies within the United States are unintended.

D. The Centers for Disease Control and Prevention (CDC) published *Recommendations to Improve Preconception Health and Health Care – United States* in 2006.

    1. Recommendation of risk assessment in addition to education and health promotion counseling as a standard of care during primary care visits to all women of reproductive age to help reduce reproductive risks and improve pregnancy outcomes

    2. Despite the recommendations from the CDC, the United States saw few improvements regarding maternal and infant mortality outcomes.

E. The American Academy of Family Physicians (AAFP) released a position paper in 2016 providing evidence-based recommendations that address reproductive healthcare.

    1. **Definition of preconception care:** Personalized healthcare for men and women during their reproductive years primarily focused on reducing maternal and fetal morbidity and mortality.

    2. Aimed to

        a. Increase chances of conception

        b. Prevent unintended pregnancies

        c. Discuss reduction of risk factors that negatively impact maternal and fetal health such as being overweight, smoking, hypertension, and diabetes mellitus.

        d. The American College of Obstetricians and Gynecologists (ACOG) and the American Society for Reproductive Medicine (ASRM) published Committee Opinion Number 762 in January 2019.

           (1) Aimed to reduce the risk of adverse health effects for the woman, fetus, and neonate while addressing modifiable risk factors and promoting education (ACOG & Committee on Gynecologic Practice, 2019).

OVERALL GOALS FOR PRECONCEPTION CARE

A. Improve the health of women of childbearing age in order to improve the outcome of any future pregnancy (Nypaver et al., 2016).

B. Improve knowledge, attitudes, and behaviors of women and men related to preconception health (Nypaver et al., 2016).

C. Create health equity and eliminate health disparities in adverse maternal, fetal, and infant outcomes (Nypaver et al., 2016).

D. Ensure that all women of reproductive age and men in the United States receive preconception healthcare services, to include screening, health promotion, and interventions (Nypaver et al., 2016; Table 12.1).

TABLE 12.1 Preconception Health Promotion and Interventions

HEALTH PROMOTION	SCREENING	INTERVENTIONS
Reproductive life plan (RLP)	Utilize a screening tool Access: http://www.healthystartepic.org/wp-content/uploads/2018/03/rep_life_planning508.pdf	• Evaluate and discuss results from screening tool • Counsel on the importance of birth spacing • Refer to CDC Medical Eligibility Criteria (MEC) for contraceptive use chart (2020) • Download app for CDC MEC from app store
Optimal weight management	Screen BMI Screen for physical activity	• Maintain optimal BMI 18.5 and 24.9 kg/m^2 • Recommend 30 minutes of moderate physical activity daily
Chronic disease management	Screen for hypertension, diabetes mellitus, depression, anxiety, seizure disorder, autoimmune disorders	• Assess medications • Counsel for untreated illness, lifestyle changes, assess for teratogenic medications, optimize risk profile of medications
Nutrition and diet	Screen for folic acid, vitamin A, essential fatty acids, vegan diet, bariatric surgery	• Recommend folic acid 400 mcg to 800 mcg • Essential fatty acids (i.e., non-high mercury fish, shellfish, walnuts, leafy vegetables)
Immunizations	Screen for immunizations	• Measles, mumps, rubella (MMR) • Varicella • Hepatitis B • Influenza • Human papillomavirus (HPV) • Tetanus, diptheria, and pertussis (T-dap) • COVID-19
Sexually transmitted infections (STI)	STI risk assessment (STIs, HIV/AIDS, cytomegalovirus) Screen with thorough history and physical exam	• Provide counseling and offer testing and treatment if indicated
Teratogen Exposure/Environmental Exposure/Occupational Exposure/Substance abuse	Assess for risk teratogen exposures Screen for opioid use using 4Ps, NIDA Quick Screen, CRAFFT (for women 26 years or younger; ACOG, 2017) Screen for substance, alcohol, tobacco use Screen medications and dietary supplements Screen for environmental exposures	• Refer to counseling and manage with multidisciplinary team if positive screen • Review of medications and consider alternative medication management and supplement management

(continued)

TABLE 12.1 Preconception Health Promotion and Interventions (*continued*)		
HEALTH PROMOTION	**SCREENING**	**INTERVENTIONS**
Family and genetic history	Screen for three-generation history and ethnic backgrounds Knowledge and screening for sickle cell, Tay-Sachs, cystic fibrosis, Fragile X, spinal muscular atrophy, Canavan disease, hemoglobinopathies, thrombophilias	• Order carrier screening labs • Refer to genetic counselor
Psychosocial risks/social determinants of health	Screen for intimate partner violence (IPV): Screen for IPV using Humiliation, Afraid, Rape, Kick (HARK); Hurt, Insult, Threaten, Scream (HITS); Extended–Hurt, Insult, Threaten, Scream (E-HITS); Partner Violence Screen (PVS); and Woman Abuse Screening Tool (WAST; U.S. Preventive Services Taskforce, 2018) Screen for access to care, financial resources, mental health (i.e., Edinburgh postnatal Depression Scale, Patient Health Questionnaire 2), food insecurity, housing insecurity using (i.e. AAFP, Social Needs Screening Tool, The Protocol for Responding to and Assessing Patients' Assets, Risks, and Experiences (PRAPARE; O'Gurek & Henke, 2018)	• Positive screen requires counseling and referral to resources within the community

E. Reduce risks among women who have had adverse perinatal outcomes through interventions in the postpartum and/or interpregnancy period (Nypaver et al., 2016).

OVERALL RECOMMENDATIONS

A. Approach *all* patient encounters of all genders with reproductive potential as an opportunity to counsel regarding current holistic wellness and healthy habits which may improve reproductive and obstetric outcomes if their intent is to plan a future pregnancy.

B. **Initiate counseling with the "one key question method":** *"Would you like to become pregnant in the next year?"* (ACOG & Committee on Gynecologic Practice, 2019)

REPRODUCTIVE LIFE PLAN

A. Approximately 45% of pregnancies in the United States are unintended.

B. This increases the risk of pregnancy complications.

C. Educational awareness regarding birth spacing and family size are essential for those who desire to initiate a family in the future.

D. Screening tools and utilizing the "one key question" (https://powertodecide.org/one-key-question) method is essential.

E. Recommended to avoid interpregnancy intervals less than 6 months; less than 6 months is associated with low birth weight, preterm birth, and small for gestational age (1B strong recommendation, moderate quality evidence; Louis et al., 2019)

F. Counseling regarding risk/benefits of interpregnancy intervals between 6 months and 18 months (2B weak recommendation, moderate quality evidence; Louis et al., 2019)

G. Short interpregnancy intervals are associated with lower rates of vaginal births after cesarean sections.

H. U.S. Medical Eligibility Criteria for Contraceptive Use and U.S. Selected Practice Recommendations may be used to facilitate contraception guidance and birth spacing.

I. Ovulatory women <35 years old without identifiable risk factors with 12 months of unprotected intercourse and women ≥36 years old after 6 months of unprotected intercourse should have comprehensive evaluation and treatment.

J. Anovulatory women and those with identifiable risk factors should be evaluated and treated without delay.

K. Referral to a fertility specialist should be considered for males and females if failed treatment and/or outside the scope of the practitioner.

L. Review past reproductive history.
  1. Previous pregnancies complicated by preterm birth, growth restriction, and adverse perinatal outcomes at risk for recurrence and risk mitigation and education regarding birth spacing, healthy habits, and medication management are essential to discuss with the patient.
  2. Maternal age and reproductive history should be reviewed and addressed.
      a. Adverse reproductive outcomes increase with maternal age (King et al., 2019).
      b. Fertility declines with increasing maternal age and comprehensive evaluation, assessment, and treatment may be indicated.

OPTIMAL WEIGHT MANAGEMENT

A. Patients should be encouraged to maintain an optimal BMI of 18.5 and 24.9 kg/m² prior to pregnancy.

B. Abnormal high or low BMI is associated with infertility, maternal and fetal complications.

C. Obesity is associated with infertility, miscarriage, birth defects, preterm delivery, gestational diabetes, gestational hypertension, cesarean delivery, thromboembolic events, stroke, heart disease, hypertension, cancer, arthritis, hyperlipidemia, and diabetes.

D. Low BMI is associated with small for gestational age, low birth weight infants.

E. Recommendation for moderate exercise 30 minutes per day, 5 days per week, for a minimum of 150 minutes of moderate exercise per week (recommended prior to pregnancy, during pregnancy, and postpartum).

CHRONIC DISEASE MANAGEMENT

A. Optimal management of chronic diseases prior to pregnancy is essential to minimize adverse maternal and fetal outcomes.

B. Referral to maternal fetal medicine may be considered.

C. **Pregestational diabetes:** Recommendation to maintain euglycemic control (HbA1C <6.5%) before and during pregnancy.
  1. Associated risks for abnormal control are congenital anomalies and pregnancy-related complications.

D. **Hypertension:** Recommendation to manage hypertension and evaluation of medications.
  1. Angiotensin-converting enzyme (ACE) inhibitors and angiotensin II receptor blockers (ARBs) are contraindicated due to increased risks of fetal malformation, oligohydramnios, fetal growth restriction, and fetal death. Hypertension increases risk of preeclampsia and intrauterine growth restriction.
  2. Consider testing for ventricular hypertrophy, retinopathy, and renal disease for longstanding hypertension or uncontrolled hypertension.

E. **Thyroid disorder:** No recommendation for universal screening
   1. Recommend risk-based screening (history of preterm delivery, history of pregnancy loss, infertility, >30 years of age, morbid obesity)
   2. Treat if thyrotropin is above the upper level of normal.
   3. Untreated hypothyroidism associated with spontaneous abortion, preeclampsia, preterm birth, placental abruption, and fetal death.
   4. Medications for hyperthyroidism may be associated with congenital anomalies.
   5. Recommend to avoid pregnancy for 6 months after receiving radioactive treatment.
F. **Mood disorders:** General consensus of benefits of treatment for mood disorders outweigh the risks.
   1. Counsel patients regarding risks of untreated mental health issues which impair maternal infant bonding, risk of maternal self-harm or neglect, increase risks of substance abuse, lower participation in prenatal care, adverse infant outcomes, higher risk of postpartum psychiatric illness, poor obstetric outcomes.
   2. Develop a strategy to treat and manage relapses of mood disorders.
G. **Autoimmune disorders:** Screen for autoimmune disorders (i.e., rheumatoid arthritis, systemic lupus erythematosus).
   1. Review of medications such as methotrexate which is considered teratogenic.
   2. NSAIDs contraindicated later in pregnancy (approximately >20 weeks gestation) because they promote premature closure of the ductus arteriosus leading to fetal pulmonary hypertension and oligohydramnios.
H. **Seizure disorders:** Women with epilepsy are at increased risk for preeclampsia, premature delivery, hemorrhage, fetal growth restriction, stillbirth, and a dramatically increased risk of maternal mortality.
   1. Multidisciplinary preconception counseling and management approach with neurology, obstetrics, and maternal fetal medicine
   2. Anticonvulsants have been known to be teratogenic. Screen for teratogenic medications.

NUTRITION AND DIET

A. Refer to recommendations from U.S. Department of Agriculture for daily allowances for vitamin A, vitamin B_{12}, vitamin B, vitamin D, and other nutrients.
B. **Folic acid:** Most women in the United States do not consume the recommended amount of folate in their diets alone.
   1. Recommendation of 400 mcg to 800 mcg of folic acid daily when planning a pregnancy or women capable of pregnancy to reduce fetal neural tube defects (King et al., 2019).
   2. Women with a history of prior neural tube disorder or women with seizure disorder should be counseled to take 4 mg folic acid daily.
C. **Vitamin D:** A level of 25-hydroxyvitamin D greater than 30 ng/mL is required to maintain a healthy level of vitamin D (Sizar et al., 2021).
   1. Universal screening is not recommended; optimal levels of 25-hydroxyvitamin D are still controversial (Sizar et al., 2021).
   2. Consideration of screening for increased risk factors such as patients who live in cold climates along northern latitudes, racial ethnic groups with dark skin, those who have routine use of sunscreen.
   3. Initial supplementation for 8 weeks with vitamin D_3 (cholecalciferol) either 6,000 IU daily or 50,000 IU weekly can be considered. Once the serum 25-hydroxyvitamin D level exceeds 30 ng/mL, a daily maintenance dose of 1,000 to 2,000 IU is recommended.
   4. Vitamin D_3 has been found to be more efficacious than vitamin D_2 (ergocalciferol) and typically the treatment of choice (Sizar et al., 2021).

D. **Vitamin A:** Not to exceed the daily recommended allowance as this has been associated with fetal malformations in the first trimester (King et al., 2019).
   1. Avoid additional supplements and multivitamins that contain added vitamin A.
E. Assess for eating disorders and refer to counseling.
F. Food safety
   1. Listeria, salmonella, L-monocytogenes, and other food borne illnesses
      a. Associated with miscarriage, stillbirth, preterm labor, preterm delivery, low birth weight infants, newborn infection.
      b. Refer to U.S. Department of Health and Human Services (foodsafety.gov) for resources for providers and patients.
   2. Fish
      a. Consume fish and seafood with low levels of mercury (e.g., salmon, pollock, catfish, canned light tuna, and shrimp).
      b. Consume cooked fish.
      c. Refer to food safety.gov for more recommendations.

IMMUNIZATIONS

A. Annual assessment Tdap, measles-mumps-rubella, hepatitis B, and varicella
B. Influenza vaccine should be administered for all eligible women of reproductive age.
C. Human papillomavirus (HPV) vaccines and cervical cancer screening should be performed according to recommendations.
D. HPV vaccine recommended for postpartum and lactating women. If the series is started prior to pregnancy, it is recommended to complete after pregnancy (ACOG, 2019).
E. **Tdap:** Recommended in pregnancy 27 to 36 weeks regardless of pre-pregnancy immunization status in order to maximize passive antibody transfer to fetus.
F. **Influenza:** Pregnant women have higher likelihood for severe illness from influenza infection and increased risk for hospitalization.
G. **COVID-19 vaccines:** COVID-19 vaccines are recommended for patients who are considering pregnancy in the future or trying to get pregnant (CDC, 2021a).
   1. Routine pregnancy tests prior to COVID-19 vaccination are not recommended.
   2. Pregnant women who are infected with COVID-19 are likely to get severely ill compared to non-pregnant women.
   3. COVID-19 vaccine may reduce severe illness and hospitalizations.
   4. COVID-19 vaccine booster is recommended prior to pregnancy and during pregnancy (CDC, 2021a).

SEXUALLY TRANSMITTED INFECTIONS

A. Screening should be performed during pre-pregnancy counseling.
B. Gonorrhea, chlamydia, syphilis, HIV screening based on age and risk factors (refer to CDC guidelines; CDC, 2021b)
C. Counsel on healthy sexual habits and protection to reduce sexually transmitted infection transmission.

TERATOGEN EXPOSURES/ENVIRONMENTAL EXPOSURES/ OCCUPATIONAL EXPOSURES

A. Environmental pollutants and workplace teratogens pose pregnancy and reproductive risks which can disrupt organogenesis.

B. Screen with thorough patient history and identification of exposure risks and counseling to avoid such toxic agents.

C. List of toxic exposures include but not limited to:

1. Lead, pesticides, solvents, phthalates, polychlorinated biphenyls, perfluorochemicals, mercury, antineoplastic drugs, bisphenol A, anesthetic gases, carbon monoxide, nitrogen dioxide, sulfur dioxide, cigarette smoke, formaldehyde, asbestos, biologics, radiation (ACOG, 2019; King et al., 2019).

SUBSTANCE/OPIOID USE

A. Smoking during pregnancy is associated with intrauterine growth restriction, placenta previa, abruptio placentae, decreased maternal thyroid function, preterm labor, premature rupture of membranes, low birth weight infants, ectopic pregnancy (ACOG, 2019).

B. Children with mothers who smoke have an increased risk of asthma, infantile colic, and childhood obesity (ACOG, 2019).

C. Screen with validated tools such as CAGE substance abuse screening tool.

D. Effective tobacco cessation models should be employed such as 5As intervention model (ACOG, 2019).

E. Screen for opioid use using 4Ps, NIDA quick screen, CRAFFT (for women 26 years or younger; ACOG, 2017).

F. Refer for counseling and manage with multidisciplinary team prior to pregnancy, during pregnancy, and after pregnancy.

FAMILY AND GENETIC HISTORY

A. Screen for family history of genetic disorders, birth defects, mental disorders, and breast, ovarian, uterine, and colon cancer.

B. Screen for cystic fibrosis and spinal muscular atrophy to all who are considering pregnancy.

C. **Family history of Ashkenazi Jewish descent:** Screen for familial dysautonomia, Tay-Sach's disease, and Canavan disease

D. Fragile X screening should be offered to women with a family history, intellectual disability suggestive of Fragile X, or women less than 40 years old with ovarian insufficiency or any patient that desires with informed consent.

E. **Hemoglobinopathies:** Screen with complete blood count and hemoglobin electrophoresis based on ethnicity (African, Mediterranean, Middle Eastern, Southeast Asian, or West Indian descent; ACOG, 2019).

F. Patients with a family history of thrombophilia such as Factor V Leiden, protein C deficiency, and antithrombin deficiency should be screened, evaluated, and treated.

1. Counseling and referral to specialist may be indicated if positive.

G. Consideration of referring to genetic counselor for further counseling and testing if positive screen.

PSYCHOSOCIAL RISKS

A. Intimate partner violence

1. More than one in three women in the United States have experienced physical and/or sexual violence, rape, or stalking by an individual they have been intimate with (ACOG, 2019).

2. Screen utilizing several screening tools: Humiliation, Afraid, Rape, Kick (HARK); Hurt, Insult, Threaten, Scream (HITS); Extended–Hurt, Insult, Threaten, Scream (E-HITS);

Partner Violence Screen (PVS); and Woman Abuse Screening Tool (WAST; U.S. Preventive Services Taskforce, 2018).

3. Normalize the screening process with all patients and inform that this screening tool is given to all patients.

4. A positive screen should be referred to resources within the community and ensuring patient safety.

SOCIAL DETERMINANTS OF HEALTH

A. Race, ethnicity, age, socioeconomic factors, education, medical insurance coverage, access to medical care, transportation, prepregnancy health are factors that affect maternal, perinatal, infant, child outcomes (Office of Disease Prevention and Health Promotion, 2021).

B. Screen for food and housing insecurity using, for example, AAFP, Social Needs Screening Tool, The Protocol for Responding to and Assessing Patients' Assets, Risks, and Experiences (PRAPARE) (O'Gurek & Henke, 2018).

C. Screen for mental health using screening tools such as Edinburgh Postnatal Depression Scale, Patient Health Questionnaire 2.

D. Positive screens should be identified, and the priority would be to maximize patient safety, refer to community resources, and development of plan for follow up and consideration of home visits.

RESOURCES

Centers for Disease Control and Prevention. (2016). *U.S. medical eligibility criteria for contraceptive use; U.S. selected practice recommendations for contraceptive use.* (Version 3.1) [Mobile app]. https://itunes.apple.com

Centers for Disease Control and Prevention. (2020). *Summary chart of U.S. medical eligibility criteria for contraceptive use.* https://www.cdc.gov/reproductivehealth/contraception/pdf/summary-chart-us-medical-eligibility-criteria_508tagged.pdf

Healthy Start Epic. (2018) *Reproductive Life Planning Screening Tools.* http://www.healthystartepic.org/wp-content/uploads/2018/03/rep_life_planning508.pdf

National Center for Immunization and Respiratory Diseases. (2011). General recommendations on immunization --- recommendations of the Advisory Committee on Immunization Practices (ACIP). *MMWR. Recommendations and reports: Morbidity and mortality weekly report. Recommendations and reports, 60*(2), 1–64.

Steinberg, J. (2020). *Preconception Care Quick Ref from the National PCHHC* (Versions 1.1) [Mobile app]. Retrieved from https://itunes.apple.com/

BIBLIOGRAPHY

American College of Obstetricians and Gynecologists. (2017). ACOG Committee Opinion, Number 711. Opioid use and opioid use disorder in pregnancy. *ACOG.Org.* https://www.Acog.Org/Clinical-Guidance-and-Publications/Committee-Opinions/Committee-on-Obstetric-Practice/Opioid-use-and-Opioid-use-Disorder-in-Pregnancy, 7

American College of Obstetricians and Gynecologists. (2019). ACOG Committee Opinion No. 762 Prepregnancy Counseling. *Obstetrics and Gynecology, 133*(1), e78–e89. https://doi.org/10.1097/AOG.0000000000003013

American College of Obstetricians and Gynecologists, & Committee on Gynecologic Practice. (2019). Prepregnancy counseling: Committee Opinion No. 762. *Fertility and Sterility, 111*(1), 32–42. https://doi.org/10.1016/j.fertnstert.2018.12.003

CDC Foundation. (2018). Building U.S. capacity to review and prevent maternal deaths. Report from nine maternal mortality review committees. https://www.cdcfoundation.org/sites/default/files/files/ReportfromNineMMRCs.pdf

Centers for Disease Control and Prevention. (2021a). *COVID-19 Vaccines for People Who Would Like to Have a Baby.* https://www.cdc.gov/coronavirus/2019-ncov/vaccines/planning-for-pregnancy.html

Centers for Disease Control and Prevention. (2021b). *Screening Recommendations and Considerations Referenced in Treatment Guidelines and Original Sources.* https://www.cdc.gov/std/treatment-guidelines/screening-recommendations.htm

Davis, N. L., Smoots, A. N., & Goodman, D. A. (2019). Pregnancy-related deaths: Data from 14 US maternal mortality review committees. *Education, 40*(36), 8–2.

Floyd, R. L., Johnson, K. A., Owens, J. R., Verbiest, S., Moore, C. A., & Boyle, C. (2013). A national action plan for promoting preconception health and health care in the United States (2012–2014). *Journal of Women's Health, 22*(10), 797–802. https://doi.org/10.1089/jwh.2013.4505

King, T. L., Brucker, M. C., Kathryn Osborne, C., & Jevitt, C. M. (2019). *Varney's Midwifery* (6th ed.). Jones & Bartlett Publishers.

Louis, J. M., Bryant, A., Ramos, D., Stuebe, A., Blackwell, S. C., & American College of Obstetricians and Gynecologists. (2019). Interpregnancy care. *American Journal of Obstetrics and Gynecology, 220*(1), B2–B18. https://doi.org/10.1016/j.ajog.2018.11.1098

Mathews, T. J., MacDorman, M. F., & Thoma, M. E. (2015). Infant mortality statistics from the 2013 period linked birth/infant death data set. *National Vital Statistics Reports, 64*(9), 1–30.

Nypaver, C., Arbour, M., & Niederegger, E. (2016). Preconception care: Improving the health of women and families. *Journal of Midwifery & Women's Health, 61*(3), 356–364. https://doi.org/10.1111/jmwh.12465

Office of Disease Prevention and Health Promotion. (2021). *Maternal, Infant, and Child Health Across the Life Stages.* https://www.healthypeople.gov/2020/leading-health-indicators/2020-lhi-topics/Maternal-Infant-and-Child-Health/determinants

O'Gurek, D. T., & Henke, C. (2018). A practical approach to screening for social determinants of health. *Family Practice Management, 25*(3), 7–12.

Sizar, O., Khare, S., Goyal, A., Bansal, P., & Givler, A. (2021). *Vitamin D Deficiency.* NCBI: Stat Pearls. https://www.ncbi.nlm.nih.gov/books/NBK532266

Tikkanen, R., Gunja, M. Z., FitzGerald, M., & Zephyrin, L. (2020). Maternal mortality and maternity care in the United States compared to 10 other developed countries. *Issue Briefs, Commonwealth Fund.*

U.S. Department of Agriculture. (2021). *U.S. Department of Agriculture Individual Dietary Assessment.* https://www.nal.usda.gov/legacy/fnic/individual-dietary-assessment

U.S. Department of Health and Human Services. (2020). *People at Risk: Pregnant Women.* https://www.foodsafety.gov/people-at-risk/pregnant-women

U.S. Preventative Services Taskforce. (2018). *Final Recommendation Statement: Intimate Partner Violence, Elder Abuse, and Abuse of Vulnerable Adults: Screening | United States Preventive Services Taskforce.* https://www.uspreventiveservicestaskforce.org/uspstf/document/RecommendationStatementFinal/intimate-partner-violence-and-abuse-of-elderly-and-vulnerable-adults-screening

Wilkes, J. (2016). AAFP releases position paper on preconception care. *American Family Physician, 94*(6), 508–510.

13

COMPLEMENTARY AND ALTERNATIVE MEDICAL THERAPIES

IRIS STENDIG-RASKIN AND R. MIMI SECOR

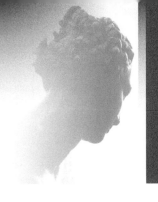

INTRODUCTION

A. The concept of complementary and alternative medicine (CAM) is not new. The attempt to blend the care of both body and mind echoes in these words penned by Plato (428-348 BCE) before the common era:

> The cure of the part should not be attempted without treatment of the whole. No attempt should be made to cure the body without the soul, and therefore, if the head and the body are to be healthy, you must begin by curing the mind. That is the first thing. Let no one persuade you to cure the headfirst until he has given you his soul to be cured.
>
> For this is the greatest error of our day in the treatment of the human body, that physicians first separate the soul from the body.

OVERVIEW

A. Many individuals are now utilizing and seeking out complementary/alternative practices as adjunct therapy to their medical care. Many have also chosen to discard traditional Western practice and solely rely upon non-mainstream therapies. While there exists a plethora of information available on the internet, it is our responsibility and obligation to provide the most up-to-date and clinically relevant, evidence-based information to those we care for.

B. As a response to the ongoing need for evidence-based clinical trials, resources, and studies, the National Institutes of Health established the Center for Complementary and Alternative Medicine in 1991. In 2014, it was re-named the National Center for Integrative and Complementary Health to better reflect its ongoing mission. The wealth of material available on the website is immense, and is highly recommended as a resource for further exploration in this area.

CATEGORIES OF COMPLEMENTARY ALTERNATIVE MEDICINE

A. Traditional alternative medicine
   1. Includes therapies that have been practiced for several centuries and have been accepted as a part of mainstream medical practice. May include such practices as:
      a. **Homeopathy:** Based on the belief that the body can cure itself based on the theory of treating "like with like." Healing responses occur by administering substances that mimic the symptoms of the disease.
      b. **Naturopathy:** A system of alternative medicine based on the theory that diseases can be successfully treated or prevented without the use of drugs via techniques such as diet, exercise, and massage. Naturopathic physicians have attended a formal 4-year training

program and several states require licensure. Traditional naturopaths have not attended a formal program.

  c. **Traditional Chinese medicine (TCM):** Based on traditions that date back over 2000 years. Sub-categories include:

    (1) **Acupuncture:** Technique in which needles are inserted through the skin by a trained and licensed practitioner. Results from studies indicate a reduction in chronic pain such as low back pain, knee pain, and carpal tunnel issues. May also relieve migraines and headaches.

    (2) **Tai chi and Qigong:** A series of gentle movements and breathwork. Has been shown to increase stability and balance in older individuals and help cope with fibromyalgia and back pain.

    (3) **Herbal medicine:** Has been used over several centuries for a variety of medical conditions. In spite of the fact that clinical studies have demonstrated no clinically significant results, one out of five Americans rely upon their usage.

B. External energy/manipulative/body-based therapies

  1. **Massage:** Massage therapy includes a variety of techniques and has been shown to decrease migraines, some fibromyalgia symptoms, supportive therapy for cancer patients if used in conjunction with aromatherapy. In 45 states, massage therapists must be licensed and certified before practicing.

  2. **Yoga:** Many different styles that incorporate a series of mental, physical, and spiritual practices. Research suggests that yoga may improve sleep health, relieve menopausal symptoms, and improve mental and physical health. May help with weight loss and smoking cessation. About one in seven Americans practice this modality.

  3. **Reiki:** A practice that originated in Japan, where the practitioner places their hands on the individual directing the flow of energy to clear blockages thereby undoing the disease state. Many hospitals are integrating this therapy for pre-op patients, pain management, and for a variety of other health conditions. Research has not been of high quality, and results have been inconsistent.

  4. **Chiropractic/osteopathic medicine:** Treatments involve stretching and sustained pressure and joint manipulations. Purpose is to improve joint motion and function. Chiropractors must pass a licensure exam and have a state license to practice.

C. When approached and questioned about any of these therapies, responses should be based on evidence-based published results. Many studies have been inconclusive in terms of proven results, and many herbs and supplements might cause an adverse reaction when used with other medication.

D. While reviewing medical history, it is the utmost importance that CAM use be reviewed at each visit. Pregnant and breastfeeding woman should consult their provider prior to utilizing any medication.

E. Many individuals seek out information regarding CAM use and menopause. While studies are ongoing, few have yielded clinical significance. Since some CAM use poses little or no risk, recommendations may be appropriate after consultation and discussion.

BRIEF OVERVIEW: COMPLEMENTARY ALTERNATIVE MEDICINE USE AND MENOPAUSAL OVERVIEW

A. Mind/body practices

  1. **Hypnosis:** Two randomized controlled studies consisting of five sessions demonstrated a clinically significant reduction in hot flashes and frequency. Also, improvement in self-reported sleep quality and sexual function. The North American Menopausal Society (NAMS) has recommended hypnosis for the treatment of menopausal symptoms with little risk posed.

2. **Bio feedback and relaxation training:** Conclusions of several small studies indicate that while relaxation and biofeedback may provide some benefit for menopausal symptom and pose low risk, more evidence is needed to draw definite conclusions.

3. **Yoga:** Moderate evidence exists for the short-term effects of yoga on psychological effects of menopause; no evidence was found for improvement in vaso-motor symptoms (VSM). Consensus is that yoga is safe and may be effective for psychological symptoms, but more research is needed for its effects on VSM and other menopausal symptoms.

4. **Tai chi/Qigong:** A series of deliberate moves and breath work resulting in increased flexibility and balance. May prevent bone loss in menopausal adults; studies are ongoing.

5. Herbal Products/Vitamins and Supplements
   a. Phytoestrogens are substances from plants that have similar properties to estrogen. Some examples are soy, flaxseed, and red clover. Studies have had inconsistent results, showing them to be no more effective than placebo use in reducing hot flashes.
   b. **Black cohosh, an herb native to North America:** Used to treat menopausal symptoms. Studies have been inconclusive; and those with any liver disorder should consult their provider before use. If abdominal pain, dark-colored urine, and jaundice occur, medication should be stopped immediately and a healthcare provider should be notified.
   c. **Dong quai:** An herb used in traditional Chinese medicine (TCM), it is used in women's health for a variety of conditions. Minimal research has been done regarding menopausal treatment. May interact with blood thinning medication, like coumadin.
   d. **Vitamin E:** Small studies have suggested that vitamin E might be helpful in reducing hot flashes. Woman taking vitamin E in large doses may increase their risk of bleeding and may have an interaction with anticoagulant use.
   e. **Pollen extract:** Made from flower pollen; showed improvement in all areas (VSM, tiredness, dizziness, mood quality, and quality of life) as compared to placebo use in a small randomized controlled study (RCT).

REASONS CITED FOR COMPLEMENTARY ALTERNATIVE MEDICINE USE

A. Natural and healing therapies: cited as natural and nontoxic

B. Sense of being in control and controlling one's healthcare

C. Reduction in symptoms/side effects

D. Distrust of traditional/conventional treatments

E. Believe in body's ability to heal itself

F. Family and cultural history of use

MEDICAL CONCERNS REGARDING COMPLEMENTARY ALTERNATIVE MEDICINE USE

A. Many studies have had inconsistent results.

B. Omission of use by patients during health history; may lead to interactions and adverse effects

C. Lack of standardization of medication/therapeutics

D. Lack of insurance/medical coverage may be a cost barrier of care to many.

E. Points to consider when talking with patients
   1. Ask about vitamins, herbal therapies, and other interventions.
   2. **Risk vs. benefits:** Many modalities (e.g., reiki, tai chi, relaxation, massage), despite the inconclusive data, pose little risk and may offer psychological benefits.
   3. Lack of regulation and standardization regarding herbals and other supplements. Actual products may not be completely disclosed due to "proprietary blends."

4. Discuss potential side effects when herbals are used with other medication.
5. Reinforce discussion with healthcare provider before utilizing herbals if medical condition exists.
6. Seek out appropriate resources to ensure knowledgeable dialogue.

ADDITIONAL RESOURCES

NIH: National Center for Complementary Health and Integrative Practice
https: www.nccih.nih.gov/health/menopausal-symptoms-in-depth
https://www.nccih.nih.gov

EVALUATION OF SPECIAL POPULATIONS

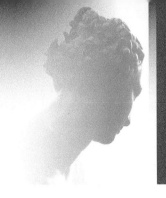

14

ASSESSMENT OF THE PREGNANT WOMAN

KATHARINE GREEN

EXPERT REVIEWER: KELLEY BORELLA

INITIAL PRENATAL EVALUATION

A. The initial evaluation of a pregnant woman should include a thorough review of the patient's medical history and a careful physical examination. This visit is a good opportunity to screen for potential complications of pregnancy that may require referral and to begin to establish a trusting relationship with the pregnant woman.

DOCUMENTATION OF PREGNANCY

A. Many practices require documentation in the chart of a positive pregnancy test result (done in the office) to verify the woman's pregnancy before beginning the comprehensive initial prenatal evaluation. Urine and serum pregnancy tests are based on levels of human chorionic gonadotropin (hCG), which is secreted into the maternal bloodstream and then excreted through the maternal urine.

B. Urine pregnancy tests
   1. Accurate greater than 97% to 99% of the time, depending on timing (98% accurate if performed when menses would be expected) and correct use of the test.
   2. Sensitive within 9 days after conception; women with high body mass indices (BMIs) may have slightly lower levels.
   3. Possible for pregnancy to be detected 5 days before first missed period. Results of home testing should be confirmed in the clinical setting as user understanding of instructions may be inaccurate and products' sensitivity may vary.
   4. Over-the-counter urine tests are inexpensive, private, and easy to obtain without a clinician order.
   5. Utilize a first morning void when possible because concentrated urine improves the pregnancy detection rate (nearly equal to that of serum).
   6. The test is specific for beta subunit of hCG (Center for Devices and Radiological Health, 2020).

C. Serum qualitative or quantitative tests do not indicate pregnancy until levels rise above baseline values (may vary by laboratory, but usually around 25 mIU/mL).
   1. hCG is detectable in serum as early as 8 to 10 days after ovulation or just after implantation at 10 mIU/mL.
   2. Serum hCG level doubles every 2 to 3 days until 8 to 11 weeks then declines and levels off. The level should be 50 to 250 mIU/dL at the time of the first missed menstrual period.
   3. The level peaks at 10 weeks at 100,000 to 200,000 mIU/mL, then decreases to approximately 20,000 mIU/mL during the first half of pregnancy, after which it remains relatively constant throughout the remainder of the pregnancy.
   4. Qualitative test results are read as positive or negative (false-positive results are rare).

5. Quantitative beta-hCG is a radioisotope test performed on a blood sample to quantify levels of hCG. It is most useful when:
   a. Serial testing is desired to monitor suspected ectopic pregnancy, molar pregnancy, or spontaneous abortion.
   b. Variable results from other tests are present.
6. Must specify qualitative or quantitative test when ordering serum hCG.
7. All urine and serum pregnancy tests should be considered presumptive and should be confirmed by exam and other labs.
   a. False-negative results may be caused by samples that are too diluted or too early in the pregnancy.
   b. False-positive results may be caused by trophoblastic diseases or certain neoplasms (Center for Devices and Radiological Health, 2020).
D. Progesterone levels
   1. Usually used to predict ovulation; not routinely performed during pregnancy.
   2. Progesterone levels rise midcycle for 6 to 10 days. If pregnancy occurs, levels do not fall and stay steady or increase to full term.
   3. Nonviable pregnancies have much lower levels than normal pregnancies.
   4. Progesterone levels are highly predictive of pregnancy outcome.
E. **Signs and symptoms of pregnancy:** The diagnosis of pregnancy is based on the following:
   a. Presumptive signs (see Table 14.1 for the signs and symptoms)
   1. Probable signs
   2. Positive signs

ESTIMATED DATE OF CONFINEMENT OR DELIVERY

A. Obtain date of the first day of the last menstrual period (LMP).
   1. Evaluate patient's surety on the date because estimated date of confinement (EDC) is based on the LMP.
   2. Conception usually occurs approximately 2 weeks after the LMP in a 28-day cycle.
B. Review menstrual cycles.
   1. **Frequency of menses:** If the woman does not have a regular 28-day cycle, adjust EDC accordingly.
   2. Duration of flow
   3. Question whether LMP was normal for the patient. If flow was exceptionally light or spotting only, the condition could be the result of syncytiotrophoblastic cells implanting in the endometrial lining at about the time the next menstrual cycle would have been expected which may cause a change in the EDC.
C. Accurate dating is important to allow for prenatal testing to be carried out at the appropriate time intervals as well as to establish the due date (EDC or EDD).
   1. Clarification of terms
      a. **Pregnancy:** 40 weeks (10 lunar months), or 280 days from LMP
      b. **Fetal calculation:** 38 weeks or 266 days from conception
   2. **Naegele's rule:** Date is estimated by adding 7 days to the first day of the LMP; then subtracting 3 months from that date to estimate the EDC.
   3. Obstetric wheels and electronic date calculators are available from many companies and online sources for calculation of EDC.
   4. A dating ultrasound with crown-rump measurements before 13 6/7 weeks of gestation is considered the most accurate technique for dating pregnancies.
      a. If an ultrasound EDC is done before 14 weeks differs from the LMP by more than 7 days, the EDC should be changed to match the ultrasound date (American College of Obstetricians and Gynecologists [ACOG], 2017).

TABLE 14.1 Signs and Symptoms of Pregnancy

SIGNS	DESCRIPTION
PRESUMPTIVE	Signs experienced by the woman that may suggest pregnancy *or* other conditions.
Cessation of menses	Uterine lining does not shed as progesterone rises. May have some spotting around the time of implantation.
Nausea, vomiting, "morning sickness"	Onset at 2 to 12 weeks of gestation; usually subsides 6 to 8 weeks later. Commonly most severe on awakening.
Frequent urination	Pressure from enlarging uterus pressing on bladder causes reduced bladder capacity.
Breast tenderness	Onset at 2 to 3 weeks of gestation; may be present throughout pregnancy. Soreness and tingling of breasts occur from hormonal stimulation and development of ducts and glands.
Perception of fetal movement, or "quickening"	Occurs at 16 to 20 weeks of gestation; should be present until delivery. A sensation of "fluttering" or motion in abdomen is perceived by the mother.
Fatigue	Common early in pregnancy; usually resolves by 20 weeks of gestation. Related to increased cardiac output.
Skin changes	Abdominal striae and increased pigmentation result from hormonal changes.
PROBABLE	Signs observable by an examiner that may suggest pregnancy or other conditions are observable by an examiner.
Enlargement of the uterus	Palpated abdominally above symphysis pubis at 12 weeks of gestation.
Hegar's sign	Occurs at 6 weeks of gestation; palpable softening of lower uterine segment.
Goodell's sign	Occurs at 8 weeks of gestation; the cervix softens (changes from consistency of the tip of the nose to that of lips).
Chadwick's sign	Occurs at 6 to 8 weeks of gestation; blue-violet hue from congestion seen on the vulva, vagina, and cervix.
Braxton–Hicks contractions	May be felt as early as end of first trimester. Irregular, painless, intermittent uterine contractions.
Pregnancy test	Test is positive 8–10 days or more after conception.
Movement	Occurs at 16–20 weeks of gestation; mother may feel movement weeks earlier but it must be verified by examiner (this is classified as a positive sign by some experts).
POSITIVE	Pregnancy is confirmed.
Ultrasound	Test shows evidence of pregnancy.
Fetal heart auscultation	Fetal heart motion detected by ultrasound at 5 weeks of or more gestation.
	Fetal heart sounds detected by Doppler by 8 to 12 weeks after conception.
Visualization of the fetus	Ultrasound can visualize fetus at 5 to 6 weeks of gestation. Ultrasound is used more frequently to establish EDC.

EDC, estimated date of confinement.

Source: American College of Obstetricians and Gynecologists (2017). Methods for estimating the due date. Committee Opinion No. 700. *Obstet Gynecol*, *129*(5), e150–4. https://doi.org/10.1097/AOG.0000000000002046

CURRENT IDENTIFYING DATA

A. These items provide general information that is current and allow the woman to answer relatively uncomplicated questions comfortably, establishing a pattern for the rest of the interview. These items should include:
1. Current name
2. Date of birth to screen for age-related complications
    a. If the woman is older than 35 years, genetic counseling should be offered.
    b. Review the risk for chromosomal abnormalities relative to maternal age (Table 14.2).
        (1) Anomalies other than aneuploidy (abnormal number of chromosomes) may be discussed
    c. Risk factors include those of chronic diseases with increased maternal age
3. **Current employment:** Screen for occupational hazards to the health of the mother and the developing fetus
4. Partner's name, if involved with patient, or support person's name
5. Partner's employment
6. **Household members:** Screen for support structure and children living in the home.
7. **Cultural background related to childbearing:** Ascertain patient preferences for care.
8. **Religion, if any:** Screen for any religious restrictions on care or nutrition, and for practices specific to childbearing.
9. Educational level

EVALUATE REACTIONS TO PREGNANCY

A. Pregnancy is the reason the patient has sought care, and it is the most important issue to the patient. It is wise to discuss early in the visit what the patient's expectations are in relation to pregnancy and to establish what care is expected. In addition, the reactions of the patient's partner and family should be explored.
B. **Feelings about pregnancy:** Whether planned or unplanned
1. Unplanned pregnancies comprise approximately 45% of all U.S. pregnancies (Finer & Zolna, 2016).
2. Risk factors for unplanned pregnancies include low socioeconomic status, substance use disorder, poor psychologic health, minority identity, being unmarried, or a history of intimate partner violence.
    a. Social support can decrease risk of unplanned pregnancy by at least 13% (Feld et al., 2021).
C. Plans for the pregnancy, including
1. To keep the baby
2. To put the baby up for adoption
3. To prevent/terminate the pregnancy; provide resources
    a. Plan B levonorgestrel (One-Step) 1.5 mg orally; Over-the-counter; taken within 72 hours of unprotected intercourse.
    b. Ulipristol (Ella) by prescription; 30 mg orally taken within 5 days of unprotected intercourse.
    c. Insert copper IUC (Paragard T-380) within 5 days of unprotected intercourse.
    d. Medical abortion with mifepristone (Mifeprex); refer to women's health provider. May be prescribed up to 70 days of pregnancy.
    e. Refer for surgical abortion (according to state law).
D. Determine if family and friends have been informed, elicit their reactions and discuss with the pregnant patient.
E. Partner's response

TABLE 14.2 Risk for Chromosomal Abnormality (at Birth) at Various Maternal Ages		
MATERNAL AGE	RISK FOR DOWN SYNDROME	TOTAL RISK FOR CHROMOSOMAL ABNORMALITIES
20	1:1,667	1:526
21	1:1,667	1:526
22	1:1,429	1:500
23	1:1,429	1:500
24	1:1,250	1:476
25	1:1,250	1:476
26	1:1,176	1:476
27	1:1,111	1:455
28	1:1,053	1:435
29	1:1,000	1:417
30	1:952	1:385
31	1:909	1:385
32	1:769	1:322
33	1:602	1:286
34	1:485	1:238
35	1:378	1:192
36	1:289	1:156
37	1:224	1:127
38	1:173	1:102
39	1:136	1:83
40	1:106	1:66
41	1:82	1:53
42	1:63	1:42
43	1:49	1:33
44	1:38	1:26
45	1:30	1:21
46	1:23	1:16
47	1:18	1:13
48	1:14	1:10
49	1:11	1:8

Note: Because sample size for some intervals is relatively small, 95% confidence limits are sometimes relatively large. Nonetheless, these figures are suitable for genetic counseling (Goetzinger et al., 2017).

CURRENT PHYSICAL SYMPTOMS

A. Include severity of symptoms, when they occurred, treatment or relief measures tried, and effectiveness of any relief measures. Table 14.3 summarizes common complaints of pregnancy and their explanation.

B. Nausea and vomiting (i.e., "morning sickness")
   1. Most common problem associated with pregnancy. Common in first trimester (80% of pregnant women); infrequent after 14 to 16 weeks of gestation. May occur any time of the day.
      a. Initial treatment for nausea and vomiting may include vitamin B_6, doxylamine, or ingestion of ginger (ACOG, 2018).

TABLE 14.3 Common Complaints During Pregnancy and Explanations

COMMON COMPLAINT	TIME IN PREGNANCY	EXPLANATION AND EFFECTS ON WOMAN'S BODY
No menses (*amenorrhea*)	Throughout	Continued high levels of estrogen, progesterone, and hCG after fertilization of the ovum allow the uterine endometrium to build up and support the developing pregnancy rather than to slough as menses.
Nausea with or without vomiting	First trimester	Possible causes include increased hCG levels or proteins, hormonal changes of pregnancy leading to slowed peristalsis throughout the gastrointestinal tract, changes in taste and smell, the growing uterus, or emotional factors. Women may have a modest (2–5 pounds) weight loss in the first trimester.
Breast tenderness, tingling	First trimester	The hormones of pregnancy stimulate the growth of breast tissue. As the breasts enlarge throughout pregnancy, women may experience upper backache from their increased weight. There is also increased blood flow throughout the breasts, increasing pressure on the tissue.
Urinary frequency (non-disease related)	First and third trimesters	There is increased blood volume and increased filtration rate in the kidneys with increased urine production. Due to less space for the bladder from pressure from the growing uterus (first trimester) or from the descent of the fetal head (third trimester), the woman needs to empty her bladder more frequently.
Fatigue	First trimester	Mechanisms are not clearly understood, but are multifactorial, including increased cardiac output.
Heartburn and constipation	Throughout	Relaxation of the lower esophageal sphincter allows stomach contents to back up into the lower esophagus. The decreased gastrointestinal motility caused by pregnancy hormones slows peristalsis and causes constipation. Constipation may cause or aggravate existing hemorrhoids.
Leukorrhea	Throughout	Increased secretions from the cervix and the vaginal epithelium due to the hormones and vasocongestion of pregnancy result in an asymptomatic milky-white vaginal discharge.
Weight loss	First trimester	If a women experiences nausea and vomiting, she may not be eating normally in early pregnancy (see Nausea previously described).
Backache (non-disease related)	Throughout, may increase in third trimester	Hormonally induced relaxation of joints and ligaments and the lordosis required to balance the growing uterus sometimes result in a lower backache. Pathologic causes must be ruled out.

hCG, human chorionic gonadotropin.

2. **Unknown cause:** Possibly related to changes in maternal hormones, proteins, or blood glucose levels.
3. Frequent and consistent vomiting, dehydration, weight loss, electrolyte imbalance, poor appetite, or food intake, or ketonuria may indicate hyperemesis gravidarum (0.5%–2% of all pregnancies).

C. Breast tenderness (mastalgia)
   1. Tenderness is related to increased levels of estrogen, progesterone, and chorionic somatomammotropin.
   2. Often, this is the first presumptive sign of pregnancy.

D. Abdominal pain or cramping
   1. May be benign or problematic. Pain is frequently associated with round ligament pain after first trimester.
   2. If present, practitioner should check for symptoms of impending miscarriage, such as preterm labor, bleeding, or for gastrointestinal disorders.

E. Vaginal discharge or bleeding
   1. Discharge may be normal or may indicate genital tract infection (sexually transmitted infections [STIs] or non-infectious vaginitis such as bacterial vaginosis [BV], or vulvovaginal candidiasis [VVC]).
   2. Spotting may be normal indicating implantation of the blastocyst, resulting from invasive chorionic villi activity in the uterine lining. Spotting may occur at approximately the time a woman would have been expecting her menses if she was not pregnant.
   3. Heavy bleeding in pregnancy is abnormal and must be evaluated further.
      a. If in the primary care setting, refer to emergency department and/or ObGyn practitioner ASAP.
      b. Obtain complete blood count (CBC), type and Rh factor, and a quantitative hCG level for later comparison.
      c. Obtain a sonogram because there is always a chance some products of conception may not have passed.
      d. If Rh negative, administer Rhogam within 72 hours of bleeding.
      e. Refer to OB/GYN practitioner for follow-up.

F. Urinary frequency associated with pregnancy
   1. Frequency may be normal due to uterine position in relation to maternal bladder in the first and third trimesters.
   2. If urination is accompanied by dysuria, it may indicate a urinary tract infection (Ailes, Summers, Tran, Gilboa, Arnold, Meaney-Delman, & Reefhuis, 2018).

G. **Headache:** Monitor for preeclampsia if persistent or after the 20th week of pregnancy.

H. **Nosebleeds:** If mild, may be considered normal; related to increased vascularity of nasal mucosa.

I. Fatigue
   1. Very common in first trimester, related to increased cardiac output.
   2. Provide reassurance that fatigue will lessen as the pregnancy progresses.

J. Heartburn
   1. Common in pregnancy, typically increases in intensity late in pregnancy
   2. Related to increased pressure in abdomen and softening of pyloric sphincter
      a. May be a warning sign of pregnancy-induced hypertension (PIH) or hemolysis, elevated liver enzymes, low platelets counts (HELLP) syndrome so this must be carefully evaluated.

K. Back pain
   1. Common

2. Should discuss relief measures, such as a good support bra, support bands for abdomen, warm soaks, erect posture, and massage if no disease is noted during examination, gentle stretching.

L. Quickening, if present (patient's first awareness of fetal movement)
   1. Assists in dating pregnancy.
   2. Quickening is usually not felt until approximately 16 to 22 weeks of gestation.
      a. Although there is some variability, quickening is typically felt later in first pregnancies and earlier in subsequent pregnancies; Bryant et al., 2021).

M. Normal skin changes may include
   1. Darkening of the areola
   2. Linea nigra (darkened, vertical line mid-abdomen)
   3. Chloasma (darkened areas on face)
   4. Breast and abdominal striae from stretching of skin

N. Ptyalism (excessive salivation)
   1. May occur with nausea and vomiting in early pregnancy or with hyperemesis gravidarum.
   2. Reassure the patient that the problem is distressing, but not indicative of poor outcomes.
   3. Attempts at treatment are largely unsuccessful, although patient should try remedies for nausea.
   4. Will resolve spontaneously usually at end of first trimester but may continue until delivery (Thaxter Nesbeth et al., 2016).

O. Absence of menses

P. Constipation
   1. Common; 11% to 38% of pregnant women are affected.
   2. Related to low-fiber diet and/or inadequate fluid intake. Also, may be precipitated by progesterone-induced suppression of bowel motility and compression of the intestine from the enlarging uterus.
   3. Hemorrhoids are common in pregnancy and are aggravated by constipation (Kuronen et al., 2021).

HISTORY OF POSSIBLE EXPOSURES SINCE CONCEPTION

A. Screen for exposure to medications or other substances that may increase risk of adverse pregnancy outcomes for the pregnant woman and/or her baby including anomalies or miscarriages.

B. Radiation exposure, including x-ray studies (even dental) without use of a shield (lead shields are usually routinely used on women of childbearing age)

C. Viral exposure
   1. Effects of viral exposure during pregnancy vary with the specific viral type, the gestational age of the fetus at exposure, and the risks to the mother. Information on viral exposures in pregnancy is evolving rapidly. Check the Centers for Disease Control and Prevention (CDC), World Health Organization (WHO), and National Institutes of Health (NIH) websites for up-to-date information and reportable status of possible or confirmed viral exposures.
      a. Among the viruses of concern in pregnancy include exposure to Zika, HIV, rubella, rubeola, influenza, herpes simplex virus (HSV), parvovirus B19 (Fifth's disease), mumps, and SARS-CoV-2 (COVID-19; CDC, 2016, 2021a).
   2. Other "childhood illnesses" the woman has been exposed to since conception or illnesses since conception.
      a. Infection in pregnancy may cause various complications or be entirely benign.

D. Fever
   1. Evaluate for date and approximate time of onset of fever and how high temperature is/has been.

2. Febrile episodes may provide a clue to first-trimester exposure to diseases that may affect pregnancy such as rubella, toxoplasmosis (from cat litter), Fifth's disease (human parvovirus B-19), or COVID-19 and the need for laboratory work to confirm exposure (CDC, 2021a).

E. Medications used since conception
   1. Inquire about the use of
      a. Over-the-counter medications
      b. Home remedies and herbal preparations
      c. Prescribed medications
      d. Progesterone in infertility patients
      e. Vitamins, folic acid, or mineral supplements, particularly calcium and iron
   2. A revised drug-labeling system for pregnancy was drafted in 2020 by the U.S. Department of Health and Human Services (DHHS) Food and Drug Administration, and includes three categories: "Pregnancy," "Lactation," and "Females and Males of Reproductive Potential."
      a. All medications taken by the pregnant person should be evaluated by the examiner in current drug references and registries to determine the individual patient's response and the expected effect on pregnancy.

F. Recalled or documented pre-gravid weight and weight gain since onset of pregnancy
   1. Overweight and obesity may be related to pregnancy complications, including higher risks of hypertension, diabetes, fetal macrosomia, fetal demise, and labor and delivery complications (Vernini et al., 2016).
   2. Underweight women may be at higher risk for preterm labor and small for gestational age infants.

MEDICAL HISTORY

A. Include diseases or conditions that could affect the woman's health or fetal well-being during pregnancy.

B. **Diabetes:** Correlates with an increased risk for multiple maternal and fetal complications, such as preterm labor, infectious illnesses, hydramnios and hypertension (maternal), congenital anomalies, fetal macrosomia, intrauterine fetal death, delayed fetal pulmonary maturation, and metabolic abnormalities.
   1. Diabetes (of any type) in pregnancy necessitates close monitoring and management, sometimes in consultation with a specialist.
   2. Screening is recommended for all pregnant women during initial history. Further screening is recommended between 24- and 28-weeks of gestation, with initial laboratory work for diabetes with 1 hour, 50-g glucola test. Testing should be done earlier if indicated by history of gestational diabetes or high-risk factors, such as morbid obesity.
      a. Detailed information on screening can be found on the U.S. Preventive Services Task Force (USPSTF) website found at: https://www.uspreventiveservicestaskforce.org/uspstf/recommendation/gestational-diabetes-screening#fullrecommendationstart
   3. Consider types of diabetes identified during pregnancy.
      a. **Insulin dependent:** Should assess age at onset and amount and type of insulin used; refer patient promptly for insulin management and close monitoring, including nutritional counseling.
      b. **Noninsulin dependent:** Refer patient promptly for management plan for close monitoring of serum glucose levels, possible use of oral hypoglycemics or insulin, and to a nutritionist for dietary counseling.
      c. **Gestational diabetes:** Diabetes during pregnancy. Higher risk for mother and fetus for diabetes later in life. Refer patient promptly for management plan for close monitoring of serum glucose levels, possible use of oral hypoglycemics or insulin, and nutritionist for dietary counseling (Randall et al., 2021; USPTFS, 2021).

C. **Hypertension:** Rates have increased markedly over the past 15 years. Consult and refer as needed.
 1. Categories include chronic hypertension, gestational hypertension, chronic hypertension with superimposed preeclampsia, preeclampsia with or without severe features, eclampsia, and postpartum hypertension.
 2. For all categories, assess for method of control including dietary and lifestyle changes and for use of antihypertensive medication.
 3. For all categories, consult or refer due to increased risks to current pregnancy.

D. Cardiac disease
 1. Functional murmurs during pregnancy are usually benign.
 2. Consultation is necessary for evaluation and possible management of suspected valvular disorders and other cardiac diseases.

E. Liver disease
 1. Assess risk factors for hepatitis and screen with blood testing as needed. Infants may require treatment with immunoglobulins soon after delivery if hepatitis is present.

F. Renal disease
 1. Urinary tract infections, including asymptomatic bacteriuria, urethritis, or cystitis, can be managed with appropriate antibiotics.
 a. Urine culture is recommended at the initiation of prenatal care to screen for asymptomatic bacteriuria.
 b. Urine culture is recommended for all suspected types of urinary tract infections in pregnant patients.
 c. Persistent or repetitive (chronic, recurrent, or refractory) urinary tract infections, pyelonephritis, or other renal diseases require referral for management (Ailes et al., 2018).

G. **Gallbladder disease:** Can be exacerbated in pregnancy.
 1. Counsel patient to eat a low-fat diet and refer as needed.

H. Stomach or bowel disease
 1. If abdominal surgery was performed, note type of surgery and location of any scarring.
 2. Consult a specialist because gastrointestinal conditions (such as cholestasis or inflammatory bowel disease) could cause deleterious effects during the antepartum or intrapartum period.

I. Pulmonary disease
 1. If asthma is present, assess which medications or inhalers the patient currently uses and frequency of use.
 2. Assess current and recent status of asthma (mild, intermittent, severe).
 3. If pulmonary disease is present, evaluate early with consultation because of possibly needing anesthesia in labor.

J. **Congenital anomalies and genetic diseases:** Must screen for risk to patient and fetus during pregnancy and labor.

K. Cancer
 1. If cancer of the cervix is treated with cone biopsy or LEEP (loop electrosurgical excision procedure), the patient is at increased risk for preterm labor. Refer or manage with OB/GYN practitioner.

L. Genitourinary tract diseases

M. **Varicosities and phlebitis:** May worsen during pregnancy.

N. Anemia
 1. Inquire about sickle cell disease and sickle cell trait as well as thalassemia.
 2. Screen with initial laboratory work, mid-pregnancy and more often as indicated.

O. Infectious diseases
 1. **Hepatitis:** Assess for type and current status.

2. Tuberculosis
3. HIV infection
    a. Inquire about history of high-risk sexual behaviors or IV drug use.
    b. Rate of transmission of HIV with retrovirals is approximately 2%.
4. Syphilis (increasing since the mid-2000s)
5. COVID (possible increased risk of miscarriage)

P. Autoimmune disorders
1. Increased rate of miscarriage in women with systemic lupus erythematosus (SLE)

Q. Neurologic disorders or any neurologic defects

R. Psychiatric disorders
1. Screen for risk factors for postpartum depression including current or past history of anxiety, depression, or other mental health issues, physical or sexual abuse, traumatic pregnancy or labor, substance use disorder, poor social support, low socioeconomic status, suicidal ideation, or eating disorders.

S. Multifetal gestation

T. Genetic diseases including anemias

U. **Allergies:** Document reaction.

OBSTETRIC AND GYNECOLOGIC HISTORY

A. Gynecologic
1. Abnormal uterine bleeding
2. History of sexually transmitted infections (STIs) in patient and/or partner
    a. STIs include human papillomavirus (HPV), herpes simplex virus (HSV), HIV, chlamydia, gonorrhea, *Trichomonas*, syphilis, and hepatitis (CDC, 2021).
    b. Note test of cures with dates, if done.
    c. Any long-term sequelae
3. Contraception
    a. Types ever used
    b. Most recently used method
    c. When contraception was most recently used
    d. If patient became pregnant while actively using contraception, the examiner may need to discuss any effects of contraceptive method on pregnancy.
4. **Gynecologic surgery:** List date, procedure, and reason for procedure or surgery.

B. Infertility treatments performed
1. Previous attempts at pregnancy, including timed intercourse
2. Include current or continuing infertility treatments, including assisted reproductive technologies (ARTs).

C. Past pregnancy history
1. Written as
    a. **Gravida:** Number of total pregnancies
    b. **Para:** Number of specific type of births (Box 14.1)
2. Include
    a. Abortions
    b. Miscarriages, ectopic, and molar pregnancies
    c. Preterm deliveries
    d. Number of living children and their current health
    e. Multifetal gestations
    f. Complications with pregnancy, labor, or delivery
    g. Cesarean deliveries

BOX 14.1 *Terminology of Pregnancy*

Gravida: Refers to the number of times a woman has been pregnant, regardless of the outcome of the pregnancy or the number of babies born from the pregnancy.

Parity: Technically means the number of pregnancies that ended with the birth of a viable fetus. In practice, used as a system of digits describing the outcome of pregnancies.

First digit: Number of term babies (>37 weeks of gestation or 2,500 g) delivered

Second digit: Number of preterm babies delivered (28–36 weeks of gestation or 1,000–2,499 g)

Third digit: Number of pregnancies ending in spontaneous or elective abortion or molar pregnancies

Fourth digit: Number of currently living children

Example: If a woman is currently pregnant and has one living child born at term, she is listed as G2 P1001.

SURGICAL HISTORY

A. Include past surgeries, types of anesthesia, and any complications.
1. List all surgical procedures. Include:
   a. Abdominal or pelvic surgeries that could affect pregnancy or delivery
   b. Scarring
   c. Complications
B. Other hospitalizations
C. Types of anesthesia ever received and any reactions
D. Blood transfusions
E. Accidents that caused injuries that may affect the woman's ability to labor or deliver

GENERAL HEALTH AND NUTRITION

A. Exercise (Box 14.2 lists recommendations)
1. Discuss amount and type currently practiced.
2. Use opportunity to discuss and encourage moderate, regular exercise during pregnancy
   a. National recommendations include 150 minutes of moderate intensity exercise per week. Examples include walking, cycling, swimming, or prenatal yoga.
B. Diet
1. Inquire about current special diet requirements.
   a. Lactose-free, gluten-free, or other intolerances
   b. Vegetarian (specify type)
   c. Food allergies
2. Check for calcium intake, and recommend supplementation as needed.
   a. Current recommendations for calcium intake are 1,000 mg daily for pregnant women over age 18 and 1,300 mg daily for pregnant women ages 14 to 18 (NIH, 2021).
   b. Adequate calcium can prevent calf cramps later in pregnancy.
3. Encourage appropriate weight gain considering woman's age, pre-pregnancy weight, and health status.
   a. Evaluate pre-pregnancy weight using standardized measure (e.g., BMI or ideal body weight [IBW]). Normal-weight women should gain 25 to 35 pounds during the course of the pregnancy; less if overweight and more if underweight at the onset of pregnancy.

> **BOX 14.2 Recommendations Relating to Exercise During Pregnancy (ACOG Committee Opinion, 2021)**
>
> - Consult with provider about current or new exercise program.
> - Avoid high-risk and high-impact sports and activities.
> - Regular, moderate exercise most days of the week is recommended.
> - If a woman is exercising regularly, maintaining current levels of exercise in pregnancy as tolerated is considered to be safe in pregnancy.
> - Wear supportive bra and shoes.
> - Exercise of any kind should not be fatiguing and should be combined with periods of rest.
> - Drink liquids before and after exercise to avoid dehydration.
> - Avoid vigorous exercise in hot weather to prevent hyperthermia.
> - Stop activity and consult provider if symptoms occur (palpitations, shortness of breath, dizziness, abdominal pain, bleeding, numbness and tingling, no fetal movement).
> - See Box 14.2 for exercise recommendations in pregnancy.
> - Avoid sitting or standing for long periods.

    b. The average additional caloric consumption to a normal diet during pregnancy is approximately 300 calories per day for women with a normal BMI at the onset of pregnancy (Marshall et al., 2019).

4. Folate
   a. For normal-weight pregnant women, the CDC recommends 0.4 mg (400 mcg) of folic acid per day during the first trimester for prevention of neural tube defects.
   b. The CDC recommends all women of reproductive age take 0.4 mg of folic acid daily to decrease the risk of neural tube defects and anencephaly in planned or unplanned pregnancies.
5. **Iron:** Evaluate hemoglobin and hematocrit levels. If iron-deficiency anemia is present, the pregnant person should supplement with 30 to 120 g/day. Not routinely recommended at onset of pregnancy unless anemic (ACOG, 2021).
   a. No specific formulation of iron supplements is recommended, and providers or patients may consider cost in choosing a ferrous supplement.

SOCIAL HISTORY

A. **Substance use disorder:** Screen for past and current use, including amount and frequency and dates of most recent use.
   1. **Use of any of the following is not recommended during pregnancy:** Tobacco (including vaping), alcohol, or use of non-prescribed substances.
   2. Inquire about amount, type, and pattern of use of
      a. Tobacco including smoking cigarettes or pipes or vaping
      b. Alcohol
      c. Non-prescription substances
   3. If patient has a substance use disorder, brief intervention techniques utilizing motivational interviewing and referral to an appropriate treatment or counseling center should be considered.
B. Physical abuse (see Chapter 35, "Intimate Partner Violence")
   1. Current and/or past
   2. Counseling received in past

3. Encourage patient to assess current safety and refer to counseling or local agencies as needed.
   a. Abuse may intensify during pregnancy.
4. Help patient develop a safety plan.

C. Financial stressors
1. Does patient have insurance coverage or private means to pay for pregnancy? If not, refer to social worker, financial aid worker, Medicaid, or local funding organizations as needed.
2. Does patient have housing and adequate food during and after pregnancy? If not, refer to Women, Infants, and Children (WIC); social services; or local agencies as needed.

D. Social support system
1. Family or friends whom the patient can rely on during her pregnancy and after delivery

E. Patient's plans for pregnancy and postpartum recovery
1. Does patient plan to attend prenatal classes?
2. What contraceptive method is patient planning after delivery?
   a. If patient plans sterilization, does patient meet criteria within state and/or institution?
3. Does patient plan to breastfeed or bottle feed the baby?
   a. If patient plans to bottle feed, is she aware of the benefits of breastfeeding?

FAMILY HISTORY

A. Used for screening for potential physical and emotional complications of pregnancy and familial patterns of health or illness. Document relationship to patient and type of condition, if known.
1. Diabetes
2. Hypertension or gestational hypertension
3. Heart disease
4. Renal disease
5. Cancer, including primary site, if known
6. Anemia
7. Other blood disorders
8. Infectious diseases; screen for patient exposure or immunization
9. Neurologic disorders
10. Psychiatric disorders
11. Congenital anomalies
12. Genetic diseases
13. Multifetal gestations or births

PHYSICAL EXAMINATION

A. A complete physical examination should be performed, including breast, abdominal, and pelvic examinations.
B. Explain to the patient what provider will be doing and what the patient may expect to feel during the examination.
C. Baseline vital signs including blood pressure, height, weight, and BMI. These will serve as baseline measurements throughout the pregnancy.
D. Breast examination (see Chapter 9, "Assessment of the Female Breast"). In addition to routine observation and palpation, the examination should include a check of the nipples' ability to evert with a gentle squeeze of the areola, to predict eversion of nipples during breastfeeding.
E. The abdominal examination should include:
1. Notation of any abdominal scarring

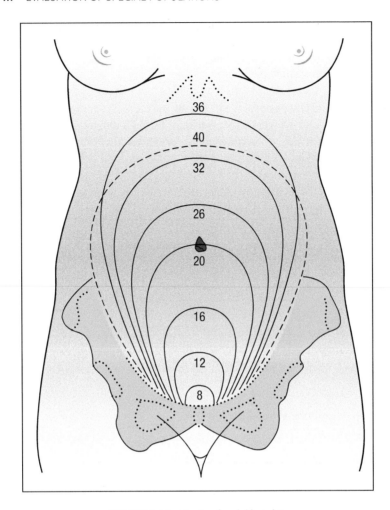

FIGURE 14.1 Uterine fundal height.

2. Estimation of size and position of the uterus
3. If fundus is palpable, fundal height in centimeters from the symphysis pubis to the top of the fundus should be noted (Figure 14.1)
4. Assessment of fetal heart tones; can be auscultated using Doppler ultrasonography or fetoscope.
    a. It is possible to assess fetal heart tones by 10 weeks of gestation with Doppler or with fetoscope by 20 weeks of gestation.
    b. Normal fetal heart rate averages 110 to 160 beats per minute.
    c. Maternal heart rate during pregnancy averages 91 to 92 beats/minute (Green et al., 2020).
5. Assess for gradual uterine and abdominal enlargement.
    a. Fundus should reach top of symphysis at 10 weeks, umbilicus at 20 weeks, then measure approximately the same number of centimeters, at weeks of gestation between 20 and 35 weeks.
F. **Pelvic examination (see Chapter 5, "The Physical Examination"):** In addition to a routine pelvic examination, evaluate:

1. **Cervical position, length, and any dilation:** Dilation or effacement (thinning of the cervical length) is abnormal until late in the third trimester.
2. Uterine size should be estimated with bimanual examination, noting congruence with LMP to estimate the current gestational age.
   a. If incongruence of size and dates is noted, ultrasonography should be considered to modify due date as needed and to assess fetal viability.
3. The adnexa should be gently palpated for tenderness or enlargement to screen for ectopic pregnancy. If fullness is noted, do not palpate too deeply as this may precipitate rupture of an ectopic pregnancy.
   a. Ectopic pregnancy occurs when the fertilized ovum is implanted outside the uterus, usually in the fallopian tube.
   b. Symptoms of ectopic pregnancy are initially those of a normal pregnancy. Further symptoms may be vague or pronounced. They may include:
      (1) Lower left or right quadrant abdominal pain
      (2) Vaginal spotting or bleeding
      (3) Syncopal symptoms (related to blood loss)
      (4) Adnexal fullness and/or tenderness
      (5) Enlarged uterus
      (6) Diarrhea
      (7) Neck or shoulder pain with rupture
   c. To confirm diagnosis, obtain a STAT quantitative baseline serum hCG and a STAT transvaginal ultrasound.
   d. Obtain OB/GYN consultation immediately if ectopic pregnancy is suspected.
   e. Treatment may be medical (methotrexate) or surgical.
   f. Risk factors are usually related to conditions that affect the lumen of the fallopian tubes or uterine cavity (Box 14.3).
4. The bony pelvis should be evaluated during bimanual examination, including:
   a. Diagonal conjugate
   b. Sacral shape
   c. Prominence of the ischial spines
   d. Coccyx mobility
   e. Angle of the pubic arch
   f. Diameter of the ischial tuberosities
5. **Chadwick's, Goodell's, and Hegar's signs:** No longer considered necessary in the diagnosis of pregnancy; however, examiners may still note:
   a. **Chadwick's sign:** A bluish color of the cervix, vagina, and vulva
      (1) Caused by increased vascularity in pregnancy at 6 to 8 weeks of gestation
   b. **Goodell's sign:** Mild softening of the cervix from the nonpregnant state
      (1) May be evident at approximately 7 to 8 weeks' gestation
   c. **Hegar's sign:** Softening and compressibility of the lower uterine segment

---

BOX 14.3 Risk Factors for Ectopic Pregnancy

- Prior tubal pregnancy
- Tubal surgery such as reversal of tubal ligation
- Pelvic inflammatory disease in which the tubes become scarred
- Endometriosis
- Intrauterine device

LABORATORY TESTS

A. Routine testing is performed to identify pregnancies at risk more clearly and to provide an opportunity to prevent problems.

B. Blood type and Rh factor
1. If patient is Rh negative and partner is Rh positive, Rh incompatibility may result.
   a. The patient should be advised that RhoGAM will likely be administered during the pregnancy within 72 hours of exposure to Rh positive blood, typically at 28 weeks, and after delivery if the baby is Rh positive.
2. If the patient's blood type is O and the partner is A, B, or AB, there may be ABO incompatibility.

C. Antibody screen (serology)
1. Antibodies are formed from major or minor blood group antigens.
2. If the test yields positive results, the antibody should be identified, and a titer should be performed.
3. Screening should be repeated at 28 weeks of gestation in the Rh-negative pregnant patient.
4. RhoGAM is usually given to prevent antibody formation in Rh negative, antibody negative pregnant patients at approximately 28 weeks of gestation or with any bleeding.

D. Complete blood count (CBC) with differential smear
1. Hemoglobin and hematocrit
   a. Blood volume increases from 30% to 50% during pregnancy, with plasma volume increasing (hemodilution) more than red blood cell (RBC) volume.
   b. A decrease in hemoglobin and hematocrit levels is normal during pregnancy.
   c. Mild anemia during pregnancy is defined as less than 11 g/dL hemoglobin; severe anemia is defined as less than 9 g/dL.
   d. Anemia during pregnancy is usually iron-deficiency anemia; however, other types may coexist.
   e. Diagnosis of anemia varies by trimester as it affects hemoglobin (Hgb) and hematocrit (Hct).
      (1) **First trimester:** Hgb <11 g/dL, Hct <33%
      (2) **Second trimester:** Hgb <10.5 g/dL and Hct <32%
      (3) **Third trimester:** Hgb <11 g/dL, Hct <33%
   f. Iron-deficiency anemia should be treated using iron supplements; severe anemia should be evaluated further, with referral as needed (ACOG, 2021).
2. A platelet count should be performed to detect thrombocytopenia.
3. **Leukocytes:** To screen for leukemia and infection. Pregnancy values may normally reach 17,000 leucocytes. RBCs and indices are used to diagnose various types of anemia.
4. The differential is used to identify types of leukocytes, erythrocytes, cell abnormalities, and platelets.

E. Rubella titer to indicate immune status for rubella

F. Serology
1. The Venereal Disease Research Laboratory (VDRL) test is usually used as a screening test for syphilis; if the test result is positive, a fluorescent treponemal antibody (FTA) test is performed to confirm diagnosis.
2. Parenteral penicillin is the only recommended treatment for syphilis during pregnancy. Dosage is dependent on stage of infection and complicating factors (CDC, 2021).

G. Hepatitis B surface antigen (HBsAg)
1. If the test is positive, the infant will require immunoprophylaxis at delivery.
2. Hepatitis B vaccination is indicated in pregnancy if HBsAg is negative.

3. Hepatitis C surface antigen; repeated at 28 weeks of gestation, along with hemoglobin and hematocrit (H/H), hepatitis B, HIV, and diagnostic medical sonography (DMS).

H. HIV screening
   1. Recommend testing for all pregnant women as early as possible in pregnancy.
   2. Treatment for HIV can substantially lower transmission to infants of infected women from 15% to 20% to less than 2%. All pregnant women with HIV should be referred for treatment during pregnancy.
   3. Breastfeeding is not recommended in HIV-positive women because of the risk of transmission through breast milk.

I. Other screening to be considered for patients at risk
   1. Urinalysis to screen for asymptomatic kidney or bladder infections (see Chapter 47, "Urinalysis and Urinary Tract Infections")
      a. The presence of bacteria, leukocytes, and erythrocytes may indicate infection.
      b. The presence of white blood cell (WBC) casts and/or RBCs may indicate pyelonephritis.
      c. Urine glucose level may be normal due to the increased glomerular filtration rate, or may be elevated, indicating possible increased risk of diabetes. If a second test result is positive, obtain blood glucose testing to screen for overt or gestational diabetes.
      d. **Protein:** Value greater than 1+ is abnormal and may be related to urinary tract infection, pregnancy-induced hypertension, or kidney disease.
   2. Sickle cell preparation or hemoglobin electrophoresis for sickle cell trait, thalassemia, or other hemoglobinopathy as indicated by history
   3. Tay–Sachs or other genetic screening for couples at risk (ACOG, 2016)
   4. Toxoplasmosis screening should be considered if the woman is exposed to cat feces, undercooked meat, or unwashed vegetables from contaminated soil.
      a. Pregnant patients should be warned not to change cat litter or work in the garden without gloves during pregnancy because of risk of toxoplasmosis. All fresh produce should be thoroughly washed, and meat should be well cooked.
   5. Cytomegalovirus screening with known exposure
   6. Tuberculosis testing
   7. Thyroid screening with thyroid-stimulating hormone (TSH) test, if symptoms are present or as indicated

J. Cervical cancer screening and STI testing
   1. Cervical cancer screening
      a. All patients should receive a cervical cancer screening test with hrHPV at age 25, then at 5-year intervals (if the tests are negative) according to the 2020 American Cancer Society screening guidelines (see Chapter 45, "Cervical Cancer Screening and Colposcopy").
   2. STI screening/testing
      a. The 2021 CDC STI screening guidelines in pregnancy recommend the following tests:
         (1) **First trimester:** Syphilis, HIV, hepatitis B and C (HCV), chlamydia and gonorrhea, if under 25 or at increased risk
         (2) **Third trimester:** Syphilis, HIV, chlamydia and gonorrhea, if under 25 or at increased risk
      b. Chlamydial infection necessitates treatment during pregnancy.
      c. If the results are positive, treat per current 2021 CDC STI treatment guidelines.
         (1) Current recommendation for treatment during pregnancy is azithromycin 1 g orally in a single dose. Alternatively, amoxicillin 500 mg orally three times per day for 7 days may be used (CDC, 2021).
      d. Repeat culture should be considered in third trimester if possibility of reinfection exists.
   3. Gonorrhea culture
      a. Gonorrheal infection requires treatment during pregnancy.
      b. If the results are positive, treat per the 2021 CDC STI treatment guidelines.

       (1) Current recommendation for treatment is ceftriaxone 500 mg IM in a single dose, if <150 kg = 330 lb. If ≥ 150 kg = 330 lb give ceftriaxone 1 g IM in a single dose. If chlamydia cannot be ruled out, give doxycycline 100 mg PO bid times 7 days. If ceftriaxone cannot be used and alternative treatment is needed, consult the 2021 CDC STI guidelines (CDC, 2021).

     c. Repeat culture should be considered during third trimester if possibility of reinfection exists (CDC, 2021).

   4. **Bacterial vaginosis:** If a patient is symptomatic and there is a positive wet mount/diagnostic test, treat the condition; treatment may lower incidence of preterm labor.

     a. Current recommendation for treatment includes metronidazole 500 mg orally two times each day for 7 days, or 1 applicator of metronidazole gel 0.75% intravaginally once daily for 5 days, or clindamycin cream 2% one full applicator (5 g) intravaginally at bedtime × 7 days (CDC, 2021).

     b. For alternative treatments, consult the 2021 CDC STI treatment guidelines.

   5. Herpes simplex virus (HSV)

     a. Women should be questioned regarding history of HSV and, if history is positive, should be asked about prodromal symptoms and symptoms of outbreaks.

     b. Testing is necessary only to confirm the diagnosis of active herpes.

     c. Vaginal delivery is preferred if the woman has no prodromal symptoms and no lesions are visible at the onset of labor. If active lesions are present, cesarean section is the preferred mode of delivery.

     d. Risk to neonate is high if woman acquires genital herpes close to the time of delivery, and low in women who have a history of recurrent herpes or who acquire the infection in the first trimester.

     e. Women should avoid any sexual contact with partners with known or suspected herpes during the third trimester.

     f. Suppression therapy may be recommended for women with history of HSV to decrease the risk of outbreaks at term to help avoid cesarean delivery starting at 36 weeks of gestation. Treatment recommendations are acyclovir 400 mg orally three times daily or valacyclovir 500 mg orally twice daily (CDC, 2021).

   6. Group B *Streptococcus* infection

     a. Screening recommended for all pregnant women at 35 to 37 weeks of gestation. Separate samples should be taken from the vagina and rectum.

     b. Treatment of choice is IV penicillin administered during labor. Susceptibility testing should be done on specimens from patients with known penicillin allergy.

   7. *Trichomoniasis*

     a. Wet mount, culture, or commercial test

     b. Current 2021 CDC recommendation for treatment is 500 mg metronidazole two times daily for 7 days (CDC, 2021).

   8. *Vulvovaginal candidiasis* infection

     a. Infections tend to be more frequent during pregnancy due to high estrogen levels causing increased vaginal production of glycogen.

     b. Topical or vaginal azoles are the only recommended treatment options during pregnancy. These include terconazole, tioconazole, miconazole, and clotrimazole. Medications that should not be used during pregnancy include fluconazole and butoconazole (CDC, 2021).

K. Other antenatal screening

   1. Use of ultrasonography

     a. Recommended for dating if unknown LMP or if there is a size/date discrepancy

     b. **Routine screening:** Frequently done at 16 to 19 weeks of gestation

       (1) May be combined with other antenatal testing.

  c. Used to identify anomalies or complications of pregnancy such as:
   (1) Multiple gestations
   (2) Molar pregnancy
   (3) Fetal anomalies
   (4) Maternal anomalies
   (5) Placenta previa
 2. Amniocentesis or other antenatal testing
  a. Amniocentesis should be performed between 15 and 19 weeks of gestation when indicated for screening of genetic abnormalities (ACOG, 2016; Goetzinger et al., 2017).
  b. Chorionic villus sampling between 10 and 13 weeks of gestation is offered when indicated for screening for genetic abnormalities when earlier results are desirable (ACOG, 2016; Goetzinger et al., 2017).
  c. The maternal serum AFP screen is performed between 15 and 22 weeks of gestation, most commonly from 16 to 18 weeks of gestation, as a screen to detect:
   (1) Neural tube defects
   (2) Selected genetic abnormalities such as Down syndrome (Goetzinger et al., 2017)
   (3) Various other defects (ACOG, 2016)
 3. **Cell-free DNA (cfDNA) and carrier screening (serology):** This testing may be offered from 10 weeks of gestation through the end of the pregnancy for women who may be at high risk for trisomy 13, 18, or 21. If positive, offer genetic counseling and referral to maternal fetal medicine for possible advanced testing.
  a. Limited sharing of public information by company; may have false-positive or false-negative results and should be offered cautiously. Despite these limitations, some practices are offering this screening to all pregnant patients.
  b. Limited utility for multifetal gestations, if patient BMI >30, or if patient is pregnant with donor egg or as gestational carrier.
  c. Ethical concerns about the genotyping of samples with potential compromise of the genetic privacy of the fetus and the birthing parent (Parobek et al., 2021)
L. Table 14.4 summarizes common laboratory tests, indicating changes with pregnancy and timing of the test.

PLANNING AN INITIAL VISIT

A. Most patients in the United States expect to be prescribed vitamins regardless of nutritional status, although utility is somewhat controversial. Prenatal vitamins are available over the counter or by prescription and for the normal pregnant woman should contain 0.4 mg of folic acid.

B. Laboratory tests should be ordered and testing necessary in first or early second trimesters should be discussed and arranged.

C. Nutrition should be discussed or refer to a nutritional service/dietician, as needed.

D. Consultation should be arranged as needed for physical or emotional problems discovered during the visit, and the patient should be referred to social services or for medical consultation as needed as soon as any issues are identified.

E. The patient should be referred for OB/GYN consultation if she is not within normal limits in any aspect of her medical, gynecologic, or obstetrical status.

F. The patient should be screened briefly with questions listed in Box 14.4 and instructed to return:

TABLE 14.4 Common Laboratory Values in Pregnancy

TEST	NORMAL RANGE (NONPREGNANT)	CHANGE IN PREGNANCY	TIMING
		SERUM CHEMISTRIES	
Albumin	3.5–4.8 g/dL	↓ 1 g/dL	Most by 20 weeks, then gradual
Calcium (total)	9–10.3 mg/dL	↓ 10%	Gradual decrease
Chloride	95–105 mEq/L	No significant change	Gradual increase
Creatinine (female)	0.6–1.1 mg/dL	↓ 0.3 mg/dL	Most by 20 weeks
Fibrinogen	1.5–3.6 g/L	↑ 1–2 g/L	Progressive
Glucose, fasting (plasma)	65–105 mg/dL	↓ 10%	Gradual decrease
Potassium (plasma)	3.5–4.5 mEq/L	↓ 0.2–0.3 mEq/L	By 20 weeks
Protein (total)	6.5 d >8.5 g/dL	↓ g/dL	By 20 weeks, then stable
Sodium	135–145 mEq/L	↓ 2–4 mEq/L	By 20 weeks, then stable
Urea nitrogen	12–30 mg/dL	↓ 50%	First trimester
Uric acid	3.5–8 mg/dL	↓ 33%	First trimester, increase at term
		URINARY CHEMISTRIES	
Creatinine	15–25 mg/kg/d (1–1.4 g/day)	No significant change	
Protein	Up to 150 mg/day	Up to 250–300 mg/day	By 20 weeks
Creatinine clearance	90–130 mL/min/1.73 m^2	40%–50%	By 16 weeks
		SERUM ENZYMATIC ACTIVITIES	
Amylase	23–84 IU/L	↑ 50%–100%	Controversial
Transaminase	5–35 mU/dL	No significant change	Glutamic pyruvic (SGPT)
Glutamic oxaloacetic (SGOT)	5–40 mU/dL	No significant change	
Hematocrit (female)	36%–46%	↓ 4%–7%	Lowest values at 30–34 weeks
Hemoglobin (female)	12–16 g/dL	↓ 1.5–2 g/dL	Lowest values at 30–34 weeks
Leukocyte count	4.8–10.8 × 10^3/mm^3	↑ 3.5 × 10^3/mm^3	Gradual
Platelet count	150–400 × 10^3/mm^3	Slight decrease	
Erythrocyte count	4.0–5.0 × 10^6/mm^3	↑ 25%–30%	Begins at 6–8 weeks
		SERUM HORMONE VALUES	
Coritsol (plasma)	8–21 mcg/dL	↑ 20 mcg/dL	Peaks at 28–32 weeks, then constant to term
Prolactin (female)	25 ng/dL	↑ 50–400 ng/dL	Gradual, peaks at term
Thyroxine, total (T_4)	5–11 g/dL	↑ 5 mg/dL	Early sustained
Triiodothyronine, total (T_3)	125–245 ng/dL	↑ 50%	Early sustained SGOT, serum glutamic–oxaloacetic transaminase; SGPT, serum glutamic pyruvic transaminase

BOX 14.4 Questions to Ask at Each Subsequent Prenatal Visit

Since Your Last Visit Have You Had Problems With:

Physical symptoms, such as:
- Headaches
- Eyes (blurred vision, blind spots, flashing lights or lines)
- Swelling of face
- Swelling of hands
- Swelling of legs or feet
- Pain in your chest
- Pain in your back
- Pain in your abdomen
- Urination (burning or pain)
- Leaking urine
- Not being able to wait to use the toilet
- Bleeding or spotting from vagina
- Leaking fluid from your vagina (watery)
- Vaginal discharge or change in discharge
- Vaginal burning, itching, or bad smell
- Increase in sores or growths in genital area
- Illnesses or fever
- Exposure to sick children or adults

Signs of labor, such as:
- Contractions
- Cramping
- Pelvic pressure
- Low backache

Any changes in the way the baby moves

Any visits to another doctor, midwife, nurse, clinic, or emergency room

Any medicines or substances you have used, including:
- Medicines (prescription, vitamins, or over the counter)
- Substance use (if any) including use of cigarettes or vaping, alcohol, or other substances
- Plants or herbs/herbal teas used to help you feel better or treat an illness
- Do you need any prenatal vitamins, iron, or other medicines?

Since Your Last Visit, Have You Had Any Accidents or Falls, Been Hit, Hurt, or Threatened?

There are many common discomforts of pregnancy. If there is one particular thing that is bothering you or that you want information about, or would like help or suggestions on how to work with or relieve the discomfort, please mark it in the following. If none of these worry or bother you, skip this section.

- Nausea (feeling sick to your stomach)
- Diarrhea
- Hemorrhoids
- Vomiting (throwing up)
- Constipation
- Numbness or tingling of hands or legs or feet
- Tired all the time (fatigue)
- Sciatica (sharp pains down your leg)
- Heart jumping, skipping, or beating very fast
- Changes in desire for sex or way sex feels
- Shortness of breath
- Not feeling hungry
- Breast tenderness
- Heartburn
- Varicose veins
- Angry or irritable
- Trouble sleeping
- Leg cramps
- Backache
- Sad or crying for "no reason"
- Unusual or intense dreams
- Any other concern not on this list

On a scale of 1 (*awful*) to 10 (*wonderful*), how are you doing right now? If things are not so good, what would help? Please tell us about anything else that is worrying you or about any information you want.

1. **1 to 28 weeks of gestation:** Every 4 weeks
2. **28 to 37 weeks of gestation:** Every 2 weeks
3. **37 weeks of gestation to delivery:** Weekly
4. Centering, or group, prenatal care may be recommended if available.
5. Telehealth prenatal care may be utilized for some low-risk patient visits.

G. The patient should be asked if there are any further questions or need for additional information.

H. The patient should be instructed to call with any questions or problems (see Table 14.5 for warning signs).
   a. Premature rupture of membranes (PROM)

I. All medications should be evaluated for their benefits versus potential risks in pregnancy.

J. Inform the patient about prepared childbirth classes.
   1. Classes are readily available throughout the United States in person or online.
   2. Provide the patient with valuable knowledge about labor and delivery to decrease anxiety.
   3. Exercise and toning in preparation for labor makes labor easier for most women.
   4. Classes are a good way to help partners or support people to be involved with the pregnancy.

K. Additional concerns
   1. Sexual intercourse
      a. May be unrestricted in normal pregnancy as long as the cervix is not significantly dilated.
      b. Avoid if vaginal bleeding, ruptured membranes, or placenta previa are present, if there is a current or past history of preterm labor, or if either partner is uncomfortable.
   2. Travel
      a. Air travel is not recommended after 36 weeks of gestation.
         (1) Patient should check travel regulations, risks and restrictions related to their pregnancy, and consider carrying a copy of prenatal records
      b. Avoid long periods of sitting, which may cause venous stasis.
      c. Patient should consider possibility that competent obstetrical care may not be immediately available in some areas.

TABLE 14.5 Warning Signs During Pregnancy

DANGER SIGN OR SYMPTOM	POTENTIAL CAUSE
Marked decrease in fetal movement	Fetal compromise, anoxia
Vaginal bleeding; abdominal pain or cramping	Impending miscarriage, spontaneous abortion, or ectopic pregnancy
Leakage of fluid from the vagina	Premature rupture of membranes (PROM)
Persistent headache	Preeclampsia or pregnancy-induced hypertension
Dizziness	Hypotension, dehydration
Spots before the eyes	Preeclampsia or vision changes
Swelling of the hands or face	May be normal, but may be symptom of preeclampsia
Elevated blood pressure	Any of the hypertensive disorders of pregnancy
Fever or chills	Infection
Recurrent vomiting	Hyperemesis gravidarum

    d. Pressurized aircraft pose no additional risk. Airlines may have restrictions on overseas flights related to gestational age.

L. Table 14.6 provides guidelines for continuing assessment during an uncomplicated pregnancy.

TABLE 14.6 Continuing Assessment During Uncomplicated Pregnancy		
SCHEDULE OF RETURN VISITS **ONCE MONTHLY, ONSET OF CARE IN FIRST TRIMESTER TO 28 WEEKS OF GESTATION**		
EVERY 2 WEEKS, 27–36 WEEKS OF GESTATION **ONCE WEEKLY, 37–40 WEEKS OF GESTATION**		
WEEKS OF GESTATION	**ASSESSMENT**	**RATIONALE**
Every visit	Weight	Evaluate fetal growth, screen for maternal edema, preeclampsia, under- and over-nourishment
	BP	Screen for PIH
	Fundal height (McDonald's rule)	Evaluate fetal growth
	Leopold's maneuvers after 32 weeks of gestation	Determine fetal position
	FHR after 10 weeks of gestation	Evaluate fetal well-being with Doppler after 10 weeks of gestation, with fetoscope if desired after 20 weeks of gestation
	Edema	Screen for PIH, fluid retention
	Symptoms	Identify problems, discomforts
	Adjustment to stage of pregnancy	Identify problems, provide support
	Nutrition	Determine adequacy of diet
10 to 13 weeks	Offer chorionic villus sampling if appropriate[a]	Detect fetal chromosomal abnormalities
15 to 19 weeks	Ultrasound if indicated	Determine fetal age, and development, and screen for anomalies
	Hgb electrophoresis[a]	Detect sickle cell, thalassemias, other hemoglobinopathies
15 to 22 6/7 weeks	AFP	Screen for fetal neural tube defects
	Amniocentesis[a]	Detect fetal genetic abnormalities
	Ultrasound if indicated	Determine fetal age, development, screen for anomalies
24 to 28 weeks	Glucose 50 mg	Screen for gestational diabetes
28 to 34 weeks	Hematocrit/Hgb	Detect anemia
36 to 42 weeks	GBS screening Pelvic examination, with STI screening, if indicated	Identify cervical changes preceding labor onset Screen for current STI infection

AFP, alpha-fetoprotein; BP, blood pressure; FHR, fetal heart rate; GBS, group B *Streptococcus*; Hgb, hemoglobin; PIH, pregnancy-induced hypertension; STD, sexually transmitted disease.

[a]For clients at risk.

CASE STUDY: Initial Prenatal Visit

Patient Situation

A 25-year-old female presents to the outpatient women's health department complaining of urinary frequency and breast tenderness. She states she "did a home pregnancy test and it was positive" and wants "to know her due date." She has a new partner as of 3 months ago. This is an unplanned pregnancy.

Subjective Data

- Gravida 3 Para 1011. Daughter, aged 2, is at home. Had one miscarriage at 7 weeks of gestation.
- States she thinks her LMP was 2 months ago.
- Feels nauseous most afternoons, but she has not gained or lost weight.
- Home medications: none
- Smokes one-half pack/day
- No medical problems. Had a normal spontaneous vaginal delivery with her first pregnancy. Had group B strep with her first pregnancy and received penicillin during labor. No known allergies.

Objective Data

- Urine pregnancy test in office is positive
- Pelvic exam: uterus 8 weeks size, adnexa WNL
- Vital signs: blood pressure 104/68, pulse 84/min, respiration 22/min
- Height: 5'6" Weight 190 lbs.

Clinical Analysis

What labs do you anticipate will be ordered, and why?
- Laboratory tests:
  - CBC to evaluate for anemia and baseline platelet count
  - Blood type and Rh to evaluate for need for Rhogam with any bleeding in pregnancy
  - Hepatitis B surface antigen and hepatitis C antibody test to screen for hepatitis infection
  - RPR to screen for syphilis
  - HIV test to screen for HIV infection
  - Rubella to screen for need for rubella immunization immediately postpartum and for risk mitigation
  - Gonorrhea and chlamydia cultures to screen for STIs
  - Ultrasound to confirm dating

Identify this patient's risk factors during pregnancy.
- BMI 30.7 at the start of pregnancy
- Smokes ½ pack per day
- History of Group B Strep in the last pregnancy

What are the priority interventions based on the patient's clinical presentation?
- Confirming patent's due date as 32 weeks from today.
- Discussing patient's feelings about pregnancy and her plans for baby.
- Evaluation of cigarette use, brief intervention utilizing motivational interviewing, and referral to a smoking cessation program.
- Nutritional consultation for plan for 15- to 25-pound weight gain during pregnancy

What else should be included in this patient's plan of care?
- Relief measures for nausea including increasing fluids in morning and ingesting ginger
- Use of condoms if not monogamous relationship
- Evaluating social support system for pregnancy and postpartum
- Group B Strep culture at 36 weeks' gestation to evaluate need for penicillin in labor.

REFERENCES

American College of Obstetricians and Gynecologists (2017). Methods for estimating the due date. Committee Opinion No. 700. *Obstet Gynecol, 129*(5), e150–4. https://doi.org/10.1097/AOG.0000000000002046

Centers for Disease Control and Prevention (CDC) (2021). *Sexually transmitted infectious treatment guidelines, 2021.* https://www.cdc.gov/std/treatment-guidelines/toc.htm.

Marshall, N., Biel, F., Boone-Heinonen, J., Dukhovny, D., Caughey, A., & Snowden, J. (2019). The association between maternal height, body mass index, and perinatal outcomes. *American Journal of Perinatology, 36*(6), 632–640. https://doi.org/10.1055/s-0038-1673395

Parobek, C., Russo, M. & Lewkowitz, A. (2021). Privacy risks in prenatal aneuploidy and carrier screening. *Obstetrics & Gynecology, 137*(6), 1074–1079. https://doi.org/10.1097/AOG.0000000000004387.

BIBLIOGRAPHY

ACOG Committee Opinion. (2021). Physical activity and exercise during pregnancy and the postpartum period: ACOG Committee Opinion Number 804. *Obstetrics & Gynecology, 135*(4), e178–e188. https://doi.org/10.1097/AOG.0000000000003772

ACOG Practice Bulletin No. 189: Nausea and vomiting of pregnancy. (2018). Committee on Practice Bulletins-Obstetrics. *Obstetrics & Gynecology, 131*(1), 190–193. https://doi.org/10.1097/AOG.0000000000002456.

ACOG Practice Bulletin, Number 233. (2021). Anemia in Pregnancy: *Obstetrics & Gynecology, 138*(2), e55–e64. https://doi.org/10.1097/AOG.0000000000004477

Ailes, E., Summers, A., Tran, E., Gilboa, S., Arnold, K., Meaney-Delman, D., & Reefhuis, J. (2018). Antibiotics dispensed to privately insured pregnant women with urinary tract infections – United States, 2014. *MMWR: Morbidity & Mortality Weekly Report, 67*(1), 18–22. https://doi.org/10.15585/mmwr.mm6701a4

American Cancer Society. (2020). Cervical cancer screening for individuals at average risk: 2020 guideline update from the American Cancer Society. *CA: A Cancer Journal for Clinicians.* https://acsjournals.onlinelibrary.wiley.com/doi/full/10.3322/caac.21628#caac21628-tbl-0001. Retrieved February, 2022. *70*(5):321–346. https://doi.org/10.3322/caac.21628.

American College of Obstetricians and Gynecologists. (2016). Prenatal diagnostic testing for genetic disorders. ACOG Practice Bulletin No. 163. *Obstetrics and Gynecology, 127*(5), e108–e122. doi:10.1097/AOG.0000000000001405

Bryant, J., Jamil, R., & Thistle, J. (2021). *Fetal movement. StatPearls Publishing; 2022 Jan-.* https://www.ncbi.nlm.nih.gov/books/NBK470566/

Center for Devices and Radiological Health (2020). *Guidance for Over-the-Counter (OTC) Human Chorionic Gonadotropin (hCG) 510(k)s - Guidance for Industry and FDA Reviewers/Staff. U.S. Department of Health and Human Services; Food and Drug Administration. Docket number* FDA-2020-D-0957. https://www.fda.gov/regulatory-information/search-fda-guidance-documents/guidance-over-counter-otc-human-chorionic-gonadotropin-hcg-510ks-guidance-industry-and-fda.

Centers for Disease Control and Prevention. (2016). *Mumps. For healthcare providers.* https://www.cdc.gov/mumps/hcp.html#pregnancy

Centers for Disease Control and Prevention. (2017). *10 Tips for preventing infections before and during pregnancy.* https://www.cdc.gov/pregnancy/infections.html

Centers for Disease Control and Prevention (CDC) (2021). *Pregnant and recently pregnant people at increased risk for severe illness from COVID-19.* https://www.cdc.gov/coronavirus/2019-ncov/need-extra-precautions/pregnant-people.html.

Feld, H., Barnhart, S., Wiggins, A. T., & Ashford, K. (2021). Social support reduces the risk of unintended pregnancy in a low-income population. *Public Health Nursing, 38*(5), 801–809. https://doi.org/10.1111/phn.12920

Finer L., Zolna M. (2016). Declines inunintended pregnancy in the United States, 2008–2011. *The New England Journal of Medicine. 374*(9):843–52. https://doi.org/10.1056/NEJMsa1506575.

Goetzinger, K. R., Shanks, A. L., Odibo, A. O., Macones, G. A., & Cahill, A. G. (2017). Advanced maternal age and the risk of major congenital anomalies. *American Journal of Perinatology, 34*(3), 217–222. https://doi.org/10.1055/s-0036-1585410

Green, L., Mackillop, L., Salvi, D., Pullon, R., Loerup, L., Tarassenko, L., Mossop, Ju., Edwards, C., Gerry, S., Birks, J., Gauntlett, R., Harding, K., Chappell, L., & Watkinson, P. (2020). Gestation-specific vital sign reference ranges in pregnancy. *Obstetrics & Gynecology, 135*(3), 653–664. https://doi.org/10.1097/AOG.0000000000003721.

Günther, V., Alkatout, I., Vollmer, C., Maass, N., Strauss, A., & Voigt, M. (2021). Impact of nicotine and maternal BMI on fetal birth weight. *BMC Pregnancy & Childbirth, 20*(1), 1–6. https://doi.org/10.1186/s12884-021-03593-z

Haque, I., Lazarin, G., Kang, H., Evans, E., Goldberg, J., & Wapner, R. (2016). Modeled fetal risk of genetic diseases identified by expanded carrier screening. *JAMA: Journal of the American Medical Association, 316*(7), 734–742. https://doi.org/10.1001/jama.2016.11139

Kuronen, M., Hantunen, S., Alanne, L., Kokki, H., Saukko, C., Sjövall, S., Vesterinen, K., & Kokki, M. (2021). Pregnancy, puerperium and perinatal constipation – an observational hybrid survey on pregnant and postpartum women and their age-matched non-pregnant controls. *BJOG: An International Journal of Obstetrics & Gynaecology, 128*(6), 1057–1064. https://doi.org/10.1111/1471-0528.16559

Medline Plus. (2020) *Pregnancy test. U.S. National Library of Medicine.* https://medlineplus.gov/lab-tests/pregnancy-test/ 11/12/21

National Institute on Drug Abuse. (2020). Substance use in women research report: Substance use while pregnant and breastfeeding. National Institutes of Health (NIH). https://www.drugabuse.gov/publications/research-reports/substance-use-in-women/substance-use-while-pregnant-breastfeeding.

National Institutes of Health (NIH), Office of Dietary Supplements. (2021). *Calcium: Fact sheet for health professionals.* https://ods.od.nih.gov/factsheets/Calcium-HealthProfessional.

Newsome, M. (2021). Drug safety in pregnancy. *New Scientist 250*(3338), 20–21. https://doi.org/10.1016/s0262-4079(21)00992-1.

Randall, D., Morris, J., Kelly, P., & Glastras, S. (2021). How has change in gestational diabetes diagnosis affected pregnancy outcomes? *International Journal of Epidemiology, 50*, 1. https://doi.org/10.1093/ije/dyab168.561

Substance Abuse and Mental Health Services Administration (SAMHSA). (2018). *Clinical guidance for treating pregnant and parenting women with opioid use disorder and their infants.* HHS Publication No. (SMA) 18-5054.

Thaxter Nesbeth, K. A., Samuels, L. A., Nicholson Daley, C., Gossell-Williams, M., & Nesbeth, D. A. (2016). Ptyalism in pregnancy—a review of epidemiology and practices. *European Journal of Obstetrics, Gynecology, and Reproductive Biology, 198*, 47–49. https://doi.org/10.1016/j.ejogrb.2015.12.022

U.S. Food and Drug Administration. (2016). *Radiation-emitting products.* Ultrasound imaging. https://www.fda.gov/radiation-emittingproducts/radiationemittingproductsandprocedures/medicalimaging/ucm115357.htm

U.S. Preventative Services Task Force (USPSTF) (2021). *Final recommendation statement: Gestational diabetes: Screening.* https://www.uspreventiveservicestaskforce.org/uspstf/recommendation/gestational-diabetes-screening. Retrieved Nov. 1, 2021.

Venkatesh, K., & Landon, M. (2021). Diagnosis and management of gestational diabetes: What every OB/GYN needs to know to manage this complication. *Contemporary OB/GYN, 66*(5), 9–15.

Vernini, J. M., Moreli, J. B., Magalhães, C. G., Costa, R. A. A., Rudge, M. V. C., & Calderon, I. M. P. (2016). Maternal and fetal outcomes in pregnancies complicated by overweight and obesity. *Reproductive Health, 13*(1), 100. https://doi.org/10.1186/s12978-016-0206-0

15

ADOLESCENT HEALTH

HANNE HARBISON AND WHITNEY TAYLOR ERIKSEN

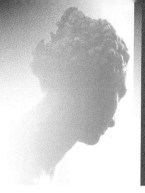

OVERVIEW

A. Adolescents experience barriers in access to sexual and reproductive healthcare, leading to a disproportionately high burden of disease and morbidity.

B. Teens and young adults may avoid or delay accessing care due to perceived or experienced bias or judgment from healthcare providers or perceived or experienced inability to access care independently.

C. Establishing positive, trusting relationships with adolescents is key to prevention and promotion of life-long health.

CONFIDENTIALITY

A. Confidentiality plays a critical role in developing strong client/provider relationships, particularly for adolescent clients. Perception of confidentiality impacts an adolescent's decision to seek care, disclose behaviors and concerns, as well as return for follow-up care (English & Ford, 2018).

B. Many professional organizations, including American College of Obstetricians and Gynecologists (ACOG, 2020), Society for Adolescent Health and Medicine (SAHM), American Academy of Pediatrics (AAP, 2016), and Association of Women's Health, Obstetric and Neonatal Nurses (AWHONN, 2017), endorse confidential adolescent healthcare.

C. Providers can facilitate expectations surrounding confidentiality for both parents and adolescents by clearly communicating policies prior to visits, noting when parents will and will not be included in the visit. This can be supported through displaying materials in the clinic space or sending emails to clients as the transition to adolescence approaches.

D. Familiarize yourself with state laws regarding consent to services by minors.
1. See Table 15.1 for details regarding age of consent for common services.
2. Services provided at Title X clinics must be confidential.

E. All 50 states require healthcare providers to report suspected child abuse (either specifically as a member of the medical community or designating all persons as mandated reporters).

PREVENTIVE HEALTH AND EDUCATION

A. Screening and counseling
1. Adolescents aged 13 to 17 years should receive the following preventive screening and applicable counseling (Ham & Allan, 2012):
   a. Height and weight (BMI)*
   b. Depression screening*, such as with the patient health questionnaire for adolescents (PHQ-A) and the Beck depression inventory–primary care version
   c. Violence/intimate partner violence (IPV)*
   d. Tobacco and alcohol use*
   e. Counseling regarding reducing skin cancer risk for fair-skinned individuals*

*Indicates Grade A/B by USPSTF.

TABLE 15.1 Age of Consent and Access to Services by State

STATE	AGE OF CONSENT	ACCESS TO STI SERVICES	ACCESS TO HIV TESTING AND TREATMENT	ACCESS TO CONTRACEPTIVE SERVICES	PARENTAL NOTIFICATION	ACCESS TO PRENATAL SERVICES	ACCESS TO ABORTION SERVICES
Alabama	16 years	12 years	Yes	If married, parent, ever pregnant, HS graduate, or 14+ years	May inform of STI care	Yes	Parental consent
Alaska	16 years	Yes		Yes		Yes	Parental notification, permanently enjoined by court order
Arizona	18 years	Yes		Yes		NEP	Parental consent
Arkansas	16 years	Yes		Yes	May inform of STI care	Yes	Parental consent
California	18 years	12 years	Yes	Yes		Yes	Parental consent, permanently enjoined by court order
Colorado	17 years	13 years	Yes	Yes	May inform of consent to HIV/AIDS treatment and if younger than 16	Yes	Parental notification
Connecticut	16 years	Yes	Yes	If married	Must report positive STI/HIV test if younger than 12	NEP, married minor has same rights as adult	

State							
Delaware	18 years	12 years	Yes	If 12+ years	May inform of STI, contraceptive, or prenatal care	Yes	Parental notification for patient under 16, may be waived in certain circumstances, other relatives allowed to consent
DC	16 years	Yes	Yes	Yes		Yes	
Florida	18 years	Yes	Yes	If married, parent, ever pregnant, or medically necessary		Yes	Parental notification and consent
Georgia	16 years	Yes	Yes	Yes	May inform of STI care	Yes	Parental notification
Hawaii	16 years	14 years		If 14+ years	May inform of STI, contraceptive, or prenatal care	14 years	
Idaho	18 years	14 years	Yes	Yes		Yes	Parental consent
Illinois	17 years	12 years	Yes	If married, parent, ever pregnant, medically necessary	May inform of STI care	Yes	Parental notification, other relatives allowed to consent
Indiana	16 years	Yes		If married		NEP, married minor has same rights as adult	Parental consent
Iowa	16 years	Yes	Yes	Yes	Must notify of positive HIV result	Yes	Parental notification, other relatives allowed to consent

(continued)

TABLE 15.1 Age of Consent and Access to Services by State (continued)

STATE	AGE OF CONSENT	ACCESS TO STI SERVICES	ACCESS TO HIV TESTING AND TREATMENT	ACCESS TO CONTRACEPTIVE SERVICES	PARENTAL NOTIFICATION	ACCESS TO PRENATAL SERVICES	ACCESS TO ABORTION SERVICES
Kansas	16 years	Yes		If mature minor	May inform of STI care	Mature minor	Parental consent from both parents
Kentucky	18 years	Yes	Yes	Yes	May inform of STI, contraceptive, or prenatal care	Yes	Parental consent
Louisiana	17 years	Yes		If married	May inform of STI care	NEP, married minor has same rights as adult	Parental consent
Maine	16 years	Yes		Yes	May inform of STI, contraceptive, or prenatal care	Yes	
Maryland	16 years	Yes		Yes	May inform of STI, contraceptive, or prenatal care	Yes	Parental consent, may be waived in certain circumstances
Massachusetts	16 years	Yes		Yes	Must inform if health or life is at risk	Yes, parent must be notified if health or life of minor at risk	Parental notification for patient under 16
Michigan	16 years	Yes	Yes	If married	May inform of STI or prenatal care	Yes	Parental consent
Minnesota	16 years	Yes		Yes	May inform of STI, contraceptive, or prenatal care	Yes	Parental notification to both parents
Mississippi	16 years	Yes	Testing, no treatment	If married or parent		Yes	Parental consent from both parents

Missouri	17 years	Yes	If married	May inform of STI or prenatal care	Yes	Parental consent, consenting parent must notify other custodial parent or guardian
Montana	16 years	Yes	Yes	May inform of STI, contraceptive, or prenatal care	Yes	Parental consent, temporarily enjoined by court order; parental notification
Nebraska	16 years	Yes	If married		NEP	Parental consent
Nevada	16 years	Yes	If married, parent, or mature minor		Mature or married minor	Parental notification, permanently enjoined by court order
New Hampshire	16 years	14 years	If mature minor		Mature minor	Parental notification
New Jersey	16 years	13 years	If married or ever pregnant	May inform of STI or prenatal care	Yes	Parental notification, permanently enjoined by court order
New Mexico	16 years	Testing, no treatment	Yes		Yes	Parental consent, permanently enjoined by court order
New York	17 years	Yes	Yes		Yes	
North Carolina	16 years	Yes	Yes	May inform of prenatal care	Yes	Parental consent, other relatives allowed to consent
North Dakota	18 years	Yes	NEP		Parental consent in 2nd and 3rd trimester	Parental consent from both parents

(continued)

TABLE 15.1 Age of Consent and Access to Services by State (*continued*)

STATE	AGE OF CONSENT	ACCESS TO STI SERVICES	ACCESS TO HIV TESTING AND TREATMENT	ACCESS TO CONTRACEPTIVE SERVICES	PARENTAL NOTIFICATION	ACCESS TO PRENATAL SERVICES	ACCESS TO ABORTION SERVICES
Ohio	16 years	Yes	Testing, no treatment	NEP		NEP	Parental consent
Oklahoma	16 years	Yes	Yes	If married or ever pregnant	May inform of STI, contraceptive, or prenatal care	Yes	Parental consent and notification
Oregon	18 years	Yes	Yes	Yes	May inform of contraceptive or prenatal care	15 years	
Pennsylvania	16 years	Yes	Yes	Yes		Yes	Parental consent
Rhode Island	16 years	Yes	Yes	NEP		NEP	Parental consent
South Carolina	16 years	Yes	Yes	If married, 16+ years, or mature minor		16 years or mature minor	Parental consent for patients under 17, may be waived in certain circumstances, other relatives allowed to consent
South Dakota	16 years	Yes	Yes	If married		NEP, married minor has same rights as adult	Parental notification
Tennessee	18 years	Yes	Yes	Yes		Yes	Parental consent
Texas	17 years	Yes	Yes	If married, state funds disallowed	May inform of STI or prenatal care	Yes	Parental consent and notification

State						
Utah	18 years	Yes		If married, state funds disallowed	Yes	Parental consent and notification
Vermont	16 years	12 years	Testing, no treatment	If married	NEP, married minor has same rights as adult	
Virginia	18 years	Yes	Yes	Yes	Yes	Parental consent and notification, other relatives allowed to consent
Washington	16 years	14 years	Yes	Yes	Yes	
West Virginia	16 years	Yes		If married or mature minor	Mature minor, married minor >16 years has same rights as adult	Parental notification
Wisconsin	18 years	Yes	NEP	NEP	NEP	Parental consent, may be waived in certain circumstances; other relatives allowed to consent
Wyoming	17 years	Yes	Yes	Yes	NEP, married minor has same rights as adult	Parental consent and notification

Yes = Explicitly allows all minors to access service.

HS, high school; NEP, no explicit policy.

Source: Adapted from the Guttmacher Institute.

    f. **Hematocrit (Hct)/hemoglobin (HgB):** once for all adolescents, annually for menstruating individuals

    g. **STI screening:** If sexually active, teens should be screened annually for chlamydia, gonorrhea, HIV, and syphilis*

    h. Hepatitis B, if at increased risk*

    i. Cholesterol, if at increased risk

    j. Vision, hearing, and dentition by appropriate providers

  2. Adolescents aged 18 years should additionally receive (Ham & Allan, 2012):

    a. Blood pressure*

    b. Hepatitis C*

    c. Substance use and abuse, including alcohol and tobacco use*

B. Other important recommendations

  1. Cervical cytology (pap smear) is not recommended until age 21.

  2. HPV testing is not recommended until age 30.*

  3. Annual breast exams are not recommended until age 45.

IMMUNIZATIONS: RECOMMENDED IMMUNIZATIONS FOR ADOLESCENTS

A. **Influenza:** One dose annually

B. **Tdap:** One dose, typically at 11 to 12 years

C. **HPV:** Two to 3 doses within 6 to 12 months depending on age, see HPV in the following for further details

D. **Meningococcal:** One dose at 11–12 years, second dose at 16 years

E. COVID-19 (data accurate as of November 2021):

  1. **Comirnaty (Pfizer-BioNTech):** Two doses 3 weeks apart. FDA emergency use authorization for ages 5 to17 and full FDA approval for ages 18+.

  2. **Spikevax (Moderna):** Two doses, 4 weeks apart. FDA emergency use authorization for ages 18+.

  3. **COVID-19 vaccine (J&J-Janssen):** One dose. FDA emergency use authorization for ages 18+.

  4. Booster shot recommendations vary by age, comorbidities, and exposure; check with the Centers for Disease Control and Prevention (CDC) for the most up-to-date information (Wodi et al., 2021).

EDUCATION ON BODY DEVELOPMENT

A. Formal education on body development and reproductive health varies widely across the United States (Lindberg & Kantor, 2021); as such, adolescents may not have a thorough, accurate understanding of the physical, developmental, and mental changes that occur in adolescence.

B. Following are some key education points to review with patients, focused on individuals with XX chromosomes (Hoffman et al., 2020).

  1. **Puberty:** The process of sexual maturation, starts between 8 and 13 years of age.

    a. Breast development occurs first, typically between ages 9 and 11. Nipples will become more prominent, areolas will darken and expand; breasts may grow at different rates. Some soreness is common, as is asymmetric growth. Use of training bras or undershirts may facilitate comfort as adolescents acclimate to a changing chest.

    b. Hair will start to grow in the underarms and vulva, followed by thickening and darkening. Body odor changes and acne may develop. New hygiene routines may need to be established during this time. Patients will see a period of significant height growth,

---

*Indicates Grade A/B by USPSTF.

commonly beginning around age 12. This is a sign that menarche is on the horizon, often within a year.

2. Median age of menarche (first period) in the United States is 12 years for non-Hispanic Black females, 12.5 years for non-Hispanic White females (Martinez, 2020).
   a. Periods may be irregular at first but will become more predictable within 2 years.
   b. Normal cycles last 21 to 35 days, with 3 to 8 days of menses and less than 80 mL of blood loss.
   c. Encourage individuals to find hygiene and management routines that best fit the needs of their cycles. Education surrounding menstrual management and use of hygiene products such as tampons, pads, and cups/discs, should include appropriate length of use of tampons (changing every 4–8 hours, alternating use with pad, using lowest absorbency) and cleaning of cups to decrease risk of toxic shock syndrome.
   d. Tracking periods with a calendar or app can support teens in anticipating menses and managing accompanying symptoms.
   e. Establishing care with a women's health provider is encouraged between 13 and 15 years of age; early visits focus on education and establishing a trusting relationship between the provider and patient (ACOG, 2020).

ATYPICAL MENSTRUAL BLEEDING IN ADOLESCENCE

A. Primary amenorrhea: When a patient has not started menstruating (a) by age 15 with normal growth and development of secondary sexual characteristics, or (b) within 3 years of breast development, or (c) has no secondary sexual characteristics by age 13, assessment for primary amenorrhea is recommended (Klein, Paradise, & Reeder, 2019).
   1. Primary amenorrhea is often the result of genetic (Turner's syndrome, androgen insensitivity) or anatomical (Mullerian agenesis, imperforate hymen) abnormalities. See Table 15.2 for a detailed list of causes of amenorrhea.
   2. Evaluation of primary amenorrhea should include (Klein et al., 2019):
      a. Detailed patient and family medical history, review of systems.
      b. Physical exam with particular attention to:

TABLE 15.2 Causes of Primary Amenorrhea

Outflow	Congenital	Complete androgen resistance Imperforate hymen Mullerian agenesis Transverse septum
	Acquired	Ashermans syndrome Cervical stenosis
Primary ovarian insufficiency	Congenital	Gonadal dysgenesis Turner syndrome
	Acquired	Autoimmune destruction Chemotherapy Radiation
Pituitary		Autoimmune disease, cocaine use, Cushing syndrome, empty Sella syndrome, hyperprolactinemia, infiltrative disease, medications (antidepressants, antihistamines, antipsychotics, opiates), pituitary or central nervous system tumor, prolactinoma, Sheehan syndrome
Hypothalamic		Eating disorder, female athlete triad, rapid weight loss, malabsorption, infection, gonadotropin deficiency, stress, traumatic brain injury, tumor

    (1) Hair patterning: Absence or sparse patterning suggestive of adrenarche or androgen insensitivity. Male pattern growth suggestive of elevated androgen levels.

    (2) Appearance of vulva and vagina: Clitoralmegaly suggestive of elevated androgens. Pale, thin, non-rugated vaginal mucosa suggestive of low estrogen levels

  c. Labs: Serum follicle-stimulating hormone (FSH), prolactin, thyroid-stimulating hormone (TSH), testosterone, dehydroepiandrosterone sulfate (DHEAS), human chorionic gonadotropin (HCG), chromosomal analysis

  d. Imaging: Ultrasound may be helpful in identifying anatomic variations in the reproductive tract, MRI can facilitate identification of tumors or diseases of the hypothalamus and pituitary gland.

  e. Testing: Progesterone withdrawal test with PO medroxyprogesterone acetate 10 mg daily for 5 to 10 days.

3. Anovulatory conditions: If the patient experiences a withdrawal bleed, suggestive of anovulatory conditions such as polycystic ovarian syndrome (PCOS)

4. If the patient does not experience a withdrawal bleed, follow with 2.5 mg of conjugated estrogen (Premarin) for 21 days and 10 mg of medroxyprogesterone acetate on days 17 to 21.

  a. If bleeding occurs, amenorrhea is due to hypoestrogenism.

  b. If no bleeding follows 21 days of hormone treatment, an anatomic abnormality (Mullerian agenesis, imperforate hymen) is indicated.

5. Treatment is dependent on etiology and patient goals and should be referred or comanaged with a physician as needed.

ABNORMAL UTERINE BLEEDING (AUB) IN ADOLESCENCE

A. Often presents as missed or skipped periods. This is most frequently the result of persistent anovulation due to immaturity or dysregulation of the hypothalamic-pituitary-ovarian (HPO) axis, which can be normal.

B. Common causes of AUB in adolescence include anovulation or polycystic ovary syndrome (PCOS), coagulopathies, pregnancy, STIs, injury, or abuse (Wilkinson & Kadir, 2010).

C. Workup should be guided by symptom presentation.

PREGNANCY IN ADOLESCENCE

A. Background

  1. Pregnancy rates among adolescents in the United States have been declining since the early 1990s; as of 2019 it was 16.7 per 1,000 females.

  2. Disparities persist among racial and ethnic groups with higher birth rates per 1,000 for American Indian/Alaska Native teens (29.2), Native Hawaiian/Pacific Islander (26.2), non-Hispanic/Latinx Black (25.8), and Hispanic/Latinx teens (25.3), compared to non-Hispanic/Latinx White teens (11.4) and non-Hispanic/Latinx Asian teens (2.7; Martin et al., 2021).

  3. The majority of pregnancies in adolescents are unplanned (Finer & Zolna, 2016).

B. Pregnancy options and emergency contraceptive counseling

  1. Prior to counseling, reflect on personal biases to facilitate provision of neutral, supportive care. Evidence shows that shaming and stigmatization does not delay or reduce sexual activity, rates of teen pregnancy, or rates of STIs; rather, these approaches have been shown to delay access to care and impair the relationship between provider and patient (Cunningham et al., 2009).

  2. Counseling with the pregnant teen should focus on active listening, establishing patient goals, and provision of accurate information (Hornberger, 2017).

3. **Abortion:** Assess patient's perceptions of abortion; clarify methods as indicated by gestational age and accessibility; inform patient of adolescent-specific considerations (see Table 15.1); refer or provide appropriate care as indicated by patient decision and applicable state laws.

4. **Adoption:** Assess patient's perceptions of adoption; clarify types of adoption (open, semi-open, closed); assess facilitators and barriers to adoption (partner support, family support, cultural or religious support); provide resources for learning about adoption and adoption services.

5. **Parenting:** Assess patient's perceptions of parenthood; discuss potential risk of health outcomes of pregnancy for patient; connect patient to resources to facilitate parenting, continuing education.

COUNSELING THE ADOLESCENT PATIENT REGARDING EMERGENCY CONTRACEPTIVES

A. Current methods do not have age restrictions for use, but access may be restricted by state law (see Table 15.1).

B. These methods, when used correctly, are very safe. They do not cause abortion if implantation has already occurred. Use of emergency contraception has not been shown to increase risky behaviors in adolescents.

C. If appropriate, review options for safe and reliable methods for preventing pregnancy that are used prior to engaging in sexual acts.

D. Options for emergency contraception include ulipristal acetate (Ella), levonorgestrel (Plan B, etc.), and copper IUD. The Yuzpe method of combining oral contraceptives for two doses of 100 mcg ethinyl estradiol and 0.5 mg levonorgestrel 12 hours apart is not recommended in the setting of other options available as it generally conveys more side effects and variable efficacy (HAEGER et al., 2018).

E. Time considerations and efficacy of the selected method

1. **Copper IUD:** Most effective at preventing pregnancy, insertion should be done within 120 hours (5 days) of unprotected sex.

2. **Ulipristal acetate (Ella):** More effective at preventing pregnancy than levonorgestrel. Take as one dose within 120 hours (5 days) of unprotected sex. Efficacy may be decreased in patients over 195 lb. Counsel patient to wait 5 days before initiating hormonal birth control and abstain or utilize another form of contraception (condoms) for 2 weeks to allow for contraceptive benefits from hormonal birth control.

3. **Levonorgestrel (Plan B, etc.):** Take as one dose, ideally within 72 hours (3 days) of unprotected sex. Considerations: Efficacy may be decreased in patients over 155 lb., available over the counter without prescription or age restriction.

CARE FOR PREGNANT ADOLESCENT

A. Pregnant teens are at increased risk for hypertension; nutritional deficiencies (anemia, poor weight gain); preterm birth and low birth weight; infant and maternal mortality; STIs and intimate partner violence; and peripartum depression (Klein, 2005).

B. Prenatal care and education for the pregnant teen should include

1. Good nutrition during pregnancy, particularly sufficient iron, folic acid, and caloric intake for fetal and maternal growth (typically approximately 300 kcal above baseline)

2. Education on avoidance of substances harmful to the growing fetus, including alcohol, tobacco, marijuana, illegal drugs, raw or undercooked meat and fish, high-mercury fish, unpasteurized foods and drinks, lunch meats, and caffeine

3. Review of over-the-counter and prescription medications and supplements, notably medications for pain, acne, anxiety and depression, and antibiotics
4. Importance of maintaining care throughout pregnancy and strategies to support attendance of prenatal visits
5. Connection to resources, such as peer support programs, educational support, family and/ or partner involvement, and employment or housing assistance, can facilitate a healthy pregnancy and continuation of educational, family, and life goals
6. Screening for STIs, intimate partner violence, peripartum depression

SEXUAL AND REPRODUCTIVE HEALTH

A. The psychosocial assessment tool HEADSSS (which stands for "home, education and/or employment, eating, activities, drugs, sexuality, suicide and/or depression, and safety") is a way to assess for many risks simultaneously (Cohen et al., 1991). See Table 15.3.
B. **STIs:** The highest rates of STIs are in adolescents and young adults ages 15 to 24 representing 25% of the population and 50% of STI infections (Boyer, 2021). Specifically, marginalized groups experience the highest rates of infections, including LGBTQ+ youth and youth of color (Workowski, 2021).
   1. Factors that contribute to STI risk include multiple partners, inconsistent use of barrier protection, having low social-economic status, and difficulty accessing care (Workowski, 2021).
   2. Confidentiality is especially important for STI services.
   3. All 50 states allow minors to consent for STI services; age at which that begins varies (see Table 15.1).
   4. No state requires parental consent for STI care.
   5. Adolescents should be seen alone by providers when discussing sexual health.
C. STI screening recommendations
   1. In 2019 only 8.6 % of 9th through12th graders had been tested for an STI (National Health and Nutrition Examination Survey [NHANES], 2019).
   2. It is recommended that all sexually active people with a uterus <25 years old should be screened at least annually for *Chlamydia trachomatis* (CT) and *Neisseria gonorrhoeae* (GC). Extragenital screening should be based on reported sexual exposure (Workowski, 2021).

TABLE 15.3 HEADSSS Tool	
Home	Where do you live, and who lives there with you?
Education/ employment	Are you in school? What are you good at in school? What is hard for you? What grades do you get?
Activities	What do you do for fun? What things do you do with friends? What do you do with your free time?
Drugs	Many young people experiment with drugs, alcohol, or cigarettes. Have you or your friends ever tried them? What have you tried?
Sexuality	Are you involved in a relationship? Have you been involved in a relationship? How was that experience for you? How would you describe your feeling toward guys or girls? How do you see yourself in terms of sexual preference (i.e., gay, straight, or bisexual)?
Suicide/ depression	Patient health questionnaire for adolescents (PHQ-A), ages and stages questionnaire (asQ)
Safety	Do you feel safe in your relationships? In your home? Has anyone forced you to do anything sexually that you did not want to do?

3. HIV screening should be offered to all adolescents (Workowski, 2021).
4. All pregnant adolescents should be screened for syphilis (Workowski, 2021).
5. Clean-catch urine samples used for the Nucleic Acid Amplification test (NAAT) have been shown to have equivalent sensitivity and specificity to diagnose CT and GC when compared to the gold standard vaginal swabs. This may make testing easier since screening for urinary tract infections also requires clean-catch urine (Pickett, 2021).
6. Cervical cancer screening should not begin until age 21 per USPSTF and ACOG.

D. HIV and PreP
1. In 2015, there were 1,729 adolescents aged 13 to 19 years with HIV infection diagnosed in the United States and six dependent areas.
2. The rate of diagnoses of HIV infection in adolescents was 5.8 per 100,000 population (NHANES, 2019).
3. HIV and PreP recommendations
   a. Tenofovir/emtricitabine (TDF/FTC) is approved for Pre-exposure Prophylaxis (PreP) by the FDA for use in adolescents weighing at least 77 pounds (CDC, 2021).
   b. All adolescents should be counseled about HIV transmission risks and prevention options and PreP should be discussed (Hosek, 2020).
   c. Adolescents at increased risk for HIV acquisition include HIV-positive sexual partner, bacterial STI in the last 6 months, history of inconsistent/no condom use (CDC, 2021).
   d. Clinical eligibility criteria: documented negative HIV test within 1 week, no signs or symptoms of HIV infection, creatinine clearance >30 mL/min, no contraindicated medications (CDC, 2021).
   e. Dosage: Tenofovir/emtricitabine (TDF/FTC) PO daily for 90 days (CDC, 2021).
   f. Follow-up every 3 months including assessment of medication adherence, STI screening for men having sex with men (MSM) and transgender women, and HIV test (CDC 2021).

E. HPV vaccination
1. Early vaccination has been shown to be extremely effective at reducing cervical cancer.
2. Women who received the Cervarix HPV vaccine at age 12 or 13 have shown an 87% reduction in cervical cancer compared to the expected rate for the unvaccinated (Falcaro, 2021).
3. Gardasil 9 vaccine is FDA approved for all females and males from ages 9 to 45 years.
   a. For ages 9 to 14 years old there is a two-dose schedule. First injection today and second injection in 6 to 12 months.
   b. There is also a three-dose schedule: first today, second in 2 months, third in 6 months.
   c. Potential side effects
      (1) Local reactions (reported in 20%–90% of recipients) include pain, redness, and swelling at the injection site.
      (2) Ten percent to 13% have reported a low-grade fever (100°F) in the 2 weeks following vaccination.
      (3) Syncope is a possibility; adolescents should lie down for 15 minutes post vaccination (Workowski, 2021).

MENTAL HEALTH

A. Top global causes of morbidity in female-identified adolescents include anxiety and depression (Guthold, 2021). It is critical for all primary care providers to screen adolescents for anxiety and depression.
B. **Screening tools:** The following tools should be used in the adolescent population. Positive screening results should be referred to mental health services.
1. The PHQ-A should be used to screen for depression in those ages 11 to 17 (Johnson, 2002).
2. The general anxiety disorder-7 (GAD-7) screening tool should be used to screen adolescents for anxiety (Lowe, 2008).

EATING DISORDERS

A. Approximately 90% of people with eating disorders identify as female, and eating disorders are the second leading cause of mental health disability (Arcelus, 2011). Eating disorders have the highest mortality rate of any psychiatric condition.

B. It is important for the APRN to be aware of common signs and behaviors that are associated with eating disorders, to screen clients for eating disorders, and to refer to the appropriate services.

1. The following is a list of common signs of a possible eating disorder
   a. Significant weight gain or loss, or failure to gain weight/height according to growth pattern
   b. Electrolyte abnormalities, including low potassium and high blood alkaline levels
   c. Low blood pressure
   d. Low body temperature
   e. A slow or irregular heartbeat
   f. Amenorrhea
   g. Cold intolerance
   h. Complaints of nausea, stomachaches, bloating, or constipation
   i. Complaints of dizziness, weakness, or fatigue
   j. Swollen salivary glands
   k. Dry, pale skin
   l. Fine hair growth on body and thinning hair on head
   m. Brittle nails and blue nail beds

2. The following is a list of behaviors that may signal a client has an eating disorder:
   a. Preoccupation with food
   b. Distorted body image or excessive worry about weight and shape
   c. Sudden significant changes to diet
   d. Avoidance of social situations involving food
   e. Aversion to tastes, smells, or textures
   f. Fear of vomiting or choking
   g. Obsessive exercise
   h. Purging by self-induced vomiting or abusing laxatives, diuretics, or diet pills
   i. Hiding or hoarding food, or eating in secret

3. The SCOFF questionnaire is a quick screening tool that providers can use (Morgan, 1999). If the client answers yes to two or more questions, there is a strong likelihood they have an eating disorder and should be referred to a specialist.
   a. Do you feel like you sometimes lose or have lost control over how you eat?
   b. Do you ever make yourself sick because you feel uncomfortably full?
   c. Do you believe yourself to be fat, even when others say you are too thin?
   d. Do food or thoughts about food dominate your life?
   e. Do thoughts about changing your body and/or your weight dominate your life?
   f. Have others become worried about your weight and/or eating?

SUBSTANCE USE

A. The American Academy of Pediatrics recommends universal screening for substance abuse in pediatric care.

1. Tobacco use among teens rose significantly between 2017 and 2019 (East, 2021), especially in the use of vaping, smokeless tobacco, and nicotine replacement products. According to the 2019 Youth Risk Behavior Survey, 6% of students currently smoke tobacco; 32.7% of

students currently use a vapor product; and 21.7% currently use marijuana. In the same survey, 29.2% of 9th to 12th graders reported currently drinking alcohol, while 13.7% reported binge drinking with even higher rates in females at 14.6% (CDC, 2019).

2. All patients 12 to 17 years old should be screened with a validated screening tool (Kelly, 2014; Levy, 2014). The most researched tool for adolescents is the CRAFFT. Adolescents are more likely to answer honestly if they answer questions themselves, rather than have the provider ask the questions. The latest version of the tool includes nicotine as well (Knight, 1999).

3. The National Institute on Drug Abuse also has two screening tools that can be administered online either by the patient or the provider.
   a. **Screening to Brief Intervention Tool (S2BI):** https://www.drugabuse.gov/ast/bstad/#
   b. **Brief Screener for Tobacco, Alcohol, and other Drugs (BSTAD):** https://www.drugabuse.gov/ast/s2bi/#

BULLYING

A. Both traditional bullying and cyberbullying have been shown to have negative health consequences including anxiety, depression, self-harm, and suicidality (Hellstrom, 2015; Myklestad, 2021).

B. APRNs are in a position to provide anticipatory guidance and screening for bullying for their adolescent clients (Moreno, 2017).

C. There are certain populations that are at higher risk for bullying, such as LGBTQ+ youth. Providers should be aware of signs of likely bullying and include screening questions in intake questionnaires and/or in-person interviews. There are limited resources about how best to screen for bullying in the healthcare setting. Asking clients if they have experienced any in-person or cyberbullying is a way to start.

D. The following are signs of potential bullying
   1. Avoiding school (more truancy and absences, leaving school due to reported health problems, less willing to attend, other academic problems)
   2. Lower self-esteem, increased depression and/or anxiety
   3. Reporting health problems (e.g., stomachaches, headaches)
   4. Trouble sleeping or frequent nightmares
   5. Detachment from friends
   6. Sudden withdrawal at home
   7. Sudden anger or rage
   8. Self-destructive behavior such as cutting

SUICIDE PREVENTION

A. Suicide is the second leading cause of death among youths between 15 and 24 years old. Teen suicide rates are consistently higher in boys than in girls (22.4 vs. 13.9/100,000 in 2019; NIMH, 2019).

B. All teens should be screened for suicide risk. Tools specific for this purpose include the PHQ-A (Johnson, 2002) and the Ask Suicide Screening Questions (asQ) (NIMH 2020).
   1. If a client screens positive for suicide risk, the next steps are as follows
      a. **Low risk:** Counsel, refer, follow-up
      b. **Moderate risk:** Counsel, refer, develop safety plan, follow-up
      c. **Severe risk:** Counsel, ensure parents/caregivers closely monitor child, remove lethal means, develop safety plan, make a crisis referral, follow-up

SOCIAL MEDIA

A. 95% of teens have access to a smartphone, and 45% say they are online almost constantly. AAP recommends that adolescents stop media use 60 minutes before bed to avoid sleep disruptions (delayed bedtimes, disruption of circadian rhythms, increased arousal; AAP, 2016).

B. Social media use has also been associated with poor mental health, self-harm, and suicidality especially among girls (Mikelstad, 2021). There appears to be a dose response relationship between time spent on social media and adverse effects (Abi-Jaoude, 2020). It is important for providers to be aware of these potential risks and to have resources for referrals.

BIBLIOGRAPHY

Abi-Jaoude, E., Naylor, K. T., & Pignatiello, A. (2020). Smartphones, social media use and youth mental health. *CMAJ: Canadian Medical Association Journal, 192*(6), E136–E141. https://doi.org/10.1503/cmaj.190434

American Academy of Pediatrics. (2016). Confidentiality protections for adolescents and young adults in the health care billing and insurance claims process. *Journal of Adolescent Health, 58*(3), 374–377. https://doi.org/10.1016/j.jadohealth.2015.12.009

American Academy of Pediatrics Council on Communications and Media. (2016). Media use in school-aged children and adolescents. *Pediatrics, 138*, e20162592. https://doi.org/10.1542/peds.2016-2592

American College of Obstetricians and Gynecologists. (2020a). Confidentiality in adolescent health care: ACOG Committee Opinion No. 803. *Obstet Gynecol, 135*, e171–7. https://doi.org/https://www.acog.org/clinical/clinical-guidance/committee-opinion/articles/2020/04/confidentiality-in-adolescent-health-care

American College of Obstetricians and Gynecologists. (2020b). The initial reproductive health visit. ACOG Committee Opinion No. 811. *Obstet Gynecol 136*, e70–80. https://doi.org/https://www.acog.org/clinical/clinical-guidance/committee-opinion/articles/2020/10/the-initial-reproductive-health-visit

Arcelus, J., Mitchell, A. J., Wales, J., & Nielsen, S. (2011). Mortality rates in patients with anorexia nervosa and other eating disorders. A meta-analysis of 36 studies. *Archives of General Psychiatry, 68*, 724–731. https://doi.org/10.1001/archgenpsychiatry.2011.74

Association of Women's Health, Obstetrics, and Neonatal Nursing. (2017). Confidentiality in adolescent health care. *Nursing for Women's Health, 21*(6), 509–510. https://doi.org/10.1016/S1751-4851(17)30329-X

Bibbins-Domingo, K., Grossman, D. C., Curry, S. J., Davidson, K. W., Epling, J. W., García, F. A., Gillman, M. W., Harper, D. M., Kemper, A. R., Krist, A. H., Kurth, A. E., Landefeld, C. S., Mangione, C. M., Phillips, W. R., Phipps, M. G., Michael, P., Pignone, M. P., & US Preventive Services Task Force. (2016). Screening for syphilis infection in nonpregnant adults and adolescents: US preventive services task force recommendation statement. *JAMA, 315*(21), 2321–2327. https://doi.org/10.1001/jama.2016.5824

Boyer, C. B., Agénor, M., Willoughby, J. F., Mead, A., Geller, A., Yang, S., Prado, G. J., & Guilamo-Ramos, V. (2021). A renewed call to action for addressing the alarming rising rates of sexually transmitted infections in U.S. adolescents and young adults. *Journal of Adolescent Health, 69*(2), 189–191. https://doi.org/10.1016/j.jadohealth.2021.05.002

Centers for Disease Control and Prevention. (2021). *US public health service: Preexposure prophylaxis for the prevention of HIV infection in the United States—2021 Update: A clinical practice guideline*. https://www.cdc.gov/hiv/pdf/risk/prep/cdc-hiv-prep-guidelines-2021.pdf.

Cohen, E., MacKenzie, R. G., Yates, G. L. (1991). HEADSS, a psychosocial risk assessment instrument: Implications for designing effective intervention programs for runaway youth. *Journal of Adolescent Health, 12*(7), 539–544. https://doi.org/10.1016/0197-0070(91)90084-Y

Cunningham, S. D., Kerrigan, D. L., Jennings, J. M., & Ellen, J. M. (2009). Relationships between perceived STD-related stigma, STD-related shame and STD screening among a household sample of adolescents. *Perspectives on Sexual and Reproductive Health, 41*(4), 225–230. https://doi.org/10.1363/4122509

Curry, S. J., Krist, A. H., Owens, D. K., Barry, M. J., Caughey, A. B., Davidson, K. W., Doubeni, C. A., Epling, J. W., Kemper, A. R., Kubik, M., Landefeld, C. S., Mangione, C. M., Silverstein, M., Simon, M. A., Tseng, C-W., John B Wong, J. B., & US Preventive Services Task Force. (2018a). Screening and behavioral counseling interventions to reduce unhealthy alcohol use in adolescents and adults: US Preventive Services Task Force recommendation statement. *JAMA, 320*(18), 1899–1909. https://doi.org/10.1001/jama.2018.16789

Curry, S. J., Krist, A. H., Owens, D. K., Barry, M. J., Caughey, A. B., Davidson, K. W., ... & US Preventive Services Task Force. (2018b). Screening for intimate partner violence, elder abuse, and abuse of vulnerable adults: US preventive services task force final recommendation statement. *JAMA, 320*(16), 1678–1687. https://doi.org/10.1001/jama.2018.14741

Davidson, K. W., Barry, M. J., Mangione, C. M., Cabana, M., Caughey, A. B., Davis, E. M., Donahue, K. E., Doubeni, C. A., Krist, A. H., Kubik, M., Li, L., Ogedegbe, G., Pbert, L., Silverstein, M., Simon, M. A., Stevermer, J., Tseng, C. W., Wong, J. B., & US Preventive Services Task Force. (2021). Screening for chlamydia and gonorrhea: US preventive services task force recommendation statement. *JAMA, 326*(10), 949–956. https://doi.org/10.1001/jama.2021.14081

East, K. A., Reid, J. L., Rynard, V. L., Hammond, D. (2021). Trends and patterns of tobacco and nicotine product use among youth in Canada, England, and the United States from 2017 to 2019. *Journal of Adolescent Health, 69*(3), 447–456. https://doi.org/10.1016/j.jadohealth.2021.02.011.

English, A., & Ford, C. A. (2018). Adolescent health, confidentiality in healthcare, and communication with parents. *The Journal of Pediatrics, 199*, 11–13. https://doi.org/10.1016/j.jpeds.2018.04.029

Falcaro, M., Castañon, M., Ndlela, B., Checchi, M., Soldan, K., Lopez-Bernal, J., Elliss-Brookes, L., & Sasieni, P. (2021). The effects of the national HPV vaccination programme in England, UK, on cervical cancer and grade 3 cervical intraepithelial neoplasia incidence: A register-based observational study. *Lancet,* 1–9. https://doi.org/10.1016/S0140-6736(21)02178-4.

Finer, L. B., & Zolna, M. R. (2016). Declines in unintended pregnancy in the United States, 2008–2011. *New England Journal of Medicine, 374*(9), 843–852. https://doi.org/10.1056/NEJMsa1506575

Grossman, D. C., Curry, S. J., Owens, D. K., Barry, M. J., Caughey, A. B., Davidson, K. W., Doubeni, C. A., Epling, J. W., Kemper, A. R., Krist, A. H., Kubik, M., Landefeld, S., Mangione, C. M., Silverstein, M., Simon, M. A., Tseng, C. W., & US Preventive Services Task Force. (2018). Behavioral counseling to prevent skin cancer: US preventive services task force recommendation statement. *JAMA, 319*(11), 1134–1142. https://doi.org/10.1001/jama.2018.1623

Grossman, D. C., Bibbins-Domingo, K., Curry, S. J., Barry, M. J., Davidson, K. W., Doubeni, C. A., Epling, J. W., Kemper, A. R., Krist, A. H., Kurth, A. E., Landefeld, S., Mangione, C. M., Phipps, M. G., Silverstein, M., Simon, M. A., Tseng, C. W., & US Preventive Services Task Force. (2017). Screening for obesity in children and adolescents: US preventive services task force recommendation statement. *JAMA, 317*(23), 2417–426. https://doi.org/10.1001/jama.2017.6803

Guthold, R. Baltag, V., Katwan, E., Lopez, G., Diaz, T., & Ross, D. A. (2021) The top global causes of adolescent mortality and morbidity by age and sex, 2019. *Journal of Adolescent Health, 69*(4), 540. https://doi.org/10.1016/j.jadohealth.2021.06.023.

Guttmacher Institute. (2021). *An overview of consent to reproductive health services by young people.* https://www.guttmacher.org/state-policy/explore/overview-minors-consent-law#

Haeger, K. O., Lamme, J., & Cleland, K. (2018). State of emergency contraception in the US, 2018. *Contraception and Reproductive Medicine, 3*(1), 1–12. https://doi.org/10.1186/s40834-018-0067-8

Ham, P., & Allen, C. W. (2012). Adolescent health screening and counseling. *American Family Physician, 86*(12), 1109–1116. https://www.aafp.org/afp/2012/1215/p1109.html

Hellström, L., Persson, L., & Hagquist, C. (2015). Understanding and defining bullying - adolescents' own views. *Archives of Public Health, 73*(1), 4. https://doi.org/10.1186/2049-3258-73-4

Hornberger, L. L. (2017). Options counseling for the pregnant adolescent patient. *Pediatrics, 140*(3). https://doi.org/10.1542/peds.2017-2274

Hosek, S. & Henry-Reid, L. (2020). PrEP and adolescents: The role of providers in ending the AIDS epidemic. *Pediatrics, 145*(1), e20191743. https://doi.org/10.1542/peds.2019-1743

Hoffman, B. L., Schorge, J. O., Halvorson, L. M., Hamid, C. A., Corton, M. M., & Schaffer, J. I. (2020). *Williams Gynecology.* McGraw Hill.

Johnson, J. G., Harris, E. S., Spitzer, R. L., & Williams, J. B. (2002). The patient health questionnaire for adolescents: Validation of an instrument for the assessment of mental disorders among adolescent primary care patients. *The Journal of Adolescent Health: Official Publication of the Society for Adolescent Medicine, 30*(3), 196–204. https://doi.org/10.1016/s1054-139x(01)00333-0

Kelly, S. M., Gryczynski, J., Mitchell, S. G., Kirk, A., O'Grady, K. E., & Schwartz, R. P. (2014). Validity of brief screening instrument for adolescent tobacco, alcohol, and drug use. *Pediatrics, 133*(5), 819–826. https://doi.org/10.1542/peds.2013-2346

Klein, D. A., Paradise, S. L., & Reeder, R. M. (2019). Amenorrhea: A systematic approach to diagnosis and management. *American Family Physician, 100*(1), 39–48. https://www.aafp.org/afp/2019/0701/p39.html

Klein, J. D. (2005). Adolescent pregnancy: Current trends and issues. *Pediatrics, 116*(1), 281–286. https://doi.org/10.1542/peds.2005-0999

Knight, J. R., Shrier, L. A., Bravender, T. D., Farrell, M., Vander Bilt, J., & Shaffer, H. J. (1999). A new brief screen for adolescent substance abuse. *Archives of Pediatrics & Adolescent Medicine, 153*(6), 591–596. https://doi.org/10.1001/archpedi.153.6.591

Krist, A. H., Davidson, K. W., Mangione, C. M., Barry, M. J., Cabana, M., Caughey, A. B., Donahue, K., Doubeni, C. A., Epling, J. W. Jr., Kubik, M., Ogedegbe, G., Pbert, L., Silverstein, M., Simon, M. A., Tseng, C. W., Wong, J. B., & US Preventive Services Task Force. (2020a). Behavioral counseling interventions to prevent sexually transmitted infections: US preventive services task force recommendation statement. *JAMA, 324*(7), 674–681. https://doi.org/10.1001/jama.2020.13095

Krist, A. H., Davidson, K. W., Mangione, C. M., Barry, M. J., Cabana, M., Caughey, A. B., Curry, S. J., Donahue, K., Doubeni, C. A., Epling, J. W. Jr., Kubik, M., Ogedegbe, G., Pbert, L., Silverstein, M., Simon, M. A., Tseng, C. W., Wong, J. B., & US Preventive Services Task Force. (2020b). Screening for unhealthy drug use: US preventive services task force recommendation statement. *JAMA, 323*(22), 2301–2309. https://doi.org/10.1001/jama.2020.8020

Krist, A. H., Davidson, K. W., Mangione, C. M., Barry, M. J., Cabana, M., Caughey, A. B., Donahue, K., Doubeni, C. A., Epling, J. W. Jr., Kubik, M., Ogedegbe, G., Owens, D. K., Pbert, L., Silverstein, M., Simon, M. A., Tseng, C. W., Wong, J. B., & US Preventive Services Task Force. (2020c). Screening for hepatitis B virus infection in adolescents and adults: US preventive services task force recommendation statement. *JAMA, 324*(23), 2415–2422. https://doi.org/10.1001/jama.2020.22980

Krist, A. H., Davidson, K. W., Mangione, C. M., Cabana, M., Caughey, A. B., Davis, E. M., Donahue, K. E., Doubeni, C. A., Kubik, M., Li, L., Ogedegbe, G., Pbert, L., Silverstein, M., Stevermer, J., Tseng, C. W., Wong, J. B., & US Preventive Services Task Force. (2021). Screening for hypertension in adults: US preventive services task force reaffirmation recommendation statement. *JAMA, 325*(16), 1650–1656. https://doi.org/10.1001/jama.2021.4987

Levy, S., Weiss, R., Sherritt, L., Ziemnik, R., Spalding, A., Van Hook, S., & Shrier, L. A. (2014). An electronic screen for triaging adolescent substance use by risk levels. *JAMA Pediatrics, 168*(9), 822–828. https://doi.org/10.1001/jamapediatrics.2014.774

Lindberg, L. D., & Kantor, L. M. (2021). Adolescents' receipt of sex education in a nationally representative sample, 2011–2019. *Journal of Adolescent Health, 70*(2), 290–297. https://doi.org/10.1016/j.jadohealth.2021.08.027

Löwe, B., Decker, O., Müller, S., Brähler, E., Schellberg, D., Herzog, W., & Herzberg, P.Y. (2008). Validation and standardization of the Generalized Anxiety Disorder Screener (GAD-7) in the general population. *Med Care, 46*(3), 266–274

Martin, J. A., Hamilton, B. E., Osterman, M. J. K., & Driscoll, A. K. (2021). Births: Final data for 2019. *National Vital Statistics Reports, 70*(2), 1–50. https://doi.org/10.15620/cdc:100472

Martinez, G. M. (2020). *Trends and patterns in menarche in the United States, 1995 through 2013–2017* (National Health Statistics Reports; no 146). National Center for Health Statistics. https://stacks.cdc.gov/view/cdc/93643

Moreno, M. A., & Vaillancourt, T. (2017). The role of health care providers in cyberbullying. *Canadian Journal of Psychiatry, 62*(6), 364–367. https://doi.org/10.1177/0706743716684792

Morgan, J. F., Reid, F., & Lacey, J. H. (1999). The SCOFF questionnaire: Assessment of a new screening tool for eating disorders. *British Medical Journal, 319*(7223), 1467–8. https://doi.org/10.1136/bmj.319.7223.1467

Myklestad, I., & Straiton, M. (2021). The relationship between self-harm and bullying behaviour: Results from a population based study of adolescents. *BMC Public Health, 21*(1), 1–15. https://doi.org/10.1186/s12889-021-10555-9

National Center for Health Statistics. (2021). *National Health and Nutrition Examination Survey.* https://wwwn.cdc.gov/nchs/nhanes/continuousnhanes/default.aspx?BeginYear=2019.

National Institute of Mental Health. (2020). *AsQ Suicide Risk Screening Toolkit.* https://www.nimh.nih.gov/research/research-conducted-at-nimh/asq-toolkit-materials

National Institute of Mental Health. (2021). *Suicide.* https://www.nimh.nih.gov/health/statistics/suicide

Owens, D. K., Davidson, K. W., Krist, A. H., Barry, M. J., Cabana, M., Caughey, A. B., Curry, S. J., Donahue, K., Doubeni, C. A., Epling, J. W. Jr., Kubik, M., Ogedegbe, G., Pbert, L., Silverstein, M., Simon, M. A., Tseng, C. W., Wong, J. B., & US Preventive Services Task Force. (2020). Primary care interventions for prevention and cessation of tobacco use in children and adolescents: US preventive services task force recommendation statement. *JAMA, 323*(16), 1590–1598. https://doi.org/10.1001/jama.2020.4679

Owens, D. K., Davidson, K. W., Krist, A. H., Barry, M. J., Cabana, M., Caughey, A. B., Curry, S. J., Doubeni, C. A., Epling, J. W. Jr., Kubik, M., Landefeld, C. S., Mangione, C. M., Pbert, L., Silverstein, M., Simon, M. A., Tseng, C. W., Wong, J. B., & US Preventive Services Task Force. (2019). Screening for HIV infection: US preventive services task force recommendation statement. *Journal of the American Medical Association, 321*(23), 2326–2336. https://doi.org/10.1001/jama.2019.6587

Owens, D. K., Davidson, K. W., Krist, A. H., Barry, M. J., Cabana, M., Caughey, A. B., Donahue, K., Doubeni, C. A., Epling, J. W. Jr., Kubik, M., Ogedegbe, G., Pbert, L., Silverstein, M., Simon, M. A., Tseng, C. W., Wong, J. B., & US Preventive Services Task Force. (2020). Screening for hepatitis C virus infection in adolescents and adults: US preventive services task force recommendation statement. *Journal of the American Medical Association, 323*(10), 970–975. https://doi.org/10.1001/jama.2020.1123

Physicians for Reproductive Health. (2021). *Provider resources in adolescent health curriculum best practices.* https://prh.org/arshep-ppts/#best-practices

Pickett, M. L., Visotcky, A., Brazauskas, R., Ledeboer, N. A., & Drendel, A. L. (2021). Can a clean catch urine sample be used to diagnose chlamydia and gonorrhea in adolescent females? *Journal of Adolescent Health,* 69 (4), 574–578. https://doi.org/10.1016/j.jadohealth.2021.02.022

Siu, A. L. (2016). Screening for depression in children and adolescents: US preventive services task force recommendation statement. *Annals of Internal Medicine, 164*(5), 360–366. https://doi.org/10.7326/M15-2957

Wilkinson, J. P., & Kadir, R. A. (2010). Management of abnormal uterine bleeding in adolescents. *Journal of Pediatric and Adolescent Gynecology, 23*(6), S22–S30. https://doi.org/10.1016/j.jpag.2010.08.007

Wodi, A. P., Ault, K., Hunter, P., McNally, V., Szilagyi, P. G., & Bernstein, H. (2021). Advisory committee on immunization practices recommended immunization schedule for children and adolescents aged 18 years or younger—United States, 2021. *Morbidity and Mortality Weekly Report, 70*(6), 189. https://doi.org/10.15585/mmwr.mm7006a1

Workowski, K. A., Bachmann, L. H., Chan, P. A., Johnston, C. M., Muzny, C. A., Park, I., Reno, H., Zenilman, J. M., & Bolan, G. A. (2021). Sexually transmitted treatment guidelines 2021. *MMWR Recommendations and Reports, 70*(4), 1–192. https://doi.org/10.15585/mmwr.rr7004a1

16

LACTATION ASSESSMENT AND MANAGEMENT

JAMILLE NAGTALON-RAMOS, HANNAH E. BERGBOWER, AND
SAMANTHA E. NOBLEJAS

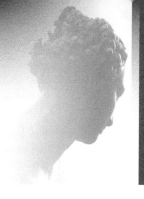

ANATOMY AND PHYSIOLOGY

A. Changes in breasts during pregnancy
1. Begins early in pregnancy
2. Ducts, lobules, and alveoli develop in response to hormones: estrogen, progesterone, human chorionic somatomammotropin (hCS), and prolactin.
B. Milk production
1. Produced in alveoli through a complex process by which substances from the mother's bloodstream are reformulated into breast milk
C. Hormones of lactation
1. Oxytocin
   a. Increases in response to nipple stimulation and causes the milk ejection reflex or let-down reflex, the release of milk from the alveoli into the ducts
   b. During feeding, the milk-ejection reflex occurs several times; some mothers have a tingling sensation of the breast when let-down occurs, and milk is expressed out of the nipples
2. Prolactin
   a. Loss of placental hormones result in increasing levels of prolactin
   b. Hormone responsible in activating milk production
D. Lactogenesis stages
1. Lactogenesis stage 1
   a. Starts in pregnancy and continues during early days after birth
   b. Colostrum (aka Liquid Gold)
      (1) Present by 16 weeks of gestation
      (2) Thick, yellow substance that is higher in protein, vitamins, and minerals than mature milk
      (3) Rich in immunoglobulins which helps protect the GI tract from infection. Immunoglobulin A establishes normal flora in the intestines and also has a laxative effect that speeds the passage of meconium (the baby's first stool).
2. Lactogenesis stage 2
   a. Begins 2 to 3 days after birth
   b. Transitional milk
      (1) Milk that gradually changes from colostrum to mature milk, appears over the next 10 days
      (2) Amount of milk increases rapidly which the patient may feel as the milk "coming in" and feels their breasts to be fuller
      (3) Immunoglobulins decrease and lactose, fat, calories increase
3. Lactogenesis stage 3
   a. Mature milk replaces transitional milk

      b. Bluish and not as thick; patients may think this milk is not "rich" or fatty enough for their infants.

      c. Still contains immunoglobulins

E. **Breast milk nutrient composition:** Protein, carbohydrates, fat, vitamins, minerals, enzymes

F. Breast milk also has infection-preventing components:

   1. Promotes growth of *Lactobacillus bifidus*, important part of intestinal flora

   2. Protects against common intestinal pathogens

   3. Leukocytes present in breast milk also help protect against infection.

   4. High amounts of immunoglobulins in colostrum

G. Physiology behind lactational amenorrhea

   1. Postpartum follicle-stimulating hormone (FSH) returns to normal levels by 4 to 8 weeks, but luteinizing hormone (LH) is disorganized and suppressed.

   2. Infant suckling stimulates nerve endings that tell the hypothalamus to trigger prolactin release which results in milk production.

   3. Suckling disrupts pulsatile gonadotropin-releasing hormone (GnRH) release which impacts LH pulsatility. The ovum cannot be released without LH surge.

   4. Breastfeeding also results in hypoestrogenic state. Estrogen levels are insufficient to trigger LH surge or rebuild uterine lining.

NEWBORN

A. Nutritional needs of the newborn

   1. Calories

      a. Breastfed 85 to 100 kcal/kg daily

      b. Formula fed 100 to 110 kcal/kg daily

      c. May lose less than 10% of birth weight

   2. Nutrients found in both breast milk and formula

      a. Carbohydrates

      b. Proteins

      c. Fats

      d. Vitamins/minerals

   3. Water

      a. Breast milk and formula have sufficient water content

      b. Avoid additional water

B. Infant stomach size

   1. **Day 1:** Size of a shooter marble or a cherry

   2. **Day 3:** Size of a ping pong ball

   3. **Day 7:** Size of an apricot

   4. **Day 30:** Size of a large chicken egg

DECIDING TO BREASTFEED

A. Risks related to not breastfeeding

   1. Otitis media

   2. Atopic dermatitis (eczema)

   3. Gastrointestinal infection

   4. Hospitalization for lower respiratory tract disease in the first year of life

   5. Asthma

   6. Childhood obesity

   7. Type 2 diabetes mellitus

   8. Sudden infant death syndrome (SIDS)

B. Contraindications to breastfeeding
   1. HIV
      a. The primary mechanism of HIV transmission in infants is mother-to-infant.
      b. One of the means of this transmission can be through breastfeeding.
      c. Both the Centers for Disease Control and Prevention (CDC) and the World Health Organization (WHO) have separate recommendations for mothers in high-income countries versus resource-limited settings. In countries like the United States, breastfeeding in HIV-positive mothers is considered unsafe independent of the mothers antiretroviral (ARV) status.
      d. In resource-limited countries, mothers on ARV therapy are recommended to exclusively breastfeed for the first 6 months.
   2. Herpes on nipple
      a. Mothers with an active herpes simplex virus (HSV) outbreak are safe to breastfeed if the herpes lesion is not located on any part of the breast and the affected area is fully covered.
      b. When herpetic lesions are present on any part of the breast, breastfeeding should be temporarily stopped and can resume once the lesion(s) is fully healed.
      c. Pumping or hand expressing from the affected breast should be discarded as it may have been exposed to active lesions.
      d. Stressing the importance of hand hygiene and making sure all areas are safely covered are critical in ensuring infants are not exposed.
   3. Varicella
      a. If a parturient developed infection within the 5 days prior to delivery or the 2 days following delivery, it is recommended for the breastfeeding person to temporarily refrain from breastfeeding.
      b. Expressed milk can be fed to the newborn.
C. Of caution
   1. COVID-19
      a. If the patient has COVID-19 and chooses to breastfeed their infant
         (1) Advise to wash hands prior to breastfeeding.
         (2) Wear a mask while feeding and whenever within 6 feet of the baby.
      b. If the patient has COVID-19 and chooses to express breast milk
         (1) Advise to use their own pump.
         (2) Wash hands before touching any pump or bottle parts.
         (3) Wear a mask while pumping.
         (4) Clean all parts of the pump that come into contact with breast milk.
         (5) Consider having a healthy, fully vaccinated, masked caregiver feed the pumped breast milk to the baby.
   2. Hepatitis B (HBV)
      a. HBV can be transmitted through body fluids including blood.
      b. Breastfeeding is considered safe for infants born to mothers with HBV with specific recommendations.
      c. The first dose of the HBV vaccine and hepatitis B immune globulin should be administered to the newborn within the first 12 hours after birth.
      d. Breastfeeding does not need to be delayed until administration is complete and can occur within the first hour of life per WHO recommendations.
      e. The second dose of the vaccine is recommended for administration at age 1 to 2 months and the third at 6 months, with HBV testing recommended on the infant at 9 to 12 months of age to ensure the vaccine was effective.
   3. Hepatitis C (HCV)
      a. Breastfeeding with a hepatitis C positive patient is considered safe, without evidence of spread.

4. Cracked or bleeding nipples with HCV/HBV
   a. If the breastfeeding person who is hepatitis B or C positive has cracked or bleeding nipple(s), it is recommended to refrain from breastfeeding during that time.
   b. To maintain milk supply, pumping is recommended.
   c. Milk obtained through pumping must be discarded for risk of infant exposure.
   d. Feeding can safely resume when cracks have healed and no bleeding occurs.
5. Tobacco use
   a. Lactation and pregnancy are considered important times to encourage smoking cessation.
   b. Breastfeeding and use of tobacco or e-cigarettes are considered safe with recommendations to minimize infant exposure.
   c. Tobacco can be passed through breastmilk and has the potential to reduce milk supply.
   d. If breastfeeding while consuming tobacco or e-cigarettes, it is recommended to only smoke outdoors with strict rules to have a smoke-free car or home; do not smoke near infant, and make sure to change clothes and wash hands after smoking and prior to resuming infant care.
   e. Tobacco exposure has been linked to increased risk for SIDS.
6. Alcohol use
   a. Alcohol can be found in breastmilk after consumption by the breastfeeding person.
   b. Specific amounts of alcohol can be considered safe while breastfeeding; however, not drinking while breastfeeding is considered safest by the CDC.
   c. Consumption of one standard drink per day is not known to be harmful to an infant, especially if waiting 2 or more hours before feeding.
   d. Thirty to 60 minutes after consumption is when the alcohol level is highest in breast milk.
   e. It is generally detectable for 2 to 3 hours per drink after consumption but can vary.
   f. The milk ejection reflex (letdown) can also be negatively impacted while alcohol levels are high in the breastfeeding person.

OVER-THE-COUNTER AND ILLICIT DRUGS, PRESCRIPTION MEDICATIONS, AND HERBS

A. Marijuana
1. Data are currently insufficient to understand whether breastfeeding while using marijuana is considered safe.
2. Discuss the risks of exposure to marijuana and benefits of breastfeeding with patients.
3. Marijuana can be passed directly to an infant through breastfeeding and, as marijuana is stored in fat cells, infants could potentially have unknown length of exposure.
4. Neurodevelopmental impacts of exposure on an infant remain unknown.

B. Narcotics
1. Most narcotics are prescribed during the immediate postpartum period for pain management and are of minimal risk to the newborn.
2. Prolonged narcotic use, once full lactation is established, can have severe side effects on the infant such as extreme drowsiness, central nervous system depression; even death has been associated with use.
3. Infant drowsiness can also have an impact on their ability to wake for feedings and for sustaining healthy lactation patterns.

C. Antibiotics
1. Antibiotics use does not indicate a need for the cessation or suspension of breastfeeding.
2. Many antibiotics can pass through breastmilk to the infant but are considered safe in short duration of exposure.
3. Specific medications can be further reviewed through the National Institutes of Health (NIH).

D. Medication-assisted therapy
1. Opioid use disorder in pregnancy has become more prevalent over the last two decades with further breastfeeding people using medication-assisted therapy (MAT) during the postpartum period.
2. All major organizations in the United States recommend exclusive breastfeeding for all using MAT, as long as they are not using other illicit substances.
3. Evidence has shown methadone to be safe in breastfeeding; however, use of buprenorphine is not well established.
4. An additional benefit to breastfeeding with the use of MAT, is the possible benefits of delayed neonatal abstinence syndrome with reduced symptoms in newborns who are immediately breastfed.

SPECIAL POPULATIONS

A. Breast reduction
1. Patients may consider "reduction mammaplasty," more commonly known as breast reduction surgery, for a variety of reasons, due to aesthetic preference or due to clinical issues like back pain caused by weight of the breasts. In any case, those who have undergone breast reduction surgery may have questions regarding whether or not they can breastfeed, and if so, the success rate of lactation outcomes following this surgery.
2. Milk ducts and nerves may be cut, and some glandular tissue may be removed as a result of breast reduction surgery.
3. Surgical techniques have been modified throughout the past century; newer surgical methods have made breastfeeding more possible.
4. Studies have shown that surgical techniques that preserve the column of subareolar parenchyma (parenchyma from the nipple areola complex to the chest wall) increase the likelihood of successful breastfeeding.
5. Patients who have either undergone or plan to undergo breast reduction surgery should discuss potential preference to breastfeed in the future with their surgeon.

B. Breast augmentation
1. Breastfeeding may still be possible even after a patient has undergone breast augmentation and the placement of silicone implants, saline implants, or fat transfer in the breasts, depending on the level of breast tissue and milk ducts that have been affected or removed.
2. Patients should consult with a lactation consultant and their plastic surgeon prior to this procedure to discuss potential impact.
3. Though more robust research is needed, existing studies do not show any clinical contraindications to infants breastfeeding from mothers with existing silicone implants.
4. According to the FDA, studies have found no increased risk of birth defects in infants born to those who have had breast augmentation procedures and implants placed.
5. As with patients who undergo breast reduction, breast augmentation procedures may affect the nerves and glands surrounding the breast, impacting lactation.
6. Patients may also have nipple sensitivity following augmentation.
7. The most important factor that can affect breastfeeding after augmentation is how the surgery was performed.
8. Typically, breast augmentation procedures utilizing surgical techniques that completely cut through the areola and nipple (and thus, affect the milk ducts) are more likely to cause a reduction in milk production.
9. Surgical incisions that are created under the breast have been less likely to interfere with breastfeeding.
10. Those who have had mastectomies and breast implant reconstructive surgeries may not be able to breastfeed due to the amount of breast tissue and milk ducts removed.

11. A majority of participants in a study that explored silicone breast implants were able to successfully breastfeed.
12. Some lactation and breastfeeding tips for those who have undergone breast reduction or augmentation surgeries.

C. Chest feeding or body feeding is when an individual feeds a baby milk from their chest.
   1. This terminology is commonly used by non-binary and transgender parents who are actively participating in human lactation.
   2. The term breastfeeding can be problematic for someone who does not have breasts but who is continuing to feed their baby through the production of their own milk.

CULTURAL AND RELIGIOUS VIEWS AND PRACTICES

A. Common breastfeeding myths and cultural practices
   1. Refraining from eating chocolate while breastfeeding
   2. Not breastfeeding past the appearance of baby's first tooth
   3. Refraining from breastfeeding in a car or a baby will be gassy
   4. Only consuming bland foods while breastfeeding
   5. Experiencing pain while breastfeeding is normal
   6. Exercising can affect the taste of breast milk

B. **Religious beliefs related to breastfeeding:** Conservative Muslims, Protestants, and other members of Christian affiliations have displayed higher rates of breastfeeding compared with unaffiliated counterparts.
   1. Islam
      a. In the Qu'ran, breastfeeding is taught as God's (or Allah's) right to the infant.
      b. Many Muslim women may attempt to breastfeed their child until 2 years of age, though other factors may exist that result in weaning before this age.
      c. Variations in choice and preference may exist depending on the preferences of the infant's parents.
      d. The father, according to the Qu'ran, should provide support to the breastfeeding mother and assist with finding alternative feeding sources (such as formula, donated breast milk, etc.) should the lactating parent be unable to or decide not to breastfeed.
      e. The mother may be given a variety of foods (depending on cultural background) to help aid in lactation, for example:
         (1) Egyptian mothers may consume "moghat," a mixture of powdered fenugreek seeds, nuts fried in sugar and butter, turmeric, and ginger.
         (2) Muslim mothers from some Middle Eastern and African countries may consume what they call "the blessed seed," also known as "black seed" or "black cumin," or *Nigella sativum.*
   2. Judaism
      a. According to the Talmud, breastfeeding is referred to as the ultimate source of nourishment for feeding infants.
      b. Many Orthodox Jewish women will opt to exclusively breastfeed.
      c. The Talmud recommends mothers breastfeed for up to 2 years, but exceptions are acceptable if other factors are present that do not make this possible.
      d. Jewish mothers are often given special treatment in the 7 days that follow after the birth of the infant, and are not encouraged to fast during holy holidays.
      e. Breastfeeding mothers are encouraged to seek the support of their communities in the postpartum period.
      f. If pumping, Orthodox Jewish mothers may not be able to pump during the *Shabbos,* so counseling should be included to save pumped milk and/or breastfeed infant during this time.

3. Catholicism
   a. One study has shown those who identify in the Catholic faith as most likely to exclusively formula-feed postpartum.
   b. More qualitative research is needed to explore possible factors behind this finding.

RACIAL AND ETHNIC DISPARITIES IN BREASTFEEDING

A. *Healthy People 2030* aims to increase breastfeeding initiation rates as well as the proportion of infants who are breastfeed exclusively through 6 months of age.

B. Clinicians can explore the possible factors and barriers leading to existing disparities and better counsel patients who identify from racial and ethnic minority groups.

C. Racial and ethnic minority women have been shown to have lower breastfeeding rates in comparison to White counterparts.

D. In the United States, Asian women are the only racial group that met the *Healthy People 2020* goal of breastfeeding initiation (81.9%); however, no racial/ethnic group met the *Healthy People 2020* objectives of exclusive breastfeeding at 6 months and 12 months.

E. In the United States, African American women have the lowest rates of both breastfeeding initiation (60%) and continuation to 6 (28%) and 12 (12%) months.

F. It is important to note that African American women are disproportionately more likely than their White woman counterparts to experience poor maternal health outcomes and more likely to suffer from chronic stress, trauma, and chronic illness, all of which can impact breastfeeding.

G. African American women are also less likely to receive adequate support and treatment for physical, emotional, and social needs.

H. Lower breastfeeding rates are reported in mothers who are young, come from a low-income background, unmarried, and participate in the Supplemental Nutrition Program for Women, Infants, and Children (WIC).

I. It is crucial to support women, especially those who identify with one or more of these factors, not only for the health of their infant, but their own health.
   1. African American and Hispanic women (in comparison to their White counterparts) have shown higher rates of obesity, cardiovascular disease, and diabetes mellitus.
   2. Breastfeeding has several benefits that can improve the health of these communities, including reduced incidence of type 2 diabetes in the mother, lower risk of obesity in childhood for the infant, increased likelihood of weight loss postpartum versus women who breastfeed non-exclusively and/or formula feed.
   3. Breastfeeding may assist in lowering the mother's risk of hypertension and cardiovascular diseases.

J. Some of these common barriers may exist:
   1. Lack of access to education and information on breastfeeding
   2. Lack of social support or cultural acceptance
   3. Lack of support in the professional setting (i.e., need for employment, limited maternity leave, and the inability to breastfeed or pump properly and/or safely in the workplace)
   4. Inadequate milk production or ineffective latch
   5. Lack of time

K. WIC participation has been tied to lower rates of breastfeeding initiation and lower rates of breastfeeding continuation.

L. It is important for clinicians to provide women with the benefits and importance of breastfeeding, while understanding the barriers and factors that exist while counseling and educating.

M. Women who identify with racial and ethnic minority groups that have shown lower rates of breastfeeding initiation and continuation, especially African American women, may benefit from targeted education, support, resources, and enhanced breastfeeding programs.

FIRST FEEDING

A. Golden hour
1. The first hour after birth is commonly known as the "golden hour," a period of time that should emphasize the drying of the infant and placement on mother's chest for skin-to-skin contact.
2. This hour should be utilized, if clinically possible, for maternal/infant bonding, skin-to-skin time, and the potential to assist the mother in breastfeeding for the first time.
3. If possible, infant assessments should be performed with the infant still on the mother.
4. Non-urgent tasks can be delayed to allow for the first 60 minutes of uninterrupted bonding time.
5. This bonding experience can result in the further release of oxytocin and, in turn, aid in lactation.
6. Providers should support and implement golden hour protocol at their facilities.
7. It is important to note that this may not be possible due to maternal or infant clinical condition, but the clinician should support the mother in their breastfeeding and bonding process as soon as clinically able.

B. Feeding cues
1. Some common infant feeding cues, or signs that the infant may be hungry include:
   a. Increased alertness
   b. Clenched hands
   c. Rooting and/or turning of the head toward the breast
   d. Smacking or puckering of the lips
   e. Putting hands to mouth
   f. Opening and closing of the mouth
   g. Crying (late sign of hunger)

C. Different positions
1. Patients should be educated on proper positioning, as well as the variety of breastfeeding positions that exist. Different positions can be utilized in order to aid in both maternal and infant comfort, as well as to aid in the improved delivery of breast milk from patient to infant.
2. For ease in breastfeeding, make sure that the patient is comfortable and well-supported with proper back support and pillow support for herself and infant.
3. To prevent pain at the nipple, the mouth of the infant should cover at least a half an inch of the areola.
4. Cradle hold (Figures 16.1A and 16.1B)
   a. Infant is lying on their side (resting on shoulder and hip), mouth at the same level as patient's nipple.
   b. The front of the infant's body should touch the front of the patient's body.
   c. Make sure that head, neck, and torso are in straight alignment.
   d. Utilize pillows and/or folded blankets to aid in supporting infant up to the height of the nipple.
   e. Support the breast in a U- or C-shaped hold.
   f. Infant's head rests on the patient's forearm, with their inner forearm and palm supporting the baby's back.
5. Cross-cradle (Figures 16.2A and 16.2B)
   a. Ideal for supporting the infant who needs more neck support and/or who have head discomfort from cephalohematoma or trauma from forceps or vacuum.
   b. Utilize pillow support to raise the infant to nipple level.

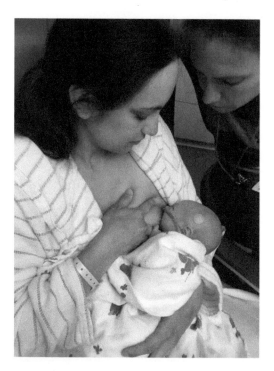

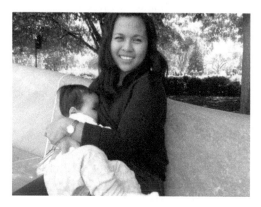

FIGURES 16.1A AND 16.1B Cradle hold: Infant's head rests on the patient's forearm, with their inner forearm and palm supporting infant's back.

c. Support the breast in a U-hold with the arm on the same side as the breast.
d. Support the infant's head with the hand on the opposite side.
e. Patient's hand under infant's ears and neck and supported with patient's index finger and thumb.

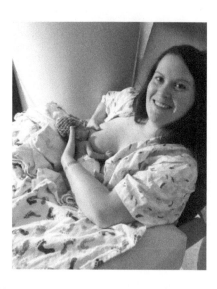

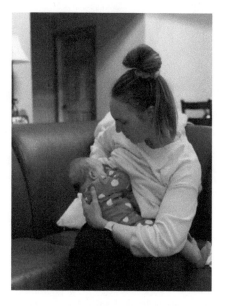

FIGURES 16.2A AND 16.2B Cross-cradle hold: Patient's hand under infant's ears and neck and supported with patient's index finger and thumb. Infant's neck should rest in the space between the index finger and thumb.

      f. Infant's neck should rest in the space between the index finger and thumb.

      g. Patient's hand touches against the infant's shoulder blades and back.

  6. Football (Figures 16.3A and 16.3B)

      a. Commonly used for patients with larger breasts and patients who have undergone a cesarean section (as it helps keep infant away from area of the surgical incision).

      b. Can also be utilized when patient has a strong milk ejection reflex, as it helps infant to better handle the amount of milk being let down.

      c. Support the infant's head with hand, infant's back should be along the arm.

      d. Infant faces patient with legs rested on back rest.

      e. Utilize pillows in order to bring the infant up to the correct height (and for patient's optimal comfort).

  7. Side-lying (Figures 16.4A and 16.4B)

      a. Patient and infant lie on their sides, facing each other.

      b. Utilize rolled blanket or pillow to support infant.

      c. Patient's forearm can cradle baby's back.

      d. Ear, shoulder, and hip of infant should be in alignment for optimal feeding and milk delivery.

  8. Proper latch (Figures 16.5A and 16.5B)

  9. LATCH tool for objective assessment (Table 16.1)

      a. The LATCH tool can be utilized to provide objective assessment of the infant's latch to the patient's breast.

      b. The tool assesses five different areas of breastfeeding (latch, audible swallowing, type of nipple, comfort, and hold) and attaches a numerical score (0, 1, or 2) to each of them.

      c. LATCH scoring should typically be done at least twice in a 24-hour time period in order to assess infant feeding.

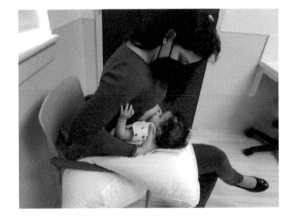
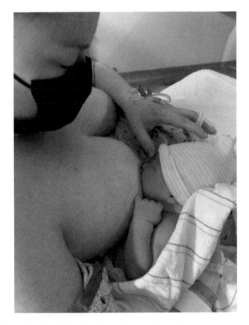

FIGURES 16.3A AND 16.3B Football hold: Infant placed like a football tucked into the patient's arm. Support the infant's head with hand; infant's back should be along the arm.

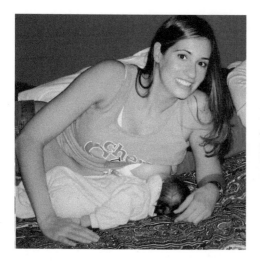
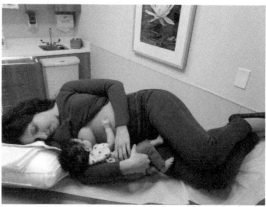

FIGURES 16.4A AND 16.4B Side-lying position: Patient and infant lie on their sides and facing each other with patient's forearm cradling infant's back.

MAINTAINING SUPPLY

A. Frequency of feeding
  1. In the first few days of life, attempt to feed every 1 to 3 hours.
  2. First few weeks to months, feeding should be attempted every 2 to 4 hours.
  3. During this time, breastfeeding will occur 8 to 12 times per day.

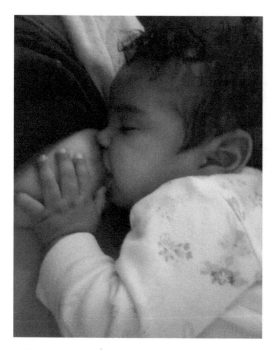
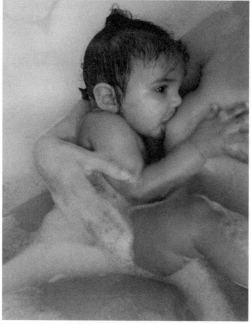

FIGURES 16.5A AND 16.5B Proper latch: Note that the infant's lips are flanged and most of the patient's areola is inside the infant's mouth.

TABLE 16.1 LATCH Tool for Objective Assessment

	0	1	2	TOTAL
L: Latch	Too sleepy; reluctant	Repeated attempts for sustained latch or suck Hold nipple in mouth Stimulate to suck	Grasps breasts Lips flanged Rhythmic sucking	
A: Audible swallowing	None	A few with stimulation	Spontaneous and intermittent	
T: Type of nipple	Inverted	Flat	Everted (after stimulation)	
C: Comfort	Engorged, pain Cracked, bleeding, blisters, bruising	Filling Reddened, small blisters	Soft Non-tender	
H: Hold	Full assist	Minimal assist	No assist	

Source: Reprinted from Jensen, D., Wallace, S., Kelsay, P. (1994). LATCH: A breastfeeding charting system and documentation tool. JOGNN 23, 27–32, with permission from Elsevier.

4. Cluster feeding occurs when the infant feeds more frequently, such as hourly, or goes longer periods while they are sleeping.
5. Infants may cluster feed every 10 to 12 days due to a possible growth spurt and need for increased milk production.
6. After 6 months, the frequency and duration of feeding will likely change as they begin to eat more table food.

NUTRITION DURING LACTATION

A. Nutritional supplements
   1. Continue taking prenatal vitamins while breastfeeding.
   2. 450 to 500 calories a day are required to make breast milk.
   3. **Fluids:** Increased water intake is recommended while breastfeeding. There are mixed recommendations regarding the exact amount, but somewhere between 12 to 16 cups of water a day is suggested by the American College of Obstetricians and Gynecologists (ACOG). Discuss urine color with patients and increase fluid intake if it is dark yellow.
B. Foods to avoid
   1. Fish with high mercury levels including bigeye tuna, king mackerel, marlin, shark, swordfish, or tilefish.
   2. All fish, including albacore tuna, should be limited to 6 oz. a week.
   3. Caffeine is considered safe up to 200 mg daily.

MILK EXPRESSION

A. Returning to work/school
   1. **Plan ahead:** Assess availability of private area for pumping/expressing milk, sink to wash pump parts, and milk storage.
B. Proper storage and preparation of breast milk

1. Prior to working with or transferring milk, it is important to always wash hands. Breast milk should be stored in either breast milk bags, food storage bags, or glass or plastic containers with a good seal.
2. Recommendations for safe storage of human milk as per the CDC (Table 16.2)
3. Obtaining a breast pump
   a. Under the Affordable Care Act (ACA) of 2010, most insurance policies are required to pay for a breast pump and supplies for members.
   b. Some insurance companies, however, with policies existing prior to March of 2010 may be "grandfathered in" and not required to provide this resource.
   c. The first step is for the patient to contact the number on the back of their insurance card and tell them they are pregnant and planning to breastfeed or that they have just delivered and need a pump.
   d. Most companies have a dedicated Maternal Child Health Specialist.
   e. Questions to ask
      (1) Do I need a prescription?
      (2) What types of pumps do you have and are upgrades possible? Hospital grade pumps are the highest quality but can also be the most expensive. If upgrades to hospital grade pumps are available, it is important for the patient to ask how much they will be required to pay.
      (3) Where will the patient need to get the pump or will it be shipped to them?
4. Employee rights and breastfeeding
   a. In 2010, the "Break Time for Nursing Mothers" law was passed as Section 4207 of the ACA, which amended Section 7 of the Fair Labor Standards Act (FLSA) of 1938 (29 U.S.C. 207). This amendment to the FLSA stated that employers must provide:
      (1) Breaktime for an employee to express milk for up to 1 year after each birth. However, employers are not required to compensate employees for this time.
   b. A place for an employee to express milk, other than a bathroom, that is (a) shielded from view and (b) free from intrusion of coworkers or the public
   c. Employers with less than 50 employees are not required to uphold these standards if the requirements would cause undue hardship to the employer.
   d. State level laws supersede this amendment if greater protections are required.

TABLE 16.2 Recommendations for Safe Storage of Human Milk as per the CDC

TYPE OF BREAST MILK	STORAGE LOCATION AND TEMPERATURES		
	COUNTERTOP 77°F (25°C) OR COLDER (ROOM TEMPERATURE)	REFRIGERATOR 40°F (4°C)	FREEZER 0°F (−18°C) OR COLDER
Freshly expressed or pumped	Up to 4 hours	Up to 4 days	Within 6 months is best Up to 12 months is acceptable
Thawed, previously frozen	1–2 hours	Up to 1 day	NEVER refreeze human milk after it has been thawed
Leftover from a feeding (baby did not finish the bottle)	Use within 2 hours after the baby is finished feeding		

Source: Centers for Disease Control and Prevention. (2021). Proper Storage and Preparation of Breast Milk. https://www.cdc.gov/breastfeeding/recommendations/handling_breastmilk.htm

SPECIAL ISSUES

A. Low milk supply
   1. Breastfeed at least 8 to 10 times each day in order to stimulate, establish, and maintain regular breast milk production.
   2. Pumping or manual hand expression after breastfeeding sessions can help empty the breasts and increase milk production.
   3. Meet with a board-certified lactation consultant to assist with best practices, feeding positioning, and effective latch.
B. Non-pharmacologic ways to increase milk supply
   1. Increase frequency and effectiveness of milk removal by hand expression or use of double breast pump.
   2. Avoid skipping feeds.
   3. Get rest, sleep, drink to satisfy thirst, and eat nutritious meals.
C. **Pharmaceutical galactagogues**: Current research on effectiveness of pharmacologic or herbal galactagogues is inconclusive. (A food or drug that increases the flow of breastmilk is known as a *galactagogue*.) The following galactagogues are not endorsed or recommended (Table 16.3).
   1. Domperidone
      a. **Suggested dose:** 10 mg tablet PO two times a day
      b. **Side effects:** Dry mouth, headache. Rare complications (found in studies not specific to lactation) of cardiac arrhythmias due to a prolonged QT interval.
      c. FDA has not approved this medication for use in lactating women.
   2. Metoclopramide (Reglan)
      a. **Suggested dose:** 10 mg tablet PO three to four times/day for 7 to 14 days
      b. Possible increase rate of milk secretion
      c. Rare reports of tardive dyskinesia (usually irreversible), causing the FDA to place a black box warning on this drug in the United States

TABLE 16.3 Pharmacologic Management of Increasing Milk Production

GALACTAGOGUES

General Comments:
- Current research on effectiveness of pharmacologic or herbal galactagogues is inconclusive.
- The galactagogues discussed in the following are not endorsed or recommended.

MEDICATION	DOSAGE: ADULT	DOSAGE: PEDIATRIC	SIDE EFFECTS/ MONITORING	COMMENTS
Domperidone	10 mg tablet PO 2x a day	Not available	Side effects: dry mouth, headache. Rare complications (found in studies not specific to lactation) of cardiac arrhythmias due to a prolonged QT interval	FDA has **not** approved this medication for use in lactating women
Metoclopramide (Reglan)	10 mg tablet PO 3–4x/day for 7–14 days	Not available	Rare reports of tardive dyskinesia (usually irreversible), causing the FDA to place a black box warning on this drug in the United States	

3. **Herbal galactagogues:** Lactating patients may be interested in the utilization of herbs to stimulate lactation and aid in their breastfeeding process. It should be noted that though studies exist, more robust controlled trials and research studies are encouraged for herbal galactagogues. It should also be noted that galactagogue use should not replace proper clinical evaluation of factors that may affect production of breast milk. Some commonly utilized herbs are highlighted in a review of galactagogues.
   a. Fenugreek (*Trigonella foenumgraceum*)
      (1) Often the main ingredient found in "mother's milk" teas sold and consumed with the goal to increase lactation
      (2) One study showed consumption of fenugreek stimulated the genes involved in increasing milk synthesis and flow and increased pituitary oxytocin expression and plasma insulin concentration in study participants.
   b. Shatavari *(Asparagus racemosus)*
      (1) Often utilized in traditional Indian medicine (Ayurveda) for a variety of clinical issues relating to gastrointestinal problems and premenstrual syndrome
      (2) Results from studies have been mixed and more rigorous research is needed on the efficacy of shatavari in lactation.
      (3) In one study, consumption of 60 mg/kg body weight of unmixed shatavari root daily induced a significant effect on serum prolactin levels and infant weight gain.
      (4) Other studies on the efficacy of shatavari lacked robust research, such as the lack of placebo control groups or the lack of significant differences in the treatment groups versus placebo groups.
   c. Garlic (*Allium sativum*)
      (1) Has been utilized as a galactogogue in Indian and Turkish culture.
      (2) Contains anti-platelet effects and should be used with caution in patients with a significant bleeding risk.
      (3) A study that involved patients' consumption of garlic capsules prior to breastfeeding showed infants stayed in the breast longer than patients given a placebo. These infants spent 30% more time at the breast than after the placebo was consumed.
      (4) Studies interpreted as infants exposed to garlic in breast milk becoming "less picky" about foods later in life.
      (5) No significant differences have been found in the increase of production of breast milk in patients consuming more garlic.
   d. Silymarin (an extract of *Silybum marianum*, also known as milk thistle)
      (1) Made of 65% to 80% of milk thistle extract
      (2) No human data are available yet on the effect of silymarin on serum prolactin levels.
      (3) One study involving the efficacy of silymarin on breastfeeding patients with normal breast milk production showed a significant increase in production in the breast milk versus the placebo group (a 64.43% baseline increase vs. 22.51% increase, respectively). This study, however, was not randomized and did not study breastfeeding duration and long-term growth of the infants.
      (4) In a study that involved the combination of silymarin and goat's rue, the total amount of milk produced and the proportion of women producing more than 200 mL of milk each day was greater in the treatment group versus the placebo group.
   e. Malunggay (*Moringa oleifera*)
      (1) Commonly used as a galactagogue in Asian countries, particularly in the Philippines
      (2) No data exist on the safety of malunggay in nursing infants.
      (3) One study displayed a higher volume of milk pumped by those in the treatment group versus the placebo group, but this study included a very small sample size, a high dropout rate, and large differences in baseline milk volumes.

D. **Common sequelae of breast pain and infections:** Nipple damage causing bacteria entry >> decreased feeding because of pain >> engorgement >> untreated and/or poorly managed >> mastitis >> if untreated/poorly managed >> abscess

1. Pain, nipple damage
   a. Generally, the result of problem with latch
   b. Pain can be caused by irritation from infant not fully latching. Pain can also be the result of concerns mentioned in the following, such as yeast or dryness.
   c. Nipple damage frequently occurs when an infant continually feeds, for significant duration, without completely latching.
   d. Damage to the nipples, such as cracks, can be a major risk factor for the possible introduction of bacteria into the ducts leading to the development of a mastitis.

2. Engorgement
   a. Most commonly occurs between days 3 and 7 postpartum but has the potential to occur at any point during the lactation journey.
   b. Occurs when both milk supply and blood flow rapidly increase in the breasts. This causes the breasts to swell and become painful and tender.
   c. Treated by complete emptying of the breasts. The challenge with engorgement, however, is that milk supply is based on meeting the demand.
   d. Overstimulation and frequent attempts to empty breasts can lead to further engorgement.
   e. Prolonged engorgement has the potential to lead to the development of an infection in a mammary called mastitis.
   f. Mastitis (Figure 16.6)
      (1) Mastitis is a blocked milk duct and can occur when milk is trapped in the breast. This is commonly due to nipple pain or damage or engorgement. Both situations often lead to the breasts not being completely emptied. Tight fitting bras can also lead to ducts becoming plugged.
      (2) Most commonly seen mastitis symptoms are localized pain, wedge-shaped red area on the breast, fever >100.4, body aches/malaise that is often described as the feeling of a "flu-like" illness.
      (3) Lactation consultation; the root of the problem must be addressed.
      (4) Pharmacologic treatment
         • Antibiotics
            ▪ Dicloxacillin 500 mg tab PO every 6 hours by mouth for 7 to 10 days
            ▪ **PCN allergy:** Erythromycin 500 mg tab PO every 6 hours for 10 days
         • Fever and pain treatment
            ▪ Acetaminophen 1g PO every 8 hours as needed
            ▪ Ibuprofen 600 to 800 mg PO every 8 hours as needed
      (5) Non-pharmacologic treatment
         • Must continue emptying breasts
         • This is a major cause of discontinuing breastfeeding; however, it is critical that breasts continue to be emptied.
         • Pumping is acceptable but direct breastfeeding has been found to be safe.
         • **Distinction between engorgement and mastitis:** Mastitis is pain localized to one area with redness, and generally symptoms are systemic with a fever and malaise. Engorgement is the experience of pain or tenderness throughout both breasts that resolves with the emptying of the breasts. Engorgement should also not be accompanied by a high-grade fever.
   g. Candidiasis/thrush
      (1) This is a very common cause of pain of the nipple and/or breast that does not resolve with improve latch or positioning
      (2) Symptoms include pain that can feel shooting and burning or itchy nipples that appear fiery red, shiny, flaky, and/or have a rash with tiny blisters.

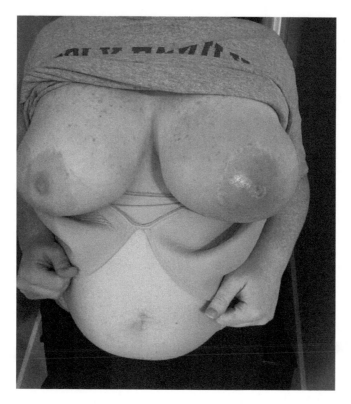

FIGURE 16.6 Mastitis: Blocked milk duct that can occur when milk is trapped in the breast.

(3) This is generally diagnosed based on symptoms. Baby's mouth should also be evaluated as they may have white patches evident.
(4) A concern is making sure both patient and infant are treated so that this does not continue to be passed back and forth as it is highly contagious.
(5) Treatment
- Topical Azole antifungal ointment to the breasts
- Nystatin suspension or Miconazole oral gel for infant's mouth
- Gentian violet (<0.5% aqueous solution) for less than 7 days. This will likely turn an infant's mouth purple if continued breastfeeding.

FAMILY PLANNING AND LACTATION

A. Refer to the CDC's *U.S. Medical Eligibility Criteria* for recommendations with family planning options and lactation.
B. Estrogen-containing methods are contraindicated if breastfeeding postpartum due to risk for decreased milk production. They are also associated with increased risk for thromboembolic event until 42 days postpartum.
C. Both hormonal and nonhormonal IUDs are considered safe with breastfeeding. If not placed during the immediate post-placental period, placement is recommended after 42 days.
D. Nexplanon, Depo Provera, and progesterone-only pills can be initiated any time during the postpartum period and are considered safe with lactation.
   1. Lactational amenorrhea method
   2. Patient must meet all three of the following criteria to ensure adequate protection from an unplanned pregnancy

      a. Amenorrhea

      b. Fully or nearly fully breastfeeding (no interval of >4–6 hours between breastfeeds)

      c. Less than 1 month postpartum

E. Lactation suppression

    1. Patients may seek out education regarding lactation suppression for a variety of reasons, from cessation of breastfeeding to perinatal or infant loss. The easiest way to stop lactation is to help stop the process of breast milk production. Clinicians should provide supportive, individualized lactation suppression education for patients experiencing loss.

    2. Avoid stimulation of the breasts and nipples (feeding, pumping, etc.).

    3. Wear a supportive bra.

    4. Advise against tight-fitting bras and binding in order to prevent mastitis and blocked ducts.

    5. Application of ice packs to the breasts.

    6. Usage of cold cabbage leaves.

    7. May reduce pain and hardness of engorged breasts due to the anti-inflammatory effect of some of the plant components of the leaves.

    8. No sufficient research evidence exists to suggest generalized use and should come along with other clinical recommendations from the provider.

COMMUNITY SUPPORT AND RESOURCES

A. Academy of Breastfeeding Medicine (https://www.bfmed.org/protocols)

B. La Leche League International (https://www.llli.org/breastfeeding-info)

C. American Academy of Pediatrics (https://www.healthychildren.org/English/ages-stages/baby/breastfeeding/Pages/default.aspx)

D. Centers for Disease Control and Prevention (https://www.cdc.gov/breastfeeding/faq/index.htm)

E. The Folklore of Breastfeeding (https://www.ncbi.nlm.nih.gov/pmc/articles/PMC1749550/pdf/bullnyacadmed00163-0078.pdf)

F. Affordable Care Act and breastfeeding (https://www.healthcare.gov/coverage/breast-feeding-benefits)

BIBLIOGRAPHY

Academy of Breastfeeding Medicine. (2018). *ABM Clinical Protocol #9: Use of Galactagogues in Initiating or Augmenting Maternal Milk Production, Second Revision 2018.* https://abm.memberclicks.net/assets/DOCUMENTS/PROTOCOLS/9-galactogoguesprotocol-english.pdf

American Academy of Pediatrics. (2018). *Breastfeeding: Support, challenges, and benefits: Provide clinical breastfeeding support, mitigate challenges, and discover developmental benefits.* American Academy of Pediatrics.

American College of Obstetricians and Gynecologists. (2021). *Breastfeeding your baby.* https://www.acog.org/womens-health/faqs/breastfeeding-your-baby

ACOG Committee Opinion No. 736: Summary: Optimizing postpartum care. (2018). *Obstetrics and Gynecology, 131*(5), 949–951. https://doi.org/10.1097/AOG.0000000000002628

ACOG Committee Opinion No. 756: Summary: Optimizing support for breastfeeding as part of obstetric practice. (2018). *Obstetrics and Gynecology, 121*(4), e187–e196. https://doi.org/10.1097/AOG.0000000000002890

Bazzano, A. N., Hofer, R., Thibeau, S., Gillispie, V., Jacobs, M., & Theall, K. P. (2016). A review of herbal and pharmaceutical galactagogues for breastfeeding. *Ochsner Journal, 16*(4), 511–524.

Beauchamp, G.K. & Mennella, J.A. (2009). Early flavor learning and its impact on later feeding behavior. *Journal of Pediatric Gastroenterology and Nutrition, 48*(1), 25–30. https://doi.org/10.1097/MPG.0b013e31819774a5

Bernard, J. Y., Rifas-Shiman, S. L., Cohen, E., Lioret, S., de Lauzon-Guillain, B., Charles, M., Kramer, M. S., & Oken, E. (2019). Maternal religion and breastfeeding intention and practice in the US Project Viva cohort. *Birth: Issues in Perinatal Care, 47*(2), 191–201. https://doi.org/10.1111/birt.12477

Boi, B., Koh, S., & Gail, D. (2012). The effectiveness of cabbage leaf application (treatment) on pain and hardness in breast engorgement and its effect on the duration of breastfeeding. *JBI Library of Systematic Review, 10*(20), 1185–1213. https://doi.org/10.11124/01938924-201210200-00001.

Burdette, A. M., & Pilkauskas, N. V. (2012). Maternal religious involvement and breastfeeding initiation and duration. *American Journal of Public Health, 102*(10), 1865–1868. https://doi.org/10.2105/AJPH.2012.300737

Candelaria, L. M., Bressler, T., & Spatz, D. L. (2019). Breastfeeding guidance for Orthodox Jewish families when new-borns require special care and continued hospitalization. *MCN: The American Journal of Maternal/Child Nursing, 44*(2), 80–85. https://doi.org/10.1097/NMC.0000000000000513

Centers for Disease Control and Prevention. (2021a). *Alcohol.* https://www.cdc.gov/breastfeeding/breastfeeding-special-circumstances/vaccinations-medications-drugs/alcohol.html

Centers for Disease Control and Prevention. (2021b). https://www.cdc.gov/breastfeeding/breastfeeding-special-circum-stances/maternal or-infant-illnesses/breast-surgery.html

Centers for Disease Control and Prevention. (2021c). *Breastfeeding and caring for newborns if you have COVID-19.* https://www.cdc.gov/coronavirus/2019-ncov/if-you-are-sick/pregnancybreastfeeding.html?CDC_AA_refVal=https%3A%2F%2Fwww.cdc.gov%2Fcoronavirus%2F2019-ncov%2Fneed-extra-precautions%2Fpregnancy-breastfeeding.html

Centers for Disease Control and Prevention. (2021d). *Contraindications to breastfeeding or feeding expressed breast milk to infants.* https://www.cdc.gov/breastfeeding/breastfeeding-special-circumstances/contraindications-to-breastfeeding.html

Centers for Disease Control and Prevention. (2021e). *Hepatitis.* https://www.cdc.gov/breastfeeding/breastfeeding-special-circumstances/maternal-or-infant-illnesses/hepatitis.html

Centers for Disease Control and Prevention. (2021f). *Herpes simplex virus.* https://www.cdc.gov/breastfeeding/breast feeding-special-circumstances/maternal-or-infant-illnesses/herpes.html

Centers for Disease Control and Prevention. (2021g). *How much and how often to breastfeed.* https://www.cdc.gov/nutrition/infantandtoddlernutrition/breastfeeding/how-much-and-how-often.html

Centers for Disease Control and Prevention. (2021h). *Human immunodeficiency virus.* https://www.cdc.gov/breastfeeding/breastfeeding-special-circumstances/maternal-or-infant-illnesses/hiv.html

Centers for Disease Control and Prevention. (2021i). *Marijuana.* https://www.cdc.gov/breastfeeding/breastfeeding-special-circumstances/vaccinations-medications-drugs/marijuana.html

Centers for Disease Control and Prevention. (2021j). *Proper storage and preparation of breast milk.* https://www.cdc.gov/breastfeeding/recommendations/handling_breastmilk.htm

Centers for Disease Control and Prevention. (2021k). *Tobacco and e-cigarettes.* https://www.cdc.gov/breast-feeding-special-circumstances/vaccinations-medications-drugs/tobacco-and-e-cigarettes.html

Centers for Disease Control and Prevention. (2016). *US medical eligibility criteria for contraception use.* https://www.cdc.gov/reproductivehealth/contraception/mmwr/mec/summary.html

Crenshaw, J. T. (2014). Healthy birth practice #6: keep mother and baby together – it's best for mother, baby, and breastfeed-ing. *The Journal of Perinatal Education, 23*(4), 211–217. https://doi.org/10.1891/1058-1243.23.4.211

Di Pierro, F., Callegari, A., Carotenuto, D., & Mollo Tapia, M. (2008). Clinical efficacy, safety and tolerability of BIO-C (micronized Silymarin) as a galactagogue. *Acta Biomedica, 79*(3), 205–210.

Drugs and Lactation Database (LactMed). (2021a). *Garlic.* National Library of Medicine. https://www.ncbi.nlm.nih.gov/books/NBK501782

Drugs and Lactation Database (LactMed). (2021b). *Milk thistle.* National Library of Medicine. https://www.ncbi.nlm.nih.gov/books/NBK501771

Drugs and Lactation Database (LactMed). (2021c). *Moringa.* National Library of Medicine. Retrieved September 20, 2021 from https://www.ncbi.nlm.nih.gov/books/NBK501899

Food and Drug Administration. (2020). *Risks and complications of breast implants.* Retrieved October 1, 2021 from https://www.fda.gov/medical-devices/breast-implants/risks-and-complications-breast-implants

Gupta, M., & Shaw, B. (2011). A double-blind randomized clinical trial for the evaluation of galactagogue activity of Asparagus racemosus willd. *Iranian Journal of Pharmaceutical Research, 10*(1), 167–172.

Hatcher, R. A. (2018). *Contraceptive Technology* (21st ed.). Managing Contraception.

Hodges, E. A., Wasser, H. M., & Colgan, B. K. (2016). Development of feeding cues during infancy and toddlerhood. *MCN: The American Journal of Maternal/Child Nursing, 41*(4): 244251. https://doi.org/10.1097/NMC.0000000000000251

Jewell, M. L., Edwards, M. C., Murphy, D. K., & Schumacher, A. (2018). Lactation outcomes in more than 3500 women following primary augmentation: 5-year data from the breast implant follow-up study. *Aesthetic Surgery Journal, 39*(8), 875–833. https://doi.org/10.1093/asj/sjy221

Johnson, A., Kirk, R., Rosenblum, K. L., & Muzik, M. (2015). Enhancing breastfeeding rates among African American women: A systematic review of current psychosocial interventions. *Breastfeeding Medicine, 10*(1), 45–62. https://doi.org/10.1089/bfm.2014.0023

Jones, K. M., Power, M. L., Queenan, J. T., & Schulkin, J. (2015). Racial and ethnic disparities in breastfeeding. *Breastfeeding Medicine, 10*(4), 186–196. https://doi.org/10.1089/bfm.2014.0152

Kraut, R. Y., Brown, E., Korownyk, C., Katz, L. S., Vandermeer, B., Babenko, O., Gross, M. S., Campbell, S., & Allan, G. M. (2017). The impact of breast reduction surgery on breastfeeding: Systematic review of observational studies. *PLoS One, 12*(10), e0186591. https://doi.org/10.1371/journal.pone.0186591

La Leche League Canada. (2015). *Newborns have small stomachs.* https://www.lllc.ca/thursday-tip-newborns-have-small-stomachs

La Leche League International. (2021). *Positioning.* https://www.llli.org/breastfeeding-info/positioning

Landon, M. B., Driscoll, D. A., Jauniaux, E. R., Galan, H. L., Grobman, W. A., & Berghella, V. (2019). *Gabbe's Obstetrics Essentials: Normal & Problem Pregnancies E-Book*. Elsevier.

Li, R., Perrine, C. G., Anstey, E. K., Chen, J., MacGowan, C. A., & Elam-Evans, L. D. (2019). Breastfeeding trends by race/ethnicity among US children born from 2009 to 2015. *JAMA Pediatrics, 173*(12), e193319. https://doi.org/10.1001/jamapediatrics.2019.3319

McKenna, K. M. & Shankar, R. T. (2009). The practice of prelacteal feeding to newborns among Hindu and Muslim families. *Journal of Midwifery & Women's Health, 54*(1), 78–81. https://doi.org/10.1016/j.jmwh.2008.07.012

McKinney, E. S., James, S. R., Murray, S. S., Nelson, K., & Ashwill, J. (2017). *Maternal-child nursing-e-book*. Elsevier Health Sciences.

Serrao, F., Corsello, M., Romagnoli, C., D'Andrea, V., & Zecca, E. (2017). The long-term efficacy of a galactagogue containing sylimarin-pharphatidylserine and galega on milk production of mothers of preterm infants. *Breastfeeding Medicine, 13*(1), 67–69. https://doi.org/10.1089/bfm.2017.0169

Sevrin, T., Boquien, C., Gandon, A., Grit, I., de Coppet, P., Darmaun, D., & Alexandre-Gouabau, M. (2020). Fenugreek stimulates the expression of genes involved in milk synthesis and milk flow through modulation of insulin/GH/IGF-1 axis and oxytocin secretion. *Genes, 11*(10), 1208. https://doi.org/10.3390/genes11101208

Swigart, T. M., Bonvecchio, A., Théodore, F. L., Zamudio-Haas, S., Villanueva-Borbolla, M. A., & Thrasher, J. F. (2017). Breastfeeding practices, beliefs, and social norms in low-resource communities in Mexico: Insights for how to improve future promotion strategies. *PLoS One, 12*(7), e0180185. https://doi.org/10.1371/journal.pone.0180185

U.S. Department of Health and Human Services. (2021). *Healthy People 2030: Increase the Proportion of infants who are breastfed exclusively through age 6 months – MICH-15*. Retrieved September 30, 2021 from https://health.gov/healthypeople/objectives-anddata/browseobjectives/infants/increase-proportion-infants-who-are-breastfed-exclusivelythrough-age-6-months-mich-15/data

United States Department of Labor. (2021). *Fact Sheet #73: Break time for nursing mothers under the FLSA*. https://www.dol.gov/agencies/whd/fact-sheets/73-flsa-break-time-nursing-mothers

Walter, M. (1975). The folklore of breastfeeding. *Bulletin of the New York Academy of Medicine 51*(7), 870.

Wambach, K., Domian, E. W., Page-Goertz, S., Wurtz, H., & Hoffman, K. (2016). Exclusive breastfeeding experiences among Mexican American women. *Journal of Human Lactation, 32*(1), 103–111. https://doi.org/10.1177/0890334415599400

World Health Organization. (2021). *Infant feeding for the prevention of mother-to-child transmission of HIV*. https://www.who.int/elena/titles/hiv_infant_feeding/en

17

ASSESSMENT AND CLINICAL EVALUATION OF OBESITY IN WOMEN

FRANCES M. SAHEBZAMANI

OBESITY IN WOMEN

A. Obesity is recognized as a complex, multifactorial, chronic disease whereby excess body fat is accumulated through complex interactions involving the environment, genetic predisposition, human metabolism, as well as neuroendocrine and behavioral factors. Given the clinical and public perceptions surrounding a lack of understanding of the term *obesity* and the integrative physiology of adipocytes on chronic disease, quality of life (QOL) and longevity, as well as an inherent stigmatization associated with the term *obesity*, the American Association of Clinical Endocrinologists (AACE) and the American College of Endocrinology (ACE) developed a chronic care model emphasizing the term *adiposity* and a complications-centric diagnostic and treatment approach to reduce confusion and stigma associated with the term obesity. This model uses a new diagnostic term *adiposity-based chronic disease* (*ABCD*) to target a more precise pathophysiological basis for diagnosis and treatment. ABCD disproportionally and differentially affects women's health across a spectrum of physical, psychological, and social conditions.

1. Although adiposity is generally thought to be attributable to an imbalance between chronic overnutrition and lower caloric expenditure, current research has shown that adiposity is influenced and regulated by the hormonal and metabolic function of adipocytes.

2. Body fat is comprised of both subcutaneous adipose tissue (gluteo–femoral weight distribution) and visceral adipose tissue (fat cells deposited into skeletal muscle and the viscera; Figure 17.1).

3. Over the past decade, research has led to a better understanding of the role of visceral adipose tissue as an active regulator of whole-body homeostasis through the production of more than 50 adipokines, hormones, and other molecules that directly affect a wide variety of psychological and physiological processes. Adipokines perform essential regulatory roles in appetite and food intake, mood, energy expenditure, reproduction, cell viability, immunity, inflammation, and cardiovascular function.

4. Adipokines release proinflammatory peptides (e.g., tumor necrosis factor [TNF]), high-sensitivity C-reactive protein (hs-CRP), interleukin-6 (IL-6), plasminogen activator inhibitor 1 (PAI-1), and vascular endothelial growth factor (VEGF) and secrete hormones (adiponectin, leptin, resistin) that contribute to a chronic low-grade inflammatory response. This chronic low-grade inflammatory state promotes metabolic aberrations highly associated with the development of atherosclerosis, autoimmune inflammatory diseases, and further weight accumulation.

5. In the clinical setting, ranges for normal weight, overweight, and obesity are determined using weight and height to calculate a surrogate measure of percentage of body fat called the *body mass index* (BMI; Table 17.1).

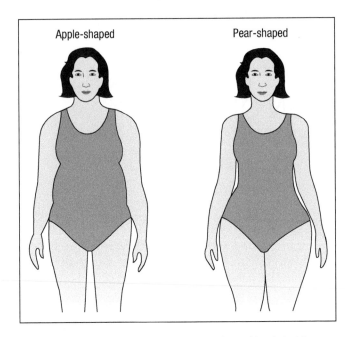

FIGURE 17.1 Apple-shaped and pear-shaped body habitus.

TABLE 17.1 Table of Body Mass Index Measurements

	120	130	140	150	160	170	180	190	200	210	220	230	240	250
4′6″	29	31	34	36	39	41	43	46	48	51	53	56	58	60
4′8″	27	29	31	34	36	38	40	43	45	47	49	52	54	56
4′10″	25	27	29	31	34	36	38	40	42	44	46	48	50	52
5′0″	23	25	27	29	31	33	35	37	39	41	43	45	47	49
5′2″	22	24	26	27	29	31	33	35	37	38	40	42	44	46
5′4″	21	22	24	26	28	29	31	33	34	36	38	40	41	43
5′6″	19	21	23	24	26	27	29	31	32	34	36	37	39	40
5′8″	18	20	21	23	24	26	27	29	30	32	34	35	37	38
5′10″	17	19	20	22	23	24	26	27	29	30	32	33	35	36
6′0″	16	18	19	20	22	23	24	26	27	28	30	31	33	34
6′2″	15	17	18	19	21	22	23	24	26	27	28	30	31	32
6′4″	15	16	17	18	20	21	22	23	24	26	27	28	29	30
6′6″	14	15	16	17	19	20	21	22	23	24	25	27	28	29
6′8″	13	14	15	17	18	19	20	21	22	23	24	25	26	28

Note: No shading = underweight, BMI <18.5; dark pink = normal, BMI: 18.5–24.9; medium pink = overweight, BMI: 25–29.9; light pink = obese, BMI: 39–39.8.

MEASURES OF OBESITY

A. BMI is calculated when height and weight are entered into a formula known as the *Quetelet index* (weight [kg]/height [m²]).

B. BMI is used in the clinical setting to assess risk for the development of adiposity-related diseases and as a metric for determining treatment interventions (see Treatment Interventions section).

C. As BMI increases, risk for visceral adiposity, metabolic dysregulation, the development of functional disorders, chronic disease, and premature death increases. As BMI approaches or exceeds 35, women have a 92-fold increased risk for the development of type 2 diabetes, compared with a 42-fold increased risk for men.

D. Research has shown that a weight loss as minimal as 3% to 5% of total body weight can improve health outcomes and reduce risk for the development of adiposity-related comorbidities (Table 17.2).

E. BMI provides an approximation of mortality and morbidity risk for obesity and is used because it correlates with the amount of body fat, but *it is not* a measurement of body fatness. An adult who has a BMI between 25 and 29.9 is considered overweight. An adult who has a BMI of 30 or higher is considered obese.

F. BMI measurements are not gender specific.

PREVALENCE OF OBESITY

A. Based on the most recent data from the National Health and Nutrition Examination Survey, in the year 2017/2018, 31.1% of adult Americans were overweight (BMI between 25 and 29.9 kg/m²) and 42.5% met the BMI diagnostic criteria for obesity (BMI ≥30 kg/m²). There were no statistical differences between men and women on prevalence of overweight or obesity.

B. Although the proportion of adults with a BMI ≥30 kg/m² has steadily increased between 2011 and 2012 (37.4%) and between 2017 and 2018 (42.5%), during this same timeframe, the proportion of obese adults with severe obesity has rapidly increased (from 6.4% to 9.2%). Severe obesity is defined as a BMI ≥40 kg/m² (class 3 obesity). Among adults classified as obese, women represent the greatest proportion of adults with severe obesity. Of women, 11.5% met the diagnostic criteria for class 3 obesity compared with 6.9% of men.

TABLE 17.2 Medical Complications of Obesity	
Diabetes mellitus (type 2)	Hypertension
High cholesterol levels	Coronary heart disease
Congestive heart failure	Angina pectoris
Stroke	Asthma
Osteoarthritis	Musculoskeletal disorders
Gallbladder disease	Sleep apnea
Respiratory problems	Gout
Bladder control problems	
Cancer(s)	

C. Severe obesity increases the risk of premature death in women and the risk for serious pregnancy complications, including an increased risk for birth defects, fetal adiposity, and the development of childhood obesity in offspring (Table 17.3).

TABLE 17.3 Reproductive Complications of Severe Obesity
MATERNAL
Gestational diabetes mellitus (GDM)
Preeclampsia
Eclampsia
Pseudotumor cerebri
Acute cholecystitis
Cesarean section
Postpartum wound infection
Operative vaginal delivery

Metabolic disturbances
  Elevated free fatty acids
  Hyperglycemia

FETAL/NEONATAL
Spontaneous abortion
Stillbirth
Fetal monitoring and imaging problems
Premature birth secondary to obstetrical and medical complications
Intra-uterine growth restriction/retardation (IUGR) second to problems such as preeclampsia
Congenital malformations
Low Apgar score
Large-for-gestational age (LGA)
Increased fetal adiposity
Hypoglycemia
NEONATAL/INFANT/CHILD
Difficulty breastfeeding
Risk of low IQ
Aggressive eating style
Risk of pediatric obesity
Type 2 diabetes

(continued)

TABLE 17.3 Reproductive Complications of Severe Obesity (*continued*)
NEONATAL/INFANT/CHILD (*CONT.*)

Metabolic syndrome
  Impaired glucose tolerance
  Dyslipidemia
  Hypertension
  Fatty liver

Asthma
Depression
Orthopedic disorders
Truancy

GDM, gestational diabetes mellitus; IUGR, intrauterine growth restriction; LGA, large for gestational age.

Source: Kral, J. G., Kava, R. A., Catalano, P. M., & Moore, B. J. (2012). Severe obesity: The neglected epidemic. *Obesity Facts, 5*(2), 254–269. https://doi.org/10.1159/000338566

D. The rates of obesity are disproportionate in ethnic groups. There is a higher prevalence of obesity among African American and Hispanic women than among White women (39.8%). Among non-Hispanic Black women, 56.9% met the diagnostic criteria for obesity compared with 41.1% of men and 43.7% of Hispanic women. In 2017 to 2018, the prevalence of obesity was higher among non-Hispanic Black, Hispanic, and non-Hispanic White women than among non-Hispanic Asian women (17.2 %; Table 17.4).

GENDER DIFFERENCES IN OBESITY

A. Gender differences in obesity and overweight are related to biological, psychological, and social issues (i.e., differences in anatomy, hormonal influences, mood disorders, stressors, and QOL issues).

B. Women are vulnerable to weight gain during reproductive milestones (i.e., puberty, pregnancy, postpartum, and menopause). Female sex hormones, specifically progesterone, as well as changes in hormones related to estrogen deficiency with menopause, influence food intake, body composition, and energy expenditure (Table 17.5).

C. Obesity has been linked to disorders of menstruation and to infertility in women. Exogenous hormones for contraception or symptoms of menopause have been shown to affect weight. Most women in developed countries live substantial portions of their lives in a postmenopausal state.

TABLE 17.4 Prevalence of Severe Obesity Among U.S. Women According to Age (2017/2018)	
AGE (YEARS)	**PREVALENCE (%)**
20–39	9.1
40–59	11.5
≥60	5.8

Note: Women may be at greater risk for severe obesity leading up to, during, and after menopause.

TABLE 17.5 Hormonal Influences Affecting Obesity Expression in Women

PREMENOPAUSAL AND EARLY POSTMENOPAUSAL YEARS	PERIMENOPAUSE, MENOPAUSE, AND POLYCYSTIC OVARY SYNDROME
Estradiol is the primary source of estrogen, which promotes gluteo–femoral adipocyte distribution	Estrone is the primary source of estrogen (estradiol is approximately one tenth of premenopausal levels)
Estrogen receptor beta more prominent in subcutaneous fat	Visceral adipocyte distribution pattern
Not associated with decreased adiponectin levels, IR, inflammatory or prothrombic factors	Estradiol deficiency promotes a shift to a reduced lean body mass
	Reduced functional activity levels
	Androgen receptors more prominent
	Highly associated with decreased adiponectin levels, IR, FFA, dyslipidemia, prothrombic and proinflammatory potential, and glucose intolerance

FFA, free fatty acid; IR, insulin resistance.

D. In the American culture, slimness is valued and rewarded. These cultural norms may promote social stigma, body-image dysfunction, and eating disorders in women.

E. Obesity affects quality and quantity of life (Table 17.6).

GENETIC CAUSES OF OBESITY

A. Approximately 112 candidate genes have been identified and associated with obesity.

1. Obesity has been shown to be primarily polygenic with each gene candidate contributing to the phenotype and with multiple genes interacting with environmental influences. Gene mutations, deletions, single nucleotide polymorphisms (SNPs), and epigenetic differences are all known to contribute to the development of obesity. Inherited genetic variations have been shown to significantly influence body mass and how the body responds to physical activity and nutrition.

TABLE 17.6 National Institutes of Health Guidelines for the Management of Obesity by Body Mass Index

TREATMENT	BMI CATEGORY				
	25–26.9 KG/M²	27–29.9 KG/M²	30–34.9 KG/M²	35–39.9 KG/M²	≥40 KG/M²
Diet, exercise, behavior therapy	With comorbidities	With comorbidities	+	+	+
Pharmacotherapy		With comorbidities	+	+	+
Surgery				With comorbidities	+

BMI, body mass index.

2. Current research on the epigenetics of obesity is investigating the influence of behavioral and environmental factors on genetic expression.

B. Monogenetic obesity is rare and usually associated with extreme obesity, the conditions of which necessitate special care and appropriate referrals for further genetic assessment, treatment, and counseling. Monogenetic causes of obesity may be identified by associated physical characteristics

   1. **Prader–Willi syndrome:** Short stature, hypogonadism, short extremities

   2. **Angleman's syndrome:** Normal stature, movement disorder, happy affect

   3. **Down syndrome:** Short stature, typical facial features, cardiac malformation, hypotonia

   4. **Bardet–Biedl syndrome:** Normal/short stature, rod/cone dystrophy, polydactyly, renal structural defects

   5. **Alstrom syndrome:** Normal/short stature, deafness, cardiomyopathy, rod/cone dystrophy

   6. **Albright's osteodystrophy:** Normal/short stature, brachydactyly (short fingers), subcutaneous ossification

   7. **Cohen syndrome:** Normal/short stature, distinctive facial features, retinochondrial dystrophy, granulocytopenia

   8. **Carpenter syndrome:** Short stature, acrocephaly, polydactyly, hypogonadism

MEDICAL CAUSES OF OBESITY

A. Hypothalamic obesity

   1. Hypothalamic obesity is rare, and results from hypothalamic damage from traumatic insult to the central nervous system (CNS). Affected structures include bilateral injury to the ventromedial hypothalamus, the paraventricular hypothalamus, or the amygdala. The pathophysiology resulting from damage to the hypothalamic structures results in the simulation of a relative state of CNS starvation through the inability to transduce afferent hormonal signals of adiposity.

   2. Symptoms consist of increased intracranial pressure (headache, vomiting, blurred vision); hypopituitarism; and neurologic problems (seizures, coma, somnolence, temperature dysregulation).

   3. Hypothalamic obesity is caused by an increase in the secretion of insulin and adipogenesis (Lustig, 2008).

B. Endocrine causes of obesity

   1. **Insulin resistance:** The metabolic dysregulation associated with insulin resistance, prediabetes, and type 2 diabetes results in insulin-resistant subcutaneous adipocytes and increased visceral adipocyte accumulation, increased risk for cardiometabolic disease, and perpetuation of weight gain.

C. Hypothyroidism

   1. Women have a twofold increased risk for hypothyroidism with risk increasing with age. Although the prevalence of hypothyroidism is low in obese individuals, overweight and obesity are associated with high normal thyroid-stimulating hormone (TSH) and low normal fT4, fT3, and total T3 levels in euthyroid individuals.

   2. High normal TSH levels have been associated with increased visceral adiposity and increased waist circumference and triglyceride levels. The mechanism linking high TSH levels within the normal range is not well understood. Hypotheses include the belief that increased TSH and elevated peripheral thyroid hormone levels (fT3 and total T3) may be an adaptation process to increase energy expenditure to reduce further weight gain. Basal metabolic rate, total energy expenditure, and sleeping energy expenditure are positively correlated with the serum total T3 or fT3 concentrations.

3. Changes in thyroid hormone concentrations may be regarded as a consequence rather than a cause of obesity. Decline in TSH has been reported after caloric restriction, leading to a 10% weight loss, or following bariatric surgical procedures.

D. Adrenal syndrome

1. Cushing's syndrome is characterized by central obesity, hypertension, and "moon faces" and associated with chronic exposure to elevated cortisol levels. Elevated cortisol levels can result from disease that results in excess cortisol, adrenocorticotropic hormone (ACTH), or corticotropin-releasing hormone (CRH), or from long-term use of glucocorticoid medications.

2. Common physical characteristics include central obesity, thin extremities, and abnormal fat deposition along the collarbone or neck (buffalo hump).

E. Polycystic ovary syndrome (PCOS) is the most prevalent heterogeneous endocrine disorder in women and is characterized by hyperandrogenism, menstrual irregularities, central adiposity, insulin resistance, and polycystic ovaries.

1. The prevalence of PCOS is estimated at 15% to 20% of women. Of women with PCOS, 30% to 50% are overweight or obese.

2. Clinical manifestations include oligomenorrhea or amenorrhea, hirsutism, infertility, and mood disorders, including depression, anxiety, and binge eating disorder (BED).

3. Insulin resistance affects 50% to 70% of women with PCOS, resulting in multiple cardiometabolic comorbidities, including metabolic syndrome, diabetes, dyslipidemia, and hypertension.

4. Weight loss has been shown to improve menstrual irregularities, fertility, and symptoms of androgen excess.

5. In addition to the management of cardiovascular risk factors, the clinical management of PCOS includes the use of oral contraceptives to normalize menstrual irregularities and reduce hirsutism and the use of spironolactone and finasteride to reduce androgen excess.

6. Proper diagnosis and management of PCOS is essential to the prevention of metabolic, endocrine, reproductive, and cardiovascular complications.

EATING DISORDERS

A. Women manifest a 2:1 higher prevalence of eating disorders than men. Common eating disorders found in overweight and obese women include binge-eating disorder (BED), night-eating syndrome (NES), and bulimia.

B. BED is thought to be a compensatory response to chronically high stress levels with subsequent heightened responsiveness to high calorie, hyperpalatable foods. Approximately 45% to 60% of obese individuals meet the *Diagnostic and Statistical Manual of Mental Disorders, Fifth Edition (DSM-5;* American Psychiatric Association [APA], 2013) diagnostic criteria for BED.

1. NES is characterized by morning anorexia, evening hyperphagia, insomnia, and depressed mood. Prevalence of NES is estimated at 9% to 15% of obese outpatients and 54% to 64% of individuals with severe obesity (class 2 or 3 obesity; Table 17.7).

2. Bulimia nervosa is characterized by frequent episodes of binge eating followed by inappropriate behaviors, such as self-induced vomiting, to avoid weight gain. *DSM-5* criteria include the criteria for BED and compensatory behaviors. Current inappropriate compensatory behaviors to prevent weight gain are described as self-induced vomiting; misuse of laxatives, diuretics, or other medications; fasting; or excessive exercise.

C. Treatment of BED, NES, and bulimia may include psychotherapy, antidepressants, and neuroleptics.

D. Psychotherapy can reduce the incidence of BED, but this treatment option has not been useful in reducing body weight.

TABLE 17.7 Proposed Diagnostic Criteria for Night-Eating Syndrome

A. Daily eating pattern of evening/nighttime hyperphagia of one or both of the following:
1. At least 25% caloric intake after the evening meal
2. At least two episodes of nocturnal eating per week
B. Awareness and recall of evening- and nocturnal-eating episodes
C. At least three of the following must be present:
1. Morning anorexia and/or skipped breakfast four or more mornings per week
2. Presence of a strong urge to eat between dinner and sleep onset and/or during the night
3. Sleep onset and/or sleep maintenance insomnia four or more nights per week
4. Presence of a belief that one must eat to return to sleep
5. Mood is frequently depressed and/or mood worsens in the evening
D. The disorder is associated with significant distress and/or impairment in functioning
E. The disordered pattern of eating is maintained for at least 3 months
F. The disorder is not secondary to substance abuse or dependence, medical disorder, medication, or another psychiatric disorder

Sources: Bray, G. A., & Greenway, F. L. (2007). Pharmacological treatment of the overweight patient. *Pharmacological Reviews, 59*(2), 151–184. https://doi.org/10.1124/pr.59.2.2; Gallant, A. R., Lundgren, J., & Drapeau, V. (2012). The night-eating syndrome and obesity. *Obesity Reviews, 13*(6), 528–536. https://doi.org/10.1111/j.1467-789X.2011.00975.x; Milano, W., De Rosa, M., Milano, L., & Capasso, A. (2012). Night eating syndrome: An overview. *Journal of Pharmacy and Pharmacology, 64*(1), 2–10. https://doi.org/10.1111/j.2042-7158.2011.01353.x

E. Pharmacotherapy with antidepressants and appetite suppressants can reduce binge or NES frequency and BMI by promoting weight loss. Newer generation neuroleptics, such as topiramate and zonisamide, have been associated with weight loss in clinical studies of epilepsy and obesity and have shown promise in the treatment of BED (Tables 17.8 and 17.9).

F. Combination therapies to include medication and cognitive behavioral therapy are significantly better than either alone.

TABLE 17.8 Pharmacotherapeutic Options for the Management of Eating Disorders

MEDICATION	OBESITY	ANOREXIA	BULIMIA	BED	NES
Topiramate	+	Not tested	++	+++	Not tested
Zonisamide	+	Not tested	Not tested	+	Not tested
SSRI	+	+/−	+	+	+
SNRI	++	+/−	+/−	+/−	+/−
Atypical	++	+/−	Not suitable	+	+/−

BED, binge eating disorder; NES, night-eating syndrome; SNRI, serotonin–norepinephrine reuptake inhibitors; SSRI, selective serotonin reuptake inhibitor.

Sources: Bray, G. A., & Greenway, F. L. (2007). Pharmacological treatment of the overweight patient. *Pharmacological Reviews, 59*(2), 151–184. https://doi.org/10.1124/pr.59.2.2; Gallant, A. R., Lundgren, J., & Drapeau, V. (2012). The night-eating syndrome and obesity. *Obesity Reviews, 13*(6), 528–536. https://doi.org/10.1111/j.1467-789X.2011.00975.x; Milano, W., De Rosa, M., Milano, L., & Capasso, A. (2012). Night eating syndrome: An overview. *Journal of Pharmacy and Pharmacology, 64*(1), 2–0. https://doi.org/10.1111/j.2042-7158.2011.01353.x

TABLE 17.9 Effects of Common Antidepressants on Weight	
MEDICATION	**EFFECT ON WEIGHT**
Amitriptyline	Gain
Nortriptyline	Gain
Imipramine	Gain
SSRIs	
Sertraline	Neutral
Fluoxetine	Neutral
Fluvoxamine	Neutral
Paroxetine	Gain
Citalopram	Neutral
NaSSAs	
Mitrazapine	Gain
SNRI	
Venlafaxine	Neutral
Sibutramine	Loss
Atypical	
Bupropion	Loss

NaSSAs, noradrenergic and specific serotonergic antidepressants; SNRIs, serotonin–norepinephrine reuptake inhibitors; SSRIs, selective serotonin reuptake inhibitors.

Source: Gallant, A. R., Lundgren, J., & Drapeau, V. (2012). The night-eating syndrome and obesity. *Obesity Reviews, 13*(6), 528–536. https://doi.org/10.1111/j.1467-789X.2011.00975.x

RISK FACTORS ASSOCIATED WITH EXOGENOUS OBESITY

A. Metabolic syndrome represents a clustering of cardiovascular and metabolic risk factors known to accelerate atherosclerosis and cardiovascular disease (Table 17.10).
   1. Visceral adipocytes and insulin resistance resulting from decreased sensitivity of insulin receptors drive the development of metabolic syndrome.
   2. Women with metabolic syndrome have a threefold to fivefold increased risk for cardiovascular disease and events.
   3. The increased release of free fatty acids impairs insulin clearance by the liver and alters peripheral metabolism.
   4. Adiponectin, a hormone secreted by adipocytes, regulates response and reduces cardiovascular risk. Adiponectin levels are inversely related to adipocyte mass.
   5. The National Cholesterol Education Panel (NCEP) Adult Treatment Program defines metabolic syndrome as the clustering of three of the following criteria:
      a. Waist circumference more than 88 cm (>35 in.)
      b. High-density lipoprotein (HDL) less than 50 mg/dL

TABLE 17.10 Factors Included for the Metabolic Assessment of Obesity

PARAMETER	MEASUREMENT	CRITICAL VALUE
Obesity	Body mass index	Up to 24.9 = normal 25–29.9 = overweight 30–34.9 = class 1 obesity 35–39.9 = class 2 obesity ≥40 = class 3 obesity
Body fat distribution	Waist circumference	Women >35 in. (89 cm)
Fasting lipid profile	HDL	Women <50 mg/dL
	Triglycerides	Women >150 mg/dL
	Low-density lipoprotein	Women >100 mg/dL
Insulin resistance	Fasting blood glucose (mmol/L)	>100 mg/dL HOMA-IR ≥5 mmol/L
	Fasting insulin	60 pmo/L
Hypertension	Blood pressure	Systolic >130 mmHg Diastolic >85 mmHg

HDL, high-density lipoprotein; HOMA-IR, homeostasis model assessment–estimated insulin resistance.

Source: Daniel, S., Soleymani, T., & Garvey, W. T. (2013). A complications-based clinical staging of obesity to guide treatment modality and intensity. *Current Opinion in Endocrinology, Diabetes, and Obesity, 20*(5), 377–388. https://doi.org/10.1097/01.med.0000433067.01671.f5

    c. Triglyceride level greater than 150 mg/dL
    d. Fasting glucose level greater than 110 mg/dL
    e. Blood pressure (systolic, diastolic, or both) greater than or equal to 130/greater than or equal to 85 mmHg

B. Reproductive milestones contributing to risk of obesity in women

1. **Puberty:** Has been shown to be a vulnerable period for the development of obesity. Studies have shown that the age of onset of menses may contribute to the development of obesity later in life. During menarche, the gonadal steroids exert strong influences on body composition related to adipose tissue growth. Early onset of puberty is associated with high adiposity in adults.

2. **Postpartum:** Retention of weight after pregnancy may be a factor in obesity in young women. The weight gain may reflect changes in the lifestyle of the woman rather than the physiologic changes associated with childbirth. After delivery, women may have a higher intake of food, have more accessibility to food during the day, and may experience decreased physical activity levels. Postpartum breastfeeding has been associated with maternal weight loss.

3. **Postmenopause:** Menopause is a period of significant physiological changes that are related to estrogen depletion and cessation of ovarian function and is associated with increased body weight, increased adiposity, and obesity-related diseases.

    a. Estrogen is thought to positively regulate body fat accumulation and weight distribution by reducing lipoprotein lipase levels in tissue and by serving as an anorectic, decreasing appetite, and affecting feeding behavior.

    b. Research evidence of the effects of postmenopausal hormone replacement therapy (HRT) on weight gain, adiposity, and distribution have been mixed, with some studies demonstrating no effect of HRT on weight gain and adiposity, whereas other studies demonstrate weight loss and a shift to less android weight distribution with HRT.

    c. Weight gain in postmenopausal women has also been attributed to the rapid decline in resting metabolic rate during menopause and to the slower decline with subsequent aging. Decreased physical activity also contributes to decreases in resting metabolic rate.

C. Menopause

   1. Studies have shown that estradiol deficiency results in a shift to a more atherogenic lipid profile characterized by increases in total cholesterol, low-density lipoproteins (LDL-C), and triglyceride and insulin levels.

   2. Research has shown that menopause is accompanied by an increase in abdominal fat distribution and a decline in gluteal/femoral distribution.

   3. Resting metabolic rate declines rapidly during menopause, suggesting an influence of estrogen on resting metabolic rate.

   4. Decreases in metabolic rate may also be associated with a loss of lean tissue mass and the loss of the luteal phase effects on an increase in energy expenditure.

   5. The ratio of androgens to estrogens shifts, thereby increasing visceral adiposity.

OBESITY-FOCUSED HEALTH HISTORY

A. An obesity-focused history allows the development of tailored recommendations and interventions to maximize treatment outcomes.

B. Components of the obesity-focused health history in women include:

   1. Past and current prescription and over-the-counter medications; weight gain is a common side effect or adverse effect of medications (Box 17.1)

   2. History of past and current comorbidities, particularly obesity-related comorbidities

   3. History of reproductive milestones and weight gain (menarche, pregnancy, breastfeeding, menopause)

   4. Change in lifestyle events; weight gain is associated with changes in lifestyle events, including marital status, employment status or occupation, illness, or caregiving responsibilities

---

BOX 17.1 Medications Associated With Weight Gain

- Glucocorticoids
- Megace
- Cyproheptadine
- Antidepressants (tricyclic, MAO inhibitors, SSRIs, mirtazapine)
- Mood stabilizers (lithium)
- Antipsychotics and phenothiazines (clozapine, olanzapine, risperidone)
- Antiepileptic medications (valproate, gabapentin)
- Hormones (contraceptives, corticosteroids, progestational steroids)
- Alpha-adrenergic–blocking drugs (beta blockers are really more of an issue; also calcium channel blockers, especially amlodipine, cause ankle edema in women, thus weight gain)
- Antidiabetic agents (sulfonylureas, insulin, thiazolidinediones, and drugs that stimulate insulin release)
- Opiates
- Asthma medications with steroids (Vanceril, Pulmicort, Azmacort, Aero-Bid)
- Osteoporosis treatments (raloxifene)
- Antihistamines, including azelastine (Astelin) and diphenhydramine (Benadryl)

MAO, monoamine oxidase; SSRIs, selective serotonin reuptake inhibitors.

TABLE 17.11 Effect of Weight Loss on Clinically Significant Versus Cosmetically Significant Outcomes

TYPE OF PROCEDURE	WEIGHT LOSS	CLINICALLY SIGNIFICANT	COSMETICALLY SIGNIFICANT
Diet/exercise	10%; from 300 to 270 pounds	Yes	No
	10%; from 200 to 180 pounds	Yes	Probably not
	10%; from 150 to 135 pounds	Yes	Yes
Liposuction	7%; from 220 to 200 pounds	No	Probably not
	7%; from 160 to 149 pounds	No	Yes
Surgery (RYGB/LB)	40%; from 264 to 165 pounds	Yes	Yes

RYGB/LB, Roux-en-Y gastric bypass/lap band.

Source: Bray, G. A., & Greenway, F. L. (2007). Pharmacological treatment of the overweight patient. *Pharmacological Reviews, 59*(2), 151–184. https://doi.org/10.1124/pr.59.2.2

5. Sleep patterns and current symptoms of sleep disorders (increased stressors, menopausal symptoms, sleep apnea, restless legs syndrome)
6. Weight gain history and velocity of weight gain (estimation of weight gain over a given period of time)
7. Current physical activity and exercise routines
8. Employment status, type of occupation, and work environment
9. Dietary recall
10. History of tobacco cessation, current use of nicotine or other tobacco products
11. History of substance abuse (illicit drugs, alcohol)
12. **Family history:** May provide insights into predisposing genetic factors
13. **Social support and financial resources:** Assess for obesity-related treatments
14. Assessment of readiness and motivation for weight loss
15. Appropriateness of the patient's expectation and weight-loss goals; educating patients regarding the differences between weight loss, which will have a cosmetic impact, versus health impact (Table 17.11).

ADIPOSITY-FOCUSED PHYSICAL EXAMINATION

A. Height, weight, and BMI
   1. Height
   2. Weight
   3. Body habitus
      a. Gynoid (pear-shaped body)
         (1) Hips wider than shoulders due to body stores of fat there; lower risk for diabetes and heart problems
      b. Android (apple-shaped body)
         (1) Body fat is stored around middle; higher risk for heart problems
         (2) Common in midlife and menopause due to decreasing levels of estrogen
B. BMI measurement
   1. BMI should be rounded to the nearest tenth (Figure 17.2).
      a. Example: 29.85 is expressed as 29.9.
      b. Example: 29.84 is expressed as 29.8.

$$\text{Body mass index (BMI)} = \frac{\text{kg of body weight}}{\text{m}^2 \text{ of body height}}$$

FIGURE 17.2 Formula for BMI, also known as the Quetelet index.

2. Example of calculation of BMI for a patient who weighs 130 pounds and is 5 ft., 4 in. tall is provided in Figure 17.3.

C. **Waist and hip circumference:** Provides an indication of trunk or visceral obesity, often associated with diabetes and heart disease. To determine the circumference:

1. The patient should stand up straight in the upright position with feet together.
2. Instruct patient to relax and stand with arms to the side.
3. Expose the waist with the undergarments pulled below the waist.
4. Find the natural waist, which is the narrowest part of the torso. This area is midway between the inferior border of the rib cage and the superior aspect of the iliac crest.
5. Place the tape measure at the measuring point and locate the point on the tape where the zero aligns with the measuring point. Record to the nearest 0.1 cm. Hold tape horizontally.
6. If necessary, ask the obese patient to elevate any sagging abdominal wall.
7. Take measurement at the end of normal expiration.

PHYSICAL FINDINGS ASSOCIATED WITH CARDIOMETABOLIC RISK

A. **Funduscopic examination:** Hypertensive or diabetic retinopathy, evidence of hyperlipidemia (xanthelasmas, corneal arcus)

B. **Neck:** Enlarged circumference

C. **Cardiovascular:** Cardiomegaly, carotid or abdominal bruit; a sustained, enlarged (>3 cm diameter) apical impulse, which may be displaced outside the midclavicular line, is characteristic of isolated left ventricular hypertrophy (LVH)

D. **Skin:** Acanthosis nigricans, acne, hirsutism

1. Convert weight from pounds to kilograms.
   Weight: 30 lb = 59.09 kg (1 lb = 2.2 kg)

2. Convert height from inches to centimeters.
   Height: 5 ft 4 in. = 64 in. × 2.54 = 162.56 cm (1 in. = 2.54 cm)

3. Convert the height to meters by dividing the number of centimeters by 100:
   162.56 cm/100 = 1.6256 (Do not round the value.)

4. Take the square of the resulting number and save it. (Do not round the value.) To get the square, multiply the number by itself.
   1.6256 × 1.6256 = 2.6425753

5. To calculate the BMI: Divide the weight by square of the height calculated in on 4. (Do not round either the weight or the square of the height.)
   59.09 kg ÷ 2.6425753 = 22.36; BMI = 22.4

FIGURE 17.3 Example of how to calculate body mass index (BMI) for a patient who weighs 130 pounds and is 5 ft., 4 in. tall.

LABORATORY TESTING

A. **Fasting blood glucose level:** Impaired fasting or impaired glucose tolerance; diagnosis of type 2 diabetes

B. Lipid panel (total cholesterol, HDL-C, LDL-C, triglycerides, hs-CRP)

C. **Electrocardiography:** LVH, evidence of myocardial ischemia

D. 2D echocardiogram to identify LVH and left ventricular function

E. **Dual-energy x-ray absorptiometry:** Accurate way to measure total body fat

F. **CT:** Can quantify the amount of visceral fat in the abdomen

G. Emerging trend is to order leptin, ghrelin, adiponectin labs, which are not necessary (per national organizations and experts).

TREATMENT INTERVENTIONS

A. Assessment of physical symptoms, functional limitations, and metabolic risk

   1. The Edmonton Obesity Staging System provides a systematic approach for determining physical symptoms, functional limitations, and metabolic risk to identify treatment options through a tailored treatment plan based on intensity of risk (Table 17.12).

   2. Provides for a complications-based approach to treatment options.

B. Behavioral strategies

   1. Assess for mood disorders (depression, anxiety, eating disorders, posttraumatic stress disorder [PTSD])

   2. Common recommendations

      a. Coping with stress

      b. Coping with frustration

      c. Compensation strategies

      d. Social environment

      e. Referral to groups

TABLE 17.12 Edmonton Obesity Staging System		
STAGE	**OBESITY-RELATED RISK FACTORS**	**PHYSICAL SYMPTOMS, PSYCHOPATHOLOGY, FUNCTIONAL LIMITATIONS, AND IMPAIRMENT OF WELL-BEING**
0	None (blood pressure, serum lipids, fasting glucose, etc.)	None
1	Subclinical (borderline hypertension, impaired fasting glucose, elevated liver enzymes, etc.)	Mild
2	Established (hypertension, type 2 diabetes mellitus, sleep apnea, osteoarthritis, reflux disease, polycystic ovary syndrome, anxiety disorder, etc.)	Moderate
3	Established end-organ damage (myocardial infarction, heart failure, diabetic complications, incapacitating osteoarthritis, etc.)	Significant
4	Severe disabilities (potentially end-stage disabilities, etc.)	Severe

TABLE 17.13 Calculating Daily Caloric Requirements

STEP 1
Estimate the recommended individual caloric requirement (kcal/day) by calculating the Resting Energy Expenditure (REE).
For adult women:
REE = 10 × weight (in kg) + 6.25 × height (in cm) − 5 × age (in years) − 161
Example = 10 × 59.09 + 6.25 × 162.56 − 5 × 36 − 161 = 1,587.9
590.9 + 1,016 − 19 = 1,587.9
Weight: 130 pounds = 59.09 kgs
Height: 5'4" = 64 in. × 2.54 = 162.56 cm

STEP 2
Multiply REE by an AF of 1.5 for women for light activity to estimate daily caloric need or by 1.6 for women for higher activity.
Example = 1,587.9 × 1.5 = 2,381.85 kcal

AF, activity factor; REE, resting energy expenditure; REE × AF, estimated total caloric need (kcal/day) to maintain weight.

     f. Referral to internet links or books

     g. Referral for psychotherapy

C. Nutritional

  1. Evidence-based dietetics practice is the use of systematically reviewed scientific evidence in making food and nutrition practice decisions by integrating best available evidence with professional expertise and patient values to improve outcomes.

  2. Common nutritional recommendations

     a. Quality and quantity of food intake

     b. Time of consumption

     c. Impact of daily calories

     d. Specific food recommendations

     e. Implementation strategies

     f. Referral to groups

     g. Referral to internet links or books

     h. Referral to dieticians

     i. Referral to commercial weight-loss programs

  3. Obtain dietary history through 24-hour or weekly recall

     a. Web-based diet diaries (Loseit.com; myfitness.pal)

  4. Computation of estimated daily caloric intake (Tables 17.13 and 17.14)

TABLE 17.14 Recommended Average Daily Energy Allowances for Women

POPULATION GROUP	AGE (YEARS)	KCAL/KG	KCAL/DAY
Women: nonpregnant, nonlactating	11–14	47	2,200
	15–18	40	2,200
	19–24	38	2,200
	25–50	36	2,200
	>51	30	1,900

Note: This is based on women engaged in light to moderate physical activity, with no underlying medical condition.

    a. BMI of 27 to 35, decrease in caloric intake of 300 to 500 kcal/day = 10% weight loss in 6 months (0.24–0.45 kg/wk)

    b. BMI >35, decrease in caloric intake of 500 to 1,000 kcal/day = 10% weight loss in 6 months (0.45–0.90 kg/wk)

D. Pharmacologic

    1. Many state boards of nursing prohibit the prescription of anti-obesity medication by an advanced practice registered nurse (APRN). Check with your state board of nursing for guidance on prescribing anti-obesity medications.

    2. Compare recommendations for pharmacologic therapies for the management of obesity in patients with metabolic dysregulation to those of metabolically healthy patients (Figure 17.4 and Table 17.15)

E. Surgical procedures

    1. Of the approximate 250,000 bariatric surgical procedures performed each year in the United States, 70% are performed on women.

    2. Types of surgical procedures

        a. Restrictive and malabsorptive bariatric procedures (metabolic surgery):

            (1) Laparoscopic gastric bypass (Roux-en-Y)

            (2) Biliopancreatic diversion (BPD)

            (3) Duodenal switch (DS) with BPD

            (4) Sleeve gastrectomy

        b. Restrictive-only bariatric procedures

            (1) Laparoscopic adjustable gastric band (LAGB)

            (2) Gastric stapling procedures

    3. The term *metabolic surgery* has emerged to describe procedures intended to treat type 2 diabetes as well as to reduce cardiometabolic risk factors.

Metabolically healthy

Stepwise approach
- Assess BMI and treatment criteria
- Behavioral interventions
- Self-selected diet
- Assess and treat mood disorders
- Primary medications
  - Phentermine
  - Topiramate
  - Zonasmide
  - Bupropion
  - Lorcaserin
- BMI >40 bariatric surgical procedure

Metabolic risk factors

Simultaneous approach
- Assess and treat:
  - Current meds
  - BMI criteria
  - CV risk factors
- Behavioral interventions
- Mediterranean diet
- Target mood disorder treatment
- Assess and treat sleep apnea
- Combination medications:

Phentermine	Orlistat
Topiramate	Metformin
Zonasmide	GLP-1
Buproprion	Pramlintide
Phe/Topa	Fiber (proxy PYY)
Lorcaserin	

- BMI >30 <35 with DM–Lap band
- BMI >35 RYGB; SG–metabolic bariartic surgical procedure

FIGURE 17.4 Pharmacologic strategies based on assessment of metabolic health: Management strategies for obesity.

BMI, body mass index; CV, cardiovascular; GLP-1, glucagon-like peptide-1; RYGB, Roux-en-Y gastric bypass; SG, sleeve gastrectomy.

TABLE 17.15 Pharmacological Management of Obesity in Women

MEDICATION	MECHANISM OF ACTION	RECOMMENDED DOSE	CONTRAINDICATIONS	SIDE EFFECTS
Adipex-P (Phentermine) Schedule IV Approved for short term use (3 months)	Appetite suppressant similar to amphetamine acts on the CNS	15–37.5 mg/day 8 mg TID	*Pregnancy (category X, ensure negative pregnancy test monthly and contraception practices in women of childbearing years),* breastfeeding, use of MAO inhibitor within 14 days, advanced cardiovascular disease, uncontrolled hypertension, hyperthyroidism, glaucoma, agitation, history of drug abuse.	Insomnia, elevated heart rate, dry mouth, taste alterations, dizziness, tremors, headache, diarrhea, constipation, vomiting, gastrointestinal distress, anxiety, restlessness
Qysmia (Phentermine/ Topiramate) Schedule IV Approved for long term use	Carbonic anhydrase inhibitor, noradrenalin releaser, and anticonvulsant that suppresses appetite, impacts satiety, stimulates thermogenesis	Initial dose 3.5/23mg *Requires dose titration schedule to initiate and to discontinue* See prescribing insert	*Pregnancy (category X, ensure negative pregnancy test monthly and contraception practices in women of childbearing years),* breastfeeding, use of MAO inhibitor within 14 days, advanced cardiovascular disease, uncontrolled hypertension, hyperthyroidism, glaucoma, agitation, history of drug abuse.	Paresthesias, headache, dizziness, taste aberations, insomnia, constipation, dry mouth, nasopharyngitis, elevation in heart rate, anxiety, depression, memory or cognitive changes, and decreased bicarbonate
Alli (Orlistat) Over the counter	Reduces fat absorption via inhibition of pancreatic lipase activity in intestine	60 mg prior to meal or up to one hour following a meal	Pregnancy, history of malabsorption digestive disorder, gallbladder disease, organ transplant, or prescribed cyclosporine	Frequent bowel movements, fatty or oily bowel movements, abdominal cramping, gas, bloating
Xenical (Orlistat) Prescription	Reduces fat absorption via inhibition of pancreatic lipase activity in intestine	120 mg prior to a meal or up to one hour following a meal	Pregnancy, history of malabsorption digestive disorder, gallbladder disease, organ transplant, or prescribed cyclosporine	Frequent bowel movements, fatty or oily bowel movements, abdominal cramping, gas, bloating
Contrave (Bupropion/ Naltraxone) Prescription	Sustained release combination of an opioid receptor antagonist and a catecholamine reuptake inhibitor thought to synergistically lead to improved energy expenditure and reduced appetite	*Requires dose titration schedule to initiate and to discontinue* Initial dose 8 mg naltrexone/90 mg Bupropion SR. Max dose 32 naltrexone/360 mg bupropion SR daily. See prescribing insert.	*Black Box Warning:* Suicidality and lowering of seizure threshold due to the bupropion component Since naltrexone antagonizes the opioid receptor, it should not be given to those on chronic opioid therapy. Neuropsychiatric reactions in patients taking bupropion for smoking cessation *Contraindicated:* Pregnancy category X Uncontrolled HTN Seizure disorders	Nausea and vomiting, Headache, dizziness, constipation, trouble sleeping, temporary high blood pressure, dry mouth

(continued)

TABLE 17.15 Pharmacological Management of Obesity in Women (*continued*)

MEDICATION	MECHANISM OF ACTION	RECOMMENDED DOSE	CONTRAINDICATIONS	SIDE EFFECTS
Saxenda (liraglutide) Wegovy (Semaglutide) Prescription	Glucagon-like peptide-1 (GLP-1) analogue	*Requires dose titration schedule from initiation through therapeutic levels.* See prescribing insert	Personal or family history of medullary thyroid carcinoma or in patients with multiple endocrine neoplasia syndrome type 2 (4, 5.1). Known hypersensitivity to liraglutide or semaglutide or any of the excipients in Saxenda or WEGOVY	Nausea, diarrhea, vomiting, constipation, abdominal pain, headache, fatigue, dyspepsia, dizziness, abdominal distension, eructation, hypoglycemia in patients with type 2 diabetes, flatulence, gastroenteritis, and gastroesophageal reflux disease

NS, central nervous system; FDA, Food and Drug Administration.

4. National Institutes of Health criteria for bariatric surgical procedures include:
   a. BMI greater than or equal to 40 kg/m² without coexisting medical problems and for whom bariatric surgery would not be associated with excessive risk
   b. Patients with a BMI greater than or equal to 35 kg/m² and one or more severe obesity-related comorbidities (Box 17.2)

BOX 17.2 Common Comorbidities Considered Medically Necessary by Third-Party Payers for Bariatric Surgical Procedures

- Type 2 diabetes
- Hypertension
- Hyperlipidemia
- OSA
- OHS
- Pickwickian syndrome (a combination of OSA and OHS)
- NAFLD
- NASH
- Pseudotumor cerebri
- GERD
- Asthma
- Venous stasis disease
- Severe urinary incontinence
- Debilitating arthritis
- Considerably impaired QOL

GERD, gastroesophageal reflux disease; NAFLD, nonalcoholic fatty liver disease; NASH, nonalcoholic steatohepatitis; OHS, obesity–hypoventilation syndrome; OSA, obstructive sleep apnea; QOL, quality of life.

Source: Mechanick, J. I., Youdim, A., Jones, D. B., Garvey, W. T., Hurley, D. L., McMahon, M. M., ... Brethauer, S. (2013). Clinical practice guidelines for the perioperative nutritional, metabolic, and nonsurgical support of the bariatric surgery patient—2013 update: Co-sponsored by American Association of Clinical Endocrinologists, the Obesity Society, and American Society for Metabolic & Bariatric Surgery. *Endocrine Practice, 19*(2), 337–372. https://doi.org/10.4158/EP12437.GL

> **BOX 17.3 Psychosocial Factors Predictive of Poor Long-Term Outcomes of Bariatric Surgery**
>
> - Unrealistically high expectations for weight loss
> - Untreated psychological disorders
> - Untreated adverse eating patterns: Grazing, night-eating syndrome, emotional or nonhungry eating, binge-eating disorder or multiple adverse eating behaviors
> - ETOH (alcohol) abuse, addictive and impulsive behaviors
> - Poor access to social support
>
> *Source*: Mechanick, J. I., Youdim, A., Jones, D. B., Garvey, W. T., Hurley, D. L., McMahon, M. M., . . . Brethauer, S. (2013). Clinical practice guidelines for the perioperative nutritional, metabolic, and non-surgical support of the bariatric surgery patient—2013 update: Co-sponsored by American Association of Clinical Endocrinologists, the Obesity Society, and American Society for Metabolic & Bariatric Surgery. *Endocrine Practice, 19*(2), 337–372. https://doi.org/10.4158/EP12437.GL

5. Gender-specific issues related to women and bariatric surgical procedures
   a. Estrogen therapy should be discontinued before bariatric surgery (one cycle of oral contraceptives in premenopausal women; 3 weeks of HRT [see Box 17.3] in postmenopausal women) to reduce the risks for postoperative thromboembolic phenomena.
   b. Weight loss through bariatric surgical procedures may increase fertility. Women should be counseled regarding reliable contraception including non-oral contraceptive options post restrictive/malabsorption procedures.
   c. Women of childbearing years are at a greater risk for malabsorption anemia post restrictive/malabsorption procedures related to menstruation.
   d. Calcium and vitamin D absorption are decreased following restrictive/malabsorption.

DEVELOPMENT OF A WEIGHT MANAGEMENT PLAN

A. An effective weight management plan based on best practice, research, and guidelines is designed to help an overweight or obese person reach and stay at a healthy body weight.
   1. The National Heart, Lung, and Blood Institute (NHLBI) panel recommends treatment for obesity for patients with a BMI of 25 to 29 kg/m² and with two or more risk factors and for patients with a BMI of 30 or more with no risk factors.
   2. The overall goals of weight management are to reduce body weight and maintain a lower body weight long term, prevent further weight gain, and control potential risk factors.
   3. Nurse practitioners should counsel their patients about dietary interventions, increasing the amount of physical activity, behavior therapy, pharmacotherapy, and a combination of all techniques available.
   4. The ability to prescribe obesity drugs varies by state. Check with your state board of nursing regarding the rules and regulations for prescribing U.S. Food and Drug Administration (FDA) anti-obesity medications (see Table 17.15).
   5. The most effective therapy for weight loss and maintenance is a combination of a low-calorie diet, an increase in physical activity, and lifestyle modifications.
   6. Using this therapy for at least 6 months and setting a goal for a 5% to 10% reduction in weight should be the initial goal for the patient. A patient's continued participation is the most important outcome in weight management.

7. Results of recent clinical trials suggested that weight management plans should be created according to a woman's current phase of life. The critical reproductive milestones that should be targeted include puberty, pregnancy, postpartum, and during menopause.
8. Internet sources are listed in Box 17.4 for further information.

BOX 17.4 Selected Web-Based Resources for Patients

American Dietetic Association: www.diet.com/g/american-dietetic-association (offers information on nutrition, healthy lifestyle, and how to find a registered dietician)

USDA Food and Nutrition Information Center: https://www.nal.usda.gov/fnic

National Heart, Lung, and Blood Institute Obesity Education Initiative: www.nhlbi.nih.gov/health/educational/lose_wt (offers information on selecting a weight-loss program, menu planning, food label reading, and BMI calculation and interpretation)

National Institute of Diabetes and Digestive and Kidney Diseases: www.niddk.nih.gov/health-information/diet-nutrition

www.fitday.com

www.myfitnesspal.com

www.loseit.com

www.sparkpeople.com

www.weightwatchers.com

Obesity-Specific Tools to Support Diagnosis, Evaluation, and Management

AACE Obesity Resource Center: obesity.aace.com/obesity-resource-toolkit

American Obesity Association: www.obesity.org

Community Health Association of Mountain/Plain States (CHAMPS) Obesity Resource List: champsonline.org/tools-products/clinical-resources/diseasecondition-specific-resources/overweight-and-obesity-treatment-and-prevention-resources

Obesity Action Coalition: www.obesityaction.org/obesity-treatments/what-is-obesity-treatment

Obesity Support Group for Bariatric Surgery: www.obesityhelp.com

Diabetes Prevention

American Diabetes Association: Meal planning, exercise, weight loss, complications: www.diabetes.org

Centers for Disease Control and Prevention: www.cdc.gov/diabetes/home/index.html

General Lifestyle Advice

Academy of Nutrition and Dietetics: www.eatright.org

Centers for Disease Control and Prevention: Healthy lifestyle: www.cdc.gov/obesity

The Center for Mindful Eating: thecenterformindfuleating.org

U.S. Department of Agriculture: Healthy food choices: www.choosemyplate.gov

American Heart Association: Heart health and healthy living: healthyforgood.heart.org

Note: fitday.com gives nutritional analysis of calories, fat, protein, carbohydrates, and fiber in table and graph form as well as offering journals, and goal-setting and activity-tracking tools.

CASE STUDY: Management of Obesity

Patient Situation (History of Present Illness)

A 72-year-old Caucasian female presents to the clinic for her yearly follow-up and medication refills.

Subjective Data

- Denies current complaints beyond her usual severe bilateral knee pain
- Reports using a wheeled walker for ambulation. Still able to drive
- Monitors blood glucose and blood pressure at home
- Widowed, lives alone, stopped smoking 1 year ago
- Admits to some symptoms of depression including fatigue, poor sleep, loss of interest in her usual activities (cooking, socializing)
- **Current medical history:** T2 diabetes, non-insulin dependent; CAD (previous MI), hypertension, dyslipidemia, hypothyroidism, COPD, peripheral neuropathy, osteoarthritis
- **Medications:** Actos 45 mg daily, Glipizide 20 mg BID, Glucophage 100 mg BID, Accupril 40 mg BID, Catapress-TTS 0.3 mg patch, Diovan 80 mg daily, Norvasc 10 mg daily, Zocor 40 mg daily, Levoxyl 200 mcg daily, Elavil 150 mg/hs, multivitamin, Vit B_{12}, ASA 81 mg daily.

Objective Data

- Antalgic gate, uses walker to ambulate
- Alert and oriented to person, place, time
- **Vital signs:** blood pressure 150/70, pulse 82/min, respiration 18/min
- **Height:** 5'2"
- **Weight:** 258 lb. BMI 51
- **Last labs:**
A1C = 7.8
Creat =1.3
LFT = WNL
TSH = 2.3

Lipids

TC = 201   TG = 210
HDL = 49   LDL = 110

Clinical Analysis

Step 1: What lifestyle interventions do you anticipate she will be able to accomplish?
- Possibly improved nutritional choices (eats at a buffet-type restaurant one time per day for main source of food, limited ability to shop for groceries, limited ability to cook)
- Possibly light upper body home strength training exercises (limited ability to ambulate, SOB with exertion due to COPD)

Step 2: Are there medications prescribed for this patient that likely contribute to her obesity and can substitutions be considered?
- Actos, Glipizide
  - Consider discontinuing Actos and Glipizide by titrating down on these medications and substituting Liraglutide titrated to a dose of 1.8 mg daily.

(continued)

CASE STUDY: Management of Obesity (*continued*)

- Elavil
  - ○ Consider substituting topiramate

Are there other clinical priorities?
- Treat the depression
  - ○ Consider treatment with Wellbutrin (bupropion)
- Improve her knee pain
  - ○ Consider physical therapy

What is the priority intervention based on the patient's clinical presentation?
- Pain management such as pain medication; skin traction as ordered to stabilize hip and prevent muscle spasms

What should be included in this patient's plan of care?
- Frequent follow-up to assess glucose levels, blood pressure, weight
- Assess response to antidepressant
- Referral to dietitian if possible
- Review patient's diet diaries to help guide nutritional choices and opportunities for intervention
- Positive reinforcement for lifestyle changes

Over the course of 12 months, patient lost 58 pounds resulting in a decrease of her BMI to 36.6

BIBLIOGRAPHY

Abrams, B., Coyle, J., Cohen, A. K., Headen, I., Hubbard, A., Ritchie, L., & Rehkopf, D. H. (2017). Excessive gestational weight gain and subsequent maternal obesity at age 40: A hypothetical intervention. *American Journal of Public Health, 107*(9), 1463–1469. https://doi.org/10.2105/AJPH.2017.303881

Agarwal, A., Agarwal, M., Garg, K., Dalai, P. K., Trivedi, J. K., & Srivastava, J. S. (2016). Metabolic syndrome and central obesity in depression: A cross-sectional study. *Indian Journal of Psychiatry, 58*(3), 281–286. https://doi.org/10.4103/0019-5545.192021

Alosco, M. L., Spitznagel, M. B., Strain, G., Devlin, M., Cohen, R., Crosby, R. D., Mitchell, J. E., & Gunstad, J. (2015). Pre-operative history of depression and cognitive changes in bariatric surgery patients. *Psychology, Health & Medicine, 20*(7), 802–813. https://doi.org/10.1080/13548506.2014.959531

American Psychiatric Association. (2013). *Diagnostic and statistical manual of mental disorders* (5th ed.). American Psychiatric Publishing.

Apovian, C. M., Aronne, L. J., Bessesen, D. H., McDonnell, M. E., Murad, M. H., Pagotto, U., Ryan, D. H., & Still, C. D.; Endocrine Society. (2015). Pharmacological management of obesity: An endocrine society clinical practice guideline. *Journal of Clinical Endocrinology and Metabolism, 100*(2), 342–362. https://doi.org/10.1210/jc.2014-3415

Bray, G. A., & Greenway, F. L. (2007). Pharmacological treatment of the overweight patient. *Pharmacological Reviews, 59*(2), 151–184. https://doi.org/10.1124/pr.59.2.2

Carwell, M. L., & Spatz, D. L. (2011). Eating disorders & breastfeeding. *MCN: The American Journal of Maternal/Child Nursing, 36*(2), 112–117; quiz 118. https://doi.org/10.1097/NMC.0b013e318205775c

Chan, J. M., Rimm, E. B., Colditz, G. A., Stampfer, M. J., & Willett, W. C. (1994). Obesity, fat distribution, and weight gain as risk factors for clinical diabetes in men. *Diabetes Care, 17*(9), 961–969. https://doi.org/10.2337/diacare.17.9.961

Cho, Y. M., Merchant, C. E., & Kieffer, T. J. (2012). Targeting the glucagon receptor family for diabetes and obesity therapy. *Pharmacology & Therapeutics, 135*(3), 247–278. https://doi.org/10.1016/j.pharmthera.2012.05.009

Clark, J. (2017). The obesity epidemic, bariatric surgery options and aftercare. *Alaskan Nurse, 68*(3), 4–5. Retrieved from http://www.aknurse.org/layouts/aknurse/files/documents/AKNURSE/The%20Alaska%20Nurse%20June-July%202017.pdf

Colditz, G. A., Willett, W. C., Rotnitzky, A., & Manson, J. E. (1995). Weight gain as a risk factor for clinical diabetes mellitus in women. *Annals of Internal Medicine, 122*(7), 481–486.

Connor, T., Martin, S. D., Howlett, K. F., & McGee, S. L. (2015). Metabolic remodelling in obesity and type 2 diabetes: Pathological or protective mechanisms in response to nutrient excess? *Clinical and Experimental Pharmacology & Physiology, 42*(1), 109–115. https://doi.org/10.1111/1440-1681.12315

Dag, Z. Ö., & Dilbaz, B. (2015). Impact of obesity on infertility in women. *Journal of the Turkish German Gynecological Association, 16*(2), 111–117. https://doi.org/10.5152/jtgga.2015.15232

Daniel, S., Soleymani, T., & Garvey, W. T. (2013). A complications-based clinical staging of obesity to guide treatment modality and intensity. *Current Opinion in Endocrinology, Diabetes, and Obesity, 20*(5), 377–388. https://doi.org/10.1097/01.med.0000433067.01671.f5

Davis, C. (2013). A narrative review of binge eating and addictive behaviors: Shared associations with seasonality and personality factors. *Frontiers in Psychiatry, 4*, 183. https://doi.org/10.3389/fpsyt.2013.00183

DeKoning, L. (2017). The clinical utility of adiposity-related hormones: The emerging role of leptin, adiponectin, and ghrelin testing. *Clinical Laboratory News, 43*(8), 12–16.

Ebrahimi-Mamaghani, M., Saghafi-Asl, M., Pirouzpanah, S., Aliasgharzadeh, A., Aliashrafi, S., Rezayi, N., & Mehrzad-Sadaghiani, M. (2015). Association of insulin resistance with lipid profile, metabolic syndrome, and hormonal aberrations in overweight or obese women with polycystic ovary syndrome. *Journal of Health, Population, and Nutrition, 33*(1), 157–167.

Flegal, K. M., Carroll, M. D., Kit, B. K., & Ogden, C. L. (2012). Prevalence of obesity and trends in the distribution of body mass index among US adults, 1999–2010. *Journal of the American Medical Association, 307*(5), 491–497. https://doi.org/10.1001/jama.2012.39

Fryar, C. D., Carroll, M. D., & Afful, J. (2020). Prevalence of overweight, obesity, and severe obesity among adults aged 20 and aver: United States, 1960–1962 through 2017–2018. *NCHS Data Brief*, (360), 1–8.

Gallant, A. R., Lundgren, J., & Drapeau, V. (2012). The night-eating syndrome and obesity. *Obesity Reviews, 13*(6), 528–536. https://doi.org/10.1111/j.1467-789X.2011.00975.x

Giandalia, A., Russo, G. T., Romeo, E. L., Alibrandi, A., Villari, P., Mirto, A. A., Armentano, G., Benvenga, S., & Cucinotta, D. (2014). Influence of high-normal serum TSH levels on major cardiovascular risk factors and Visceral Adiposity Index in euthyroid type 2 diabetic subjects. *Endocrine, 47*(1), 152–160. https://doi.org/10.1007/s12020-013-0137-2

Goracci, A., Casamassima, F., Iovieno, N., di Volo, S., Benbow, J., Bolognesi, S., & Fagiolini, A. (2015). Binge eating disorder: From clinical research to clinical practice. *Journal of Addiction Medicine, 9*(1), 20–24. https://doi.org/10.1097/ADM.0000000000000085

Gustafson, B., & Smith, U. (2015). Regulation of white adipogenesis and its relation to ectopic fat accumulation and cardiovascular risk. *Atherosclerosis, 241*(1), 27–35. https://doi.org/10.1016/j.atherosclerosis.2015.04.812

Hill, J. O., & Wyatt, H. (2002). Outpatient management of obesity: A primary care perspective. *Obesity Research, 10*(Suppl. 2), 124S–130S. https://doi.org/10.1038/oby.2002.205

Hruby, A., Manson, J. E., Qi, L., Malik, V. S., Rimm, E. B., Sun, Q., Willett, W. C., & Hu, F. B. (2016). Determinants and consequences of obesity. *American Journal of Public Health, 106*(9), 1656–1662. https://doi.org/10.2105/AJPH.2016.303326

Hung, S. P., Chen, C. Y., Guo, F. R., Chang, C. I., & Jan, C. F. (2017). Combine body mass index and body fat percentage measures to improve the accuracy of obesity screening in young adults. *Obesity Research & Clinical Practice, 11*(1), 11–18. https://doi.org/10.1016/j.orcp.2016.02.005

Jakicic, J. M. (2002). The role of physical activity in prevention and treatment of body weight gain in adults. *Journal of Nutrition, 132*(12), 3826S–3829S. https://doi.org/10.1093/jn/132.12.3826S

Johnson, D. B., Gerstein, D. E., Evans, A. E., & Woodward-Lopez, G. (2006). Preventing obesity: A life cycle perspective. *Journal of the American Dietetic Association, 106*(1), 97–102. https://doi.org/10.1016/j.jada.2005.09.048

Ken, F. (2017). Pharmacologic therapy for obesity management. *Clinical Advisor, 20*(5), 41–48

Khorassani, F. E., Misher, A., & Garris, S. (2015). Past and present of antiobesity agents: Focus on monoamine modulators. *American Journal of Health-System Pharmacy, 72*(9), 697–706. https://doi.org/10.2146/ajhp140034

Klauer, J., & Aronne, L. J. (2002). Managing overweight and obesity in women. *Clinical Obstetrics and Gynecology, 45*(4), 1080–1088.

Knerr, S., Bowen, D. J., Beresford, S. A., & Wang, C. (2016). Genetic causal beliefs about obesity, self-efficacy for weight control, and obesity-related behaviours in a middle-aged female cohort. *Psychology & Health, 31*(4), 420–435. https://doi.org/10.1080/08870446.2015.1115503

Kral, J. G. (2004). Preventing and treating obesity in girls and young women to curb the epidemic. *Obesity Research, 12*(10), 1539–1546. https://doi.org/10.1038/oby.2004.193

Kral, J. G., Kava, R. A., Catalano, P. M., & Moore, B. J. (2012). Severe obesity: The neglected epidemic. *Obesity Facts, 5*(2), 254–269. https://doi.org/10.1159/000338566

Kushner, R. F. (2012). Clinical assessment and management of adult obesity. *Circulation, 126*(24), 2870–2877. https://doi.org/10.1161/CIRCULATIONAHA.111.075424

Kushner, R. F., Calanna, S., Davies, M., Dicker, D., Garvery, W. T., Goldman, B., Lingvay, I., Thomsen, M., Wadden, T.A., Wharton, S., Wilding, J. P. H., & Rubino, D. (2020). Semaglutide 2.4 mg for the treatment of obesity: Key elements of the STEP Trials 1 to 5. *Obesity, 28*(6), 1050–1061. https://doi.org/10.1002/oby.22794.

Lustig, R. H. (2008). Hypothalamic obesity: Causes, consequences, treatment. *Pediatric Endocrinology Reviews, 6*(2), 220–227.

Lyznicki, J. M., Young, D. C., Riggs, J. A., & Davis, R. M.; Council on Scientific Affairs, American Medical Association. (2001). Obesity: Assessment and management in primary care. *American Family Physician, 63*(11), 2185–2196.

Mechanick, J. I., Apovian, C., Brethauer, S., Garvery, W. T., Joffee, A.M., Kim, J., Kushner, R. F., . . ., & Still, C. D. (2019). Clinical practice guidelines for the perioperative nutritional, metabolic, and nonsurgical support of patients undergoing bariatric procedures – 2019 Update: Cosponsored by American Association of Clinical Endocrinologists/American College of Endocrinology, the Obesity Society, and American Society for Metabolic & Bariatric Surgery, Obesity Medicine Association, and American Society of Anesthesiologist – Executive Summary. *Endocrine Practice, 25*(12), 1346–1359. https://doi.org/10.4158/GL-2019-0406

Messina, G., Viggiano, A., De Luca, V., Messina, A., Chieffi, S., & Monda, M. (2013). Hormonal changes in menopause and orexin-a action. *Obstetrics and Gynecology International, 2013*, 209812. https://doi.org/10.1155/2013/209812

Milano, W., De Rosa, M., Milano, L., & Capasso, A. (2012). Night eating syndrome: An overview. *Journal of Pharmacy and Pharmacology, 64*(1), 2–10. https://doi.org/10.1111/j.2042-7158.2011.01353.x

National Cholesterol Education Program Expert Panel. (2001). *Third report of the National Cholesterol Education Program (NCEP) Expert Panel on detection, evaluation, and treatment of high blood cholesterol in adults (Adult Treatment Panel III): Executive summary.* National Institutes of Health. Retrieved from https://www.nhlbi.nih.gov/files/docs/guidelines/atp3xsum.pdf

National Research Council. (1989). *Recommended dietary allowances.* (10th ed.). National Academies Press.

Norman, R. J., Noakes, M., Wu, R., Davies, M. J., Moran, L., & Wang, J. X. (2004). Improving reproductive performance in overweight/obese women with effective weight management. *Human Reproduction Update, 10*(3), 267–280. https://doi.org/10.1093/humupd/dmh018

Office of Disease Prevention and Health Promotion. (2018). *Healthy people.* Retrieved from http://www.health.gov/healthypeople

Østbye, T., Peterson, B. L., Krause, K. M., Swamy, G. K., & Lovelady, C. A. (2012). Predictors of postpartum weight change among overweight and obese women: Results from the active mothers postpartum study. *Journal of Women's Health, 21*(2), 215–222. https://doi.org/10.1089/jwh.2011.2947

Özcan Dağ, E., & Dilbaz, B. (2015). Impact of obesity on infertility in women. *Journal of the Turkish-German Gynecological Association, 16*(2), 111–117. https://doi.org/10.5152/jtgga.2015.15232

Panteliou, E., & Miras, A. D. (2017). What is the role of bariatric surgery in the management of obesity? *Climacteric: The Journal of the International Menopause Society, 20*(2), 97–102. https://doi.org/10.1080/13697137.2017.1262638

Reig García-Galbis, M., Rizo Baeza, M., & Cortés Castell, E. (2015). Indicators of success in the dietary management of overweight and obesity: Weight, body fat loss and quality. *Nutricion Hospitalaria, 32*(3), 1009–1016. https://doi.org/10.3305/nh.2015.32.3.9248

Ruiz-Tovar, J., Boix, E., Galindo, I., Zubiaga, L., Diez, M., Arroyo, A., & Calpena, R. (2014). Evolution of subclinical hypothyroidism and its relation with glucose and triglycerides levels in morbidly obese patients after undergoing sleeve gastrectomy as bariatric procedure. *Obesity Surgery, 24*(5), 791–795. https://doi.org/10.1007/s11695-013-1150-5

Ryan, D. H., & Stewart, T. M. (2004). Medical management of obesity in women: Office-based approaches to weight management. *Clinical Obstetrics and Gynecology, 47*(4), 914–927; discussion 980–1. https://doi.org/10.1097/01.grf.0000135359.63019.22

Tsujimoto, T., Kajio, H., & Sugiyama, T. (2016). Obesity, diabetes, and length of time in the United States: Analysis of National Health and Nutrition Examination Survey 1999 to 2012. *Medicine, 95*(35), e4578. https://doi.org/10.1097/MD.0000000000004578

Wing, R. R., & Hill, J. O. (2001). Successful weight loss maintenance. *Annual Review of Nutrition, 21*, 323–341. https://doi.org/10.1146/annurev.nutr.21.1.323

18

LESBIAN HEALTH (DON'T ASK...WON'T TELL: LESBIAN WOMEN AND WOMEN WHO HAVE SEX WITH WOMEN)

YVETTE MARIE PETTI

EXPERT REVIEWER: MEGHAN E. WHITFIELD

INTRODUCTION AND OVERVIEW

A. Lesbian women, or women who have sex with women (WSW), experience health disparities in terms of prevention screening and desired health outcomes as compared to heterosexual women.

B. Often, lesbian women avoid care due to perceived and lived experiences of homophobia from healthcare providers and healthcare institutions and systems.

C. Lesbian women are less likely to seek care due to:
   1. Stigma associated with being identified as lesbian
   2. Previously experienced negative encounters with healthcare providers

D. Lesbian women are at further risk for delayed care and reduced healthcare screening related to variables such as:
   1. Poor insurance coverage or lack of health insurance
   2. Lack of provider awareness regarding needs of this population
   3. Lack of understanding of health risks
   4. Health system design issues

E. One of the largest gaps identified in the literature that contributes to reduced screening and provider bias is the lack of curriculum addressing the healthcare needs of lesbian women.

SCREENING RECOMMENDATIONS FOR SEXUAL-MINORITY WOMEN (LESBIAN, BISEXUAL, AND WOMEN WHO HAVE SEX WITH WOMEN)

A. Breast cancer screening
   1. Lesbian women have lower rates of mammograms and higher rates of breast cancer than heterosexual women.
   2. This has been cited as caused by a lack of access to care because of a lack of insurance coupled with health behaviors such as smoking, null parity, obesity, and alcohol consumption.
   3. Lesbian women are less likely to participate in breast self-awareness via monthly self-breast exams, so be inclusive in offerings of mammography and in reviewing breast self-awareness with lesbian patients as a standard of care.

4. Exploring any reluctance that a lesbian patient may have about self-touch and explain the importance of self-breast exams in identifying risk for breast cancer. These are opportunities to offer her appropriate education and screening.

5. Share with the patient community resources offering support for screening as lesbian women may be underinsured or have no insurance.

B. Cervical cancer screening and human papillomavirus (HPV)

1. Lesbian women's rates of cervical cancer screening are lower than those for heterosexual women due to:

   a. Barriers to access to care (lack of health insurance, lack of access to a knowledgeable provider)

   b. Provider naivety

   c. Fear of examination

   d. Health disparities compounded with racial/ethnic disparities

2. A significant percentage of lesbian women have reported a history of having intercourse with a cis-male partner at some time and many continue to have intercourse with men.

3. Lesbian women are at greater risk for higher rates of abnormal cervical cancer screening tests due to delayed screening and intervention.

4. Lesbian women and WSW are not immune to human papillomavirus (HPV) and other factors leading to cervical cancer.

5. The current cervical cancer screening guidelines should be followed when providing care to lesbian women and WSW.

6. Be sensitive to the likely possibility that a lesbian patient has had sexual trauma and/or negative provider experience by conveying compassion and creating a safe environment for her to participate in this recommended screening examination. Think creatively and offer to let a care partner hold the patient's hand; they can listen to music and can even self-insert the speculum if they wish.

C. Screening for sexually transmitted infections (STIs)

1. Lesbian women and WSW are at risk for STIs, such as trichomoniasis, gonorrhea, chlamydia, genital herpes, human papillomavirus, hepatitis C, syphilis, and HIV. Follow the Centers for Disease Control and Prevention (CDC) recommended testing guidelines.

2. Exposure to STIs (like all women) is related to sexual practices, partner's risks, and number of partners. Box 18.1 lists high-risk sexual practices of lesbian and WSW persons.

3. Lower risk sexual practices include kissing and rubbing genitalia on her partner's body. Lesbians may not be using barrier protection via dental dams or condoms on sexual toys; this is an opportunity for education about barrier use.

4. Lesbian women and WSW can transmit trichomoniasis and other infections to one another.

BOX 18.1 High-Risk Sexual Practices of Lesbian Women and Women Who Have Sex With Women

- Oral-to-vaginal contact
- Genital-to-genital contact
- Digital stimulation
- Oral-to-anal contact
- Sharing of sex toys

5. Including a thorough sexual history of gender of partner, age of partner(s), number of partners, and type of sexual practices; including an oral/pharyngeal external (or internal as needed) rectal examination during the screening for HPV is critical due to the association of HPV with oral and rectal cancers
6. Include discussion of whether she and her partner(s) use condoms and/or dental dams and practice washing their hands and sex toys after penetrative sexual contact.
   a. Offer and discuss screenings for STIs candidly with lesbian patients.
7. Understand your own beliefs and work to remove bias when having candid discussions with patients regarding sexual practices and behaviors.
8. Use inclusive language and communicate in a neutral, matter-of-fact manner.

USING INCLUSIVE LANGUAGE

A. Use words that "open the door," are neutral, and are expressed in an unbiased manner.
B. When asking about a patient's socioeconomic profile, the use of the word "partnered" conveys openness to the patient.
C. When asking about partners, express the question in a manner that gives control back to the patient, and, in a neutral tone, ask "male," "female," or "both male and/or female."
D. Avoid using the term "sexually active" as this may have an ambiguous meaning. Rather, ask the patient, "Are you having sex with males, females, or both?"
E. Use the following to preface the beginning of your inquiry regarding her sexual history: "I am going to ask you some questions about your sexual health. These questions provide information that will help me identify what health screening and care you may need."
F. Ask, "Are you sexually active with males, females, and/or both males and females?"
G. Do not presume that your patient is having sex with only one person, so use "partner" and "partners" sequentially when you are asking about the patient's sexual history.
H. Inquire regarding fertility plans and review contraceptive options if desired. Review menstrual cycles to evaluate for excess menstrual flow, cycle irregularities, symptoms of dysmenorrhea and offer options for treatment.
I. Be sure to include a question during the sexual history interview regarding safety. An example of how to assess the safety of your patient with her partner(s) is to ask, "Do you feel safe in your relationship with your partner(s)?" or "Do you ever feel forced or coerced to engage in sexual activity with any partners?"
J. Many self-identified lesbians have experienced physical, emotional, and sexual assault during their lives, and the health screening examination provides an opportunity to assess for domestic and other types of violence to your patient.
K. Offer the option of a self-collected or urine sample specimen for STI testing if the patient is uncomfortable with a GYN exam.
L. Examples of questions to include in your sexual history with lesbian women and WSW are presented in Box 18.2.

APPROACH TO PATIENT AND PROVIDER COMMUNICATION

A. Variables identified in the literature as barriers to the promotion and health screening of self-identified lesbians are lack of trust of the provider and/or healthcare system, lack of health insurance, provider insensitivity, and biases of traditional healthcare delivery systems.
B. The three main influences related to sexual minority women's disclosure to their providers are sexual identity experience, perceived risk of disclosure, and the quality of relationship to provider.

BOX 18.2 Suggested Sexual History Questions

"I am going to ask the following questions to identify your care needs."
- Have you ever had sex forced on you by your partner, partners, or anyone?
- Do you have a sexual partner or partners at this time? Are they male, female, or both?
- Do you feel safe in your relationship with your partner or partners at this time?
- Do you have any concerns about your sexual relationship with your partner or partners?
- Do you participate in oral-to-vaginal contact with your partner or partners?
- Do you participate in oral-to-anal contact with your partner or partners?
- Do you participate in penile-to-vaginal intercourse with your partner or partners?
- Do you have any difficulty reaching orgasm with your partner or partners?
- Do you use sex toys (vibrators, strap-on penis, pelvic balls)? If so, do you share these with your partner or partners? Do you thoroughly clean your sex toys after each use?
- Have you ever had an STI, such as trichomoniasis, gonorrhea, chlamydia, genital herpes, genital warts, HPV, HIV, hepatitis C, syphilis, PID? When and how was it treated?

HPV, human papillomavirus; PID, pelvic inflammatory disease; STI, sexually transmitted infection.

C. Make your language inclusive so as to convey a neutral and safe environment for your lesbian patient to discuss her health and sexual history.

D. Use a nonjudgmental and neutral tone when asking about sexual practices and/or addressing sexual concerns. Do not assume pronouns, inquire regarding preferred name and pronouns. Box 18.3 lists some terminology used among lesbian women to describe their sexual practices.

RISK ASSESSMENT AND REDUCTION

A. The Gay and Lesbian Medical Association (GLMA) offers health and behavioral topics that all lesbian women should discuss with their provider.
   1. Breast cancer
      a. Lesbians have disproportionately higher rates compared with heterosexual women.
   2. Ovarian cancer
      a. Lesbians have higher rates of ovarian cancer compared with heterosexual women; one risk factor is nulliparity.
   3. Depression/anxiety
      a. Lesbians have higher rates of mental distress and depression
         (1) Due to chronic stress related to barriers to disclosure of sexual orientation/practices
         (2) Due to lack of social support
         (3) Due to social and institutional discrimination

BOX 18.3 Definitions for Selected Sexual Acts

- **Giving face or going down:** Oral to genital/vaginal contact
- **Fisting:** Using a fist and/or several fingers introduced into the vagina and/or rectum for digital stimulation
- **Rimming:** Rectal/anal stimulation with partner's tongue

    b. Fewer care-seeking behaviors

    c. Include depression screenings

      (1) The Patient Health Questionnaire-2 (PHQ-2)

      (2) The Patient Health Questionnaire-9 (PHQ-9)

4. Cardiovascular health

    a. Ask about participation in physical activity, stress levels, nutrition, sleep.

    b. Screen fasting lipids and glucose.

    c. Include alcohol, substance, and tobacco use

    d. Include family history of heart disease

5. Gynecologic cancer

    a. Lesbian and bisexual women are at higher risk for ovarian and endometrial cancer.

      (1) Thought to be due to higher rates of obesity, smoking, and lack of adequate screening, low parity (for ovarian cancer).

      (2) Ask about last date and results of cervical cancer screening.

    b. Educate about the importance of yearly well-women examination, which may include pelvic examination.

6. Fitness

    a. Rates of physical activity have been identified as lower than heterosexual women in some populations of lesbian women.

    b. Include physical activity in the assessment; type of exercise, frequency, duration, intensity, tolerance of exercise (excessive fatigue, injuries).

7. Tobacco and alcohol use

    a. Rates of tobacco and alcohol use are higher among lesbian and bisexual women.

    b. Offer tobacco-cessation intervention.

8. Substance use

    a. Rates of substance use/abuse are higher among young self-identified lesbians and bisexual women.

9. Intimate partner violence

    a. Lesbian women, bisexual women, and WSW experience intimate partner violence.

    b. Include questions about safety in your assessment.

    c. Resources are cited in Box 18.4 for women identified at risk.

10. Sexual health

    a. Ask about sexual practices, partner(s) gender.

    b. Inquire about fertility plans.

    c. Review menses history.

    d. Ask about history of sexual trauma.

    e. Ask about history of STIs.

BOX 18.4 Resources for Women at Risk

- **Gay and Lesbian Medical Association:** Top 10 things lesbians should discuss with their healthcare provider: http://www.glma.org/index.cfm?fuseaction=Page.viewPage&page-ID=691
- **Domestic Violence Resource:** info@thenetworklared.org
- **National Domestic Violence Hotline:** 1-800-799-SAFE (7233), Available 24 hours in English and Spanish, TDD: 800-787-3224

      f. Inquire regarding HPV vaccine series, recommend starting or completing series if needed.

      g. Ask about sexual concerns (vaginal dryness, dyspareunia, anorgasmia, changes in libido).

      h. Ask about use of sex toys.

        (1) Ask about shared sex toys with partner(s).

        (2) Ask how they clean and store sex toys. Provide education as needed.

B. Other age/subpopulation screenings

  1. Osteoporosis

    a. Include dietary assessment of calcium intake and vitamin D.

    b. Ask about family history of osteoporosis.

    c. Ask about prolonged use of medroxyprogesterone acetate (Depo-Provera)/levonorgestrel-containing intrauterine device (Mirena or Kyleena), or corticosteroids.

    d. Ask about early menopause/surgical menopause.

    e. Order a dual-energy x-ray absorptiometry (DXA) scan as appropriate by presentation and history.

  2. Colorectal cancer screening

    a. Ask about family history.

    b. Ask about anal receptive intercourse with men (risk of HPV associated with development of anal/rectal cancer). Anal cancer screening with hrHPV may be considered if a history of anal receptive intercourse or a history of moderate-to-severe dysplasia (CIN [cervical intraepithelial neoplasia] 2–3).

    c. Offer the national recommended screenings to all women—including fecal occult blood testing and/or colonoscopy screening as appropriate.

    d. Offer a list of community resources for these screenings.

APPROACH TO THE GYNECOLOGIC EXAM

A. Allow time for questions and discussion prior to the GYN exam. Offer therapeutic options such as music, to have a caregiver present, self-insertion of speculum.

B. Offer a word or phrase that will immediately end the exam if the patient is uncomfortable.

C. Allow patient to get redressed before continuing further with the subjective history or conversation regarding healthcare needs or education.

CASE STUDY: Identifying Risks and Opportunities

Lena, 49-year-old self-identified lesbian, calls for an appointment to establish care. She tells your receptionist that she has not had a provider for over 10 years, and she is "concerned about her health." Your receptionist transfers her to your registered nurse care manager (RNCM) as she feels that further triage is needed. Your rRNCM speaks with Lena, who states that she thinks that she is going through "the change" as her period has been irregular and she is having difficulty sleeping. Your RNCM determines that she should be scheduled for an evaluation within the next few weeks, and she is scheduled with you for a comprehensive women's wellness exam.

1. What information about her past care experiences should you obtain?
2. What may be some assumptions/biases about Lena that could influence her care?
3. Does she need cervical cancer or STI screening and other screenings such as mammography or colonoscopy?
4. Can she become pregnant? How will you determine this?

BIBLIOGRAPHY

Agenor, M., Krieger, N., Austin, S. B., Haneuse, S., & Gottlieb, B. R. (2013). Sexual orientation disparities in Papnicolau test among US women: The role of sexual and reproductive health services. *American Journal of Public Health, 16*, e1–e6. https://doi.org/10.2105/AJPH2013.30154

Alba, B., Lyons, A., Waling, A., Minichiello, V., Hughes, M., Barrett, C., Fredriksen-Goldsen, K., & Edmonds, S. (2021). Older lesbian and gay adults' perceptions of barriers and facilitators to accessing health and aged care services in Australia. *Health and Social Care Community, 29*(4), 918–927. https://doi.org/10.1111/hsc.13125. Epub 2020 Aug 5. MPID: 32761706

Blosnich, J., Foynes, M. M., & Shipherd, J. C. (2013). Health disparities among sexual minority women veterans. *Journal of Women's Health (2002), 22*(7), 631–636. https://doi.org/10.1089/jwh.2012.4214

Breiding, M. J., Chen, J., & Walters, M. L. (2013). National Intimate Partner and Sexual Violence Survey (NISVS): 2010 findings on victimization by sexual orientation. Supported by the National Center for Injury Prevention and Control–U.S. Division of Violence Prevention. Retrieved from http://stacks.cdc.gov/view/cdc/12362

Brown, J. P., & Tracy, J. K. (2008). Lesbians and cancer: An overlooked health disparity. *Cancer Causes & Control, 19*(10), 1009–1020. https://doi.org/10.1007/s10552-008-9176-z

Douglas-Brown, L. (2013). CDC: Lesbian, gay domestic violence rates same or higher than heterosexuals. *Gay Voice, 11*(3). Retrieved from http://www.thegavoice.com/news

Eliason, M. J. (2009). *Best practices for lesbian/bisexual women with substance use disorders.* Retrieved from http://static1.1.sqspcdn.com/static/f/622579/8208856/1282271659100/09+report+women.pdf?token=GXKNQo SMRUuyMx9EaWNgSOPnZ54%3D

Fredriksen-Goldsen, K. I., Kim, H. J., Barkan, S. E., Muraco, A., & Hoy-Ellis, C. P. (2013). Health disparities among lesbian, gay, and bisexual older adults: Results from a population-based study. *American Journal of Public Health, 103*(10), 1802–1809. https://doi.org/10.2105/AJPH.2012.301110

Gruskin, E. P., Hart, S., Gordon, N., & Ackerson, L. (2001). Patterns of cigarette smoking and alcohol use among lesbians and bisexual women enrolled in a large health maintenance organization. *American Journal of Public Health, 91*(6), 976–979. https://doi.org/10.2105/ajph.91.6.976

Hutchinson, M. K., Thompson, A. C., & Cederbaum, J. A. (2006). Multisystem factors contributing to disparities in preventive health care among lesbian women. *Journal of Obstetric, Gynecologic, and Neonatal Nursing, 35*(3), 393–402. https://doi.org/10.1111/j.1552-6909.2006.00054.x

Johns, M. M., Pingel, E. S., Youatt, E. J., Soler, J. H., McClelland, S. I., & Bauermeister, J. A. (2013). LGBT community, social network characteristics, and smoking behaviors in young sexual minority women. *American Journal of Community Psychology, 52*(1–2), 141–154. https://doi.org/10.1007/s10464-013-9584-4

McNair, R. P., Hegarty, K., & Taft, A. (2012). From silence to sensitivity: A new identity disclosure model to facilitate disclosure for same-sex attracted women in general practice consultations. *Social Science & Medicine (1982), 75*(1), 208–216. https://doi.org/10.1016/j.socscimed.2012.02.037

Marrazzo, J. M., Coffey, P., & Bingham, A. (2005). Sexual practices, risk perception and knowledge of sexually transmitted disease risk among lesbian and bisexual women. *Perspectives on Sexual and Reproductive Health, 37*(1), 6–12. https://doi.org/10.1363/psrh.37.006.05

Mosack, K. E., Brouwer, A. M., & Petroll, A. E. (2013). Sexual identity, identity disclosure, and health care experiences: Is there evidence for differential homophobia in primary care practice? *Women's Health Issues, 23*(6), e341–e346. https://doi.org/10.1016/j.whi.2013.07.004

National LGBT Health Education Center: A Progra.m of the Fenway Institute. Addressing Social Determinants of Health for Sexual and Gender Minority (SGM)

Polek, C., & Hardie, T. (2010). Lesbian women and knowledge about human papillomavirus. *Oncology Nursing Forum, 37*(3), E191–E197. https://doi.org/10.1188/10.ONF.E191-E197

Schulman, J. K., & Erickson-Schroth, L. (2019). Mental health in sexual minority and transgendered women. *Med Clinics of North America, 103*(4), 723–733. https://doi.org/10.1016/j.mcna.2019.02.005.PMID: 31078203 Review.

Silva, A. D. N., & Gomes, R. (2021). Access to health services for lesbian women: a literature review. *Cien Saude Colet. 26* (suppl 3), 5351–5360. https://doi.org/10.1590/1413-812320212611.3.34542019. eCollection. PMID: 34787224 Review. English, Portuguese.

Simenson, A. J., Corey, S., Markovic, N., & Kinsky, D. (2020). Disparities in chronic health outcomes and health behaviors between lesbian and heterosexual adult women in Pittsburgh: A longitudinal study. *Journal of Womens Health (Larchmt), 29*(8), 1059–1067. https://doi.org/10.1089/wjh.2019.8052. Epub 2020 Jul7. PMID: 32639182.

Snyder, M. (2019). Health care experiences of lesbian women: A metasynthesis. *Advances in Nursing Science, 42*(1), E1–E21. https://doi.org/10.1097/ANS.0000000000000226. PMID: 30325742 Review

U.S. Department of Health and Human Services, Health People 2020. Understanding Social Determinants of Health

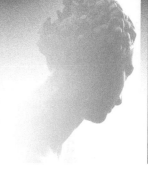

19

TRANSGENDER HEALTHCARE

MEGHAN M. WHITFIELD AND TERI BUNKER

INTRODUCTION AND OVERVIEW

A. Individuals who identify as transgender or gender incongruent experience health disparities at a higher rate than gay, lesbian, or bisexual individuals. This is multifactorial: fear of trauma/threats experienced during previous medical visits, inadequate or no insurance coverage, struggling with mental health symptoms, less access to medical providers, or suboptimal care provided by inexperienced medical providers. Persons providing medical or nursing care have an ethical duty to reduce barriers to healthcare for all persons and frequently assess, identify, and address marginalization and discrimination of all patient populations.

B. Not all transgender or gender incongruent persons will choose to take gender affirming medications and many patients may have not had gender affirming surgery. Choosing gender affirming medications, surgery, both, or neither is a highly individualized decision and does not negate identifying as transgender or gender incongruent.

C. Several resources are available for guidelines for gender affirming medication treatment and best practices. The following resources provide education and guidance for medications, routes, and dosage ranges.

1. **University of California San Francisco Gender Affirming Health Program:** https://transcare.ucsf.edu/

2. **Fenway Health in Boston:** https://fenwayhealth.org/care/medical/transgender-health/

3. **Endocrine Society Treatment of Gender-Dysphoric/Gender-Incongruent Persons Clinical Practice Guidelines:** https://core.ac.uk/reader/153399329?utm_source=linkout

4. **World Professional Association for Transgender Health (WPATH):** https://wpath.org/

D. Great care should be taken by medical clinics and providers to make the office as welcoming and gender neutral as possible. Studies have shown that gender-affirming education can be integrated into medical education/instructional programming with positive effects on employee/clinician attitudes and inclusion of transgender patients.

1. Train all staff with gender-affirming care education, including front desk staff, non-nursing or medical personnel such as billing specialists and practice managers, nursing and certified medical assistants, lab technicians, radiology, administrative staff, and environmental services (Box 19.1).

2. Nursing staff may benefit from utilization of River's *Gender Affirming Nursing Care Model* during training.

3. Involve technical support/medical record specialists in training and discuss options for correcting gender, name, and pronouns as indicated in the electronic medical record (EMR).

4. Evaluate artwork, brochures in clinic for gender neutrality; remove items with offensive language.

5. If unable to provide certain services to a patient, have alternate community resources available, including counseling and peer support groups.

BOX 19.1 Gender Terminology and Definitions

Gender identity: A person's individual sense of their gender

Gender expression: Outward expression of gender, including clothing and hairstyle. May be androgynous, masculine, or feminine qualities

Gender nonconforming: Gender identity differs from sex assigned at birth but may be more fluid on the feminine/masculine spectrum than transgender persons

Transgender: Gender identity differs from sex assigned at birth

Trans-masculine: On the masculine spectrum gender identity, may have female sex listed on original documents

Trans-feminine: On the feminine spectrum gender identity, may have male sex listed on original documents

Pronouns: They/them/their, he/him/his, she/her/hers, ze/zir/zirs, xe/xem/xyr (not an exhaustive list)

Cis-gender: Gender identity is congruent with sex assigned at birth

Source: Adapted from UCSF Transgender Care, *Terminology and definitions.*

SCREENING RECOMMENDATIONS FOR TRANSGENDER INDIVIDUALS

A. Transgender men

1. **Cervical cancer screening:** Follow American Society for Colposcopy and Cervical Pathology (ASCCP) guidelines for testing and management. All persons with a cervix 21 years of age and older are recommended for routine testing. If unable to tolerate a speculum exam, consider allowing a self-collected vaginal swab screening for human papillomavirus (HPV). The new 2020 American Cancer Society recommendations for cervical cancer screening with hrHPV should start at age 25 and be repeated every 5 years through age 65 unless the patient has certain high-risk history.

2. **Mammography:** The ACS recommends mammography for persons assigned female at birth starting at age 45 to 54. Follow ACS mammography guidelines for persons who have not undergone top surgery (chest tissue removal or male chest contouring) or only had a reduction of chest tissue. Mammography in persons who have had a full mastectomy may be technically unfeasible.

3. **Clinical chest or self-chest exam:** Unclear evidence to support continuing annual chest wall exams in persons who have had a mastectomy. Transgender men with partial chest tissue reduction or no top surgery should continue monthly self-chest wall exams. NOTE: The ACS no longer recommends routine clinical chest exams or monthly self-chest wall exams. However, high-risk individuals should have yearly clinical chest exams or as recommended based on their individual risk profile.

4. **Pregnancy:** Assess last monthly bleeding and for sexual activity with cis-male partners. Testosterone is not an effective contraceptive.

5. **Endometrial and ovarian cancer:** Evaluate unscheduled bleeding with vaginal speculum, bimanual exam, and further workup as needed. Signs of ovarian cancer such as bloating, lower pelvic pain, or pelvic mass should be evaluated with imaging and applicable workup. Risk of endometrial and ovarian cancer increases with age particularly post menopausally. Ovaries should not be palpated in post-menopausal individuals with ovaries.

B. Transgender women

1. **Clinical chest or self-chest exam:** Discuss chest health with patient. Clinician and self-chest exams have not been shown to be effective screening tools, rely on mammography per the following.

2. **Mammography:** University of California, San Francisco (UCSF) guidance recommends mammography after the age of 50 and with 5 to 10 years of feminizing hormonal medication use.

3. **Prostate cancer:** Prostate-specific antigen (PSA) levels are unreliable in persons taking feminizing medications. Fenway Institute recommends a digital rectal exam after age 50, and earlier as indicated by family history. If the patient has undergone genital surgery with neo-vagina construction, the prostate is more easily accessible via bimanual exam through neo-vagina.

C. All patients

1. Screen for tobacco use, encourage smoking cessation and support as needed with nicotine patches.

2. Screen for substance abuse and support cessation as indicated.

3. Screen for mental health concerns, may use evidence-based surveys such as PHQ9 or GAD7.

4. **Sexual health testing:** Follow CDC testing recommendations based on current anatomy, test more frequently if in a high-risk population. Test for gonorrhea and chlamydia at all sexual exposure sites (pharyngeal, genitalia, rectal). HIV, syphilis, and genital herpes testing should be based on level of risk.

5. Screen for abuse, safe housing, discrimination, and assess for social supports.

6. **Anal cancer screening:** Anal pap smears; insufficient data, no clear recommendations but discuss screening with trans-women who may receive anal sex, persons living with HIV, and the immunocompromised.

7. Encourage applicable vaccines such as HPV, hepatitis A and hepatitis B vaccine series.

8. **Osteoporosis:** Unclear guidance, begin bone density screening at age 65. May screen between ages 50 to 64 with established risk factors for osteoporosis. Transgender persons of all ages who have undergone gonadectomy and have a 5-year history of no hormone replacement would likely also benefit from bone density screening.

PATIENT AND PROVIDER COMMUNICATION

A. Establishing rapport from the initial greeting is paramount. "What name would you like me to call you?" "What pronouns do you prefer, and may I use them with any caregivers who are with you during this visit?"

B. Prepare in advance prior to initial visit with patient to assess any provider biases to improve communication. Review content supplied by resource rich websites such as UCSF, Fenway, Callen Lorde, and WPATH. Assess the clinical environment to ensure it is a welcoming space.

C. Introduce self and preferred pronouns; ask the patient if they would like to share their name and pronouns. Be aware name spoken may not be the name in the electronic medical record (EMR), make every effort to amend this to preferred name and include preferred pronouns. Use preferred name and pronouns when addressing the patient.

D. If needing to discuss chest/breast tissue or genitalia, ask the patient their preferred terms for these body parts and use these preferred terms. Practice cultural humility by asking and not assuming you know preferred terms.

E. Determine goals for the visit. Medical history and physical exam during the visit should be pertinent to visit type.

F. Primary care providers who are up to date on treatment methods and options can take an active role in managing gender-related care using an informed consent pathway. Involve the expertise of a subspecialist such as endocrinology, as needed.

G. Making a diagnosis of gender dysphoria (F64)

1. Confirm gender identity, verify persistent history of gender dysphoric feelings.

2. Assess support of community, family, peers, or friends.

3. Discuss the impact of gender nonconformity on mental health.

H. Criteria to start hormone therapy
   1. **Persistent, consistent, and insistent:** Well-documented gender dysphoria
   2. Mentally capable to make a fully informed decision and to consent to starting gender affirming medications.
   3. Of legal age in the residing state
   4. Any significant medical or mental health illness should be reasonably well controlled.

TAKING A MEDICAL AND SEXUAL HISTORY

A. Assess for family history of cancer, cardiovascular disease, diabetes, clotting disorders, and liver disease. Understanding family history allows for more thorough screening and risk discussion with a patient but does not warrant withholding or discontinuing use of gender-affirming medications. Use trauma-informed care approach.

B. Personal history of heart or vascular disease, venous thromboembolism, metabolic syndromes, liver disease, hypertension, breast or gynecologic cancers, pituitary adenomas, diabetes

C. **Mental health:** Screen for anxiety and depression as well as other mental concerns such as eating disorders, self-harm, posttraumatic stress, and substance use.

D. Social history including social support

E. Current or previous medications
   1. **Feminizing medications:** Estradiol (oral, injectable, topical), spironolactone or finasteride (oral). Estradiol dose varies based on route (Table 19.1).
   2. **Masculinizing medications:** Testosterone (injectable or topical cream, gel, or patches). Testosterone dose varies based on route (Table 19.2).
   3. Progesterone (Provera) has not been shown to be an essential component of feminizing medication therapy and has been associated with concerning syndromes such as cardiovascular disease and breast cancer. However, anecdotal reports of improved breast development, mood, and increased libido have been reported by patients taking progesterone. Discuss the role of progesterone and possible side effects carefully with patient.

F. Inquire regarding previous surgeries (include dates) including genital reconstruction, mastectomy, and cosmetic procedures such as silicone filler injections or other body modifications.

TABLE 19.1 Pharmacologic Management of Feminizing Medication Options and Dosages

HORMONE	DOSAGE: INITIAL OR LOW DOSE	DOSAGE: TYPICAL OR AVERAGE DOSE	DOSAGE: MAXIMUM
Estradiol oral/sublingual	1 mg/day	2–4 mg/day	8 mg/day
Estradiol transdermal	50 mcg	100 mcg	100–400 mcg
Estradiol valerate IM	<20 mg IM q 2 weeks	20 mg IM q 2 weeks	40 mg IM q 2 weeks
Estradiol cypionate IM	<2 mg q 2 weeks	2 mg IM q 2 weeks	5 mg IM q 2 weeks
Spironolactone[a]	25 mg q day	50 mg bid	200 mg bid
Finasteride	1 mg q day	2 mg q day	5 mg q day

[a]Monitor potassium level and blood pressure readings with each dose increase of spironolactone.

Source: Adapted from UCSF Transcare for Feminizing Medication Therapy.

TABLE 19.2 Pharmacologic Management of Masculinizing Medication Options and Dosages

ANDROGEN	LOW OR INITIAL DOSING	TYPICAL DOSE	MAXIMUM DOSE
Testosterone cypionate	20 mg/week IM/SQ	50 mg/week IM/SQ	100 mg/week IM/SQ
Testosterone topical gel 1%	12.5–25 mg Q AM	50 mg Q AM	100 mg Q AM
Testosterone topical gel 1.62%	20.25 mg Q AM	40.5–60.75 mg Q AM	103.25 mg Q AM
Testosterone patch	1–2 mg Q PM	4 mg Q PM	8 mg Q PM
Testosterone topical cream	10 mg	50 mg	100 mg
Testosterone axillary gel 2%	30 mg Q AM	60 mg Q AM	90–120 mg Q AM
Considerations: Monitor hematocrit level with each testosterone dose alteration.			

Source: Adapted from UCSF Transcare Guidelines for Masculinizing Medication Therapy.

G. **Transmen:** Assess for last monthly bleeding, and recent past pattern of menses.

H. Review tucking/binding, inquire regarding skin integrity if practicing binding/tucking frequently

I. **Sexual history:** Use a nonjudgmental attitude when taking a sexual history. Ask simple questions, clarify answers as needed. A sexual history should help determine risk reduction techniques, identify opportunities for sexual health testing, and enable offering helpful information to a patient.
   1. Inquire if patient is sexually active. If not, can conclude risk related questions and discuss sexual identity, desire for sexual activity, or answer questions as applicable. Support and refer to sexual-health/gender-affirming counselors as applicable. Not all persons are interested in sexual activity and this may not be a source of distress.
   2. If sexually active, inquire regarding gender of partner, discuss sites which may have been exposed during sexual activity. Ask "When you have sex, how does your partner identify?" "Which areas of your body are exposed when you have sex, such as your mouth, genitalia, or anus?"
   3. Inquire regarding safety concerns during sexual activity, any forced or coerced sexual activity, and offer resources as needed.
   4. Review pregnancy prevention method or fertility plans. Testosterone is not a contraceptive for transmen.
   5. Discuss previous sexual transmitted infection testing and assess need for testing per 2021 CDC STI guidelines.
   6. Sexual history is a good time to review, initiate, or complete HPV vaccinations.
   7. Assess for condom/dental dam use. Encourage consistent barrier use. Remind patients to wash sex toys after use and to change condoms on sex toys being shared between partners.
   8. Discuss HIV prevention prophylaxis (PrEP) with persons at risk for HIV exposure via IV drug use or sexual activity.
   9. Assess for sexual dysfunction, satisfaction with sexual activity. Offer resources as needed.

APPROACH TO A PHYSICAL AND OR GENITAL EXAM

A. Communication with the patient is paramount.
   1. Exam must be based on necessity to address visit type or concern.
   2. Breast/chest and genital exams are not necessarily needed prior to initiating gender-affirming medications.

TABLE 19.3 Timeline of Expected Effects of Masculinizing Medications	
Acne	1–6 months
Facial and body hair growth	3–6 months
Increased muscle strength	6–12 months
Body fat redistribution	3–6 months
Cessation of menses	2–6 months
Clitoral enlargement	3–6 months
Vaginal atrophy	3–6 months
Voice changes, lowering	3–12 months

Source: Adapted from the Endocrine Society and WPATH, 3/18/22.

3. Explain what components of the exam will be conducted prior to starting the exam; use clear language and previously identified preferred body part terms.
4. A chaperone during the physical exam may be helpful or harmful; discuss with the patient. If necessary due to clinic guidelines, explain and offer alternative option to the patient such as delaying exam or allowing the patient to choose which clinic staff may escort during the procedure.
5. Allow comfort measures, such as music, care partner, therapy animal, or meditation as desired by the patient. Pre-exam medication may also be offered.
6. Make it clear that the exam may be stopped at any time by the patient.
7. Some patients may prefer to return at another time for non-crucial, routine exam components, such as cervical cancer screenings, chest wall exams, or prostate exams. Most persons with a vagina can successfully self-insert a speculum if that alleviates anxiety. A speculum is not required to collect an HPV cervical cancer screening sample (clinician or patientself-collected).
8. Be aware of typical effects of hormonal changes on various body parts (Tables 19.3 and 19.4).
9. Use adequate amounts of lubrication with speculum exams in transmen taking testosterone and transwomen with neovaginas.
10. The prostate is more easily palpated via bimanual exam in transwomen with neovaginas (surgical reconstruction of genitalia).

TABLE 19.4 Timeline of Expected Initial Effects of Feminizing Medications	
Body fat redistribution	3–6 months
Decreased strength	3–6 months
Skin softening	3–6 months
Decreased libido/spontaneous erections	1–3 months
Breast/chest growth	3–6 months
Decreased testicular size	3–6 months
Decreased sperm production	Varies
Slowed growth of body and facial hair	6–12 months

Source: Adapted from the Endocrine Society and WPATH, 3/18/22.

TABLE 19.5 Risks of Testosterone/Estrogen Therapy

RISKS OF TESTOSTERONE THERAPY	RISKS OF ESTROGEN THERAPY
Lower high-density lipoprotein (HDL) levels, increased triglycerides	Venous thrombosis or thromboembolism
Increased homocysteine levels	Weight gain
Hepatotoxicity	Decreased libido
Polycythemia	Increased triglycerides
Chronic pelvic pain	Elevated blood pressure
Increased risk of sleep apnea	Increased risk of diabetes
Insulin resistance	Gallbladder disease

Source: Adapted from Fenway Health The Medical Care of Transgender Persons, 3/18/22.

RISK REDUCTION AND MONITORING (TABLE 19.5)

A. Labs
  1. Guidance regarding routine lab monitoring differs among the various guidelines. A couple of lab recommendations are consistent:
     a. Check hemoglobin and hematocrit for persons taking testosterone therapy every 3 months for the first year then annually thereafter.
     b. Monitor kidney function in persons taking an androgen blocker such as spironolactone or finasteride every 3 months and then annually thereafter.
     c. Follow U.S. Preventive Services Task Force recommendations for additional labs such as HgbA1C, lipids.
     d. Other labs to consider as indicated by medical history, symptoms, or medical exam include prolactin, testosterone, estrogen, liver function tests, and electrolytes. Refer to lab monitoring guidelines for gender-affirming medications.
  2. After taking hormone replacement therapy for >6 months, use the lab result range which is normal for the patient's gender. For example: Transmen taking testosterone for >6 months will have the same normal range for a CBC as a cisman.
  3. Consider monitoring estradiol levels more often in transwomen taking PrEP.
B. Post-surgery considerations
  1. Assess and monitor for complications such as infection, impaired healing, urinary incontinence, urinary retentions, urinary tract infections, bleeding, pelvic floor dysfunction, sexual concerns, tissue necrosis, and abscess formation.
  2. Inquire regarding the use of dilators for transwomen post neovagina formation.
C. **Referrals:** Have references available for patients regarding knowledgeable counselors, support groups, mental health professionals, medical professionals, and experienced surgeons for top or genitalia reconstruction surgeries. This is part of preparing for the visit.
D. Sensitive situations
  1. Discuss potential patient concerns prior to ordering EKGs, ultrasounds, or any testing which may require clothing removal or touching sensitive areas.
  2. Allow self-collection of sexual health testing; many testing platforms are approved for self-collection.
  3. Remind patient to limit tucking or binding for 8 to 12 hours at a time, wash binders frequently.

CASE STUDY

Zay, preferred pronouns she/her/hers, is a 60-year-old transwoman who presents to discuss vaginal bleeding that started a couple of weeks ago. She reports that she has a history of a hypertension and had an open reduction internal fixation (ORIF) of her left hip 2 months ago due to fracture after a fall during an argument with her partner. Zay tells your nurse that she has not been taking any medication for the past 10 years due to lack of health insurance and has no drug allergies. She is tearful often while speaking to your nurse and often avoids making eye contact.

1. What additional information regarding Zay's medical and surgical history is needed?
2. What health maintenance items and screenings are indicated for Zay at this time?
3. What social concerns do you have for Zay? How can you support or advocate for Zay today?
4. Does Zay need a speculum exam today? What is your approach to this type of exam for this patient?

BIBLIOGRAPHY

Camacho, P. M., Petak, S. M., Binkley, N., Diab, D. L., Eldeiry, L. S., Farooki, A., Harris, S. T., Hurley, D. L., Kelly, J., Lewiecki, E. M., Pessah-Pollack, R., McClung, M., Wimalawansa, S. J., & Watts, N. B. (2020). American association of clinical endocrinologists/American college of endocrinology clinical practice guidelines for the diagnosis and treatment of postmenopausal osteoporosis-2020 update. *Endocrine Practice, 26*(1), 1–46. https://doi.org/10.4158/GL-2020-0524SUPPL

Cavanaugh, T., Hopwood, R., Gonzalez, A., & Thompson, J. (2015). The medical care of transgender persons. *Fenway Health.* https://www.lgbtqiahealtheducation.org/wp-content/uploads/COM-2245-The-Medical-Care-of-Transgender-Persons-v31816.pdf

Centers for Disease Control and Prevention. (2021). Screening recommendations and considerations referenced in treatment guidelines and original sources. *Sexually transmitted infections treatment guidelines.* https://www.cdc.gov/std/treatment-guidelines/screening-recommendations.htm

Coleman, E., Bockting, W., Botzer, M., Cohen-Kettenis, P., DeCuypere, G., Feldman, J., . . . & Zucker, K. (2012). Standards of care for the health of transsexual, transgender, and gender-nonconforming people. *International Journal of Transgenderism, 13*(4), 165–232. https://doi.org/10.1080/15532739.2011.700873

Davis, W. D., Patel, B., & Thurmond, J. K. (2021). Emergency care considerations for the transgender patient: Complications of gender-affirming treatments. *Journal of Emergency Nursing, 47*(1), 33–39. https://doi.org/10.1016/j.jen.2020.07.009

de Brouwer, I. J., Elaut, E., Becker-Hebly, I., Heylens, G., Nieder, T. O., van de Grift, T. C., & Kreukels, B. P. (2021). Aftercare needs following gender-affirming surgeries: Findings from the ENIGI multicenter European follow-up study. *The Journal of Sexual Medicine, 18*(11), 1921–1932. https://doi.org/10.1016/j.jsxm.2021.08.005

Denby, K. J., Cho, L., Toljan, K., Patil, M., & Ferrando, C. A. (2021). Assessment of cardiovascular risk in transgender patients presenting for gender-affirming care. *The American Journal of Medicine, 134*(8), 1002–1008. https://doi.org/10.1016/j.amjmed.2021.02.031

Deutsch, M. B. (2016). *Guidelines for the primary and gender-affirming care of transgender and nonbinary people.* UCSF Gender Affirming Health Program. https://transcare.ucsf.edu/guidelines

De Vries, E, Kathard, H., & Muller, A. (2020). Debate: Why should gender-affirming health care be included in health science curricula? *BMC Medical Education, 20*(51). https://bmcmededuc.biomedcentral.com/articles/10.1186/s12909-020-1963-6

Hembree, W. C., Cohen-Kettenis, P. T., Gooren, L., Hannema, S. E., Meyer, W. J., Murad, M. H., Rosenthal, S. M., Safer, J. D., Tanpricha, V., & T'Sjoen, G. G. (2017). Endocrine treatment of gender-dysphoric/gender-incongruent persons: An endocrine society clinical practice guideline. *Journal of Clinical Endocrinology and Metabolism, 102*(11), 3869–3903. https://core.ac.uk/reader/153399329?utm_source=linkout

Kerckhof, M. E., Kreukels, B. P., Nieder, T. O., Becker-Hebly, I., van de Grift, T. C., Staphorsius, A. S., Kohler, A., & Heylens, G. (2019). Prevalence of sexual dysfunctions in transgender persons: Results from the ENIGI follow-up study. *The Journal of Sexual Medicine, 16*(12), 2018–2029. https://doi.org/10.1016/j.jsxm.2019.09.003

Klein, A., & Golub, S. A. (2020). Enhancing gender-affirming provider communication to increase health care access and utilization among transgender men and trans-masculine non-binary individuals. *LGBT Health, 7*(6), 292–304. https://doi.org/10.1089/lgbt.2019.0294

Klein, D. A., Paradise, S. L., & Goodwin, E. T. (2018). Caring for transgender and gender-diverse persons: What clinicians should know. *American Family Physician, 98*(11), 645–653. https://www.aafp.org/afp/2018/1201/p645.html

Krempasky, C., Harris, M., Abern, L., Grimstad, F. (2020). Contraception across the transmasculine spectrum. *American Journal of Obstetrics and Gynecology, 222*(2), 134–143. https://doi.org/10.1016/j.ajog.2019.07.043

Liszewski, W., Ananth, A. T., Ploch, L. E., & Rogers, N. E. (2014). Anal pap smears and anal cancer: What dermatologists should know. *Journal of the American Academy of Dermatology, 71*(5), 985–992. https://doi.org/10.1016/j.jaad.2014.06.045

Macapagal, K., Bhatia, R., & Greene, G. J. (2016). Differences in healthcare access, use, and experiences within a community sample of racially diverse lesbian, gay, bisexual, transgender and questioning emerging adults. *LGBT Health, 3*(6), 434–442. https://doi.org/10.1089/lgbt.2015.0124

Rivera, D., Jukkala, A., & Rohini, T. (2021). Introduction to River's gender affirming nursing care model: A middle-range theory. *Journal of Holistic Nursing, 40*(3), 255–264. https://doi-org.ezproxy3.lhl.uab.edu/10.1177/08980101211046747

Stryker, S. D., Pallerla, H., & Pickle, S. (2019). Considerations on medical training for gender-affirming care: Motivation and perspectives. *International Journal of Transgender Health, 21*(1), 79–88. https://doi.org/10.1080/15532739.2019.1 689880

20

WOMEN VETERANS:
When the Woman Was a Warrior

PATRICE C. MALENA

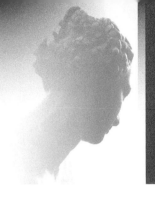

INTRODUCTION

A. Women comprise 15% of the armed forces. Since the recent military reduction in force, there are more military men and women exiting the armed forces and transitioning to civilian life. The fastest growing sub-population of veterans is women veterans. The military experiences of women veterans can and often do impact the remainder of their lives, physically and mentally. Many women veterans access healthcare through the Veterans Health Administration (VHA) via their local Veterans Affairs (VA) healthcare systems. However, most women veterans are seen in civilian medical care facilities. Healthcare providers need to recognize that the woman they are seeing today may have been in the military and is a former woman warrior.

B. You may be caring for women veterans in your practices, and don't even know it. This chapter is intended to address this problem by raising awareness so women veterans can receive excellent care in all settings (military and non-military).

C. Consider asking all female patients, "Are you a veteran?" Since many do not self-identify as veterans, asking, "Did you serve in the military?" may elicit a positive response. In addition, you can determine specific details on their service: branch (Army, Navy, Air Force, Coast Guard), dates of service, rate (what they did), stations (where they served), and combat exposure. All these factors can impact their current health.

SPECIFIC AREAS OF CONCERN

A. Primary care
   1. **Obesity:** Many women gain weight after leaving the military. As civilians, they no longer are required to stay physically fit, and no longer have superiors ordering them to physical training (PT). This may set them up for developing chronic conditions such as diabetes, heart disease, and hypertension.
   2. **Musculoskeletal:** Increased risk for joint disorders, particularly in lower extremities. It is not uncommon for women veterans to have to utilize uniforms, boots, and equipment not designed for women's bodies. In full battle gear, a female soldier may carry an extra 50 to 70 pounds on her body.
   3. **Tobacco use:** Nicotine addiction is widespread among female soldiers and can lead to multiple long-term health problems.
   4. **Cardiovascular:** Lipid deposition disorder (obesity); combining stress hormones, sleep deprivation, contraceptive choices, and prolonged sitting at computers
      a. Suboptimal nutrition (calories per meal based on male requirements)

    b. Eating habits (access to cafeteria/chow hall, canteens, shiftwork)

    c. Lack of continued physical training once separated from the military

  5. Neurologic

    a. Combat or near-combat exposure puts female soldiers at risk for brain injuries such as traumatic brain injury (TBI).

    b. Pain syndromes post injury or repetitive stress

  6. **Exposures:** Serving in certain military venues can mean exposures to toxic substances, such as Agent Orange during Vietnam. These exposures can affect multiple body systems, including respiratory and dermatologic.

  7. Reproductive

    a. Contraceptive and STI challenges during active duty

    b. Pregnancy protections

    c. Infertility

B. Mental health (most common conditions):

  1. Depression

  2. Anxiety

  3. Posttraumatic stress disorder (PTSD; https://ptsd.va.gov)

  4. Intimate partner violence (IPV)

  5. Military sexual trauma (MST) (https://mentalhealth.va.gov/mst)

  6. Suicidal ideation (New Suicide Prevention Hotline, 988.)

  7. Substance abuse

C. Trauma-informed care (TIC)

  1. TIC is the approach that assumes the woman is more likely than not to have a history of trauma. This history of trauma may have a huge impact on the woman veteran's life.

  2. Since many women veterans experienced trauma (physical, mental, emotional) during their time in the armed forces, it is best to approach each woman during each visit with the understanding that she may have not reported the experiences, or she may not correlate her current responses to her military duty.

D. Accessing care within the VHA/VA

  1. Women may not know they are eligible for VA care. Many women do not consider themselves veterans (cross-generational, all ages, all branches of the military, all years of service).

  2. Women may be concerned about the care they might receive at a VA facility (e.g., safety, respect, dignity, availability of gender-specific services).

  3. The VA may not be easily accessible. There are over 150 VA hospitals across the United States, and there are over 800 associated Community-Based Outpatient Clinics (CBOCs), extending the reach of the VA hospitals. https://www.va.gov/find-locations

  4. Military retirement provides access to care through military insurance Tricare. Many women veterans obtain dual care, accessing both civilian and VA services.

E. Veterans Health Administration (VHA) and Veterans Affairs (VA)

  1. **Eligibility:** Women who have an honorable discharge and served at least 2 years are eligible for some healthcare at the VA. There may be income restrictions. Women with a general discharge or dishonorable discharge may be eligible for acute mental health needs, and for care for military sexual trauma (MST). They can access assistance through the benefits office of VA, or local Veterans Service Organizations (VSO) such as Disabled American Veterans (DAV). https://www.ebenefits.va.gov/ebenifits/homepage

  2. Each VA hospital across the United States has a dedicated staff member called the Women Veterans Program Manager (WVPM) to assist women veterans in navigating the sometimes complicated VA system. Locate the closest WVPM at https://www.womenshealth.va.gov/WOMENSHEALTH/programoverview/wvpm.asp

3. Anyone with questions concerning women veterans and VA care can contact the toll free Women Veterans Call Center (WVCC) at 855-829-6636 via phone call or text.

4. The VA website for women veterans is https://www.womenshealth.va.gov/WOMENSHEALTH/index.as

5. VA offers specific services to women who are separating from the military to assist in their transition to civilian life. Transition and care management, especially for those who were involved in combat arenas, may be eligible. Veterans who served in post-9/11 combat venues may be eligible for 5 years of free healthcare. https://www.oefoif.va.gov

6. Women veterans are seen in primary care through Patient Aligned Care Teams (PACT) which may include providers, nurses, social workers, pharmacists, and laboratory staff. Primary care is provided by designated Women's Health Care-Primary Care Providers (WHC-PCPs) who have specialized training in comprehensive women's care, and the special needs of women veterans. They are able to provide basic reproductive healthcare. The primary care team assists in case management and referrals to other specialties. In addition, they have access to primary care integrated mental health providers who are networked into primary care clinics.

7. Due to high volume and the often complex needs of all veterans, the federal government expanded care in the community to improve access. Should there be a significant delay in accessing care or obtaining appointments, veterans can request to see a local community provider. Veterans may find, however, the delay for an appointment at the VA may be shorter than appointments in the community.

8. **Mental health needs:** Many VAs have inpatient mental health, and some of them have separate wings exclusively for women veterans. Outpatient mental health services include group therapy (gender-specific available) and individual therapy. Many VA facilities are moving toward the team approach called Behavioral Health Interdisciplinary Programs (BHIP).

9. **Pain management:** May include physical therapy, occupational therapy, chiropractic treatment, rheumatology, neurology, primary care, orthopedics, steroid injections, and complementary and alternative health practice such as acupuncture, massage, and yoga. In addition, there may be spiritual counseling and recreational therapy available.

F. Reproductive

1. VA provides the usual preventive screenings such as cervical cancer and breast cancer screenings. Ask about future family plans, current and future contraceptive needs. Many VA facilities have gynecologic providers, including nurse practitioners, physicians, or physician assistants, all of whom are skilled in the reproductive needs of women veterans.

2. **Preconceptual health:** Assist a woman who is preparing to consider pregnancy. She will want to be in excellent physical and mental health. The VA can assist with needed screenings, immunizations, testing, counseling, and folic acid recommendations (400 mcg) as she prepares to conceive.

3. **Obstetric care:** All registered women veterans are eligible for maternity care, offered through Care in the Community (CITC). There is generally no cost for women veterans for routine obstetrical care, including prenatal care, hospital labor and delivery, newborn care (for first 7 days only), and postpartum care. Any additional (non-routine) care or testing, such as amniocentesis, must be preauthorized, and is often covered. Medication prescriptions can be sent directly to their VA pharmacy to be filled. Lactation supplies such as breast pumps, nipple care cream, nursing bras, milk storage bags, and breast pads are provided. Most VA medical centers have a maternity care coordinator to assist the veteran navigate their care.

4. **Contraceptive needs:** The VA offers full gynecology services in most VA medical centers, provided by nurse practitioners, physicians, and physician assistants. Most contraceptive methods are available, and often at no cost to the veteran. In addition, women's health providers are skilled at providing basic contraception during routine primary care.

5. **Infertility and in vitro fertilization (IVF):** Infertility care may be covered. This is a complex situation and requires specific considerations and processes to be eligible. The woman veteran must have a service-connected reason for her infertility. Attempts are made to coordinate care with the Department of Defense as women transition from active duty to civilian healthcare. https://www.womenshealth.va.gov/WOMENSHEALTH/OutreachMaterials/ReproductiveHealth/Infertility.asp
6. **STI care:** Screening and treatment for sexually transmitted infections (STI) can be obtained through primary care and/or gynecology.

CONCLUSION

A. Women veterans deserve high quality compassionate care in a safe, secure environment. The VA is committed to providing excellence in care to these women warriors who served us and who now deserve the best care we can provide to them.

ACKNOWLEDGMENT

Special thanks to Ms. Shenekia Williams-Johnson, RN, VISN 6 Regional Women Veterans Program Manager, Durham, North Carolina.

BIBLIOGRAPHY

Haskell, S. G. (2021, September 01). Listen to your body–MSK conditions in women Veterans. *VAntage.* htts://blogs.va.gov/VAntage/93750/listen-to-your-body-msk-conditions-in-women-veterans

Malena, P. C. (2016). When the warrior is a woman. *Women's Healthcare, 4*(2). https://www.npwomenshealthcare.com/when-the-warrior-is-a-woman

U.S. Department of Veterans Affairs. (2015). *Veterans health administration.* Women Veterans Health Care. FAQs.

U.S. Department of Veterans Affairs. Office of Public Affairs. (2015). *Federal benefits for veterans, dependents and survivors.*

U.S. Department of Veterans Affairs. Office of Public and Intergovernmental Affairs. (2013). *VA hires more mental health professionals to expand access for veterans.*

U.S. Department of Veterans Affairs. Office of Public Affairs Media Relations. (2014). *Women veterans health care fact sheet.*

U.S. Department of Veterans Affairs. Report of the Under Secretary for Health Workgroup. (2008). *Provision of primary care to women veterans.*

U.S. Department of Veterans Affairs. Sourcebook: Women Veterans in the Veterans Health Administration, Volume 2. (2012). *Sociodemographics and use of VHA and Nnon-VA care (Fee).*

U.S. Department of Veterans Affairs. Veterans Health Administration. (2008). *Women Vveterans health strategic health care group. Guide to moving forward in providing comprehensive health care to women veterans.*

U.S. Department of Veterans Affairs. Veterans Health Administration. (2019). *Women's health transition training handbook.*

U.S. Department of Veterans Affairs. Women Veterans Health Strategic Health Care Group. (2012.) *A profile of women veterans today. Rethink veterans: Who is the woman veteran?*

U.S. Department of Veterans Affairs. Women Veterans Health Strategic Health Care Group. (2011). *On the frontlines of VA women's health: Enhancing services for women veterans.*

U.S. Department of Veterans Affairs. Women Veterans Health Strategic Health Care Group, Office of Patient Care Services. (2012). *Gender differences in performance measures VHA 2008–2011.*

21

MALE SEXUAL AND REPRODUCTIVE HEALTH

RANDEE L. MASCIOLA

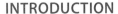

INTRODUCTION

A. Male sexual and reproductive health includes the screening, diagnosis, and management of sexual transmitted infections (STI), family planning, infertility, and sexual dysfunction.

B. Not all people who were assigned male at birth identify as a male or as a man, and it is important to provide safe, holistic, and individual sexual and reproductive health to all people.

C. Male sexual health has a significant impact on relationships, family, and chronic mental and physical health outcomes (Warner & Frey, 2013).

ANATOMY AND PHYSIOLOGY (FIGURE 21.1)

A. Penis

   1. Glans; head

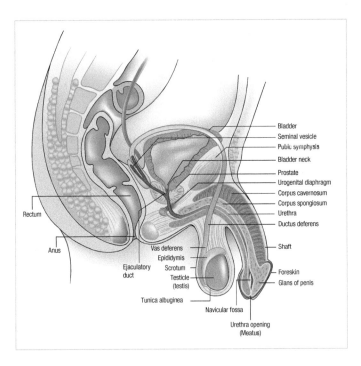

FIGURE 21.1 Male genital anatomy.

Source: From Singleton, JK. Primary Care – An Interprofessional Perspective, Second Edition. 2015, Springer Publishing Company. (Ball, 2019 and Bickley, 2020)

2. Foreskin (prepuce)
   a. Protective function and increases sensation of sexual activity
   b. May be surgically removed with circumcision
3. Shaft
   a. Must be erect for sperm to expel
   b. Houses channel for sperm and urine to leave the body
4. Frenulum
   a. Small tag of sensitive skin on underside
   b. Elastic band which helps the foreskin (when present) to contract over the glans, connecting the foreskin to mucosa

B. Scrotum
   1. Sack which houses testes away from body
C. Rectum/anus
   1. Storage and elimination of stool
D. Testes
   1. Sperm production in seminiferous tubules
   2. Testosterone production by Leydig cells
      a. Small amount also produced in adrenal gland
      b. Stimulates the development of male characteristics
E. Epididymis
   1. Rest posteriorly on each teste
   2. Sperm maturity and sperm storage
F. Vas deferens
   1. Tubes that store and transport sperm from the testes
   2. Contract to squeeze the sperm toward the base of the penis
G. Seminal vesicles
   1. Secrete seminal fluid which coagulates sperm
H. Prostate gland
   1. Secrete prostate fluid (components of semen)
   2. Muscles of the prostate gland propel this seminal fluid into the urethra during ejaculation
I. Cowper's gland
   1. Makes pre-ejaculate
J. Urethra
   1. Transportation of urine outside body
K. Cremaster
   1. Muscle that moves organs closer to body during cold or fear

ASSESSMENT

A. History
   1. Standard health history
      a. Medical, surgical, social, family, medications, allergies, and immunizations
      b. Cardiac, endocrine, mental health, and neurologic issues can affect sexual health.
      c. Nicotine, substance abuse, and environmental exposure can have effects on sexual risk, health, and function.
      d. Sexual health (Workowski et al., 2021)
   2. Five Ps assessment
      a. **Practice:** Oral, anal, vaginal
      b. **Partners:** Numbers, sex, frequency

BOX 21.1 HITS Screening Tool

- Does your partner physically Hurt you?
- Does your partner Insult you?
- Does your partner Threaten you with harm?
- Does your partner threaten or Scream at you?

Source: Rabin, R. F., Jennings, J. M., Campbell, J. C., & Bair-Merritt, M. H. (2009). Intimate partner violence screening tools: A systematic review. *American Journal of Preventive Medicine, 36*(5), 439–445. e4. https://doi.org/10.1016/j.amepre.2009.01.024

---

    c. **Prevention:** Contraception plans if needed
    d. **Protection:** Condom use frequency
    e. **Past:** Personal and partner disease history
  3. Sexual function
    a. Ask "Do you have any difficulty with intercourse/problems when having sex?" (Marcell, 2014)
    b. Ask about issues with erection, ejaculation, libido, or pain.
  4. Intimate partner and sexual violence
    a. About 25% of males experience sexual violence at some point in their lives (Smith, 2018).
    b. Hurt, Insult, Threaten, and Scream (HITS) screening tool (Box 21.1)
      (1) Most studied evidence-based screening tool for domestic violence with men
      (2) A "yes" to any of the HITS questions is a positive screen and requires follow-up.
  5. Reproductive life plan
    a. One key question (Bellanca & Hunter, 2013)
      (1) "Would you like to become pregnant in the next year?" can be adapted to "Would you like to *conceive a child* in the next year?"
      (2) Provides an opportunity for education or referral to counseling and contraceptive care.
    b. Fertility assessment
      (1) Have they ever conceived a child or had trouble conceiving a child?
B. Physical assessment (Ball, 2019; Bickley, 2020)
  1. **Vital signs:** BMI, weight, height, blood pressure
  2. Secondary sex characteristics
    a. Assess Tanner stage (Figure 21.2)
    b. Growth of body hair, including facial, underarm, abdominal, chest and pubic hair
    c. Enlargement of larynx and deepening of voice
    d. Increased muscle development, bone structure, and stature
  3. Breasts
    a. Breast exam if complains of enlargement (gynecomastia), mass, nipple discharge, or pain
  4. Pulses
    a. Palpate for femoral and peripheral pulses
  5. HEENT
    a. Signs of infection; redness, lesions, discharge
    b. Inspect mouth and throat
    c. Palpate inguinal lymph nodes bilaterally for enlargement or tenderness.
  6. Integumentary
    a. Visual inspection for rash, lesions, bruising, scratches
  7. Neurologic exam
    a. Specifically for erectile dysfunction workup

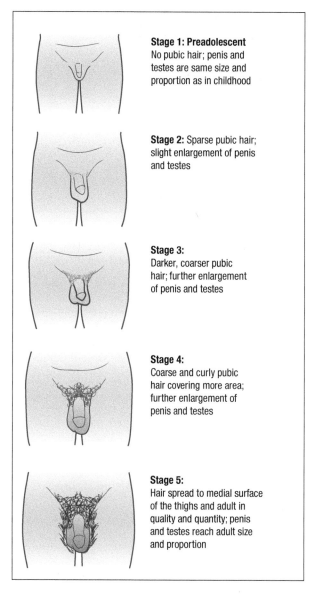

Stage 1: Preadolescent
No pubic hair; penis and testes are same size and proportion as in childhood

Stage 2: Sparse pubic hair; slight enlargement of penis and testes

Stage 3:
Darker, coarser pubic hair; further enlargement of penis and testes

Stage 4:
Coarse and curly pubic hair covering more area; further enlargement of penis and testes

Stage 5:
Hair spread to medial surface of the thighs and adult in quality and quantity; penis and testes reach adult size and proportion

FIGURE 21.2 Tanner Stages of Pubic Hair and Genital Development in Boys.

Source: Chiocca, E. M. (2019). *Advanced pediatric assessment*. Springer Publishing Company.

8. Musculoskeletal
   a. Assess for costovertebral tenderness (CVT)
9. Abdominal exam
   a. Ask patient to cough and/or bear down while standing to evaluate for bulging to rule hernia.
10. Reproductive
   a. Patient should be in supine or standing position
   b. Inspect and palpate penis
   c. Any rashes/lesions/bumps/edema/tumor?
   d. Prepuce (foreskin)
      (1) Retract if not circumcised to assess for lesions/ulcers/discharge/masses.
      (2) If retracted and not easily returned to original position, can be emergent (paraphimosis).

    e. Urethral meatus
      (1) Note location (usually tip, but can be at shaft)
        • Epispadias; located on dorsal side
        • Hypospadias; located on ventral side
      (2) Slightly squeeze to evaluate for discharge.
    f. Plaques on shaft
    g. Potential Peyronie's disease
      (1) Scar tissue on penis
      (2) Significant bend to shaft with erection
      (3) Complaints of pain, including with intercourse
      (4) **Cause:** Repeated injury/trauma
    h. Testes/scrotum
      (1) **Inspection:** Evaluate for lesion/bumps/tumor/edema/size
        • Right often higher then left
      (2) Palpate for mass or swelling
        • Normal includes smooth, form, mobile, and equal size
      (3) Epididymis
        • Palpate for pain or masses using gentle pressure; include vas deferens.
        • Two fingers on posterior sac with thumb on anterior aspect and move fingers distally
  i. Anal/rectal
      (1) **Inspect:** Skin assessment for rash, lesions, masses, or drainage
      (2) If history of anal intercourse, digital anorectal examination (DARE) is recommended to assess for masses; should be smooth.
      (3) Prostate (Schuilling, 2022)
        • Patient should be leaning over table or lying on side.
        • Insert gloved finger as far as possible and rotate index finger left and right to evaluate for masses.
        • Rotate finger 180 degrees to palpate prostate gland.
        • **Palpate:** Note size, consistency, and tenderness; normal is smooth, nontender and about the size of a walnut.

PATHOPHYSIOLOGY

A. Testicular/scrotal
  1. Hydrocele
    a. Most common testicular issue
    b. Swelling and pain caused by fluid trapped in sheath around testicle caused by inflammation or injury/trauma.
    c. Often resolves on its own, refer to urologist for management.
  2. Testicular cancer (American Cancer Society [ACS], 2021)
    a. About 9,470 new cases and 440 deaths a year
    b. Mass in testes, often asymptomatic; can have dull pain and heaviness
    c. Most commonly affects young and middle-aged men, 50% in men between 20 and 34 years old
    d. Risk factors
      (1) **Main:** History of cryptorchidism (undescended testicle)
      (2) **Other:** Age, African American/Asian American, family history/personal history
  3. Testicular torsion
    a. Sudden, acute, unilateral pain; can have nausea and vomiting
      (1) Very rarely chronic pain (weeks)

b. Medical emergency if no medical attention in 12 hours of symptoms increasing need to have teste removed due to lack of blood flow
c. Most common in puberty and in cases of trauma
d. **Treatment:** Surgery to untwist

4. Varicocele (Asafu-Adjei, 2020)
   a. Patient often complains of fullness and dull to sharp pain without radiation
   b. Evaluated with inspection and palpation
      (1) Nontender, soft scrotal mass separates from testicle with dilated veins ("bag of worms"); usually left side
      (2) More pronounced and palpable when patient is standing and performs the Valsalva maneuver; can be unpalpable when in supine position
      (3) Grading system
         • Grade 3 is visible on inspection
         • Grade 2 when felt with easy palpation
         • Grade 1 when only palpable with Valsalva maneuver
   c. Color Doppler ultrasound is standard to evaluate mass and rule out cancer and other testicular mass differentials.
   d. Surgery indicated for symptoms (pain) and fertility issues.
      (1) 30-minute procedure, 2 to 3-week recovery, over 90% successful to decrease pain and increase sperm concentration
   e. Spermatocele
      (1) Abnormal mass which is a fluid-filled sac in epididymis
      (2) Noncancerous and usually painless
      (3) **Transillumination test:** Flashlight on scrotum to identity fluid versus solid mass
      (4) Rarely needs treatment
   f. Cryptorchidism
      (1) Undescended testes at birth that doesn't move into place after 3 months of life (usually diagnosis in first year of life through adolescence)
      (2) Teste never grows or functions properly
      (3) Increase risk of infertility and cancer
      (4) Refer to urologist

B. Prostate
   1. Prostate cancer
      a. The Centers for Disease Control and Prevention (CDC) reported that in 2018 in the United State there were 211,893 new cases of prostate cancer and 31,488 males died (U.S. Cancer Statistics Working Group, 2021).
      b. **Risk factors:** Age, African American, family history
      c. Symptoms include urinary abnormalities, pain, or bleeding with ejaculation, and/or pelvis/back/hip pain
         (1) Can be asymptomatic even in advanced stages
      d. Any mass palpated with digital ano-rectal examination (DARE) should be referred to a urologist and evaluated for cancer.
      e. Biopsy is the gold standard for diagnosis.
   2. Prostatitis (proctocolitis and enteritis)
      a. Inflammation of rectal lining which can be acute or chronic
      b. Symptoms include pain, diarrhea, bleeding, discharge/mucus, sensation to have bowel movement
      c. Need to rule out sexually transmitted infection (STI), GI disorder, and history of radiation treatment
      d. **Labs:** Complete blood count (CBC) to assess hemoglobin (anemia) and white blood cells (WBC; infection), stool test for blood, and STI screenings (most common cause)

    e. Management dependent upon on causative factor

      (1) Presumptive therapy

      (2) Management recommendation from 2021 CDC guidelines: ceftriaxone 500 mg IM in a single dose for persons weighing less than 150 kg (330.7lb.) OR 1 g if weighing more than 150 kg

  3. Benign prostatic hypertrophy/hyperplasia (BPH; Edwards, 2008)

    a. Terms used interchangeably with similar assessment and management; common hormonal changes as males age causing:

      (1) Hypertrophy—increased size of existing cells

      (2) Hyperplasia—increased quantity of normal size cells

    b. **Urinary systems:** frequency, urgency, weak stream, chronic urinary infections, nocturia, and incontinence

      (1) Hematuria should be evaluated for bladder cancer

    c. Emergent if acute urinary retention, requires medical attention immediately.

    d. Ask "Does this effect your quality of life?"

      (1) If not, can wait and continue monitoring under supervision of healthcare provider

    e. American Urological Association Symptom Index is an evidence-based tool that can be used to assess symptom severity.

    f. DARE and urinalysis should be performed

    g. Management includes

      (1) Referral to urologist

      (2) Medications: Alpha blockers or 5-alpha reductase inhibitors

      (3) Surgical: Transurethral resection, newer laser techniques, many outpatient options

SEXUAL HEALTH SCREENING AND IMMUNIZATION

A. Sexually transmitted infections (STIs)

  1. Imperative to follow most recent CDC screening recommendations (Workowski et al., 2021)

  2. Human immunodeficiency virus (HIV)

    a. Testing options

      (1) Nucleic acid tests (NATs)

      (2) Antigen/antibody combination tests

      (3) Antibody tests

    b. Screening recommended for all males ages 13 to 64 years old, all males who seek STI evaluation, and all men who have sex with men (MSM) annually (every 3–6 months if high risk).

  3. Gonorrhea (GC) and chlamydia (CHL)

    a. Anal, urethral, and/or throat swab dependent on sexual practices

    b. Screening for MSM annually

      (1) Every 3 to 6 months if increased risk (previous infection, partners have multiple partners)

      (2) First morning urine preferred test as ease of use and less invasive, and equal sensitivity and specificity at nucleic acid amplification test (NAAT)

  4. Hepatitis

    a. **Hepatitis B:** Screen males at increased risk and annually for MSM.

      (1) Serological testing for HBsAg, HBV core antibody, and HBV surface antibody

    b. **Hepatitis C:** All males should be screened once in their lifetime.

      (1) Serological testing HCV RNA annually in MSM with HIV infection

    5. Syphilis
      a. More common in males than females
      b. Screen annually for MSM
      c. Presumptive diagnosis requires two positive serologic tests:
        (1) If Venereal Disease Research Laboratory (VDRL) or Rapid Plasma Reagin (RPR), then confirmation required with fluorescent treponemal antibody test absorption test (FTA-ABS).
    6. Human papilloma virus (HPV)
      a. Immunization recommended:
        (1) All males ages 9 to 26 years old
        (2) Males ages 27 to 45 years old, shared decision-making of potential benefits
      b. DARE exam for MSM
      c. Diagnosis with visual inspection, palpation of warts, and/or biopsy of growths
    7. Men having sex with men (MSM)
      a. More frequent screening if multiple or unknown partners
      b. Recommend hepatitis B vaccine
      c. DARE exam to identify masses/polyps annually
      d. Possible anal pap if symptoms suggest
        (1) Data insufficient to offer routine screening
B. Prostate Cancer Screening (U.S. Preventive Services Task Force [USPSTF], 2018)
    1. Risk assessment
      (1) Discussion of risks/benefits for each individual male
      (2) Older, African American, and family history are most significant risk factors
    2. Prostate-specific antigen (PSA)
      (1) Age 55 to 69, the decision to be screened annually should be individual.
      (2) Age 70+, screening not recommended
    3. Digital rectal exam
      (1) Not recommend as screening test (USPSTF, 2018)
C. Testicular cancer screening
    1. Provider and self-exam not recommended for screening (USPSTF, 2011)

FAMILY PLANNING

A. Male-specific contraceptives (Hatcher, 2018)
    1. Male condom
      a. Barrier method (latex, synthetic, or "natural" lamb caecum)
      b. Extensive education on when and how to use condoms for pregnancy prevention and STI prevention
      c. Low cost, widely available, easy to use, and minimal side effects
      d. Typical use failure rate is 13%
      e. Spermicide with nonoxynol-9 not recommended because increase risk of skin irritation/ulcer which creates entry point for infections
    2. Coitus interruptus (withdrawal or pull-out method)
      a. Typical use 80% effective
      b. Pre-ejaculate can fertilize an egg
      c. Lack of self-control to withdraw every time
    3. Sterilization (vasectomy or vas surgery)
      a. Cutting or including vas deferens eliminating sperm from ejaculate
      b. 99% effective
      c. Counseling is critical.

(1) Should be considered permanent
- Regret is number one side effect; most common in men under 30 years old without children.
- Reversal is possible and successful pregnancies result 38% to 89% of the time if reversal done within 10 years.

(2) Procedure not immediately effective and back-up method should be used until follow-up semen analysis 3 months after procedure.

d. Requires referral to urologist for options of approach.

(1) Incisional versus non-scalpel

e. Post-operation directions include scrotal support, ice, avoid ejaculation for 7 days, avoid strenuous activity/exercise for 7 days.

B. Preconception
1. Expectation to assess need for screening of all males at every primary care visit
2. Men should receive much of the same preconception screens and education as female partners.
   a. STI risk, screening, and prevention
   b. Advise to avoid toxic (environmental) substances such as tobacco/nicotine, "street drugs" or illegal prescriptions, and alcohol.
   c. Healthy weight
   d. Yearly physical to identify any health issues that could affect fertility
   e. Report any genetic disease with self or family, screen for mental health and safety, and counsel on partner support.
3. Factors that may affect sperm quality
   a. Medications, age, surgery on reproductive organs, stress, unhealthy weight, and use of tobacco, drugs, and alcohol can all effect the viability, quantity, and morphology of sperm (Warner & Frey, 2013).

SEXUALLY TRANSMITTED (AND OTHER) INFECTIONS

A. Most common symptoms requiring further evaluation, testing, and management based on most recent CDC guidelines (Workowski et al., 2021)
1. Pain
2. Lesions
3. Dysuria
4. Penile discharge
5. Malaise/fever

B. Gonorrhea
1. Majority of men will have symptoms.
2. Highest risk among African Americans, Hispanics, MSM, teens, and those living in southeastern United States
3. Dysuria and mucopurulent discharge from urethra most common symptom
4. **Management recommendation:** Ceftriaxone 500 mg IM in a single dose for persons weighing less than 150 kg (330.7 lb.) OR 1 g if weighing more than 150 kg

C. Chlamydia
1. Asymptomatic in 50% of men
2. Can cause urinary symptoms of pain and frequency or urethral discharge
3. **Management recommendation:** Doxycycline 100 mg orally 2 times/day for 7 days

D. Nongonococcal urethritis (NGU)
1. Cluster of symptoms associated with inflammation/infection of urethra
2. **Non-specific diagnosis:** Must rule out gonorrhea for treatment

3. **Lab:** NAAT for GC/CHL (add trichomonas for areas with high prevalence)
4. **Management recommendation:** Doxycycline 100 mg orally 2 times/day for 7 days

E. Epididymitis
1. Infection of epididymis
   a. **Common cause:** Gonorrhea and chlamydia
   b. **Symptoms:** Unilateral testicular pain, fever, swelling, and discharge
2. Presumptive therapy
3. Objective diagnosis includes positive finding of one of the following:
   a. Gram stain of urethral secretions identifying more than two white blood cells (WBC) per oil immersion field
   b. Positive leukocyte esterase test on first-void urine
   c. Microscopic examination of sediment from a spun first-void urine demonstrating more than 10 WBC per high power field.
4. Management recommendation
   a. **If GC/CHL suspected:** Ceftriaxone plus doxycycline 100 mg orally 2 times/day for 7 days
   b. **If enteric organisms (men who practice incentive anal sex) suspected:** Levofloxacin 500 mg orally once daily for 10 days

INFERTILITY

A. Inability for male partner to conceive with female partner after 12 months of unprotected intercourse
B. Causes
1. Hormonal
   a. **Hypogonadism:** Severe deficiency in gonadotropin-releasing hormone (GnRH) which leads to decrease release of testosterone
   b. Pituitary tumors
   c. Congenital lack of luteinizing hormone/follicle-stimulating hormone (LH/FSH; pituitary problem from birth)
   d. Anabolic (androgenic) steroid abuse
2. Gonadal disorders
   a. Varicocele
   b. Hypospadias
   c. Cryptorchidism
   d. Retrograde ejaculation
      (1) Sperm enters bladder instead of exiting through penis due to weak bladder neck.
         • **Causes:** Nerve damage secondary to other medical illness, medication from benign prostatic hyperplasia (BPH), or bladder surgery
      (2) Not harmful but decreases fertility opportunities
      (3) **Diagnostic test:** Post-ejaculation urinalysis
         • Identifies and measures sperm in urine after ejaculation.
   e. Sperm health (analysis described in the following)
   f. Blockage of sperm transport
      (1) Prostate-related problems
      (2) Absence of vas deferens
      (3) Vasectomy
   g. Environmental and lifestyle choices
      (1) Exposure to smoking, drugs, chemicals, toxins, or medications
      (2) Bicycling, overheat, and trauma

TABLE 21.1 Normal Semen Analysis

CHARACTER	LOWER LIMIT
Volume	1.5 mL
pH	7.2
Concentration	15 x 106 spermatozoa/mL
Quantity	39 x 106 spermatozoa/ejaculate
Mobility	40%
Forward progression	32%
Normal morphology	4%
Agglutination	Absent
Viscosity	Less than 2

Source: American Society for Reproductive Medicine. (n.d.) Semen analysis. https://www.asrm.org/topics/topics-index/semen-analysis/

    h. Aging

    i. STIs

    j. Torsion (twisting of the testis in scrotum)

    k. Overheating of testicle (hot tubs and tight underwear)

    l. Mental health issues

C. Semen analysis (Table 21.1)

    1. Most common lab test for male infertility to assess sperm health

    2. Abnormal test requires repetition in 4 to 6 weeks

    3. Usually collected by patient through masturbation

       a. Can be given instructions and cup at office and done at home, but must be kept warm and returned to office/lab within 60 minutes

    4. Must be abstinent for 2 days prior to test

D. Other lab tests to consider

    1. **Hormone testing:** Prolactin and thyroid

    2. **Genetic testing:** Rule out chromosomal disorder.

    3. **Testicular biopsy:** When a semen analysis is abnormal, sperm and other tests are negative for cause.

    4. **Transrectal ultrasound:** Imaging of the prostate, seminal vesicles, and vas deferens to differentiate congenital versus acquired obstruction issue

SEXUAL DYSFUNCTION

A. Normal physical responses to sexual activity

    1. Erection of the penis

    2. Testicular swelling

    3. Scrotal tightening

    4. Secretion of lubricating liquid

    5. Many of same non-organ responses as women:

       a. Increased vital signs (increased heart rate, respiratory rate, and blood pressure)

       b. Skin changes (flushing)

       c. Muscle tension

B. Potential causes of dysfunction (often multifactorial)

1. Endocrine/hormonal (labs based on history and assessment)
    (1) Fasting glucose
    (2) Hemoglobin A1C
    (3) Thyroid stimulating hormone (TSH)
    (4) Prolactin
    (5) Testosterone
    (6) **LH/FSH:** Inverse relationship with testosterone could indicate hypogonadism.
    (7) Testosterone deficiency
2. Neurological
    a. Dysfunction on central nervous system and nerves that innervate penis (i.e., stroke, epilepsy, spinal cord trauma)
3. Cardiovascular
    a. Decrease efficiencies and occlusions of vascular system
4. Mental health
    a. Depression, posttraumatic stress disorder, anxiety and/or history of sexual assault
5. Medications
    a. Antihypertensives, antidepressants, and antiandrogens
6. Lifestyle
    a. Caffeine, nicotine, drugs, alcohol, and obesity
7. Ejaculation issues (premature/retrograde/delayed)
8. **Health event:** Medical or psychosocial
9. Benign prostatic hyperplasia

C. Validated male sexual screening tools
    1. Sexual Health Inventory for Men (SHIM)
    2. Ageing Male Symptoms (AMS) scale
    3. Erectile Dysfunction Inventory of Treatment Satisfaction (EDITS)
    4. Erection Hardness Scale (EHS)
    5. International Index of Erectile Function (IIEF)
    6. Index of Premature Ejaculation (IPE)
    7. Premature Ejaculation Diagnostic Tool (PEDT)
    8. Quality of Erection Questionnaire (QEQ)
    9. Self-Esteem and Relationship Questionnaire (SEAR)
    10. Sexual Quality of Life-Men (SQOL-M)

D. Management strategy
    1. Order appropriate tests and labs.
    2. Assess and treat for infections (STIs).
    3. Assess and treat any sexual health pathophysiology.
    4. Hormone treatment if indicated
    5. Discuss lifestyle changes.
        a. Weight, smoking, increase frequency of intercourse, timing of sex, avoid lubricants, activities causing increase in temperature or pressure to testicles
        b. Educate on coping techniques, stress management, support, resources, and communication strategies.
    6. Referral options
        a. Assisted reproductive technology
        b. Urologist
        c. Mental health

E. Updated *Diagnostic and Statistical Manual of Mental Disorders, Fifth Edition (DSM-5)* criteria for all Sexual Dysfunction Disorders (American Psychiatric Association [APA], 2013)
    1. Gender specific
    2. Must experience condition 75% to 100% of the time

3. Minimum duration of 6 months
4. Disorder must have caused "significant distress"
5. The disorder should not be better explained by:
   a. Nonsexual mental disorder
   b. Consequence of severe relationship distress (e.g., partner violence)
   c. Other significant stressors
6. **Specifiers used:** Mild, moderate, or severe
7. Approved *DSM-5* diagnosis for male sexual dysfunction
   a. Male hypoactive sexual desire disorder
      (1) Frequent deficient (or absent) sexual fantasies and/or desire for sexual activity
      (2) Caused by psychosocial issues, medications, low testosterone, in conjunction with other sexual health issue, partner issues, and/or drugs/alcohol
      (3) Diagnosis
         • **History:** Almost always secondary
      (4) Management options
         • Lifestyle modifications
         • Psychotherapy with selective serotonin reuptake inhibitor (SSRI)
         • Alter medications
         • Add bupropion if already on SSRI
         • Change antihypertensive
         • Manage chronic opioid use
         • Considering adding testosterone
   b. Delayed ejaculation (Abdel-Hamid, 2018)
      (1) Unable to ejaculate during sexual activity specifically after 25 minutes to 30 minutes of continuous sexual stimulation
      (2) **Criteria:** Occurs almost all the time, over at least 6 months, causes individual distress; rule out secondary to other medical/surgical condition, medications, psychological issues including drug/alcohol abuse
      (3) Uncommon, not much research
      (4) Diagnosis
         • **History:** Self-reported
         • Lifelong versus acquired and general versus situational
      (5) Check prolactin/thyroid-stimulating hormone (TSH) to rule out hormonal issue
      (6) Management
         • Psychological intervention
            ▪ Performance anxiety
            ▪ Relationship issues
            ▪ Stress
            ▪ Traumatic event
            ▪ Environmental issues
         • Review medications and treat any underlying medical conditions
         • Medication options
            ▪ None currently FDA approved
   c. Premature ejaculation (Althof, 2014)
      (1) **Cause:** Psychological (anxiety) or biogenic (less defined)
      (2) Define as three criteria
         • Early ejaculation during vaginal intercourse, inability to delay or control, and marked distress
      (3) Unable to control orgasm, and climaxes in less than 1 minute after vaginal penetration
      (4) Only defined as a disorder in the case of vaginal intercourse as a time duration for oral or manual stimulation has not been established

(5) Diagnosis
  - Acquired (psychological) versus lifelong (genetic)
  - Global versus situational
(6) **Management:** None approved by the FDA for premature ejaculation; research, mounting evidence and off label options:
  - **SSRI:** Often first line (dapoxetine)
  - Tramadol
  - **Topical anesthetics:** Lidocaine
  - Prostaglandin cream
  - Phosphodiesterase-5 inhibitors
  - Non-pharmacologic:
    - Behavioral and psychological therapy
    - Acupuncture
d. Erectile dysfunction
  (1) **Define:** Recurrent inability to achieve or maintain an adequate erection during partnered sexual activities
  (2) Diagnosis based on history
  (3) **Causes:** Blocked blood flow to penis
  (4) **Risk factors:** Age and co-existing medical conditions (i.e., cardiovascular, depression, diabetes)
  (5) Management
    - **First line:** Start phosphodiesterase-5 inhibitors (PDE-5)
    - Erectile dysfunction Pharmacologic Management Chart (Table 21.2)
    - Behavioral and psychotherapy

TABLE 21.2 Pharmacologic Management of Erectile Dysfunction

PHOSPHODIESTERASE-5 INHIBITORS (PDE-5)

General Comments:
- MOA: Inhibits relaxation of blood vessel smooth muscle and increases blood flow to penis
- Contraindicated: Nitrates
- Use with caution: Alpha-adrenergic and alpha-blockers
- Side effects: Low blood pressure, Indigestion, Flushing, Headaches, Vision abnormalities, and hearing irregularities
- Medical emergency: Priapism, which is an erection lasting more than 4 hours

GENERIC/BRAND AVAILABILITY	DOSAGE: ADULT	COMMENTS
Sildenafil/Viagra Availability (Tabs): 25 mg, 50 mg, and 100 mg	• Only once a day • Can be taken 30 min to 4 hr prior to sexual activity	• Longest safety record • Take with food • Most side effects reported
Tadalafil/Cialis Availability (Tabs): 2.5 mg, 5 mg, 10 mg, and 20 mg	• 30 min prior to sexual activity • Can be taken daily without regard of timing for sexual activity	• Lowest dosing • Longest duration (36 hours) • With or without food
Avanafil/Stendra Availability (Tabs): 50 mg, 100 mg, and 200 mg	• 200 mg can be taken 15 minutes before sexual activity • Lower doses 30 min before sexual activity • Do not exceed more than one dose/day	• Newest on market • Fastest onset • With or without food • Shortest duration

Source: Khera, M. (2021). Treatment of male sexual dysfunction. In K.A. Martin (Ed.), *UpToDate.* https://www.uptodate.com/contents/treatment-of-male-sexual dysfunction?topicRef=6840&source=see_link#H19736901

PATIENT EDUCATION AND RESOURCES

A. **SSM:** International Society for Sexual Medicine
B. **SMSNA:** Sexual Medicine Society of North America
C. **ASRM:** American Society for Reproductive Medicine
D. **AASECT:** American Association of Sex Educators, Counselors and Therapists
E. **SSTAR:** Society for Sex Therapy and Research
F. **CDC:** Centers for Disease Control and Prevention-STIs

CASE STUDY

Patient Situation

A 30-year-old married male presents to the sexual health clinic complaining of severe pain in his left testicle. He is in acute pain, and states "I was reaching for a vase on the top shelf in the kitchen and the pain hit me fast and hard."

Subjective Data

- Rates pain today as 5/10 (with 10 being the worst pain possible)
- Occasional left testicular discomfort last 5 years, dull, comes and goes, rates 2/10
- Actively trying to conceive with female partner x2 years (no treatment)

Objective Data

- Vital signs: Blood pressure 145/85, pulse 88/min, respiration 16/min
- Height: 5'6" Weight 176 lbs.
- Left testicle slightly enlarged with Valsalva maneuver (Grade 1)
- Pain with light palpation of left testicle

Clinical Analysis

What diagnostics do you anticipate that will be ordered, and why?
- Scrotal ultrasound (color Doppler)
- Need to rule out solid mass, measure venous dilatation, and degree of reflux
- Grading classification system: 1 (none) through 5 (reflex at rest)

Identify this patient's modifiable and nonmodifiable risk factors.
- None

What is the priority intervention based on the patient's clinical presentation?
- Surgical management for pain management and fertility preservation
- Procedure to dilate the veins of the pampiniform plexus is currently the gold standard for treatment to improve venous drainage.
- Referral needed to urologist.

After receiving the results of the diagnostics, the patient is scheduled for surgical intervention. What should be included in this patient's plan of care?
- Pain management
- Short-term lifting restrictions
- Semen analysis to evaluate post-procedure sperm quality

BIBLIOGRAPHY

Abdel-Hamid, I. A., & Ali, O. I. (2018). Delayed ejaculation: Pathophysiology, diagnosis, and treatment. *The World Journal of Men's Health, 36*(1), 22–40. https://doi.org/10.5534/wjmh.17051

Althof, S. E., McMahon, C. G., Waldinger, M. D., Serefoglu, E. C., Shindel, A. W., Adaikan, P. G., Becher, E., Dean, J., Giuliano, F., Hellstrom, W. J., Giraldi, A., Glina, S., Incrocci, L., Jannini, E., McCabe, M., Parish, S., Rowland, D., Segraves, R. T., Sharlip, I., & Torres, L. O. (2014). An update of the international society of sexual medicine's guidelines for the diagnosis and treatment of Premature Ejaculation (PE). *Sexual Medicine, 2*(2), 60–90. https://doi.org/10.1002/sm2.28

American Cancer Society. (2021). *Surveillance, Epidemiology, and End Result (SEER) 18 registries, National, Cancer Institute, 2020.* Retrieved November 18, 2021 at https://www.cancer.org/cancer/testicular-cancer/about/key-statistics.html

American Psychiatric Association, DSM-5 Task Force. (2013). *Diagnostic and statistical manual of mental disorders: DSM-5* (5th ed.). American Psychiatric Publishing, Inc.

Asafu-Adjei, D., Judge, C., Deibert, C. M., Li, G., Stember, D., & Stahl, P. J. (2020). Systematic review of the impact of varicocele grade on response to surgical management. *Journal of Urology, 203*(1), 48–56. https://doi.org/10.1097/JU.0000000000000311

Ball, J., Dains, J., Flynn, J. A., Solomon, B. S., & Stewart, R. W. (2019). *Seidel's guide to physical examination: An interprofessional approach* (9th ed.). Mosby. ISBN-13: 978-0323481953. ISBN-10: 9780323481953

Bellanca, H. K., & Hunter, M. S. (2013). ONE KEY QUESTION®: Preventive reproductive health is part of high quality primary care. *Contraception, 88*(1), 3–6. https://doi.org/10.1016/j.contraception.2013.05.003. Epub 2013 May 11. PMID: 23773527.

Bickley, L. S., Szilagyi, P. G., Hoffman, R. M., & Soriano, R. P. (2020). *Bates' guide to physical examination and history taking* (13th ed.). Wolters Kluwer Health/Lippincott Williams & Wilkins.

Chiocca, E. M. (2019). *Advanced pediatric assessment.* Springer Publishing Company.

Edwards, J. L. (2008). Diagnosis and management of benign prostatic hyperplasia. *American Family Physician, 77*(10), 1403–1410. PMID: 18533373.

Hatcher, R. (2018) *Contraceptive technology* (21st ed.). Ardent Media, Inc.

Khera, M. (2021). Treatment of male sexual dysfunction. In K. A. Martin (Ed.), *UpToDate.* https://www.uptodate.com/contents/treatment-of-male-sexual-dysfunction?topicRef=6840&source=see_link#H19736901

Marcel, A. V. (2014). Male training center for family planning and reproductive health. *Preventive Male Sexual and Reproductive Health Care: Recommendations for Clinical Practice.* maletrainingcenter.org/wp-content/uploads/2014/09/MTC_White_Paper_2014_V2.pdf

Practice Committee of the American Society for Reproductive Medicine. (2015). Diagnostic evaluation of the infertile male: A committee opinion. *Fertility and Sterility, 103*(3), e18–e25. https://doi.org/10.1016/j.fertnstert.2014.12.103.

Rabin, R. F., Jennings, J. M., Campbell, J. C., & Bair-Merritt, M. H. (2009). Intimate partner violence screening tools: A systematic review. *American Journal of Preventive Medicine, 36*(5), 439–445.e4. https://doi.org/10.1016/j.amepre.2009.01.024

Schuiling, K. D., & Likis, F. E. (2022). *Gynecologic health care with an introduction to prenatal and postpartum care* (4th ed.). Jones and Bartlett Publishers.

Smith, S. G., Zhang, X., Basile, K. C., Merrick, M. T., Wang, J., Kresnow, M., & Chen, J. (2018). *The National intimate partner and sexual violence survey: 2015 data brief – updated release.* Centers for Disease Control and Prevention.

Warner, J. N., & Frey, K. A. (2013). The well-man visit: Addressing a man's health to optimize pregnancy outcomes. *The Journal of the American Board of Family Medicine, 26*(2), 196–202. https://doi.org/10.3122/jabfm.2013.02.120143. PMID: 23471934.

Workowski, K. A., Bachmann, L. H., Chan, P. A., Johnston, C. M., Muzny, C. A., Park, I., Reno, H., Zenilman, J. M., & Bolan, G. A. (2021). Sexually transmitted infections treatment guidelines, 2021. MMWR. Recommendations and Reports: Morbidity and Mortality Weekly Report. Recommendations and reports/ Centers for Disease Control, 70(No. RR-4), 1–187.

U.S. Cancer Statistics Working Group. (2021). *U.S. Cancer Statistics Data Visualizations Tool, based on 2020 submission data (1999–2018).* U.S. Department of Health and Human Services, Centers for Disease Control and Prevention and National Cancer Institute. www.cdc.gov/cancer/dataviz

U.S. Preventive Services Task Force. (2011). Screening for testicular cancer: U.S. preventive services task force reaffirmation recommendation statement. *Annals of Internal Medicine, 154*(7), 483–486. https://doi.org/10.7326/0003-4819-154-7-201104050-00006. PMID: 21464350.

U.S. Preventive Services Task Force, Grossman, D. C., Curry, S. J., Owens, D. K., Bibbins-Domingo, K., Caughey, A. B., Davidson, K. W., Doubeni, C. A., Ebell, M., Epling Jr. J. W., Kemper, A. R., Krist, A. H., Kubik, M., Landefeld, C. S., Mangione, C. M., Silverstein, M., Simon, M. A., Siu, A. L., & Tseng, C. W. (2018). Screening for prostate cancer: US preventive services task force recommendation statement. *JAMA, 319*(18), 1901–1913. https://doi.org/10.1001/jama.2018.3710. Erratum in: JAMA. 2018 Jun 19;319(23):2443. PMID: 29801017.

Unit IV

EVALUATION OF SPECIAL GYNECOLOGIC PROBLEMS

22

ASSESSMENT OF MENOPAUSAL STATUS

DIANE TODD PACE, LAURA REED, AND R. MIMI SECOR

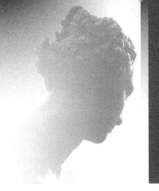

MENOPAUSE EXPLAINED

A. Spontaneous or natural menopause is marked by the end of the reproductive stage of a woman's life. It is a period of transition, and for most women is a normal, physiological, and developmental life event often perceived differently across various cultures.

1. Personal attitudes, lifestyle, and even social and demographic factors may influence one's perception of menopause. Many studies have found that attitudes toward menopause overall are mostly positive or neutral rather than negative.

2. This change in reproduction has often been medicalized, and indeed some women have symptoms such as vasomotor symptoms affecting their quality of life (QOL). It is mainly these women who seek out interventions from their primary care providers. Additionally, 80% of participants in recent surveys of postmenopausal women reported symptoms of Genitourinary Syndrome of Menopause (GSM) have a negative effect on their lives as well as 25% reported a lowered QOL. However, in other studies, women experiencing menopause reported no decrease in QOL, and only about 10% of peri- and postmenopausal women reported feelings of despair, irritability, or fatigue during this transitional time.

B. In the United States, it is estimated that 1.3 million women become postmenopausal each year.

1. Natural menopause typically occurs between the ages of 40 and 58. The number of women expected to be at age 50 by the year 2060 is approximately 90 million.

2. Today, a woman of age 54 years can expect to reach age 84.3 years and spend one third of her life in the period known as *postmenopause*.

C. A woman's health evaluation around the time of menopause should be similar to her health evaluation throughout her life span. There is no single menopause syndrome, and it is important to stress individualization with each woman as an important focus when assessing and developing a plan of care. At the time of the initial visit:

1. Determine menopausal status.

2. Discuss her view of menopause and her desire for intervention of bothersome symptoms affecting her QOL.

3. Discuss health-promotion/risk-reduction options.

4. Counsel on healthy behaviors such as smoking cessation, weight management, and exercise.

5. Using shared decision-making, consider interventions for managing bothersome symptoms.

   a. **Pharmacologic interventions:** Review risks/benefits of the options, stratifying her individual risks.

      (1) Hormone therapy (HT)/estrogen therapy (ET)

      (2) Non-HT options

   b. Nonpharmacologic/alternative/complementary options

D. **Definition:** Menopause is the permanent cessation of menses after 12 consecutive months of amenorrhea, or when follicle-stimulating hormone (FSH) levels are consistently elevated (greater than 30 mIU or mIU/mL) in the absence of other obvious pathologic causes.

TABLE 22.1 Menopause-Related Definitions	
Perimenopause/menopause transition	Occurs around menopause, beginning in the early transition, ending 12 months after the FMP
Premature menopause	General term used to describe menopause occurring before 40 years of age. It may occur spontaneously or be induced as a result of a medical intervention, such as oophorectomy, chemotherapy, or radiation therapy
Early menopause	Natural menopause occurring well before the average age, less than or equal to 45 years of age; includes premature menopause
Menopause	Permanent cessation of menses after 12 consecutive months of amenorrhea, or consistently elevated FSH (greater than or equal to 30 mIU) in absence of other obvious pathologic causes
Postmenopause	From FMP (natural or induced) extending through late menopause ending with death

FMP, final menstrual period; FSH, follicle-stimulating hormone.

1. This event usually results from loss of ovarian follicular function due to aging or can be induced by medical intervention, such as surgery (hysterectomy with bilateral oophorectomy), chemotherapy, or radiation.
2. On average, natural menopause occurs around 51 years of age but may range between 40 and 58 years of age.
3. Menopause-related definitions are summarized in Table 22.1.

E. The menopause transition represents the time when menstrual cycle, endocrine, and central nervous system changes occur.
1. In 2001, a group of scientists from multiple countries and disciplines met to propose nomenclature to stage the reproductive aging cycle in a female's life to the time of menopause (Stages of Reproductive Aging Workshop [STRAW+10]). The mModel may be viewed in the executive summary accessed at www.menopause.org/docs/default-document-library/straw10.pdf?sfvrsn=2). In 2010, STRAW+10 reconvened to review the advances in the changes in the hypothalamic–pituitary–ovarian function and update the criteria. In view of the continuing lack of international standardization of biomarker assays for clinical diagnosis, the scientists considered the menstrual cycle criteria to remain the most important criteria for staging.
2. Further delineation of the early postmenopausal years, stages +1a, +1b, +1c, were extended because research indicates FSH levels continue to increase and estradiol levels continue to decrease until approximately 2 years after the final menstrual period (FMP), when levels begin to stabilize. Symptoms, most commonly vasomotor flushes, are reported during these stages.
3. Stage +1c represents a period of stabilization for most women. The usual time frame of the early postmenopause period for most women averages 5 to 8 years.
4. Late postmenopause, during which further endocrine changes occur, is named stage +2. During this stage, the processes of aging, such as vaginal dryness and urogenital atrophy, are more prevalent.
5. The menopause transition may be further divided into stages according to the nomenclature summarized in Table 22.2.

PHYSIOLOGY OF MENOPAUSE

A. The menopause transition, also referred to as *perimenopause*, is associated with fluctuating hormone secretion causing irregular menstrual cycles and ultimately, permanent cessation of menses.

TABLE 22.2 STRAW+10 Stages of Menopause

−2 Stage = Early perimenopause	Onset of menstrual variability Duration: Variable Menstrual cycle: Variable
−1 Stage = Late perimenopausal transition 0 = FMP	Significant menstrual variability Duration: 1–3 years Menstrual cycle: Interval of amenorrhea of greater than 60 days Symptoms: Vasomotor symptoms likely
+1a Stage = Early postmenopause +1b Stage = Early postmenopause +1c Stage = Early postmenopause	Duration: FMP–1 year Symptoms: Vasomotor symptoms most likely Duration: 1 year Duration: 3–6 years
+2 Stage = Late postmenopause	Remaining life span until death

FMP, final menstrual period; STRAW, Stages of Reproductive Aging Workshop.

B. At birth, women have 1 to 2 million follicles. Accelerated follicular atresia (egg death) occurs in perimenopause and by menopause only a few hundred to a few thousand follicles remain.

C. A year before the FMP, a marked increase in FSH (more than 30 mIU/mL) occurs and plateaus within 2 years of the FMP. This is due to the rapid loss of follicles, resulting in reduced inhibin B, which increases FSH levels.

D. For a brief period, higher levels of FSH produce more follicles, causing overproduction of estradiol. This may cause a range of perimenopausal symptoms, including irritability, bloating, mastalgia, menorrhagia, growth of fibroids, and endometrial hyperplasia.

E. Irregular cycles and reduced fertility are associated with the menopause transition. However, it is critical to note and discuss with the woman that pregnancy is possible until menopause occurs (12 months since FMP).

F. The ovary is the major source of estrogen (during the reproductive years), with reductions occurring in the late menopausal transition, and major reductions in estrogen secretion throughout the first year of postmenopause (first 12 months after FMP). After this, a gradual decline occurs over the following several years.

MENOPAUSE INTRODUCTION AND CLINICAL ISSUES

A. Women often will present to the clinic requesting baseline and/or intermittent hormone testing to determine whether they are menopausal.
   1. This visit provides an opportune time to discuss the nature of menopause as being a time of gathering a careful history and examining her menstrual and symptom history.
   2. Menopause is actually a diagnosis made by retrospectively determining 12 consecutive months have passed without consecutive occurrence of menses.
   3. Baseline testing is seldom necessary and unwarranted and is often financially challenging unless the results would truly affect the interventions.
   4. In most cases, the interventions can be initiated based on the presentation of symptoms and the desire of the woman, following an in-depth history and physical.

B. Only two major early symptoms are directly attributed to menopause: change in menstrual cycles and vasomotor symptoms.
   1. Menstrual changes

    a. Variability in increasing flow and frequency leading to amenorrhea is considered the hallmark change of menopause. Approximately 90% of women will experience this change in menstrual cycle for a period of 4 to 8 years before the FMP.

    b. Changes vary from light bleeding, heavy blood loss, increased duration of bleeding, skipped cycles, to no changes until a final cycle.

    c. Until menopause is reached, pregnancy can still occur and should be considered during assessment in perimenopausal women not using contraception.

    d. Endometrial hyperplasia and carcinoma are more prevalent with age. Any bleeding in a postmenopausal woman always warrants further evaluation.

2. *Vasomotor-related symptoms* (VMS) is a global term referring to hot flashes, hot flushes, and night sweating.

    a. The second most frequently reported symptoms of menopause transition, VMS are experienced by up to 75% of all perimenopausal women in the United States.

    b. Prevalence varies among ethnic and racial groups as follows: African American (46%), Hispanic (35%), White (31%), Chinese (21%), Japanese (18%).

    c. In the Study of Women Across the Nation (SWAN), VMS persisted on average 7.4 years. African American women were most likely to report VMS and reported the longest duration (median: 10.1 years) with Asian women reporting a median of 5 years. Women who experienced the earliest onset of hot flashes had the longest total VMS duration (median: >11.8 years). In addition, a longer duration of VMS was experienced in women who were younger, had a lower educational level, greater perceived stress and symptom sensitivity, and those with higher depressive symptoms or anxiety when first reporting symptoms of their VMS.

    d. Fluctuations in estrogen and progesterone occurring in perimenopause and early menopause are commonly associated with vasomotor symptoms.

    e. VMS are thought to result from these fluctuations in estrogen and progesterone, but the precise mechanism and trigger of these symptoms are still not fully understood.

    f. Hot flashes are transient, recurrent symptoms of flushing and a sudden sensation of heat usually involving the upper body and face and often followed by chills. Heart rate increases of about 7 to 15 beats per minute occur at approximately the same time. Night sweats occurring during sleep hours are often associated with excessive perspiration, feeling overheated, and disrupted sleep.

    g. Frequency of hot flashes varies widely among women, ranging from occurring multiple times an hour, hourly, daily, weekly, or monthly. Within a 24-hour period, the greatest number of hot flashes occurs during the early evening hours. Individual episodes of hot flashes usually range from 1 to 5 minutes.

    h. Most hot flashes are mild to moderately severe; however, 10% to 15% of women have severe and/or very frequent hot flashes.

    i. Surgically induced menopause is associated with potentially severe and frequent VMS.

    j. Nearly 25% of U.S. women experience significant symptoms and seek intervention from their healthcare providers.

    k. Available pharmacologic/nonpharmacologic options offer symptomatic relief. The goal of therapy is to individualize options to the woman's needs after assessment for treatment-related risks and to evaluate her personal attitudes about menopause and treatment options. For women choosing HT/ET as an option, it should be noted that VMS may recur once HT is stopped.

C. Although VMS are common during menopause, it is important to rule out other medical conditions that may mimic VMS but are not associated with menopause (Box 22.1). Clinical evaluation of VMS should be conducted as a part of the clinical evaluation of the menopausal patient described in the following text.

BOX 22.1 Differential Diagnosis of Vasomotor Symptoms

- Hyperthyroidism
- Autoimmune disorders
- Cancer
- Hypertension (new onset)
- Cardiovascular disease (new risk)
- Medications such as tamoxifen, raloxifen
- Tuberculosis, infection, lymphoma

D. Additional physical and psychological symptoms include moodiness, headaches, memory changes, sleep disturbances, anxiety and depression, urinary symptoms, dry eyes, vaginal and vulvar irritation, dyspareunia, sexual concerns (i.e., desire, arousal, orgasm), hair and/or skin changes, weight gain, and joint pain.

E. Potential changes and possible late-onset symptoms include:
   1. Genitourinary syndrome of menopause and vulvovaginal atrophy
   2. Osteoporosis

F. Additional differential diagnoses should be considered during the initial assessment because other health issues may resemble menopausal symptoms
   1. Thyroid disorders
   2. Diabetes
   3. Cardiovascular disease (CVD)
   4. Anemia
   5. Depression
   6. Cancer

G. Symptoms and potential concerns that may be addressed during the workup are summarized in Box 22.2.

BOX 22.2 Symptoms Related to Menopause

- Vasomotor symptoms of hot flashes, night sweats, flushing
- Weight changes with weight gain most common
- Skin changes—dry skin, grey hair
- Cardiovascular concerns
- Urinary problems, including incontinence and overactive bladder
- Atropic vaginitis, dyspareunia
- Pelvic pain
- Decline in fertility
- Pregnancy
- Sexual function effects, notably reduced libido, reduced lubrication, and dyspareunia
- Alterations in sleep patterns
- Headache
- Cognition challenges
- Psychological concerns such as moodiness and anxiety
- Arthritis
- Dental and oral changes
- Ocular changes
- Hearing problems

H. Disease risks, including cancer risks and modifiable risk factors, should be identified by the clinician, and addressed with the patient.

HEALTH EVALUATION

A. The goal of the clinical health evaluation is to identify menopause and age-related health issues, to provide preventive care, anticipatory guidance, education, counseling, and support, and to diagnose and manage health problems.

B. A comprehensive nine-page menopause health questionnaire to assist clinicians in assessing the menopausal patient is available at the North American Menopause Society (NAMS) website: www.menopause.org/publications/clinical-practice-materials/menopause-health-questionnaire

C. Regular health examinations are recommended and should include:

1. Comprehensive health, past medical, psychosocial, and family history
2. Complete physical examination, including vital signs, height, weight, body mass index (BMI), thyroid, breast, pelvic and rectovaginal examinations
3. Laboratory testing as indicated
4. Other age- and risk-appropriate tests (bone density, mammogram, skin and colon cancer screening, visual and auditory screening)

D. Comprehensive history

1. Symptom history

   a. Menopause-related symptoms should be elicited and evaluated regarding frequency, severity, and duration. Also, note any associated symptoms:
      (1) Vasomotor symptoms during the day
      (2) Night flushes
      (3) Sleep disturbances
      (4) Moodiness, anxiety, depression.
      (5) Memory issues/brain fog
      (6) Vaginal dryness, irritation
      (7) Sexual issues: dyspareunia, low libido, arousal disorder
      (8) Weight change
      (9) Hair/skin changes
      (10) Joint pain

   b. Investigate what management options patient has used to manage menopausal symptoms: nonpharmacologic (exercise, yoga, acupuncture, fans, Chillow pillow, etc.); pharmacologic, including prescription HT and non-hormonal as well as over-the-counter menopausal supplements and vitamins. Investigate effectiveness and satisfaction.

2. Gynecologic history

   a. Menstrual history, age of menarche, menses pattern over the years, perimenopausal menstrual pattern, last menstrual period (LMP), first menstrual period, abnormal vaginal bleeding, vaginal discharge or pruritus, urinary symptoms

   b. Uro-gynecological issues, including a history of ovarian cysts, polycystic ovarian syndrome (PCOS), fibroids, infertility, endometriosis, premenstrual syndrome (PMS), premenstrual dysphoric disorder (PMDD), sexually transmitted infections (STIs), Pap history, diethylstilbestrol (DES) exposure in pregnancy, gynecologic surgery, history of UTIs, and urinary urge and stress incontinence

   c. The dates of last breast exam and Pap test and other screening tests, including mammogram, bone density, and most recent laboratory results

   d. Sexual history

(1) Sexuality is an important topic to address at midlife. It is often not a topic initiated by the woman, yet studies show it is a topic that women want their provider to initiate with them. To obtain a complete sexual history requires the clinician to interact with the woman in a comfortable, nonjudgmental conversation, placing the patient at ease so she can discuss her concerns openly. The sexual history should not assume a heterosexual bias and should be conducted in a supportive, confidential manner. The question could be posed, "Are you currently involved in a sexual relationship and are you having sex with men, women, or both?"

(2) Include the date of last sexual activity/coitus, number of lifetime sexual partners, history of STIs, complaints of low libido, dyspareunia, history of unprotected sex, orgasm issues.

(3) Inquire whether the patient or partner are having any sexual difficulties or concerns about sex they would like to discuss. Preface these questions with information that many women often experience vaginal dryness and changes in sexual desire around the time of menopause.

e. Contraceptive history

(1) Menopause is confirmed by retrospectively confirming 12 months without a menstrual cycle around the average age of menopause (51 years). If the LMP is less than 12 months, the woman continues in menopause transition. Although a decline in fertility due to varying fluctuations in hormones and changes in menstrual cycles may diminish the chances for a pregnancy, an unintended pregnancy may still occur. Unprotected coitus and current use of contraceptives, duration of use, doses, effectiveness, side effects, and reason for stopping should be discussed. Options to prevent an unintended pregnancy should be discussed as appropriate.

3. Obstetric history
   a. Number of pregnancies, full-term births, premature babies, abortions, living children, age of first birth, complications during pregnancy or childbirth, current age of children
4. Medical history
   a. Emphasis on cardiovascular disease (CVD), diabetes mellitus (DM), cancer, osteoporosis, and other relevant significant medical conditions, including hospitalizations should be addressed
   b. Identify modifiable risk factors (Box 22.3) and educate regarding measures to prevent or decrease symptoms of menopause.
   c. Assess for potential risk of developing medical conditions that may occur during menopause (Box 22.4). Screen where appropriate.

BOX 22.3 Modifiable Lifestyle-Related Risk Factors

- Weight gain
- Substance use and abuse
- Cigarette smoking
- Caffeine intake
- Alcohol consumption
- Prescription drug abuse
- Lack of exercise
- Sleep problems
- Stress
- Suboptimal nutrition
- Abuse (physical, sexual, mental)

BOX 22.4 Medical Conditions

- Gallbladder disease
- Cardiovascular conditions such as heart attack or stroke
- Asthma
- Cancers of the reproductive tract
- STIs
- Pregnancy/infertility
- Incapacitating VMS symptoms
- DM—metabolic syndrome
- Adverse effects of traditional and alternative therapies

DM, diabetic mellitus; STIs, sexually transmitted infections; VMS, vasomotor-related symptoms.

---

5. Surgical history
   a. Surgeries and any complications
   b. Hysterectomy; note whether with ovarian conservation or with oophorectomy
6. Medication history
   a. Current prescription medications (doses, routes, and timing). Discuss patient's adherence. Investigate patient's past use of relevant hormones.
   b. Over-the-counter medications, supplements (e.g., black cohosh, ginkgo, soy, yams)
   c. Complementary therapies (e.g., acupuncture, yoga, tai chi, meditation/guided imagery, reiki, massage)
   d. Allergies
7. Psychological history
   a. History of psychotherapy, mental health issues especially depression, anxiety, sleep issues, mood-related conditions, premenstrual syndrome (PMS), premenstrual dysphoric disorder (PMDD), postpartum depression, personality type, coping skills
      (1) Women who have a past history of mental health issues may have exacerbation of these issues in the menopause transition and need more intervention (see NAMS publication "Guidelines for the evaluation and treatment of perimenopausal depression": https://www.menopause.org/docs/default-source/default-document-library/meno-d-18-00170-final.pdf Maki et al, 2018).
   b. Developmental challenges include adolescent and/or college-aged children, empty nest, midlife crises, aging parents, retirement, grandchildren, changing spousal relations and roles.
   c. Attitude and beliefs about menopause
8. Social history
   a. Occupation, marital status, living situation, financial status
   b. History of abuse, including current or past history of verbal, physical, or sexual abuse
      (1) Ways to approach your patient:
         - "I talk to all of my patients about their sexual health and safe and healthy relationships because it can have such a large impact on health."
      (2) Sample questions:
         - "Have you been hit, kicked, punched, or otherwise hurt by someone within the past year? If so, by whom?"
         - "Do you feel safe in your current relationship?"
         - "Has your partner ever forced you to do something sexually that you did not want to do?"
         - "Is there a partner from a previous relationship who is making you feel unsafe now?"

  c. Nutritional history

   (1) Calcium; vitamin D; fruit; vegetable; protein; carbohydrate intake, including fiber, junk food, high fat, types of fat, omega-3 fatty acid intake; alcohol; soda; artificial sweeteners; herbal preparations; and vitamins

  d. Lifestyle

   (1) Exercise, sleep, work, recreation, stressors, spirituality, and social network of family and friends

 9. Family history

  a. There has been some research showing a correlation with mother's age of menopause.

  b. Osteoporosis, heart disease, cancers (especially history of breast, ovarian, and colon), Alzheimer's disease, coagulopathies, and other significant conditions

10. Review of system update with focus on menopausal health concerns

11. Diagnostic and laboratory testing

  a. As previously discussed, menopause is a clinical diagnosis based on cessation of menses for 12 months (FMP). At present, there is no single test of ovarian function that will predict or confirm menopause. Usually, a woman's medical and menstrual history and symptoms are sufficient to confirm menopause. Serum hormone level testing is *not* recommended for determining menopausal status.

  b. Laboratory confirmation may be considered if natural menses has been interrupted by hormonal contraceptives.

   (1) FSH is recommended if using hormonal contraceptives that interfere with normal menses. Test day 7 of pill-free interval. If results are unclear, repeat 1 month after discontinuing contraceptive.

   (2) Recommend condom use until laboratory results are known.

   (3) FSH greater than 30 mIU/mL suggests menopause.
    • Not necessary to diagnose menopause

   (4) Effective contraception should be used for an additional 12 months at which point FSH should be repeated. If still elevated, then contraception may be discontinued, and the patient is considered menopausal.

   (5) Estradiol less than 20 pg/mL suggests menopause.
    • Not necessary to diagnose menopause

   (6) Testosterone level
    • Indicated if rapidly virilizing symptoms, or suspected tumor, or pathology.
    • With age, androgen levels decline in women, but do not change across the menopause transition. Androgen levels are significantly lower in women with primary ovarian insufficiency and following bilateral oophorectomy.
    • Not indicated for routine menopausal screening.

  c. Routine diagnostic tests to consider based on age, history, and guidelines

   (1) Fasting lipid profile

   (2) Cervical cancer prevention/Pap test with co-testing/primary screening based on guidelines

   (3) Thyroid testing

   (4) Blood glucose

   (5) Comprehensive metabolic panel (CMP)

   (6) Urine screening

   (7) Hepatitis C virus (HCV)

   (8) Per the Centers for Disease Control and Prevention (CDC) 2021 STI Guidelines, STI testing as needed (e.g., rapid plasma regain [RPR]; HIV; gonorrheal culture [GC]/chlamydia)

   (9) Serum hydroxy vitamin D, per National Osteoporosis Foundation (NOF) guidelines

    d. Age- and risk-related screenings

      (1) **Bone density:** For low-risk women, screen for osteoporosis in women 65 years or older per the U.S. Preventive Services Task Force (USPSTF; see FRAX at www.sheffield.ac.uk/FRAX; for women with risk factors).

      (2) Mammogram

      (3) Skin assessment

      (4) Colon cancer screening now starting at age 45 years (per American Cancer Society [ACS])

      (5) Appropriate cultures or smears with suspicion of infection

      (6) Glaucoma

      (7) Hearing testing

      (8) Immunization update

    e. Other testing as appropriate for the evaluation of health concerns. Endometrial biopsy if irregular menses and heavy bleeding should occur, particularly if it has been more than a year since last menses. *Note:* Any vaginal bleeding occurring in postmenopause should be investigated.

E. Physical examination of the menopausal patient

  1. Height

  2. Weight and BMI

  3. Blood pressure

  4. HEENT (head, eye, ear, nose, and throat)

  5. Lungs

  6. Cardiac/neck for carotids/extremity pulse evaluation

  7. Breast examination

  8. Abdomen

    a. Note tenderness, rebound, and other abnormalities.

  9. Pelvic examination

    a. This vaginal exam should be conducted yearly to assess for signs of GSM, benign lesions, lesions such as Lichen sclerosis/planus, and perhaps malignancy.

      (1) Explain to the patient the difference between a "pelvic exam" and "Pap smear" as older women are often told they no longer need a female exam and equate the two as the same exam.

      (2) Current guidelines suggest cervical cancer screening (see Chapter 45, "Cervical Cancer Screening and Colposcopy") be discontinued for women over 65 who still have a uterus and who have a history of negative screenings. However, in a recent study, two thirds of women in that age range did not qualify to end screening under that criterion since findings from over a half million insurance claims found most women over age 55 years were not getting adequately screened for cervical cancer. Clinicians are urged to establish quality measures in their practices to ensure women over 65 years continue to be screened until they meet the guidelines (Mills et al., 2021).

        • External genitalia

          ▪ Thinning and/or greying of hair, loss of landmarks, tissue pallor, erythema, lesions, fissures, tenderness, urethral caruncle, introital shrinkage or laxity, cystocele, and rectocele

        • Vagina

          ▪ Introital laxity and loss of tone with Kegel and Valsalva maneuver (note cystocele, rectocele, and grade of condition)

          ▪ Erythema, pallor, petechiae, flattening of rugae, abnormal discharge (scant to variable), infection, lesions, shortening and narrowing of vagina, loss of elasticity, and tenderness

- In the absence of infection, vaginal pH greater than 5.0 secondary to reduced estrogen in menopause
- Change in vaginal maturation index (VMI) due to decreasing estrogen leads to a decrease in superficial cells and increase in parabasal cells replacing normal vaginal epithelium and leading to these changes which can be visually seen by clinician.
b. Cervix
(1) Erythema, friability, bleeding, tenderness, flattening, shortening, and stenosis of cervical os (small)
c. Uterus
(1) Size, shape, especially asymmetry (associated with fibroids that usually shrink in menopause), diffuse enlargement associated with pregnancy or pathology such as hyperplasia, tenderness, sometimes fibroids, and so forth
d. Pelvic floor
(1) Note cystocele, rectocele, introital tone with Kegel and Valsalva maneuver.
e. Ovaries
(1) In menopause, ovaries may not be palpable.
10. Colorectal evaluation
a. Rectocele, lesions, hemorrhoids, bleeding, tarry stools, guaiac testing
11. Extremities
a. Including feet
12. Skin
a. Note new or changing lesions
b. Evaluate yearly, especially with a history of excessive sun exposure.

INTERVENTIONS

A. Treatment options should be collaborative utilizing shared decision-making between the patient and the provider. Dependent upon various factors including:
1. Risk/benefit evaluation
2. Patient preference
3. Costs of intervention
4. Side/adverse effects
B. Nonpharmacologic options
1. Nonhormonal therapies include:
a. Dress in cool layers.
b. Avoid smoking, which has some effect on estrogen metabolism and increases risk of flushes; some studies have also shown exercise reduces VMS.
c. Avoid personal hot-flash triggers (hot drinks, caffeine, spicy foods, ETOH [alcohol], and/or emotional reactions).
d. Reduce stress through paced respirations, mind/body techniques, and use of cognitive behaviorial therapy.
e. Use devices such as cooling pillows (e.g., Chillow pillow), bed fan, wicking clothing/pajamas, and/or wicking sheets/pillowcases.
f. In small, limited studies, exercise, yoga, and acupuncture have shown some improvements in hot flashes and sleep disturbances.
g. Herbals have been found effective for some women including:
(1) **Black cohosh (brand name Remifemin):** Study results are mixed on whether black cohosh effectively relieves menopausal symptoms. National Center for Complementary and Integrative Health (NCCIH)-funded study found black cohosh, whether used alone or with other botanicals, compared to placebo, failed to relieve vasomotor flushes and night sweats in perimenopausal women or those approaching

menopause. In general, clinical trials of black cohosh for menopausal symptoms have not found serious side effects.

(2) **Phytoestrogens (brand name Equelle):** Modestly effective in relieving VMS. Supplements providing higher proportions of genistein or S(Y)-equol may provide more benefits. More clinical studies are needed to compare outcomes among women who have ability to convert daidzein to equol with those who lack that ability.

(3) **Swedish pollen extract (brand name Relizen):** Available in the United States for approximately the last 5 years/available in Europe for more than 15 years for the treatment of VMS. Nonallergenic derivative of flower pollen, shown in several small randomized clinical trials to have no estrogenic effects/no endometrial activity. Mechanism of action: Serotonergic; subpharmacologic levels of phytoestrogens. Randomized controlled trial (RCT) of 54 women: 65% had decreased VMS compared to 38% in control group. Dose: 2 per day; available online without prescription.

PHARMACOLOGIC OPTIONS

A. Menopausal hormon therapy (HT) is the most effective pharmacological treatment for vasomotor symptoms associated with menopause.

1. **Terminology:** The term *hormone replacement therapy* is no longer used as appropriate terminology because it is considered a misnomer. The Food and Drug Administration (FDA) declared the word *replacement* can no longer be used by the marketing industry for products in the United States because postmenopausal levels of HT do not replace premenopausal hormonal levels. The correct terminology for therapies is listed as follows:

   a. **Hormone therapy:** HT (encompassing both ET and combined estrogen–progestogen therapy)
   b. **Estrogen therapy only:** ET
   c. **Combined estrogen–progestogen therapy:** EPT
   d. **Progestogen therapy:** Encompassing both natural progesterone and synthetic progestins

B. Refer to the Hormone Therapy Position Statement published by the North American Menopause Society for evidence-based data on prescribing HT at http://www.menopause.org/docs/default-source/2017/nams-2017-hormone-therapy-position-statement.pdf or the NAMS app "Menopro."

C. Before the age of 60 years or within 10 years after menopause, benefits of HT/ET are more likely to outweigh risks for symptomatic women.

D. The option of initiating HT/ET should be reached through shared decision-making between the woman and her provider in terms of QOL issues and health priorities as well as personal risk factors such as age, time since menopause, and the women's individual risks of venous thromboembolism, stroke, ischemic heart disease, and breast cancer.

1. Patients may be quick to say "My grandmother died of breast cancer and I am afraid to take estrogen," or "I hear hormone therapy causes breast cancer." It is important to normalize and recognize their concern by saying that the risk is a complex issue.

2. Tell the woman that this fear has been prompted from a large study (WHI) released in 2002, but we know over the past 20 years the data have provided more favorable information giving us comfort in understanding the risk.

3. Providers should understand that estrogen alone showed a non-significant reduction in breast cancer risk after an average of 7.2 years of randomization, with 7 fewer cases of invasive breast cancer per 10,000 person-years, which remained for up to a median 13 years. In WHI, the attributable risk of breast cancer (mean patient age, 63 years) randomized to CEE and MPA is less than 1 additional case of breast cancer diagnosed per 1,000 users annually.

4. It is helpful to explain to women that the risk is slightly greater than that observed with drinking one daily glass of wine, and less than drinking two daily glasses of wine. The risk is *similar* to the risk reported with obesity, low physical activity, and other medications (Chen et al., 2006; Li et al., 2013; Manson et al., 2013).

E. Risks may differ depending on the type, dose, duration of medication use, and the route of administration, and the timing of initiation and health risks.

F. Estrogen therapy only is prescribed for patients who have had a hysterectomy. Women with a uterus should also be treated concomitantly with a progestogen because of estrogen stimulation on the endometrium and potential for causing hyperplasia/cancer.

G. Many options are available for prescribing including oral, transdermal, or a systemic vaginal ring. Additionally, many options are available in dosing and cycling/administration. Refer to the NAMS textbook or position statement for more detailed information (Crandall, 2019; NAMS 2017 HT Position Statement).

NON-HORMONAL PHARMACOLOGIC OPTIONS

A. A number of non-hormonal pharmacologic options are available that may help reduce VMS. Most have shown in clinical studies some degree of efficacy in symptomatic menopausal women, although FDA indication for this purpose is not approved (Crandall, 2019).

1. Selective serotonin reuptake inhibitors (SSRI)/serotonin–norepinephrine reuptake inhibitor (SNRI):
   a. Paroxetine (Brisdelle) one 7.5 mg capsule taken at bedtime (FDA approved in 2013); contains a lower dose of paroxetine than that used for psychiatric conditions
   b. Venlafexine (Effexor XR) 37.5 mg a day—titrate as needed; commonly 75 mg/day
   c. Desvenlafaxine (Pristiq) 50 to 100 mg/day
   d. Escitalopram (Lexapro) 10–20 mg/day
2. **Gabapentin:** Indicated in treatment of partial seizures and post herpetic neuralgia; studied in hot flash reduction three times a day (TID) at 900 mg/day up to 1200 mg/day. Increasing doses associated with adverse effects (i.e., dizziness and somnolence).
3. **Clonidine:** 0.05 mg PO (by mouth) BID (twice a day; may require an increase to 0.1 mg BID daily); modest effect on symptoms, adverse side effects (insomnia, dry mouth, constipation, drowsiness); may be a good choice for patients with hypertension (HTN).
4. **Oxybutynin:** Dose: 2.5–15 mg; used primarily for treatment of urge urinary incontinence; antimuscarinic, anticholinergic, and antispasmodic effects.

CASE STUDY

Patient Situation

Subjective Data

- **Chief Complaint:**
  "I would like the 'natural hormones' I saw on television."
- **History of Present Illness:**
  A 51-year-old African American female presents to your office stating she would like the "natural hormones" that Suzanne Somers recommends. She tells you her LMP was at age 48, and she is experiencing 9 to 10 vasomotor symptoms a day that she rates as moderate to severe. She awakens one to two times/night most nights. She states, "I can't deal with the sweating when I am at work, I can't sleep, and I can't think anymore/I'm just in a fog

(*continued*)

CASE STUDY (*continued*)

most of the time." She reports, "I don't want to have sex anymore because it hurts down there, and I am dry as the Sahara Desert and have a prickly feeling like cactus. I have some white vaginal discharge with an odor. I just have to make myself do it to keep my marriage together. I have tried that menopausal black cohosh from the drugstore, but it is not working."

- **Medical History:**
  Hypertension – controlled
  Mammogram 18 months ago: Benign with heterogeneously dense breasts
  No colonoscopy
  Has had all appropriate vaccinations including COVID
- **Surgical History:**
  Bilateral tubal ligation, age 35
- **Current Medications:**
  Hydrochlorothiazide 12, 5 mg daily
  OTC black cohosh daily
  Vitamin D 1000 IU gel cap daily
- **Reproductive History:**
  LMP at age 48
  Sexually active with vaginal penetrative sex; in "good" monogamous relationship of 27 years with husband. See HPI. No history of STDs
  G2P2; normal vaginal deliveries
  Last Pap smear: 3 years; no history of abnormal Pap smears but unsure if had HPV co-testing
  Used oral contraceptives throughout early reproductive years without adverse effects
- **Family Medical History:**
  Mother: Type 2 diabetes; coronary artery disease – died age 60
  Maternal grandmother: Breast cancer – died age 65
  Father: Medical history unknown
  Son: Age 27 – healthy
  Daughter: Age 25 – healthy
- **Social History:**
  Married for 27 years. Lives with husband.
  Employed full time as a high school teacher.
  Denies tobacco use, alcohol use, illicit drug use.

Objective Data

- **Vital signs:** Blood pressure 124/72, pulse 76/min, respirations: 18 bpm, BMI 30.2
- **Physical Exam:**
  HEENT: No abnormal findings, thyroid normal
  Cardiac: No carotid bruits, heart sounds regular, rhythm regular, no murmur noted
  Respiratory: Breath sound clear to auscultation
  Abdomen: Soft, nontender, BS present in all 4 quadrants
  Genitourinary:
      External genitalia: Thinning/greying hair, tissue pale appearing, no fissures, no lesions, no cystocele/rectocele
      Vaginal exam: Discomfort on insertion of speculum; mucosa pale, flattened rugae, small amount grey discharge; pH 5.4

(*continued*)

CASE STUDY (*continued*)

- Lab results from PCP
  UA dipstick: Urine color: cloudy; Leukocytes 1+, Trace blood
  Urine C&S: Negative/normal urogenital flora
  Total cholesterol: 250/LDL = 120/TG = 160
  CMP: Electrolytes normal
  LFTs: Normal
  TSH: Normal
  HgbA1C: 5.8

Clinical Analysis

- What diagnostic testing would you plan to order and why?
  - Would not order serum/saliva testing. She is obviously menopausal by definition and symptoms. Discuss with patient since she is probably expecting this from reading Somer's book. NAMS, ACOG, and Endocrine Society do not recommend testing. Treat the symptoms.
  - No further lab testing since she is being followed by PCP and labs such as TSH and HgbA1C have been checked.
  - Pap smear with co-testing; consider appropriate cultures (BV, chlamydia/gonorrhea, candidiasis, trichomoniasis...).
  - Consider RPR, hepatitis C, and HIV if have not been checked.
  - Screening mammogram
- How would you approach the plan of care for this patient?
- Ask patient for her visit goals
  - Set realistic outcomes
  - Explain shared decision-making
  - Suggest future visits
- Investigate patient's knowledge and source of knowledge
  - Suzanne Somers' book "Forever Health"
  - Certified behavioral health technician (CBHT)
  - Internet
  - Friends
- Educate patient/clear myths with evidence-based information
  - Identify physiological and socio-emotional changes that occur at menopause resulting from moderate/severe vasomotor symptoms and GSM affecting the woman's QOL
  - Discuss patient's challenges/risks
  - Provide resources
- Develop a plan using shared decision-making for VMS and GSM which will help the woman effectively manage her symptoms
  - Non-pharmacologic/alternative/complementary
  - Pharmacologic: Hormonal
  - Pharmacologic: Non-hormonal
  - Resources: NAMS Consumer book; NAMS handouts; www.MiddlesexMD.com: ACOG; EB handouts as appropriate

BIBLIOGRAPHY

Alexander, I. M., & Andrist, L. C. (2013). Menopause. In K. D. Schuiling & F. E. Likis (Eds.), *Women's gynecologic health* (2nd ed., pp. 285–328). Jones & Bartlett.

Avis, N. E., Crawford, S. L., Greendale, G., Bromberger, J. T., Everson-Rose, S. A., Gold, E. B., Hess, R., Joffe, H., Kravitz, H. M., Tepper, P. G., & Thurston, R. C. (2015). Duration of menopausal vasomotor symptoms over the menopause transition. *Journal of the American Medical Association Internal Medicine, 175*(4), 531–539. https://doi.org/10.1001/jamainternmed.2014.8063

Ayers, B., Forshaw, M., & Hunter, M. S. (2010). The impact of attitudes towards the menopause on women's symptom experience: A systematic review. *Maturitas, 65*(1), 28–36. https://doi.org/10.1016/j.maturitas.2009.10.016

Bachmann, G. A., & Nevadunsky, N. S. (2000). Diagnosis and treatment of atrophic vaginitis. *American Family Physician, 61*(10), 3090–3096.

Carcio, H. A. (1999). The maturation index. In *Advanced health assessment of women* (Vol. 12, pp. 226–228). Lippincott.

Carcio, H. A. (2009). Urogenital atrophy: A new approach to vaginitis diagnosis. *Advance for Nurse Practitioners, 10*(10), 40–47.

Centers for Disease Control and Prevention. (n.d.). *Adult immunization schedules—United States, 2017.* Retrieved from https://www.cdc.gov/vaccines/schedules/downloads/adult/adult-combined-schedule-bw.pdf

Chen, W. Y., Manson, J. E., Hankinson, S. E., Rosner, B., Holmes, M. D., Willett, W. C., & Colditz, G. A. (2006). Unopposed estrogen therapy and the risk of invasive breast cancer. *Archives of Internal Medicine, 166*(9), 1027–1032.

Crandall, J. C. (Ed.). 2019. *Menopause Practice: A clinician guide* (6th ed.). The North American Menopause Society. ISBN 978-0-578-53228-8

Harlow, S. D., Gass, M., Hall, J. E., Lobo, R., Maki, P., Rebar, R. W., Sherman, S., Sluss, P. M., & de Villiers, T. J. (2012). Executive summary of the stages of reproductive aging workshop + 10: Addressing the unfinished agenda of staging reproductive aging. *Menopause, 19*(4), 387–395. https://doi.org/10.1097/gme.0b013e31824d8f40

Kingsberg, S., Iglesia, C., Kellogg, S., & Krychman, M. (2011). *Handbook on female sexual health and wellness.* Association of Reproductive Health Professionals. http://www.arhp.org/uploadDocs/ARHP_ACOG_SexualityHandbook.pdf

Kingsberg, S. A., Wysocki, S., Magnus, L., Krychman, M. L. (2013). Vulvar and vaginal atrophy in postmenopausal women: Findings from the REVIVE (REal Women's VIews of Treatment Options for Menopausal Vaginal ChangEs) survey. *Journal of Sexual Medicine, 10*(7), 1790–1799. https://doi.org/10.1111/jsm.12190

Li, C. I., Daling, J. R., Tang, M. T., Haugen, K. L., Porter, P. L., & Malone, K. E. (2013). Use of antihypertensive medications and breast cancer risk among women aged 55 to 74 years. *JAMA Internal Medicine, 173*(17), 1629–1637. https://doi.org/10.1001/jamainternmed.2013.9071

Lindau, S. T., Dude, A., Gavrilova, N., Hoffmann, J. N., Schumm, L. P., & McClintock, M. K. (2018). Prevalence and correlates of vaginal estrogenization in postmenopausal women in the United States. *Menopause, 24*(5), 536–545. https://doi.org/10.1097/GME.0000000000000787

Maki, P. M., Kornstein, S. G., Joffe, H., Bromberger, J. T., Freeman, E. W., Athappilly, G., Bobo, W. V., Rubin, L. H., Koleva, H. K., Cohen, L. S., Soares, C. N. On behalf of the Board of Trustees for The North American Menopause Society (NAMS) and the Women and Mood Disorders Task Force of the National Network of Depression Centers. (2018). Consensus recommendations: Guidelines for the evaluation and treatment of perimenopausal depression: Summary and recommendations. *Menopause: The Journal of The North American Menopause Society, 25*(10), 1069–1085. https://doi.org/10.1097/GME.0000000000001174

Manson, J. E., Chlebowski, R. T., Stefanick, M. L., Aragaki, A. K., Rossouw, J. E., Prentice, R. L., . . . Robert B Wallace, R. B. Menopausal hormone therapy and health outcomes during the intervention and extended post stopping phases of the Women's Health Initiative randomized trials. *JAMA, 310*(13), 1353–1368. https://doi.org/10.1001/jama.2013.278040.

Mills, J. M., Morgan, J. R., Dhaliwal, A., & Perkins, R. B. (2021). Eligibility for cervical cancer screening exit: Comparison of a national and safety net cohort. *Gynecologic Oncology, 162* (2), 308–314. https://doi.org/10.1016/j.ygyno.2021.05.035.

Modi, M. & Dhillo, W. S. (2019). Neurokinin 3 receptor antagonism: A novel treatment for menopausal hot flushes. *Neuroendocrinology, 109*(3), 242–248. https://doi.org/10.1159/000495889

North American Menopause Society. (2014). *Menopause practice: A clinician's guide* (5th ed.). Author.

North American Menopause Society. (2017a). *Nonhormonal management of menopause-associated vasomotor symptoms: 2015 position statement of the North American Menopause Society.* http://www.menopause.org/docs/default-source/professional/pap-pdf-meno-d-15-00241-minus-trim-cme.pdf

North American Menopause Society 2017 Hormone Therapy Position Statement Advisory Panel. (2017). The 2017 hormone therapy position statement of the North American Menopause Society. *Menopause, 24*(7), 728–753. https://doi.org/10.1097/GME.0000000000000921

North American Menopause Society. (2020). The 2020 genitourinary syndrome of menopause position statement of the North American Menopause Society. *Menopause, 27*(9), 976–992. https://doi.org/10.1097/GME.0000000000001609.

Pandya, K. J., Raubertas, R. F., Flynn, P. J., Hynes, H. E., Rosenbluth, R. J., Kirshner, J. J., Pierce, H. I., Dragalin, V., & Morrow, G. R. (2000). Oral clonidine in postmenopausal patients with breast cancer experiencing tamoxifen-induced hot flashes: A university of rochester cancer center community clinical oncology program study. *Annals of Internal Medicine, 132*(10), 788–793. https://doi.org/10.7326/0003-4819-132-10-200005160-00004

Simon, J. A., Gaines, T., & LaGuardia, K. D., Extended-Release Oxybutynin Therapy for VMS Study Group. (2016). Extended-release oxybutynin therapy for vasomotor symptoms in women: A randomized clinical trial. *Menopause, 23*(11), 1214–1221. https://doi.org/10.1097/GME.0000000000000773

Stuenkel, C. A., Gass, M. L., Manson, J. E., Lobo, R. A., Pal, L., Rebar, R. W., & Hall, J. E. (2012). A decade after the Women's Health Initiative—The experts do agree. *Menopause, 19*(8), 846–847. https://doi.org/10.1097/gme.0b013e31826226f2

U.S. Preventive Services Task Force. (2016). *Final update summary: Hepatitis C: Screening.* https://www.uspreventiveservicestaskforce.org/Page/Document/UpdateSummaryFinal/hepatitis-c-screening

Welcome to FRAX®. (n.d.). http://www.sheffield.ac.uk/FRAX

23

OSTEOPOROSIS AND EVALUATION OF FRACTURE RISK

NANCY R. BERMAN, CAITLIN M. VLAEMINCK, CATHY R. KESSENICH, AND RICHARD S. POPE

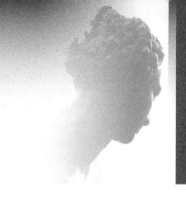

SCOPE OF THE PROBLEM

A. Osteoporosis is a disease of low bone mass and compromised bone strength that leads to increased risk of fracture.

B. Low bone mass can be quantified through bone density testing and is reported along a continuum from mild to moderate loss, called *osteopenia,* and to severe loss, called *osteoporosis.*

C. Fracture risk is significantly increased when low bone mass reaches the severity of osteoporosis, but the majority of fractures occur in women with mild to moderate low bone density (osteopenia) as there are more women in that range.

D. Bone density testing will identify women with osteoporosis who should be treated with medication for fracture prevention based on their level of bone loss. This is in accordance with the Bone Health and Osteoporosis Foundation (BHOF; formerly National Osteoporosis Foundation [NOF]) and the World Health Organization (WHO).

E. Using a 10-year fracture-risk assessment tool called *FRAX*— which incorporates demographics and the bone density at the femoral neck, additional women are identified who reach a diagnosis of osteoporosis and would benefit from pharmacologic therapy to reduce fracture risk. In the United States, osteoporosis is diagnosed in patients when the 10-year probability for major osteoporotic fracture is ≥20% or the 10-year probability of hip fracture is ≥3%.

F. Because most women with osteoporosis will not have symptoms, bone densitometry is a way to recognize those women who have the potential to develop fractures and those who do not have an increased fracture risk.

G. Bone mass measurements provide a quantitative value so that a low bone density diagnosis can encourage the patient to modify her lifestyle, diet, and consider the option of Food and Drug Administration (FDA)-approved medications for treatment.

H. Central dual-energy x-ray absorptiometry (DXA) scanning is the accepted methodology to test bone density. It is highly reproducible and accepted by multiple organizations, including WHO, BHOF, and the American Association of Clinical Endocrinology (AACE).

I. Bone mass densitometry (BMD) predicts the risk for fracture even more accurately than hypertension predicts risk for stroke.

J. Many clinicians will be treating women with increased fracture risk. It is imperative that they understand the indications for BMD and the implications of treatment.

K. Not all fractures can be prevented, but interventions can significantly reduce fracture risk.

L. Once a fracture occurs, the risk of a subsequent fracture is increased; therefore, it is important to prevent the first fracture.

OSTEOPOROSIS EXPLAINED

A. Definition
1. *Osteoporosis* is defined as a skeletal disorder characterized by compromised bone strength predisposing a person to increased risk for fracture.
2. It is a condition of porous bones that is underdiagnosed because it has a silent disease process.
3. Osteoporosis is a generalized disease that affects all skeletal sites.
4. Diagnosis is established by BMD measurement, FRAX 10-year fracture risk calculation, or the occurrence of adulthood fragility fractures that were not due to major trauma.
5. Most serious fractures are those of the hip because they contribute substantially to morbidity rate, mortality rate, and healthcare costs.
6. Vertebral fractures are also significant and can lead to disability and chronic pain.
7. There is an increased risk for osteoporosis with advancing age; it begins at the wrist and progresses to the vertebrae and last to the hip.
8. The bone density test creates a T-score that is determined by comparing that individual's bone density at multiple sites to a young adult's average bone density. The score is reported in standard deviations (SDs) from the young-adult average.
9. The T-score is normal up to −1.0; osteopenia or low bone mass is −1 to −2.5.
10. Osteoporosis is diagnosed by bone densitometry as a T-score of −2.5 or lower at any site.
11. The risk for fracture is increased with low bone density and other factors such as age and fall risk.

B. Related statistics
1. Osteoporosis causes approximately 2.3 million fractures annually at a cost of more than $23 billion in the United States and Europe.
2. One in two women older than 50 years will suffer a fracture secondary to osteoporosis, or nearly 25 million postmenopausal American women are affected.
3. Seventy-five percent of women between the ages of 45 and 75 years have never talked to their clinician about osteoporosis.
4. A woman's relative risk for hip fracture is equal to her combined risk for breast, uterine, and ovarian cancers.
5. Vertebral fractures are the most common (700,000 annually), whereas the occurrence of hip fractures is 300,000 annually.
6. All races and ethnic groups can be affected, including African Americans, Mexicans, and Asians, as well as Caucasians.

C. Guidelines from the BHOF, ISCD (International Society for Clinical Densitometry), and the North American Menopause Society (NAMS) recommend when to initiate bone density testing and how often to repeat this testing. It is prudent to screen women at risk for osteoporosis (Box 23.1).

D. Some facts related to hip fractures
1. Equal in number to wrist fractures
2. More expensive than wrist fractures because of immobility and prolonged hospitalization
3. The mortality rate associated with hip fractures is 12% to 20% during the year after injury.
4. Fewer than 50% of patients with a hip fracture ever return to their pre-fracture level of function.
5. One in seven women experiences osteoporosis-induced hip fractures.

E. Some facts related to vertebral fractures
1. They are twice as common as hip fractures.
2. They are less readily diagnosed because up to two thirds are asymptomatic and painless.
3. Successive fractures lead to a loss in height.

> **BOX 23.1 Risk Factors for Osteoporosis**
>
> - Adults with fragility fractures
> - Dietary- and weight-related factors
> - Slight build with loss of body fat
> - High caffeine intake
> - Excessive alcohol consumption
> - Lifetime low intake of dietary calcium (lactose intolerance)
> - Lack of weight gain since age 25 years
> - Eating disorder
> - Estrogen deficiency
> - Early menopause
> - Nulliparity
> - Family history of osteoporosis, including paternal and maternal hip fracture
> - Present smoking
> - Lack of exercise
> - Inability to rise from a chair without using the armrest for support
> - Immobility
> - Other conditions and medications may also increase the risk such as hyperthyroidism or hyperparathyroidism
> - Long-term steroid therapy (prednisone 5 mg or more for more than 3 months) especially in those women with rheumatoid arthritis or chronic lung disease
> - Heparin treatment
> - Intestinal malabsorption, such as gastric bypass surgery, celiac disease, and other conditions
> - Discontinuation of estrogen therapy
> - Cushing's disease
> - Type 1 diabetes

    a. A loss of 1.5 inches is suggestive of osteoporotic spinal fractures.
    b. Figure 23.1 visually shows how fractures can lead to loss of height throughout the life span.

MEASUREMENT OF BONE DENSITY

A. Bone density is measured in grams per square centimeter.
    1. Bone density differs throughout the body due to variations in cortical and trabecular bone distribution.
    2. The bones of the vertebrae are mainly composed of trabecular bone, whereas the bones of the femoral neck are mostly made of cortical bone.
    3. Bone density is used to define osteoporosis in terms of SDs from the average peak bone mass.
    4. SD is a statistical term used to express the average amount by which an individual's bone density varies from the norm.
    5. Values are matched against average bone density for young adult women when bone mass generally is at its peak.
B. **Parameters for diagnosis:** Both WHO and Bone Health and Osteoporosis Foundation (BHOF) (formerly NOF) categorize a patient's bone density using SD.

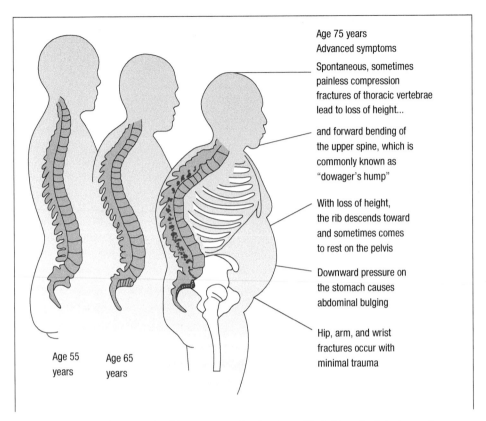

Age 75 years
Advanced symptoms

Spontaneous, sometimes painless compression fractures of thoracic vertebrae lead to loss of height...

and forward bending of the upper spine, which is commonly known as "dowager's hump"

With loss of height, the rib descends toward and sometimes comes to rest on the pelvis

Downward pressure on the stomach causes abdominal bulging

Hip, arm, and wrist fractures occur with minimal trauma

Age 55 years

Age 65 years

FIGURE 23.1 Silent vertebral fractures can lead to loss of height and related symptoms.

1. WHO scale
   a. **Low risk of osteoporotic fracture:** An SD of 0 to −1.0 below peak bone density is normal.
   b. **Greater risk of fracture:** Patients with an SD between −1 and −2.5 are diagnosed with osteopenia (low bone mass).
   c. **Have osteoporosis:** Patients with an SD greater than −2.5 are diagnosed with osteoporosis, even though they have not had a bone fracture.
   d. Using these criteria, WHO classifies 30% of postmenopausal women in the United States as having osteoporosis.
   e. WHO and BHOF recommend that all individuals who are categorized with osteoporosis should be treated.
   f. BHOF criteria would classify 45% of postmenopausal women as osteoporotic
2. **Z scores:** BMD reporting in females before menopause
   a. An SD of 0 to −1.0 below peak bone density is normal, the same as that used by WHO.
   b. **Osteoporosis:** An SD of −2.5 or less than that of a young adult in the reference population indicates osteoporosis.
3. Low BMD at the spine, hip, or forearm is sufficient for a diagnosis of osteoporosis.
4. One SD at the spine or hip increases the risk of fracture approximately twofold.
C. **T-score:** Reports the BMD in SDs compared to the young-adult average. See Table 23.1 for a summary of the SD categories of bone density. See Table 23.2 for AACE diagnostic criteria for osteoporosis in postmenopausal women.

TABLE 23.1 Summary of Bone Density T-Score Categories	
DIAGNOSIS	**BMD T-SCORE: NUMBER OF SDs BELOW MEAN IN HEALTHY YOUNG WOMEN**
Normal	No lower than −1
Osteopenia (low bone mass)	Between −1 and −2.5
Osteoporosis	−2.5 or less
Severe osteoporosis	−2.5 or less with fragility fractures

BMD, bone mass densitometry; SD, standard deviation.

1. **Normal:** −1.0 and higher
2. **Low bone mass (osteopenia):** T-score between −1.0 and −2.5
3. **Osteoporosis:** T-score at or less than −2.5
4. **Severe or established osteoporosis:** T-score at or less than −2.5 with one or more fractures

D. Vertebral imaging
   1. Vertebral fracture assay (VFA) can be performed at the same time as BMD on certain machines.
      a. This is a scan of the spine that evaluates vertebral height and has no increase in the risk of radiation. Also known as *lateral vertebral assay (LVA).*
      b. If VFA is not available, then a dorsal spine and/or lumbar spine x-ray is helpful to identify compression fractures.
      c. These tests should be ordered when there is height loss of more than 1.5 inches and can be performed easily at the time of DXA scanning.
E. Diagnosis and therapeutic intervention can be based on this assessment. In addition to BMD testing, vertebral imaging is recommended in individuals with a risk of vertebral fracture.
   1. Individuals at risk for vertebral fracture include:
      a. All women aged 70 years and older
      b. Women aged 65 to 69 years if BMD T-score is −1.5 or less
      c. Postmenopausal women aged 50 to 64 years with specific risk factors
         (1) Low trauma fracture
         (2) Historical height loss of 1.5 in. or more (4 cm)
         (3) Recent or ongoing long-term glucocorticoid treatment

THE PROCEDURE

A. Assess and monitor various disease states and conditions.
   1. Evaluate those women at risk for fracture who are unsure whether to initiate therapy.
   2. Detect low bone mass (osteopenia) and assess its severity.

TABLE 23.2 2020 American Association of Clinical Endocrinologists/American College of Endocrinology Diagnosis of Osteoporosis in Postmenopausal Women
1. T-score −2.5 or below in the lumbar spine, femoral neck, total proximal femur, or 1/3 radius
2. Low-trauma spine or hip fracture (*regardless of bone mineral density*)
3. T-score between −1.0 and −2.5 **and** a fragility fracture of the proximal humerus, pelvis, or distal forearm
4. T-score between −1.0 and −2.5 **and** high FRAX (or if available, TBS-adjusted FRAX®) fracture probability based on country-specific thresholds

3. Evaluate patients with metabolic bone disease that affects the skeleton, including comorbid conditions associated with risk for fractures. These secondary causes of the bone disease include hyperparathyroidism, vitamin D deficiency, and other conditions.
4. Monitor the effectiveness of prevention or treatment measures for osteoporosis.
5. Monitor a patient undergoing long-term glucocorticoid therapy.
6. Evaluate a patient with a hip, radial, or vertebral compression fracture.
7. Establish baseline BMD for future measurements in those with prior osteoporotic fracture.

B. Contraindications to BMD evaluation
   1. Pregnancy is the only absolute contraindication.
   2. Spinal deformity. Use radius and hip. The diagnosis can be established by testing the wrist. For patients with hyperparathyroidism, the wrist is best used for diagnosis and monitoring.
   3. The presence of orthopedic hardware. Use another location away from the hardware. Note: BMD results can be affected by the presence of metal objects such as a belt, button, or corset. It also can be affected by the patient's recent ingestion of calcium-containing tablets.

C. **Accuracy:** Generally good (90%–95%)

D. The DXA scan
   1. When BMD is indicated, central DXA is the preferred technique, not peripheral.
   2. DXA measures the density of bone at major sites.
      a. Hip
      b. Spine
      c. Forearm
   3. **Accuracy:** Within 3% to 5%
   4. **Precision:** Within 0.5% to 2.0%
   5. Best correlation to predict the risk of fractures at the hip
   6. Process takes 10 to 15 minutes, with the woman lying on a table while an imager passes over her body.
   7. A computer calculates the density of the patient's bones and compares this with normal bone at peak mass, as well as the average bone density for individuals of the patient's age.
   8. Results are expressed in grams per square centimeter in SD of the peak value of matched controls.
   9. Bones with normal mineralization produce a higher reading in grams per centimeter than does osteoporotic bone.
   10. Arthritis in the lumbar spine can make the T-scores falsely higher than they actually are.
   11. Limitations of the DXA
      a. There is a precision error that is part of the test. Be sure that regular testing of phantoms is performed, and the software is up to date. The testing center will be able to provide this information.
      b. It is preferable to use the same machine, same location, and same technologist. Measuring patients on different machines and/or using equipment made by different manufacturers can be misleading as error rates are difficult to calculate.

E. Diagnosis at single or multiple bone sites is controversial.
   1. Some studies have determined that there is not a great difference in bone density at different sites.
   2. Other studies reported that BMD at several sites increased the predictive accuracy.

F. **Biochemical tests:** Blood and urine tests measure the rate of bone remodeling.
   1. These tests indicate a high rate of bone turnover, which may indicate rapid bone loss.
   2. Commonly used in research but not in clinical practice except in uncommon instances.

DIAGNOSTIC ASSESSMENT

A. BHOF diagnostic guidelines for BMD testing
1. In women 65 years and older and men 70 years and older recommend BMD testing.
2. In postmenopausal women and men aged 50 to 69 years, recommend BMD testing based on the risk-factor profile.
3. To determine the degree of disease severity, recommend BMD testing and vertebral imaging to those who have had a fracture.
4. **Note:** BMD testing should be performed at DXA facilities using accepted quality assurance.

LIFETIME MONITORING RECOMMENDATIONS

A. The BHOF recommends follow-up intervals for bone density testing.
1. Perform BMD testing 1 to 2 years after initiating therapy to reduce fracture risk and every 2 years thereafter. More frequent testing may be warranted in certain clinical situations.
2. Perform BMD testing every 2 to 5 years in untreated postmenopausal women.
B. Dietary recommendations are listed in Table 23.3.
C. Women who are diagnosed with osteoporosis should be treated to prevent fracture.
1. BMD T-scores –2.5 or worse should be treated.
2. Guidelines for treatment choices are available from BHOF, AACE, and NAMS.
D. Preventive therapy may be indicated for women at high risk of fracture who do not have T-scores of –2.5 or lower. Examples include those on long-term steroid therapy, those with rheumatoid arthritis, or other inflammatory arthritis-associated conditions, and women on aromatase inhibitors.
1. FRAX was developed to identify those individuals who would benefit from treatment.
   a. The FRAX tool was developed by WHO to evaluate the fracture risk for patients.
   b. It is based on individual patient models and integrates the risks associated with clinical risk factors and BMD at the femoral neck.
   c. FRAX is a calculation tool that incorporates patient demographics and the bone density at the femoral neck in a computer calculation.
   d. FRAX addresses factors, such as age, height, weight, family history of hip fractures of either parent, history of the previous fracture as an adult, current smoking, glucocorticoid use, and chronic disease, such as rheumatoid arthritis, that contribute to fracture risk. The calculator also provides a list of other medical causes of secondary osteoporosis that are associated with a high risk for fracture.
   e. FRAX recognizes that the risk of fracture may be greater than the T-score suggests and allows for a diagnosis of osteoporosis based on 10-year fracture risk and when the initiation of therapy is indicated.

TABLE 23.3 Daily Recommendations for Dietary Supplements

SUPPLEMENT	AGE (YEARS)	DAILY REQUIREMENTS
Calcium	<50	1,000 mg
Calcium	>50	1,200 mg
Vitamin D	<50	400–800 IU
Vitamin D	>50	800–1,000 IU

    f. The algorithms give the 10-year probability of fracture.

      (1) Osteoporosis is diagnosed when the 10-year risk of a major osteoporotic fracture is ≥20% and treatment is indicated.

      (2) Osteoporosis is diagnosed when the 10-year risk of a hip fracture is ≥3% and treatment is recommended.

    g. The tool is found at www.sheffield.ac.uk/FRAX.

TREATMENT CHOICES

A. No pharmacologic therapy should be initiated without continuous reassessment of the need to continue treatment.

B. After the initial 3 to 5 years of treatment, a comprehensive risk assessment should be performed.

C. Evidence suggests that there are risks from bisphosphonates in medications that increase with long-term use.

    1. **Osteonecrosis of the jaw:** A problem of the exposed jawbone that may be more common in individuals with dental procedures while on antiresorptive treatments and cancer in patients receiving IV infusion of bisphosphonate.

    2. **Atypical subtrochanteric fractures:** Fractures of the femur that may occur even without trauma.

      a. All patients on therapy should be assessed for hip, groin, or upper leg pain.

D. Addressing long-term use of bisphosphonates

    1. Controversy continues regarding the length of treatment

    2. Limited evidence at this time

    3. "Drug holiday" of 1 to 2 years not taking medication is considered after years of use based on the risk for fracture as determined by bone density and other risk factors

      a. **Mild risk:** May consider a 1- to 2-year drug holiday after 5 years of treatment

      b. **High risk:** May consider a drug holiday after 6 to 10 years of stability

      c. For zoledronic acid, may consider a drug holiday after 3 years for high-risk patients but up to 6 years in very-high-risk patients.

      d. Ending a drug holiday should be based on individual patient situations:

        (1) Decrease in BMD

        (2) Increase in bone turnover markers

        (3) Increase in fracture risk

      e. Drug holidays should never be initiated with non-bisphosphonates.

E. Current pharmacologic agents FDA approved for the prevention and treatment of osteoporosis (Table 23.4)

    1. Anti-resorptive agents

      a. **Bisphosphonates:** All bisphosphonates can affect renal function and are contraindicated in patients with an estimated glomerular filtration rate (GFR) less than 30 to 35 mL/min.

        (1) Weekly oral alendronate (Fosamax)

        (2) Weekly or monthly risedronate (Actonel)

        (3) Monthly, oral, or quarterly IV ibandronate (Boniva)

        (4) Once yearly infusion of zoledronic acid (Reclast)

        (5) Should not be used in patients with creatinine clearance less than 35 mL/min or in patients with renal impairment.

      b. Rank ligand inhibitor

        (1) Denosumab (Prolia)

          • May cause hypocalcemia.

          • Serum calcium levels should be monitored.

TABLE 23.4 Pharmacological Management of Osteoporosis

CLASS	GENERIC NAME	BRAND NAME	DOSE/ FREQUENCY/ ROUTE	CONSIDERATIONS
Bisphosphonates	Alendronate	Fosamax	70 mg once a week oral	Not recommended with severe renal impairment, avoid oral therapy with esophagus problems, GERD, trouble swallowing, inability to remain upright for 30 minutes.
	Risedronate	Actonel/ Altevia	150-mg oral dose once a month	Rare complications include ONJ and atypical subtrochanteric fracture
	Ibandronate	Boniva	150 mg oral dose monthly or 3 mg IV every 3 months	Fracture risk reduction in lumbar spine
	Zoledronic acid	Reclast	5 mg IV once yearly	
Rank ligand inhibitor	Denosumab	Prolia	60-mg injection every 6 months	Caution with severe renal diseases. Rare complications include ONJ and atypical subtrochanteric fracture
PTH	Teriparatide	Forteo	20 mcg SC once daily for maximum 2 years	Should not be prescribed for people who are at increased risks for osteosarcoma. This includes those with Paget's disease of bone or unexplained elevations of serum alkaline phosphate, open epiphysis, or prior radiation therapy involving the skeleton
	Abaloparatide	Tymlos	80 mcg SQ once daily for maximum 2 years	Orthostatic hypotension: Instruct patients to sit or lie down if symptoms develop after administration of the dose
				• Hypercalcemia: Avoid use in patients with pre-existing hypercalcemia and those known to have an underlying hypercalcemic disorder, such as primary hyperparathyroidism
				• Hypercalciuria and urolithiasis: Monitor urine calcium if pre-existing hypercalciuria or active urolithiasis are suspected
Anti-sclerostin agent	Romosozumab	Evenity	210 mg SQ monthly for a maximum 1 year	• Can be considered initial therapy for high-risk patients • Should not be used in patients at high risk for cardiovascular events or who have had a recent myocardial infarction or stroke

(continued)

TABLE 23.4 Pharmacological Management of Osteoporosis (*continued*)

CLASS	GENERIC NAME	BRAND NAME	DOSE/ FREQUENCY/ ROUTE	CONSIDERATIONS
			SELECTIVE ESTROGEN	
Receptor modulator (SERM)	Raloxifene Evista	60 mg orally once daily		FDA approved for the prevention of vertebral fractures.
				Increased risk of venous thromboembolism and death from stroke
Hormonal therapy	Estrogen	Oral, transdermal		FDA approved for prevention only. May consider for women who have a contraindication for all other osteoporosis treatments

FDA, Food and Drug Administration; GERD, gastroesophageal reflux disease; IV, intravenous; ONJ, osteonecrosis of the jaw; PTH, parathyroid hormone; SERM, selective estrogen receptor modulator; SQ, subcutaneous.

- Serious infections have been reported.
- Denosumab should never be discontinued due to the risk for multiple vertebral fractures.
  c. Calcitonin (Miacalcin)
   (1) Intranasal spray
   (2) Helps with bone pain
  d. Estrogen agonist/antagonist (selective estrogen receptor modulators [SERMs])
   (1) Raloxifene (Evista)
    - Can increase the risk of deep vein thrombosis and may cause hot flashes in a small percentage of patients.
  e. Anabolic agents
   (1) Parathyroid hormone
    - Teriparatide (Forteo)
    - Abaloparatide (Tymlos)
  f. Estrogen/hormone therapy
   (1) These agents are only approved for the prevention of osteoporosis along with the treatment of vasomotor symptoms.
  g. Antisclerostin agent
   (1) Romosozumab (Evenity) can be used in patients with prior radiation exposure.

BIBLIOGRAPHY

Adler, R. A., El-Hajj Fuleihan, G., Bauer, D. C., Camacho, P. M., Clarke, B. L., Clines, G. A., Compston, J. E., Drake, M. T., Edwards, B. J., Favus, M. J., Greenspan, S. L., McKinney, R. Jr., Pignolo, R. J., & Sellmeyer, D. E. (2016). Managing osteoporosis in patients on long-term bisphosphonate treatment: Report of a task force of the American Society for Bone and Mineral Research. *Journal of Bone and Mineral Research, 31*(1), 19–35. https://doi.org/10.1002/jbmr.2708

Adult positions. (2021). *ISCD.* Retrieved October 19, 2021, from https://iscd.org/learn/official-positions/adult-positions.

Bray, V. J. (2012). *Osteoporosis screening guidelines.* http://www.iscd.org/publications/osteoflash/osteoporosis-screening-guidelines

Camacho, P. M., Petak, S. M., Binkley, N., Diab, D. L., Eldeiry, L. S., Farooki, A., Harris, S. T., Hurley, D. L., Kelly, J., Lewiecki, E. M., Pessah-Pollack, R., McClung, M., Wimalawansa, S. J, & Watts, N. B. (2020). American Association of Clinical Endocrinologists/American College of Endocrinology Clinical Practice Guidelines for the Diagnosis and Treatment of Postmenopausal Osteoporosis-2020 Update. *Endocrine Practice, 26*(1), 1–46. https://doi.org/10.4158/GL-2020-0524SUPPL

Cosman, F., Crittenden, D. B., Adachi, J. D., Binkley, N., Czerwinski, E., Ferrari, S., Hofbauer, L. C., Lau, E., Lewiecki, E. M., Miyauchi, A., Zerbini, C. A., Milmont, C. E., Chen, L., Maddox, J., Meisner, P. D., Libanati, C., & Grauer, A. (2016). Romosozumab treatment in postmenopausal women with osteoporosis. *New England Journal of Medicine, 375*(16), 1532–1543. https://doi.org/10.1056/NEJMoa1607948

Cosman, F., de Beur. S. J., LeBoff., M. S., Lewiecki, E. F., Tanner, B., Randall, S., & Lindsay, R. (2014). Clinician's guide to prevention and treatment of osteoporosis. *Osteoporosis International, 25*(10), 2359–2381. https://doi.org/10.1007/s00198-014-2794-2

Cosman, F., Nieves, J. W., & Dempster, D. W. (2017). Treatment sequence matters: Anabolic and antiresorptive therapy for osteoporosis. *Journal of Bone and Mineral Research, 32*(2):198–202. https://doi.org/10.1002/jbmr.3051

Crandall, J. C. (Ed.). (2019). *Menopause practice: A clinician guide* (6th ed.). The North American Menopause Society. ISBN 978-0-578-53228-8

Diab, D., & Watts, N. (2014). Use of drug holidays in women taking bisphosphonates. *Menopause, 21(2)*, 195–197. https://doi.org/10.1097/GME.0b013e31829ef343.

National Osteoporosis Foundation. (2013). *Clinician's guide to prevention and treatment of osteoporosis.* Author. https://my.nof.org/bone-source/education/clinicians-guide-to-the-prevention-and-treatment-of-osteoporosis

Nelson, H. D., Haney, E. M., Chou, R., Dana, T., Fu, R., & Bougatsos, C. (2010). *Screening for osteoporosis: Systematic review to update the 2002 U.S. Preventive Services Task Force Recommendation. Evidence Synthesis No. 77* (AHRQ Publication No. 10-05145-EF-1). Agency for Healthcare Research and Quality.

North American Menopause Society. (2010). Management of osteoporosis in postmenopausal women: 2010 position statement of the North American Menopause Society. *Menopause, 17*(1), 25–54. https://doi.org/10.1097/gme.0b013e3181c617e6

Qaseem, A., Forciea, M. A., McLean, R. M., & Denberg, T. D. (2017). Treatment of low bone density or osteoporosis to prevent fractures in men and women: A clinical practice guideline update from the American College of Physicians. *Annals of Internal Medicine, 166*(11), 818–839. https://doi.org/10.7326/M15-1361

Siris, E., & Delmas, P. D. (2008). Assessment of 10-year absolute fracture risk: A new paradigm with worldwide application. *Osteoporosis International, (19)*4, 383–384. https://doi.org/10.1007/s00198-008-0564-8

Szulc, P., & Delmas, P. D. (2008). Biochemical markers of bone turnover: Potential use in the investigation and management of postmenopausal osteoporosis. *Osteoporosis International, 19*(12), 1683–1704. https://doi.org/10.1007/s00198-008-0660-9.

Tsourdi, E., Langdahl, B., Cohen-Solal, M., Aubry-Rozier, B., Eriksen, E. F., Guañabens, N., Obermayer-Pietsch, B., Ralston, S. H., Eastell, R., & Zillikens, M. C. (2017). Discontinuation of denosumab therapy for osteoporosis: A systematic review and position statement by ECTS. *Bone, 105*, 11–17. https://doi.org/10.1016/j.bone.2017.08.003

Wagner, E. H., Williams, C. A., Greenberg, R., Kleinbaum, D., Wolf, S. H., & Ibrahim, M. A. (2009). Simply ask them about their balance—Future fracture risk in a national cohort study of twins. *American Journal of Epidemiology, 169*, 143. https://doi.org/10.1093/aje/kwn379

Welcome to FRAX®. (n.d.). https://www.sheffield.ac.uk/FARX

24

GENITOURINARY SYNDROME OF MENOPAUSE AND VULVOVAGINAL ATROPHY

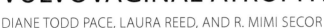

DIANE TODD PACE, LAURA REED, AND R. MIMI SECOR

GENITOURINARY SYNDROME OF MENOPAUSE EXPLAINED

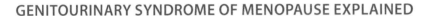

A. Epidemiology
   1. In the United States, it is estimated that 1.3 million women become postmenopausal each year. Natural menopause typically occurs between the ages of 40 to 58. The number of women expected to be at age 50 by the year 2060 is approximately 90 million.
   2. Today, a woman of age 54 years can expect to reach age 84.3 years and spend one third of her life in the period known as *postmenopause.*
   3. Of all post-menopausal women, 45% to 50% will experience symptoms of genitourinary syndrome of menopause (GSM) with greater than 64 million menopausal women in the United States suffering from GSM.
   4. Previously known by the term vulvovaginal atrophy (VVA) or vulvovaginitis, the term genitourinary syndrome of menopause (GSM) was recommended by the boards of the North American Menopause Society (NAMS) and the International Society for the Study of Women's Sexual Health (ISSWSH) in 2014.
      a. GSM is a comprehensive term that includes symptomatic vulvar and vaginal atrophy. ISSWSH and NAMS concluded that the commonly used terms VVA and atrophic vaginitis did not accurately encompass the full breadth of menopausal symptoms associated with physical changes of the vulva, vagina, and lower urinary tract associated with estrogen deficiency.
      b. Additionally, the organizations determined the terms did not clearly communicate the constellation of symptoms that include but are not limited to the genital symptoms of dryness, burning, and irritation; the sexual symptoms, including lack of lubrication, discomfort or pain, and impaired function; and the urinary symptoms of urgency, dysuria, and recurrent urinary tract infections.

PATHOPHYSIOLOGY

A. Atrophic urogenital changes can occur not only during postmenopause, but also during perimenopause, often well in advance of cessation of menses. Vulvovaginal mucosal tissues contain many estrogen receptors that are commonly affected by lower levels of estrogen (Box 24.1).

B. As the vaginal walls become thinner, there is decreased support of the pelvic organs, adjacent muscles, and ligaments.

C. The drop in estrogen causes a decrease in glycogen-reducing lactobacilli resulting in an elevation in vaginal pH (from acid to alkaline). This is frequently associated with overgrowth of various pathogenic bacteria such as *Gardnerella vaginalis*, mycoplasma, streptococci, and other bacterial organisms (Figure 24.1).

BOX 24.1 Causes of Urogenital Atrophy

Antiestrogen medications
- Leuprolide (Lupron)
- Clomiphene (Clomid)
- Medroxyprogesterone (Provera)
- DMPA (DepoProvera) contraceptive injection
- Nafarelin acetate (Synarel)
- Tamoxifen citrate (Nolvadex)
- Danazol (Danocrine)

Postpartum: Precipitous drop in estrogen
Breastfeeding: Antagonistic action of prolactin on estrogen
Premenopausal: Premature ovarian failure
Perimenopausal: Variable estrogen levels
Menopause: Low estrogen levels

Other causes
- Surgery (oophorectomy)
- Chemotherapy
- Radiation
- Heavy smoking: Reduced estrogen levels
- Reduced sexual activity
- Inadequate systemic estrogen replacement therapy: Often inadequate for treatment of VVA/GA

DMPA, depot medroxyprogesterone acetate; GA, genital atrophy; VVA, vulvovaginal atrophy.

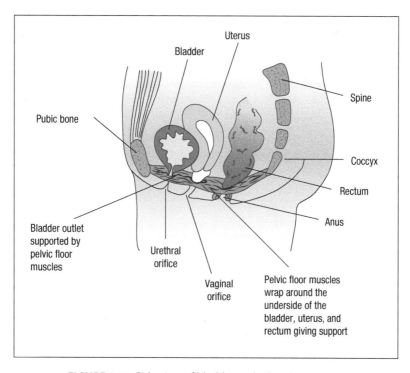

FIGURE 24.1 Side view of bladder and related structures.

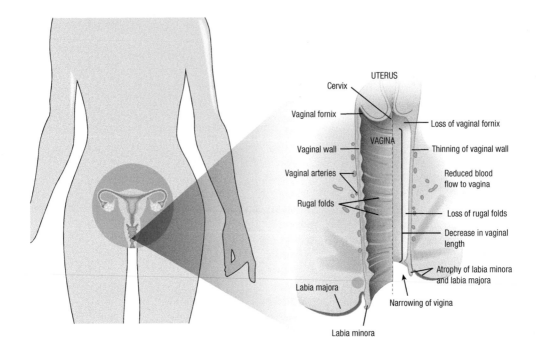

FIGURE 24.2 Changes in vaginal anatomy associated with atropy after menopause.
Source: TherapeuticsMD.

D. Reduced estrogen may also result in a reduced blood flow, loss of collagen, elasticity, and muscle tone (Figure 24.2). Thinning of the urogenital epithelium leads to various symptoms associated with GSM, including dyspareunia and pruritus.

E. Similar tissue changes may involve the urinary tract and contribute to dysuria, incontinence, urinary frequency, and increased risk of urinary tract infections.

F. Symptoms and signs of GSM may develop slowly, over many months or years, or may be a more rapid onset.

G. Symptoms vary and are influenced by factors such as an individual's estrogen levels and response to these levels.

H. Change in Vaginal Maturation Index (VMI)

1. With the decrease in estrogen during menopause, there is a change in the ratio of four vaginal epithelial cell types (Figures 24.3 and 24.4). The changes in ratio of these cell types can be measured by the vaginal maturation index (VMI). The VMI provides an objective assessment of the estrogen status of the vaginal epithelium and related genital structures (vulva, urethra, bladder). The types of cells are:

   a. **Basal:** Least mature; less differentiated; rarely visible; round in circumference

   b. **Parabasal:** Adjacent/above the basal cells; nucleus fills a larger portion of cells; round in circumference; often becomes top layer in thin, atrophic vagina replacing normal mature epithelial cells

   c. **Intermediate:** Nucleus becomes smaller and cytoplasm increases; becomes flatter and more cuboidal

   d. **Superficial:** Line the well-estrogenized vagina; represent a mature, well-differentiated epithelium; composed of larger, flat, squared-off cells with even smaller nuclei and increasing amounts of cytoplasm. Normally shed in latter half of menstrual cycle and comprise normal vaginal discharge. Represent outer layer of cells most commonly visible on a routine cytolytic examination.

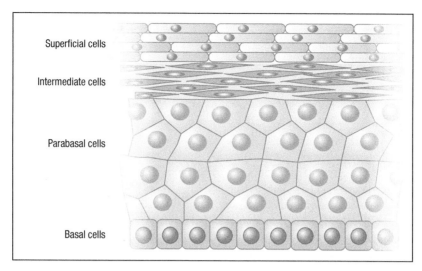

FIGURE 24.3 Layers of the vaginal epithelium. Note how cells layer on top of each other from bottom to top, thickening the vaginal wall.

2. The higher the number of mature cells, the higher the maturation index or "estrogen" effect on the vaginal mucosa.
3. In menopause with decreasing estrogen, there is an increase in parabasal cells and a decrease in the mature superficial cells. This leads to changes that can be visualized on the physical exam (discussed earlier).
4. A cytological examination can be performed to evaluate the ratio.

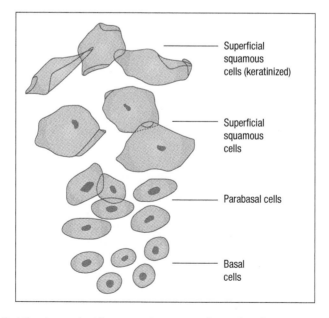

FIGURE 24.4 Note that the size evolves from round to square, the nucleus becomes smaller and the amount of cytoplasm increases, until the top layer of superficial squamous cells do not even have a nucleus.

INDICATIONS FOR EVALUATION

A. The complaint of urogenital symptoms is an indication for a thorough workup.

B. A detailed medical history that includes a sexual health history that identifies signs or symptoms of GSM.

ASSESSMENT

A. **Subjective:** A history of symptoms may include the following:
1. Vulvovaginal symptoms
    a. Vulvar dryness, lack of lubrication, pruritus, irritation, and vaginal discharge
2. Vaginal bleeding
    a. Due to tissue thinning and friability, vaginal spotting is often a presenting symptom. The source of bleeding must be determined and, if necessary, a transvaginal ultrasound and/or a biopsy should be performed. According to an American College of Obstetricians and Gynecologists (ACOG) statement, when the results from the transvaginal ultrasound reports an endometrial echo of ≤4mm, an endometrial biopsy is not required. An endometrial biopsy may be indicated and/or a referral to gynecology may also be appropriate.
    b. Bleeding may be noticed after sex or after wiping with toilet tissue.
3. Dyspareunia
    a. Also known as *painful intercourse*, dyspareunia may result from stretching or tearing of the thin, narrowed introital mucosa, or from stretching of the dry, less elastic, thinner, and shorter vagina. Dyspareunia may be superficial, with symptoms occurring at the vaginal opening, or "deep" with symptoms occurring inside the vagina.
    b. These changes are less likely to occur if sexual relations are maintained during perimenopause and beyond (the "use it or lose it" phenomenon).
4. Low libido and other sexual complaints, such as lack of lubrication, dyspareunia, and distress, may be associated with atrophic and/or sexual complaints.
5. Urinary symptoms
    a. The lower urinary tract and pelvic musculature contain estrogen receptors and are under the influence of estrogen and share a common embryologic origin with the vagina.
    b. Squamous epithelium of the trigone and urethra becomes thin and blood flow decreases when estrogen levels are low.
    c. Urinary symptoms related to low estrogen levels include dysuria, hematuria, frequency, nocturia, urinary incontinence (usually stress type), sensation of a dropped bladder, and history of frequent urinary tract infections.
6. Hematuria is commonly associated with GSM and must be thoroughly evaluated. Although uncommon, it can be a symptom of bladder cancer.

B. Gynecologic history may include
1. Menstrual history, including last menstrual period (LMP), first menstrual period (FMP), abnormal bleeding, history of hot flashes, night sweats, or flushing
2. Age of biological mother or sisters at time of menopause onset
3. Date of last Pap test, results, history of abnormal Pap, and management
4. Sexual history, including dyspareunia, dryness, sexual partner (gender), date of last sex, frequency of sexual activity, kinds of activities engaged in, use of lubricants, distress related to symptoms, relationship status/issues
5. Total hysterectomy is often associated with moderate to severe GSM and symptoms may be severe due to the sudden reduction in estrogen levels.

C. Medical history may include diabetes, cardiovascular disease, thyroid issues, anemia, psychiatric disorders.

D. Medication history may include psychiatric medications such as selective serotonin reuptake inhibitors (SSRIs) benzodiazepines, tricyclics; hormonal agents including oral contraceptives; cardiovascular agents such as beta blockers, digoxin, clonidine; and other medications including Dilantin, ketoconazole, and indomethacin.

BOX 24.2 Physical Examination: Characteristics of Genitourinary Syndrome of Menopause

The physical examination should include (Box 24.2 summarizes the characteristic symptoms of urogenital atrophy):

Labia (majora and minora)
- Less prominent, flattened
- Fusion of labia minora
- Lax and wrinkled (lack of subcutaneous fat)
- Thinning cell layer
- Prominent sebaceous glands
- Positive "sticky glove" sign
- Easily traumatized (fissures, erythema, excoriations)
- Irritation due to continuous use of pads for urinary incontinence

Clitoris
- Less prominent
- Retracts beneath the prepuce
- Slight atrophy

Subcutaneous fat
- Diminished

Pubic hair
- Thinning
- Less coarse

Vaginal wall epithelium
- Thin (a few layers thick)
- Friable
- Shiny
- Small ulcerations
- Patches of granulation tissue
- Petechial spots (resemble trichomoniasis)
- Fissures
- Ecchymotic areas from exposed capillaries (mottling appearance)
- Loss of rugae
- Decreased vascularity (pale)
- Less lubrication (dryness)
- Loss of distensibility, elasticity
- Decreased or increased discharge may occur

(continued)

BOX 24.2 Physical Examination: Characteristics of Genitourinary Syndrome of Menopause (*Continued*)

Vagina
- Introital stenosis (less than two fingers in diameter)
- Shortened
- Shrinkage of fornices
- Less elasticity
- Possible cystocele, rectocele, or pelvic prolapse

Discharge
- *Variable quantity and quality*
- *Watery to thick, white, yellow/green*
- *May be serosanguineous from friable surfaces*

Maturation index
- Predominance of parabasal and basal cells, few superficial cells

Vaginal wet mount/microscopy
- Elevated pH
- Negative amine/KOH whiff test
- Reduced LB, increased WBCs, negative for clue cells, trichomoniasis, yeast

Cervix
- Shrinks, flattens into vaginal wall
- Os often becomes tiny, may even be difficult to identify
- Squamocolumnar junction recedes up the cervical canal and may become stenotic

Uterus
- Smaller
- Endometrium thins—less glandular, atrophic
- Uterine stripe less than 4 mm
- Fibroids may shrink (due to low estrogen)

Perineum
- Minor fissures or superficial lacerations within the posterior fourchette, perineum

Urethra
- Caruncle—red, berry-type protrusion, often friable
- Atrophy
- Polyps
- Prolapse/eversion of urethral mucosa

Pelvic floor
- Muscle tone diminishes
- Cystocele
- Rectocele

Ligaments and connective tissue
- Loss of strength and tone

Bladder mucosa and urethra
- Decreased tone

KOH, potassium hydroxide; LB, lactobacilli; WBC, white blood cells.

A. Annual wellness exam

B. Menopausal woman physical exam
1. External genitalia examination
   a. Note thinning of hair and tissues, pallor, erythema, lesions, fissures, loss of architectural landmarks, introital shrinkage, vulvar atrophy, pallor, erythema (diffuse vs. focal), and tenderness.
   b. Vulvar dryness and/or positive "sticky glove" sign, which occurs when the examiner's glove adheres temporarily and is considered diagnostic for GSM.
   c. Urethral caruncle
      (1) Small friable polyp of urethral mucosa that protrudes from the inferior border of the urethral meatus (Figure 24.5)
      (2) Associated with symptoms of dysuria, frequency, and may be the cause of vaginal bleeding in the menopausal woman.
2. Vaginal examination
   a. Cystocele, rectocele, and grade
   b. Tenderness with palpation or during speculum insertion and/or examination
   c. Note vaginal pallor, erythema, lesions, loss of rugae (flattening), lesions, shortening of vagina, loss of elasticity, tenderness
   d. **Discharge:** Variable quantity ranging from scant to copious, and variable quality ranging from thin to thick, clumpy, smooth, and varying color from white to yellow/green and possibly malodorous
   e. **Cervix:** Erythema, lesions, friability, bleeding, tenderness, flattening and shortening, stenosis of cervical os (small)
3. Bimanual examination
   a. Uterus

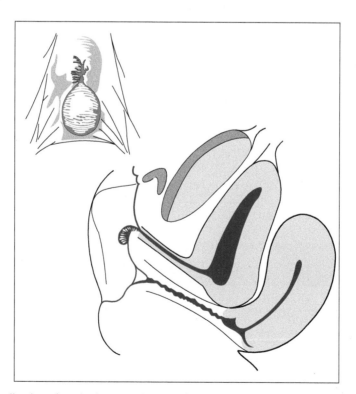

FIGURE 24.5 Small polyp of urethral mucosa in sagittal section and shown protruding from the inferior border of the urethral meatus.

      (1) Size, shape, especially asymmetry (associated with fibroids that usually shrink in menopause); diffuse enlargement associated with pregnancy or pathology such as hyperplasia, tenderness, sometimes fibroids

  b. Pelvic floor

      (1) Note cystocele, rectocele, introital tone with Kegels, and Valsalva maneuver.

  c. Ovaries

      (1) In menopause, ovaries should *not* be palpable.

      (2) If ovaries are palpable, a timely and thorough workup is indicated.

DIAGNOSTIC TESTING AND DIFFERENTIAL DIAGNOSIS

A. Differential considerations (Table 24.1)

  1. Vaginal pH

    a. Atrophic vaginitis is associated with a significantly elevated vaginal pH, usually greater than 5.

      (1) A normal vaginal pH (4.0–4.6) indicates normal circulating estrogen levels and rules out VVA.

      (2) A high pH is due to the lack of LB, which produce lactic acid.

    b. Many factors can alter the vaginal pH results (Box 24.3).

  2. Amine testing with potassium hydroxide (KOH)

    a. If negative, bacterial vaginosis (BV) is unlikely, and GSM must be considered, especially if the vaginal pH is also elevated.

  3. Vaginal microscopy

    a. Note reduced or absent LB.

    b. Note the immature epithelial cells indicating low estrogen.

    c. Rule out trichomoniasis. If microscopy is equivocal for the identification of *Trichomonas*, a trichomoniasis culture or office test (i.e., Affirm or Osom tests) should be done. Trichomoniasis may be asymptomatic for decades and reactivate in perimenopause or postmenopause. The clinical presentation may mimic that of GSM. Prevalence of trichomoniasis in women older than 40 years may be as high as 10% to 15% according to recent research.

    d. Genital herpes, a lifelong viral infection, is often an unrecognized infection and shed intermittently by persons unaware that they have the infection or who are asymptomatic when transmission occurs. The vesicular or ulcerative lesions classically associated with the disorder are often absent/not visualized in many infected persons at the time of the clinical exam.

    e. If white blood cells (WBCs) are noted, this is most likely related to atrophic effects, which will usually resolve when local estrogen (or an agent that acts like estrogen such as oral ospemifene or vaginal DHEA) is administered and maintained.

TABLE 24.1 Differential Considerations in the Diagnosis of Genitourinary Syndrome of Menopause

DIFFERENTIAL	PH	KOH	MICROSCOPY
VVA	≥5.0	Negative	Few LB, WBCs variable, immature ECs
Trichomoniasis	>5.0	Negative	Trichomonads, WBCs, immature ECs, few LB
BV	>4.7	Positive	Clue cells, few WBCs, few LB

ECs, epithelial cells; KOH, potassium hydroxide; LB, lactobacilli; VVA, vulvovaginal atrophy; WBCs, white blood cells.

BOX 24.3 Factors Affecting Vaginal pH

- Menses (pH 7.2)
- Semen (pH ≥ 7)
- Cervical mucus (pH ≥ 7)
- Lubricant from speculum and/or gloves
- Intravaginal medication
- Tap water

---

    f. Sexually transmitted infections (STIs) must be ruled out, especially if WBCs are noted. STIs are increasing in older adults, so assessing risk is important and should include clinical assessment (history and examination), determining age of sexual partners, use of condoms, and sexual behaviors.

TREATMENT CONSIDERATIONS

A. According to the NAMS GSM position statement, the focus of clinical treatment for women is to alleviate symptoms, and a stepwise approach might be appropriate, depending on the severity of the disorder. First-line interventions include use of non-prescription, non-scented, non-warming vaginal moisturizers/lubricants. Moisturizers can be used three times a week, whereas lubricants are used during sexual penetration to reduce friction for dry, irritated vaginal tissue. The World Health Organization recommends products with an osmolarity of <1,200 milliosmoles/kg of water since *hyper-osmotic* moisturizers can pull moisture out of cells, actually drying the tissue, and those that are *hypo-osmotic* can cause cells to pull water out of the moisturizer/lubricant, causing them to swell and rupture. Additionally, other lifestyle modifications can be suggested to help with vaginal health such as regular sexual activity to promote blood flow to the genital area and to help maintain vaginal health and non-penetrative sexual activity such as massage or oral stimulation. Also suggest avoiding scented panty liners and smoking.

B. Because GSM pathology is based on decreasing estrogen occurring in menopause, these first line interventions will not prevent or treat the disorder.

C. Currently there are three FDA-approved pharmacologic options available to treat GSM.
    1. Estrogens
        a. All systemic estrogens are indicated for treating VVA/GSM as well as managing vasomotor symptoms (VMS) and preventing osteoporosis. However, if the woman only needs intervention for GSM, topical vaginal estrogen is preferred to systemic and is considered safer with less risk/side effects due to lower/no systemic absorption of the drug. Some women, however, on systemic estrogen may also require additional topical vaginal estrogen to treat severe symptoms of GSM in addition to systemic management of VMS.
        b. The "environment" of the vagina is affected by decreasing estrogen changes of menopause which may lead to recurrent UTIs, candidiasis, and bacterial vaginosis. Administration of estrogen can reverse changes by reducing vaginal pH and increasing production of lactobacilli.
        c. Low-dose vaginal estrogens include creams, a tablet, a low-dose ring, and a vaginal insert. Patients often complain creams are "messy" and the tablet must be inserted by an applicator which often is uncomfortable when a woman is highly symptomatic.

d. The newer vaginal soft-gel insert can be inserted without an applicator at any time of the day and adheres to the vaginal mucosa which prevents disruption of daily activities and is not "messy." Two doses are available: a low dose and ultra-low dose. Initial dosing is daily for 2 weeks then two times a week as maintenance.

e. The low-dose estrogen ring is inserted into the upper third of the vagina and releases approximately 7.5 mcg per day for 90 days, then replaced. The clinician should be aware there are two vaginal rings and ensure they prescribe the low dose versus the higher dose systemic estrogen used for managing VMS symptoms.

f. Two vaginal creams are available (conjugated equine estrogen/CEE or estradiol): Recommended dosing is 0.5–1.0 g intravaginally once daily for 2 weeks, followed by a maintenance dose of 0.5 g two to three times weekly. This can be administered by an applicator or by applying a small/pea-sized amount of the cream by the finger to the introital area.

g. The low dose vaginal tablet is dosed at daily for 2 weeks then 1 tablet twice a week. It must be administered by an applicator.

h. Research has demonstrated that serum estradiol levels in menopausal women using low-dose vaginal estrogen therapy remains within post-menopausal range (no systemic effect). Because of this finding, a concomitant progestogen with low-dose vaginal estrogen is not needed for women who have a uterus.

i. A 2020 online survey identified gaps in provider awareness of the boxed warning and comfort level in counseling women about low-dose vaginal estrogen. The boxed warning is linked to the *class effect* of estrogen from the large Women's Health Initiative Study, however research has failed to show its application to the low dose topical vaginal estrogen due to its very low/no systemic absorption. Women must be adequately counseled on the warning so they are not anxious about using the product.

j. Survivors of breast cancer, particularly individuals treated with aromatase inhibitors, often have significant complaints of GSM. Treatment with estrogen is a complex issue. Because data have not demonstrated an increased risk of recurrence in survivors with use of vaginal estrogen, both NAMS and ACOG have endorsed the use of low dose vaginal estrogen for treatment of GSM in collaboration with the patient's oncologist.

k. If BV is present with GSM, either local estrogen alone may be used, or BV may be treated initially then followed by local estrogen. If estrogen has been stopped and BV recurs, local estrogen should be restarted (or a nonestrogen equivalent, such as oral ospemifene or vaginal DHEA, daily without taper) and used daily for 2 to 6 weeks, then twice weekly for long-term maintenance to prevent BV. Estrogen supports the regrowth and maintenance of LB, which is thought to help prevent recurrent BV infections and recurrent GSM postmenopause.

2. DHEA

a. Vaginal dehydroepiandrosterone (DHEA), also FDA approved for the treatment of GSM as Prasterone, is a vaginal insert administered daily at bedtime by an applicator. It is a steroid hormone which is transformed by the vaginal mucosal cells to estradiol and androgens including testosterone.

b. DHEA does not have a boxed warning. However, it has not been studied in the breast cancer population and should be used with caution until further data can be obtained. It should be reassuring to clinicians, however, that in the American Society of Clinical Oncology Clinical Practice Guideline Interventions to Address Sexual Problems in People with Cancer, a recommendation was included for use of this therapy in treatment of GSM for women with current or history of breast cancer and on aromatase inhibitors who have not responded to previous interventions.

3. Selective estrogen receptor modulator (SERM)
   a. The only FDA approved oral prescription option for treating GSM is ospemifene, a selective estrogen-receptor modulator (SERM) administered daily.
   b. This drug has the same outcomes as estrogen through increasing superficial cells, decreasing parabasal cells, and reducing vaginal pH thereby relieving both moderate to severe vaginal dryness and moderate to severe dyspareunia due to menopause. The side effect profile is favorable; however, warnings should be reviewed with the patient when considering this medication. Vasomotor symptoms were the most common adverse event.

D. Other treatment options
   1. Vaginal dilators/vibrators
      a. Ideally, if a menopausal woman has not had penetrative intercourse for several years, she may need counseling regarding vaginal dilators to help in stretching the vagina. Encourage her to moisturize/lubricate before using dilators. They can be used alone or with a partner.
      b. Vibrators may help older women before and during partnered sex or for self-stimulation, to help a woman reach orgasm by increasing genital sensation, and to maintain healthy vaginal tissues between sexual encounters and/or sexual partners.
   2. Vulvovaginal energy-based devices
      a. Devices include lasers and radio-frequency devices being used by clinicians as treatments for GSM. Although they have been marketed for treatment of GSM, as of 2021 however, none have FDA approval for this indication. The procedures are relatively expensive, require multiple interventions, and insurance may or may not cover the cost of the therapy.
      b. These devices induce collagen formation, angiogenesis, and epithelial thickening which in turn is found to improve vaginal health.
      c. Safety of these devices has been questioned as there have been complaints of discomfort and findings of vaginal scarring, lacerations on resumption of intercourse, and persistent or worsening dyspareunia.
      d. Currently there are some published studies including randomized controlled trials on efficacy and safety and continuing studies are in progress. However, additional trials still are needed before these therapies can be routinely recommended for treatment of GSM.

E. Pelvic floor physical therapy
   1. Often unremitting vaginal or pelvic pain occurs alongside GSM. The physical exam can help in determining the cause of such pain and if other treatment is needed for such causes such as infection. However, considering a referral to a pelvic floor physical therapist is such an asset in helping in the care of the patient with GSM having pelvic pain, incontinence, and other causes of dyspareunia. The pelvic floor physical therapist uses hands-on therapy to stretch, strengthen, and relax muscles in the lower pelvis and massage-like technique, known as myofascial release, to help stretch and release fascia.

F. ASSECT certified therapists
   1. During the history taking of women during menopause, it is important to obtain a sexual history. Research has demonstrated less than 81% of clinicians initiate this conversation although sexuality is a quality-of-life issue, and women with GSM often experience dyspareunia which may lead to other sexual issues. The VIVA and REVIVE trials both showed that women reported that symptoms of GSM often had an approximately 75% negative effect on their "sex lives." If investigation of these issues is reported, and resolving the clinical issues of GSM does not resolve the issues, consider referring the woman to an ASECT certified sex therapist. These therapists are licensed mental health professionals, specialized in treating clients with sexual issues and concerns.

FOLLOW-UP

A. Follow-up visits may range from 2 weeks to 3 to 12 months based on the severity of the patient's problem, response to therapy, and clinician recommendation.

RESOURCES

- Menopro App (Care of postmenopausal women; NAMS)
- The North American Menopause Society (NAMS): www.menopause.org
- www.MiddlesexMD.com
- AASECT: https://www.aasect.org/aasect-certified-sex-therapist-0

BIBLIOGRAPHY

American College of Obstetricians and Gynecologists. (2018). ACOG Committee Opinion NO. 734: The role of transvaginal ultrasonography in evaluating the endometrium of women with postmenopausal bleeding. *Obstetrics and Gynecology, 131*(5), e124–e129. https://doi.org/10.1097/AOG.0000000000002631

Alshiek, J., Garcia, B., Minassian, V., Iglesia, C. B., Clark, A., Sokol, E. R., Murphy, M., Malik, S. A., Tran, A. & Shobeiri, S. A. (2020). Vaginal energy-based devices. *Female Pelvic Medicine & Reconstructive Surgery, 26*(5), 287–298. https://doi.org/10.1097/SPV.0000000000000872.

Chen, F., Dagur, G., Smith, N., Cali, B., & Khan, S. A. (2016). Genitoruinary syndrome of menopause: An overview of clinical manifestations, pathophysiology, etiology, evaluation and management. *American Journal of Obstetrics and Gynecology, 215*(6), 704–711. https://doi.org/10.1016/j.ajog.2016.07.045

Crandall, J. C. (Ed.). (2019). *Menopause Practice: A clinician guide* (6th ed.). The North American Menopause Society. ISBN 978-0-578-53228-8

Edwards, D., & Panay, N. (2016). Treating vulvovaginal atrophy/genitourinary syndrome of menopause: How important is vaginal lubricant and moisturizer composition? *Climacteric, 19*(2), 151–161. https://doi.org/10.3109/13697137.2015.1124259

Hodges, A. L., Holland, A. C., Dehn, B., & Pace, D. T. (2018). Diagnosis and treatment of genitourinary syndrome of menopause. *Nursing for Women's Health, 22*(5), 423–430. https://doi.org/10.1016/j.nwh.2018.07.005

Kagan, R., Kellogg-Spadt, S., & Parish, S. J. (2019). Practical treatment considerations in the management of genitourinary syndrome of menopause. *Drugs & Aging, 36*(10), 897–908. https://doi.org/10.1007/s40266-019-00700-w

Kingsberg, S. A., & Krychman, M. L. (2013). Resistance and barriers to local estrogen therapy in women with atrophic vaginitis. *Journal of Sexual Medicine, 10*, 1567–1574. https://doi.org/10.1111/jsm.12120.

Kingsberg, S. et al. (2016). The Women's EMPOWER Survey: Identifying women's perceptions on vulvar and vaginal atrophy (VVA) and treatment. *Menopause. 23*, 1363–1407.

Kingsberg, S. A., Krychman, M., Graham, S., Bernick, B., & Mirkin, S. (2017). The Women's EMPOWER Survey: Identifying women's perceptions on vulvar and vaginal atrophy and its treatment. *Journal of Sexual Medicine, 14*(13), 413–424. https://doi.org/10.1016/j.jsxm.2017.01.010

Krychman, M. L., Shifren, J. L., Liu, J. H., Kingsberg, S. L., & Utian, W.H. (2015). Laser treatment safe for vulvovaginal atrophy? *Medscape.* https://www.medscape.com/viewarticle/846960.

Labrie, F., Archer, D. F., Koltun, W., Vachon, A., Young, D., Frenette, L., . . . Moyneur, É.; VVA Prasterone Research Group. (2016). Efficacy of intravaginal dehydroepiandrosterone (DHEA) on moderate to severe dyspareunia and vaginal dryness, symptoms of vulvovaginal atrophy, and of the genitourinary syndrome of menopause. *Menopause, 23*(3), 243–256. https://doi.org/10.1097/GME.0000000000000571

Labrie, F., Derogatis, L., Archer, D. F., Koltun, W., Vachon, A., Young, D., . . . Moyneur, É.; Members of the VVA Prasterone Research Group. (2015). Effect of intravaginal prasterone on sexual dysfunction in postmenopausal women with vulvovaginal atrophy. *Journal of Sexual Medicine, 12*(12), 2401–2412. https://doi.org/10.1111/jsm.13045

Pace, D. T., Chism, L. A., Graham, S., & Amadio, J. (2019). How nurse practitioners approach treatment of genitourinary syndrome of menopause. *The Journal for Nurse Practitioners, 16*(2), https://doi.org/10.1016j.nurpra.2019.11.019

Pinkerton, J. V., Kaunitz, A. M. & Manson, J. E. (2018). Not time to abandon use of local vaginal hormone therapies. *Menopause, 25*(8), 855–858. https://doi.org/10.1097/GME.0000000000001142.

Portman DJ, Gass ML (2014). Vulvovaginal atrophy terminology consensus conference panel. Genitourinary syndrome of menopause: New terminology for vulvovaginal atrophy from the international society for the study of women's sexual health and the North American Menopause Society. *Menopause, 21*(10), 1063–1068. https://doi.org/10.1097/GME.0000000000000329

Portman, D. J., Bachmann, G. A., & Simon, J. A.; Ospemifene Study Group. (2013). Ospemifene, a novel selective estrogen receptor modulator for treating dyspareunia associated with postmenopausal vulvar and vaginal atrophy. *Menopause, 20*(6), 623–630. https://doi.org/10.1097/gme.0b013e318279ba64

Santen, R. J., Pinkerton, J. V., Liu, J. H., Matsumoto, A. M., Lobo, R. A., Davis, S. R., & Simon, J. A. (2020). Workshop on normal reference ranges for estradiol in postmenopausal women (September, 2019, Chicago, Illinois). *Menopause, 27*(6), 614–624. https://doi.org/10.1097/GME.0000000000001556.

Shifren, J. L. (2018). Genitourinary syndrome of menopause. *Clinical Obstetrics and Gynecology, 61*(3), 508–516. https://doi.org/10.1097/GRF.0000000000000380

Shifren, J. L., & Gass, M. L. (2014). The North American Menopause Society recommendations for clinical care of midlife women. *Menopause, 21*(10), 1038–1062. https://doi.org/10.1097/GME.0000000000000319

Simon, J. A., Kokot-Kierepa, M., Goldstein, J., & Nappi, R. E. (2013). Vaginal health in the United States: Results from the vaginal health: Insights, views & attitudes survey. *Menopause, 20*(10), 1043–1048. https://doi.org/10.1097/GME.0b013e318287342d

Spadt, S. K. & Larkin, L. C. (2021). Genitourinary syndrome of menopause. *Menopause, 28*(4). https://doi.org/10.1097/GME.0000000000001701.

The North American Menopause Society. (2020). The 2020 genitourinary syndrome of menopause position statement of the North American Menopause Society. *Menopause, 27*(9), 976–992. https://doi.org/10.1097/GME.0000000000001609.

25

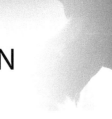

ASSESSMENT OF PELVIC PAIN

BETH R. STEINFELD, SAMANTHA DEBRA IERVOLINO, AND
AMY MANDEVILLE O'MEARA

PELVIC PAIN

A. Definition
1. Pelvic pain refers to pain in the region of a woman's internal reproductive organs.
2. It may be a symptom of infection or may arise from pain in the pelvic bone area or in nonreproductive internal organs, such as the bladder or colon.
3. It can very well be an indication that there may be a problem with one of the reproductive organs in the pelvic area (uterus, ovaries, fallopian tubes, cervix, or vagina).
4. It is important to do a thorough health history assessment and focused physical examination (see Chapter 3, "The Health History" and Chapter 5, "The Physical Exam").

PELVIC PAIN ASSESSMENT

A. Symptom review (Box 25.1)
1. Location of pain
2. **Description of pain:** Sharp, dull, throbbing, intermittent, and continuous
3. Does pain radiate?
4. What activities, if any, make the pain worse?
5. What measures, if any, relieve the pain?
6. Any unintentional or recent weight gain or loss?
7. Rate pain on a scale of 1 to 10, 10 being the worst.
8. Has similar pain occurred before?
9. Presence of urinary or gastrointestinal symptoms or systemic symptoms of fever, fatigue, etc.
    a. Diarrhea or blood in stool or urine
10. Vaginal bleeding or discharge
11. Pain with intercourse; specify superficial, deep or both
12. Timing in relation to menses, change in character

BOX 25.1 Pelvic Pain Assessment: COLDERR

- Character: What does the pain feel like (sharp, dull, crampy)?
- Onset: Does the pain come on suddenly or gradually? Is it cyclic or constant?
- Location: Is the pain localized or diffuse?
- Duration: How long has the pain been present and how has it changed over time?
- Exacerbation: What activities or movements make it worse?
- Relief: What medication, activities, and positions make it better?
- Radiation: Does the pain radiate anywhere (back, groin, flank, shoulder)?

---

13. Sexual history
    a. Exposure to sexually transmitted infections (STIs)
    b. Change in sexual partner
    c. Unprotected intercourse
    d. Change in contraception
    e. Use of sex toys
14. Pelvic surgery, especially in past 12 to 24 months

B. Abdominal assessment
   1. Scars indicate previous surgery or injury; penetration of the peritoneum may result in adhesions.
   2. Bowel sounds may be altered by paralytic ileus, peritonitis, intestinal obstruction, diarrhea.
   3. Percussing
      a. Tympany may suggest intestinal obstruction.
      b. Dullness may suggest enlarged liver or spleen, distended bladder, pregnancy, or tumor.
   4. Palpation
      a. **Light palpation:** Persistent involuntary muscle spasm with relaxation suggests peritoneal inflammation (acute abdomen).
      b. **Deep palpation:** Sources of masses include tumors, pregnant uterus, bowel obstruction, abdominal aortic aneurism.
   5. **Pain mapping:** A process by which the patient and provider identify and document the exact location and intensity of pain; patients may also do this outside of the office visit if pain is not active at that time.

C. Pelvic examination (see Chapter 5, "The Physical Exam")
   1. Pelvic muscles (see Chapter 31, "Pelvic Organ Prolapse")
   2. Visualize vagina and cervix
   3. Assess uterine size, mobility, cul-de-sac nodularity
   4. Ovaries (*Note:* should be non-palpable in post menopause.)

D. Cervical motion tenderness (Chandelier sign)
   1. Traditionally associated with pelvic inflammatory disease (PID) and may also be seen in the following:
      a. Present in 28% of patients with appendicitis (*Note:* Usually limited to right side with appendicitis, and is usually bilateral with PID.)
      b. Ectopic pregnancy
      c. Endometriosis
      d. Ovarian cysts
      e. Degenerating uterine fibroids
      f. Ovarian torsion

E. Rectal examination
   1. Assess for masses, lesions, tenderness, discharge.

F. Figure 25.1 shows the pain sites within the abdominal and pelvic cavities.

ACUTE PELVIC PAIN

A. Most common type of pelvic pain, often experienced by patients after surgery or other soft tissue traumas and tends to be immediate, severe, and short lived.

B. Pregnancy related
   1. Spontaneous abortion
      a. **Inevitable abortion:** Cervix is dilated, bleeding occurs, and cramping is intense.
      b. **Incomplete abortion:** Heavy bleeding and cramping occur with passage of products of conception (POC).

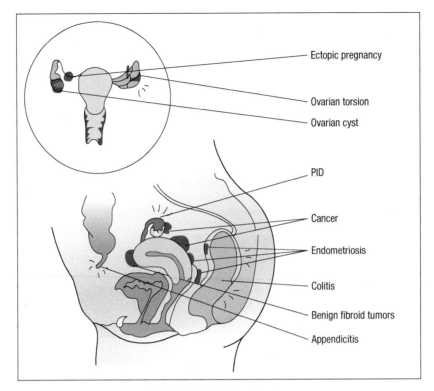

FIGURE 25.1 Pelvic pain sites.

PID, pelvic inflammatory disease.

    c. **Complete abortion:** Cramping and bleeding decrease, cervix closes.

    d. **Missed abortion:** Amenorrhea is the only symptom; no cramping, bleeding, or cervical changes.

    e. **Septic abortion:** An abortion complicated with an upper genital tract infection.

    f. **Labs/imaging:** Perform ultrasound and serial quantitative serum beta human chorionic gonadotropin (hCG), Rh, and complete blood count (CBC) testing as indicated.

  2. Ectopic pregnancy

    a. Should *always* be in the differential diagnosis for acute pelvic pain (APP).

      (1) Risk factors

- History of PID
- Prior tubal surgery
- Current intrauterine contraception (IUC) use
- Prior ectopic pregnancy
- If the patient has had one ectopic pregnancy, the chance of a second is 10% to 20%.

    b. Imaging/labs

      (1) **Ultrasound:** Gestational sac should be visible by ultrasound at 5.5 weeks and/or beta hCG of 1,500 to 2,400 mIU/mL.

      (2) **Serial quantitative serum beta hCG:** Levels should increase by at least 50% every 2 days.

 C. Gynecologic, infectious

  1. PID

    a. Treat all women with pelvic or lower abdominal pain who, on examination, have cervical motion tenderness *or* uterine tenderness *or* adnexal tenderness.

      (1) Leukocytes in vaginal secretions (most women with PID will have this); its absence argues strongly against PID.

TABLE 25.1 Pharmacologic Management of Outpatient Pelvic Inflammatory Disease Treatment

MEDICATIONS	NOTES
Ceftriaxone 250 mg IM single dose PLUS Doxycycline 100 mg PO BID for 14 days WITH (per CDC 2021 guidelines) metronidazole 500 mg BID for 14 days	Patient should return to clinic within 3 days to monitor care/assess progress Patient should return again after treatment for evaluation

BID, twice a day; IM, intramuscular; PO, per os.

(2) Cervical exudates/mucopus

(3) Cervical friability

(4) Temperature greater than 101°F (38.3°C)

(5) Labs:
- Elevated sedimentation rate
- Elevated C-reactive protein
- Gonorrhea and chlamydia bacterial vaginosis

(6) Outpatient PID treatment detailed in Table 25.1

2. PID indications for hospitalization

a. Surgical emergency (e.g., appendicitis) cannot be ruled out.

b. Patient is pregnant.

c. Patient does not respond to oral antibiotics.

d. Patient is unable to follow or tolerate oral medications.

e. Severe illness combined with high fever, nausea, and vomiting.

f. See tubo-ovarian abscess discussion, which follows.

g. **Note:** Advisability of routine removal of intrauterine device (IUD) with PID has not been established and is not a currently recommended practice by the Centers for Disease Control and Prevention (CDC). Consider Ob/Gyn consult if considering removal of IUC.

3. Tubo-ovarian abscess

a. Occurs in 15% to 34% of cases of PID.

b. May spread to other structures, such as the bladder.

c. Diagnosis made by bimanual examination, ultrasound, or laparoscopy.

d. Surgical management is indicated, so prompt referral to Ob/Gyn is recommended.

4. **Endometritis:** Pregnancy-related inflammation of endometrium

a. Occurs after 1% to 3% of normal spontaneous vaginal deliveries (NSVDs) and after 13% to 90% of cesareans.

b. Unlike PID, endometritis is not associated with infertility or chronic pelvic pain (CPP).

c. Presentation

(1) Fever, usually within 36 hours of delivery (100.4+°F) but within 10 days of delivery, 101.6+°F within first 24 postpartum hours

(2) Uterine tenderness

(3) Lower abdominal pain

(4) Foul-smelling lochia

(5) Abnormal vaginal bleeding and/or discharge

(6) Malaise

5. Dysmenorrhea

a. Recurrent, crampy, suprapubic pain during first few days of menses

b. Typically occurs for the first time within 2 years of menarche

c. More commonly a cause of CPP than APP

d. Caused by overproduction of or heightened response to endometrial prostaglandins

      e. Dysmenorrhea after years of pain-free menses is suggestive of endometriosis

         (1) Major causes of secondary dysmenorrhea

- Endometriosis
- Adenomyosis
- PID
- Adhesions
- Uterine fibroids
- Cervical stenosis (stenosis without obstruction is a very rare cause)
- Inflammatory bowel disease
- Irritable bowel syndrome (IBS)
- Psychogenic disorders
- Uterine polyps
- Cancer: endometrial, cervical, ovarian, fallopian "bladder/renal," and colon.

         (2) Treatment (Box 25.2)

  6. Uterine fibroids

    a. Most commonly present with pain after 35 years of age

    b. Present in approximately 20% to 25% of women of reproductive age

       (1) Typically presents as feeling of chronic pressure. May be acute pain with fibroid degeneration or torsion of pedunculated fibroid.

       (2) On examination, uterus may feel firm, nontender, irregularly enlarged, textured.

       (3) Ultrasound is diagnostic.

    c. Medication treatment (Table 25.2)

  7. Ovarian cysts

    a. Physiologic cysts

       (1) Should not cause pain unless there is rupture, torsion, or hemorrhage. Most physiologic cysts will resolve spontaneously in 1 to 2 months.

    b. Ovarian cysts, rupture

       (1) Release of fluid from a follicular cyst.

       (2) Fluid may irritate the peritoneum.

       (3) Pain onset may be sudden and severe but resolves spontaneously within 24 to 48 hours.

    c. Ovarian cysts, hemorrhage

       (1) Rupture of a corpus luteum cyst

       (2) Highly vascular, may lead to severe hemorrhage and pain similar to that of ectopic pregnancy

       (3) May be managed by watchful waiting, or surgery may be indicated

  8. Adnexal torsion

    a. Presents as sudden unilateral, colicky, lower abdominal pain. Nausea and vomiting in two thirds of cases.

    b. Enlarged, tender adnexa occurs in 90% of patients.

    c. Adnexa twists along utero-ovarian ligament; may involve fallopian tube as well.

BOX 25.2 DYSMENORRHEA TREATMENT

- NSAIDs: 800 mg ibuprofen every 6 hours for up to 2 days. Take with food.
- Combined oral contraceptives
- Heat applied to lower abdomen (hot water bottle, heating pad, etc.)
- Exercise (not during acute pain)

NSAIDs, nonsteroidal anti-inflammatory drugs.

TABLE 25.2 Initial Pharmacologic Management of Fibroids and Endometriosis		
NSAIDs	Ibuprofen	400–600 mg every 4–6 hr
	Naproxen base	500 mg initial dose; 250 mg every 6–8 hr
	Indomethacin	25 mg TID
	Meloxicam	7.5 mg QD
Combined oral contraceptive	Estrogen–progestin pill OR Transdermal patch OR Vaginal ring	Continuous cycling more effective than cyclic use
Progestin therapy	DMPA	150 mg IM every 3 months OR 104 mg SQ every 3 months
	Norethindrone acetate	2.5–15 mg PO QD
	Etonogestrel implant	Device implanted inside of upper arm
	Levogestrel intrauterine device	Device introduced into uterus

SPECIALTY MEDICAL INTERVENTIONS

Progesterone receptor modulators (*Note:* This treatment applies to fibroids but not to endometriosis)	Ullipristal acetate	5 mg or 10 mg for 13 weeks
GnRH agonists (use of these medications typically includes add-back therapy with norethindrone 5 mg PO daily to minimize hypoestrogenic effects)	Leuprolide acetate	3.75 mg IM monthly OR 11.25 mg IM every 3 months
	Nafarelin acetate	Intranasal 200 mcg BID
GnRH antagonists	Elagolix	150 mg PO QD OR 200 mg BID
Androgen therapy	Danazol	100–400 mg PO BID
Aromatase inhibitors	Anastrozole	1 mg PO QD
	Letrozole	2.5 mg PO QD

BID, twice a day; DMPA, depot medroxyprogesterone acetate; GnRH, gonadotropin-releasing hormone; IM, intramuscular; NSAID, nonsteroidal anti-inflammatory drug; PO, per os; QD, every day; SQ, subcutaneous; TID, three times a day.

    d. Is typically preceded by enlargement of ovary by cyst or neoplasm. (*Note:* Ovaries should not be palpable in post menopause.)

    e. Low-grade fever may be present.

    f. Hemorrhage may rarely lead to anemia, and necrosis resulting in infection may manifest as leukocytosis.

    g. Requires acute referral and management.

  9. Gastrointestinal, acute

    a. Appendicitis

    b. Gastroenteritis

    c. Diverticulosis/diverticulitis

    d. See chronic pelvic pain (CPP), section E (approximately 49% of CPP as well)

    e. Inflammatory bowel disease

    f. Bowel obstruction

    g. Mesenteric lymphadenitis

    h. Constipation

    i. See CPP, section C

10. Urinary tract, acute

    a. See Chapter 47, "Urinalysis and Urinary Tract Infections"

    b. Interstitial cystitis (IC)

    c. Pyelonephritis

    d. Nephrolithiasis

        (1) Symptoms

- Pain of differing degrees that comes and goes in waves
- Pain with urination
- Frequent urge to urinate
- Pink, red, or brown urine
- Nausea and vomiting
- Foul smelling, cloudy urine

        (2) Medication treatment (Table 25.3)

    e. Renal/bladder cancer. (*Note:* persistent hematuria and/or UTIs. Higher risk if >40 years old with history of cigarette smoking.)

D. Box 25.3 summarizes the differentials in the diagnosis of APP.

CHRONIC PELVIC PAIN

A. To be considered chronic, pelvic pain must last for 6 or more months. 15% to 20% of women aged 18 to 50 years have CPP for 1 or more years. Box 25.4 lists those historical factors that increase the risk for CPP. Table 25.4 discusses the interdisciplinary treatment options for CPP.

TABLE 25.3 Pharmacologic Management of Nephrolithiasis		
ACUTE TREATMENT		
Note: All patients should be instructed to strain urine for stones and bring them to the provider for analysis that will inform preventive treatments.		
Analgesics	Ibuprofen	400–600 mg every 4–6 hr
	Naproxen base	500 mg initial dose; 250 mg every 6–8 hr
	Indomethacin	25 mg TID
	Meloxicam	7.5 mg QD
	Ketorolac	20 mg initial dose; then 10 mg every 4–6 hr (maximum daily dose 40 mg/day)
Stone passage (for stones <10 mm in diameter)	Tamsulosin	0.4 mg QD for 4 weeks
	Silodosin	8 mg/day
	Tadalafil	10 mg/day

QD, every day; TID, three times a day.

BOX 25.3 Acute Pelvic Pain Differential Diagnoses

APP Differential by Quality
Abrupt and severe pain
   Perforation (ectopic pregnancy)
   Strangulation (ovarian torsion)
   Hemorrhage (ovarian cysts)
Crampy pain
   Dysmenorrhea
   Miscarriage
Colicky pain (comes in waves)
   Ovarian torsion
   Nephrolithiasis
Burning or aching pain
   Inflammatory process
   PID
   Appendicitis

APP Differential by Age: Menarche to 21 Years
Dysmenorrhea
PID
Ovarian cysts
   Rupture
   Hemorrhage
   Torsion
Pregnancy
   Miscarriage
   Ectopic pregnancy
Appendicitis
IBS

APP Differential by Age: 21 to 35 Years
Ovarian cysts
   Hemorrhage
   Torsion
   Rupture
Endometriosis
Pregnancy
   Miscarriage
   Ectopic pregnancy
PID
IBS

APP Differential by Age: 35 Years to Menopause
Uterine fibroids
Endometriosis
Ovarian tumor benign or malignant
Various cancers: including colon, endometrial, cervical, ovarian tumor

(continued)

BOX 25.3 Acute Pelvic Pain Differential Diagnoses *(continued)*

Pregnancy
 Miscarriage
 Ectopic pregnancy
Nephrolithiasis
IBS
Diverticulitis
Hernias
PID

APP Differential by Onset: Seconds to Minutes
Ovarian cysts
 Rupture
 Hemorrhagic
 Torsion
Tubo-ovarian abscess
Abdominal aortic aneurysm
Ectopic pregnancy
Aortic dissection
Nephrolithiasis
Appendicitis

APP Differential by Onset: Hours to Days
Diverticulitis
Herpes zoster
Gastroenteritis
Mittelschmerz
Primary dysmenorrhea
Miscarriage

APP Differential by Onset: Days to Weeks
Neoplasms
Cystitis
Pyelonephritis
Ectopic pregnancy
PID
Diverticulitis
Miscarriage
Abdominal aortic aneurysm

APP by Associated Symptom
With nausea, vomiting, anorexia
 Peritoneal irritation
 Hemoperitoneum
 Ovarian cyst rupture or hemorrhage
 Appendicitis

(continued)

BOX 25.3   Acute Pelvic Pain Differential Diagnoses *(continued)*

PID
  Tubo-ovarian abscess
With vaginal bleeding
  Pregnancy-related disorders
  PID
  Neoplasm
  Fibroids
  Polyps

APP, acute pelvic pain; IBS, irritable bowel syndrome; PID, pelvic inflammatory disease.

B. Endometriosis
  1. The number one leading cause of gynecologic pelvic pain
  2. Occurs in 7% to 10% of women in the United States; four out of 1,000 hospitalized annually.
  3. The presence of endometrial mucosa implanted in sites other than uterine cavity
  4. The tissue responds to normal hormonal cycling, causing bleeding, an inflammatory response, and so forth.
  5. Implants found on ovaries, fallopian tubes, inside and outside bowel, inside and outside urinary bladder, kidney, spleen, nasal mucosa, spinal canal, breast.
  6. The amount of ectopic tissue does not appear to have any correlation with severity of symptoms.
  7. Risk factors
      a. Delayed childbearing
      b. Long duration menses
      c. Short menstrual cycle
      d. Early menarche
      e. Family history (10-fold increased incidence)
      f. Structural defects
      g. Iron deficiency
      h. Because it is estrogen dependent, primarily seen before menopause
      i. Seen in 20% to 50% of infertile women
      j. Endometriosis found in 20% to 50% of asymptomatic women

---

BOX 25.4   Historical Factors That Increase the Risk of Chronic Pelvic Pain

- Physical or sexual abuse (40%–50% of women with CPP have a history of abuse)
- PID (18%–35% of women with PID will develop CPP)
- Endometriosis (seen laparoscopically in 33% of women with CPP)
- IC (38%–85% of women with CPP may have IC)
- IBS (symptoms seen in 50%–80% of CPP)

CPP, chronic pelvic pain; IBS, irritable bowel syndrome; IC, interstitial cystitis; PID, pelvic inflammatory disease.

TABLE 25.4 Interdisciplinary Treatment Options for Chronic Pelvic Pain

PHARMACOLOGIC TREATMENT	CBT (COGNITIVE BEHAVIORAL THERAPY)	MPT (MYOFASCIAL THERAPY)	NON-INVASIVE PROCEDURES AND TREATMENTS	INVASIVE SURGICAL PROCEDURES
Intended to treat the pain related to inflammation and neuropathy	Intended to treat and control the malfunction of pain perception related to psychological factors	Intended to allow optimal functioning of pelvic floor muscles, strengthen weak muscles, and reduce discomfort	Intended to address neurological dysfunction that causes pain in the pelvic floor	Intended to be a last resort when all other treatments fail to improve pain but is often exploratory. Surgical interventions may not improve pain and occasionally make it worse.
Analgesics To decrease mild pain and inflammation • NSAIDs (Motrin, Anaprox) • Acetaminophen	*Techniques to relax pelvic muscles* Yoga, exercise *Deep Breathing* Guided imagery, meditation, creative visualization *Bladder training* Delayed and timed urination, limiting fluids at certain times of day	*Botulinum toxin* Used as a neuromuscular blockade to decrease pelvic floor spasm	*Nerve block and neuromodulation* Weak evidence for success in treatment, should be part of a broader treatment plan and performed by a chronic pain management specialist	*Hysterectomy and bilateral salpingo-oophorectomy* Option for patients where there is an underlying gynecologic cause of the CPP
Neuropathic agents To decrease pain, reduce symptoms of depression and improve sleep • Tricyclic antidepressants (amitriptyline and imipramine) • Anticonvulsants that act as calcium-channel blockers (gabapentin and pregabalin) • SNRIs/SSRIs (venlafaxine and duloxetine)	*Sexual counseling* Individual and couples therapy to help clients understand their bodies, the pain they are experiencing, and if any underlying sexual dysfunction is related	*Pelvic floor physical therapy* Electric muscle stimulation, biofeedback treatment, manual manipulation, acupressure, muscle coordination training focus on pelvic floor, hips, back and abdominal wall muscles	*Destroy the bladder nerves* Decrease urologic symptoms of pain	*Lysis of adhesions* Option for patients who have endometriosis that is the cause of their CPP
Opioids If all other reasonable treatments have failed Must screen patients for opioid dependence and must be prescribed by a chronic pain management specialist			*Electrical stimulation* To electrically stimulate nerve roots to suppress nociceptive processing of pain signals	*Vestibulectomy* Option for patients experiencing vestibulodynia; mucous membrane of the vagina, the hymen, and some glands in the area are removed

8. Symptoms
   a. New-onset dysmenorrhea
   b. Dyspareunia
   c. Pain with urination and bowel movements
9. Endometriosis, examination
   a. Fixed, retroverted uterus
   b. Nodularity and/or tenderness in the cul-de-sac and uterosacral ligaments
   c. Ovarian enlargement
      (1) Surgery diagnostic
10. Medication treatment for endometriosis is the same as that for fibroids (Table 25.2).

C. **Adenomyosis:** Endometrial tissue within the myometrium
   1. Most often asymptomatic
   2. **Average onset:** 40 years of age
   3. Increased parity may be a risk factor.
   4. May cause long heavy periods, dyspareunia, dyschezia, dysmenorrhea.
      a. Uterus diffusely enlarged, soft, tender during menses; movement of uterus not restricted.

D. Pelvic adhesions
   1. Webs of intra-abdominal scar tissue
   2. Most often have history of previous pelvic surgery or injury.
   3. Noncyclic pain may be increased with intercourse or activity.
   4. Chronic pain may be related to restriction of bowel mobility, distention, and even bowel obstruction.

E. Pelvic congestion
   1. Varicosities of pelvic veins
   2. Signs and symptoms
      a. Bilateral abdominal and back pain, secondary dysmenorrhea, dyspareunia, chronic fatigue, IBS
      b. Uterus may be bulky, and ovaries enlarged with multiple cysts.
      c. Tenderness of pelvic ligaments
      d. **Labs/imaging:** Transuterine venography, pelvic ultrasound, MRI, laparoscopy

F. Irritable bowel syndrome
   1. Accounts for 60% of referrals for pelvic pain
   2. Thirty-five percent of people with IBS have CPP
   3. Diagnosis (Box 25.5)
   4. Treatment (Table 25.5)

G. Interstitial cystitis/painful bladder syndrome (IC/PBS)
   1. Main GU (genital/urinary) cause of CPP
   2. There are currently no biological markers for use in diagnosis; the diagnosis remains one of exclusion.
   3. Symptoms commonly start in a woman's 30s and may not be diagnosed until her 40s.
   4. Associated with remissions and exacerbations; may spontaneously disappear in 9 months (50%).
   5. Symptoms
      a. Pelvic pain, pressure, or discomfort related to the bladder, typically associated with a persistent urge to void or urinary frequency in the absence of infection or other pathology
         (1) Urinary frequency is usually more than eight times the normal rate.
         (2) Nocturia
      b. Present for more than 6 weeks
      c. Pain often increases with bladder filling; may diminish during voiding.
      d. Worse before or during menstruation

BOX 25.5 Diagnosis of Irritable Bowel Syndrome

Rome Criteria for IBS
- Recurrent abdominal pain or discomfort[a] at least 3 days/month in the last 3 months. Associated with two or more of the following:
  - ○ Improvement with defecation
  - ○ Onset associated with a change in frequency of stool
  - ○ Onset associated with a change in form (appearance) of stool
  - ○ Criteria must be fulfilled for the prior 3 months with symptom onset at least 6 months prior to diagnosis.

IC clinical management principles
- Treatments must be from most to least conservative; surgery is the last intervention.
- Initial treatment depends on severity of symptoms, patient preference, and clinical judgment.
- Multiple treatments may be offered concurrently.
- Ineffective treatments should be stopped.
- Pain management should be implemented throughout therapy while minimizing side effects.
- Diagnosis should be reconsidered if no improvement is noted.

[a]*Discomfort* refers to an uncomfortable sensation not described as pain.

IBS, irritable bowel syndrome; IC, interstitial cystitis.

TABLE 25.5 Initial Pharmacological Management of Irritable Bowel Syndrome

- Reassurance and education
- Stress reduction
- Low FODMAP diet
- Exclusion of high gas-producing foods
- Avoidance of lactose and gluten for those who are intolerant
- Use bulk-forming agents such as psyllium or ispaghula
- Increased physical activity

ADJUNCTIVE MEDICATIONS

PROBLEM	MEDICATION	DOSING
Constipation refractory to psyllium or ispaghula	PEG 3350	Miralax: 17 g in 4–8 oz of liquid daily for up to 7 days
Diarrhea	Loperamide	2 mg 45 min before meals
Abdominal pain	Antispasmodics	Dicyclomine 20 mg PO up to 4x daily PRN OR Hyoscyamine 0.125–0.25 mg PO or SL 3 to 4x daily PRN
	Tricyclic antidepressants (use cautiously in patients with constipation)	Amitriptyline 10–25 mg PO HS OR Nortriptyline 10–25 mg PO HS OR imipramine 10–25 mg PO HS OR Desipramine 12.5–25 mg PO HS

FODMAP, fermentable oligosaccharides, disaccharides, monosaccharides, and polyols; HS, at bedtime; IBS, irritable bowel syndrome; IM, intramuscular; PEG, polyethylene glycol; PO, by mouth; PRN, as needed; SL, sublingual.

BOX 25.6 Initial Treatment of Interstitial Cystitis

- Heat (e.g., hot water bottle, heating pad)
- Avoidance of trigger foods and beverages (common triggers include caffeine, citrus, spicy foods, tea, alcohol, artificial sweeteners, and chocolate)
- Pelvic physical therapy
- Fluid intake management

    e. Flares with intercourse, either during or 1 to 2 days after
    f. Women with IC also may suffer from seasonal allergies
    g. Palpable bladder tenderness
6. Etiology
    a. Abnormal bladder epithelial permeability ("leaky bladder theory")
    b. Neurogenic abnormalities
    c. Inflammatory process—mast cells released
    d. Autoimmune disorders
7. Rule out labs and procedures as indicated
    a. Urinalysis, culture—usually negative
    b. Urine cytology, particularly in the presence of hematuria and smoking to rule out bladder cancer
    c. Postvoid residual—capacity is usually less than 350 mL
        (1) Imaging
        (2) Simple cystometrogram (CMG; see Chapter 57, "Simple Cystometrogram") to rule out overactive bladder
        (3) Vaginal and cervical culture to rule out PID, herpes
        (4) Potassium sensitivity test
        (5) Cystoscopy to assess for Huhner's ulcers (present 10% of the time) and rule out bladder cancer
8. Initial treatment (Box 25.6)
9. Interdisciplinary treatment options for chronic pelvic pain (Table 25.4)

BIBLIOGRAPHY

Al-Abbadey, M., Liossi, C., & Graham, C. A. (2019). The Impact of Female Chronic Pelvic Pain Questionnaire (IF-CPPQ). *The Clinical Journal of Pain, 35*(7), 602–610. https://doi.org/10.1097/AJP.0000000000000703.

Bickley, L. (2017). *Bates' guide to physical examination and history taking (12th ed.).* Wolters Kluwer.

Bonnema, R., McNamara, M., Harsh, J., & Hopkins, E. (2018). Primary care management of chronic pelvic pain in women. *Cleveland Clinic Journal of Medicine, 85*(3), 215–223. https://doi.org/10.3949/ccjm.85a.16038. PMID: 29522389.

Chey, W. D., Kurlander, J., & Eswaran, S. (2015). Irritable bowel syndrome: A clinical review. *Journal of the American Medical Association, 313*(9), 949–958. https://doi.org/10.1001/jama.2015.0954

Ford, A. C., Bercik, P., Morgan, D. G., Bolino, C., Pintos-Sanchez, M. I., & Moayyedi, P. (2013). Validation of the Rome III criteria for the diagnosis of irritable bowel syndrome in secondary care. *Gastroenterology, 145*(6), 1262.e1–1270.e1. https://doi.org/10.1053/j.gastro.2013.08.048

George, S. E., Clinton, S. C., & Borello-France, D. F. (2013). Physical therapy management of female chronic pelvic pain: Anatomic considerations. *Clinical Anatomy, 26*, 77–88. https://doi.org/10.1002/ca.22187

Glazer, H., Rodke, G., Swencions, C., Hertz, R., & Alexander, W. (1995) Treatment of vulvar vestibulitis syndrome with electromyographic biofeedback of pelvic floor musculature. *Obstetrical & Gynecological Survey, 50*, 658–659. https://doi.org/10.1097/00006254-199509000-00015.

Grinberg, K., Granot, M., Lowenstein, L., Abramov, L., & Weissman-Fogel, I. (2017). A common pronociceptive pain modulation profile typifying subgroups of chronic pelvic pain syndromes is interrelated with enhanced clinical pain. *Pain, 158*(6), 1021–1029. https://doi-org.newproxy.downstate.edu/10.1097/j.pain.0000000000000869

Grinberg, K., Sela, Y., & Nissanholtz-Gannot, R. (2020). New insights about Chronic Pelvic Pain Syndrome (CPPS). *International Journal of Environmental Research and Public Health, 17*(9), 3005. MDPI AG. Retrieved from http://dx.doi.org/10.3390/ijerph17093005

Hanno, P. M., Burks, D. A., Clemens, J. Q., Dmochowski, R. R., Erickson, D., FitzGerald, M. P., ... Faraday, M. M. (2011). *Diagnosis and treatment interstitial cystitis/bladder pain syndrome.* http://www.auanet.org/guidelines/interstitial-cystitis/bladder-pain-syndrome-(2011,amended-2014)

Hanno, P. M., Erickson, D., Moldwin, R., Faraday, M. M., & American Urological Association. (2015). Diagnosis and treatment of interstitial cystitis/bladder pain syndrome: AUA guideline amendment. *Journal of Urology, 193*(5), 1545–1553. https://doi.org/10.1016/j.juro.2015.01.086

Hawkins, J. W., Roberto-Nichols, D. M., & Stanley-Haney, J. L. (2015). *Guidelines for nurse practitioners in gynecologic settings* (11th ed.). Springer Publishing.

Hoffman, B. L., Schorge, J. O., Halvorson L. M., Hamid, C. A., Corton, M. M., & Schaffer, J. I. (Eds.). (2020). *Williams Gynecology, 4e.* McGraw Hill. https://accessmedicine.mhmedical.com/content.aspx?bookid=2658&sectionid=217599855

Ingimarsson, J. P., Krambeck, A. E., & Pais, V. M. (2016). Diagnosis and management of nephrolithiasis. *Surgical Clinics of North America, 96*(3), 517–532. https://doi.org/10.1016/j.suc.2016.02.008

Kavoussi, S. K., Lim, C. S., Skinner, B. D., Lebovic, D. I., & As-Sanie, S. (2016). New paradigms in the diagnosis and management of endometriosis. *Current Opinion in Obstetrics & Gynecology, 28*(4), 267–276. https://doi.org/10.1097/GCO.0000000000000288

Kotarinos, R. K. (2003). Pelvic floor physical therapy in urogynecologic disorders. *Current, Women's Health Reports, 3,* 334–339.

Kotarinos, R. K. (2015) Myofascial pelvic pain: Rationale and treatment. *Current Bladder Dysfunction Reports, 10,* 87–94. https://doi.org/10.1007/s11884-014-0287-y.

Rosenbaum, T. Y., & Owens, A. (2008). The role of pelvic floor physical therapy in treatment of pelvic and genital pain related sexual dysfunction. *The Journal of Sexual Medicine, 5,* 513–523. https://doi.org/10.1111/j.1743-6109.2007.00761.x.

Ryan, S. A. (2017). The treatment of dysmenorrhea. *Pediatric Clinics of North America, 64*(2), 331–342. https://doi.org/10.1016/j.pcl.2016.11.004

Schuiling, K. D., & Likis, F. E. (2016). *Women's gynecologic health* (3rd ed.). Jones & Bartlett.

Speer, L. M., Mushkbar, S., & Erbele, T. (2016). Chronic pelvic pain in women. *American Family Physician, 93*(5), 380–387.

Varney, H., Kriebs, J. M., & Gegor, C. L. (2018). *Varney's midwifery* (6th ed.). Jones & Bartlett.

26

ASSESSMENT OF VULVAR PAIN AND VULVODYNIA

CHRISTY MARTIN, DEBORAH A. LIPKIN, AND
AIMEE CHISM HOLLAND

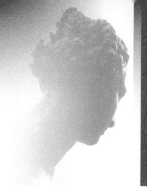

VULVAR PAIN

A. In the late 1880s, Skene identified "excessive sensitivity" of the vulva. Vulvar pain was officially recognized by the International Society for the Study of Vulvovaginal Disease (ISSVD) in 1976 at which time the term *burning vulva syndrome* was used. It was not until the early 1980s that vulvar pain was covered in the literature (Moyal-Barraco & Lynch, 2004).

1. In 2003, the ISSVD revised the classification of vulvar pain disorders. In 2015, this classification system was further expanded by consensus with the International Society for the Study of Women's Sexual Health (ISSWSH), and the International Pelvic Pain Society (IPPS).

   a. Vulvar pain that is related to a specific disorder (infectious, inflammatory, neoplastic, or neurologic).

   b. Vulvar pain in the absence of relevant visible finding or clinically identifiable disease. This is termed *vulvodynia.*

   c. Both vulvar pain secondary to known disorders and vulvodynia can be further described as localized, generalized (or mixed), provoked, spontaneous (or mixed), primary or secondary onset, or by temporal pattern (intermittent, persistent, constant, immediate, delayed).

2. Many vulvar conditions can cause soreness, rawness, irritation, and burning.

3. It is important to recognize that these conditions can be debilitating not only physically, but also emotionally. They can have an enormous impact on functioning in everyday activities, as well as psychosexual functioning.

4. The most successful treatment involves a multimodal approach of one or all the following: medical management of identifiable underlying conditions, management of pain, psychological support, sexual therapy, and physical therapy.

5. Despite appropriate therapy and remission of symptoms, approximately half of all women have relapsing symptoms.

B. Demographics

1. Quantitative research shows 16% of woman report chronic vulvar pain including burning, soreness, throbbing, and pain on contact with or without itching lasting 3 months or longer and it affects 25% of women in their lifetime.

2. Incidence may be much higher. Women are reluctant to disclose their symptoms because of embarrassment, shame, lack of response from multiple clinicians, or well-meaning clinicians who do not have the knowledge to manage or correctly assess these conditions or who diagnose by phone. One study showed that 39% of women who suffer from vulvar symptoms do not seek treatment.

C. Presentation

1. Pain may range from mild to severe and debilitating; it may be chronic, intermittent, provoked, or unprovoked.

2. It may involve other systems; most often, the urinary tract or the bowel.
3. Pain descriptors include sharp, burning, shooting, lancinating, or aching.
4. Mild to severe itching may be present.
5. Symptoms may be associated with position (sitting, standing).
6. Irritants may be problematic, including certain types of fabric (e.g., "Lycra"), personal hygiene products, or laundry detergent.
7. Sexual-related symptoms include pain to touch and/or penetration.
8. Discharge and/or odor may be present. Complaints of one or both are common, often with negative wet prep and potassium hydroxide (KOH).
9. Pelvic floor dysfunction (PFD).
   a. Many women with vulvar pain are likely to have contractile characteristics of the pelvic floor musculature. Occasionally, this is the initial source of pain, but more often it is a secondary source of pain. It is common for women to have no awareness of the tension held within the pelvic floor; they can contract their muscles when asked to "Kegel," but they are unable to release or "drop down" the muscles of the pelvic floor. Hypertonicity of these muscles is often overlooked during examination.
   b. Symptoms of PFD include pinching, burning, or aching.

D. Box 26.1 summarizes causes of vulvar pain.

E. Pathogenesis of pain may be explained by the following:
1. Pain is a complex mechanism that may be caused by stimulation of nerve endings, with nonmyelinated sensory nerve fibers (type C nerve fibers) responsible for sensations of itching and light pain; myelinated sensory nerve fibers (type A nerve fibers) are responsible for sensations of deep pain, pressure, and warmth
2. Increased numbers of intraepithelial nerve fibers, causing the thresholds for temperature and pain to be lowered, increase blood flow and erythema.
3. Increased inflammatory substances in the vulvar tissue
4. Immunologic changes
5. Genetic susceptibility

BOX 26.1 Common Causes of Vulvar Pain

- Infection (e.g., recurrent yeast, herpes)
- Genetic factors
- Immune factors
- Neuropathway involvement
- Injury or trauma
- Laser treatments
- Early and frequent intercourse
- Atrophic vaginitis secondary to menopause or breastfeeding
- Oral contraceptives (started at 16 years of age or younger and taken for more than 3 years)
- Dermatoses (lichen sclerosus, lichen planus)
- Dermatitis
- STI
- Metabolites
- Childbirth
- Cryotherapy
- Chemotherapy

STI, sexually transmitted infection.

6. **Localized vulvodynia:** May be due to nociceptors (C-nerve fibers) or neuropathic pain
   a. Trauma or chronic inflammation of C-nerve fibers may cause the inflammatory cytokines that surround them to fire repeatedly.
   b. Mechanoreceptors develop allodynia (pain elicited by nonpainful stimuli) secondary to central sensitization. Neuropathic pain is caused by injury to the sensory nervous system itself.
7. **PFD:** Many women with vulvar pain show pelvic floor abnormalities that may be the cause of pain or may worsen existing pain.

ASSESSMENT OF A WOMAN WITH VULVAR PAIN

A. **History:** The patient history is very important.
   1. A patient with vulvar pain may present with symptoms listed in Box 26.2.
   2. What triggers symptoms? Is pain associated with intercourse or touch, tight clothing, orgasm?
      a. Was onset gradual or was there one precipitating event?
      b. How long have the symptoms been present and are they constant/intermittent/cyclic?
      c. What are the characteristics of the symptoms? Descriptions might include itching, soreness, sharp, stabbing, prickly, raw, irritated, burning, throbbing.
      d. Is the location general or very specific? In other words, is the pain located over the whole vulva; only at the introitus, anus, or perineum; or elsewhere?
      e. Are there associated skin symptoms, such as bumps, rash, cracks, splitting/fissuring?
      f. Are there associated vaginal symptoms, such as discharge or bleeding?
      g. If pain is associated with intercourse, is it present at initial penetration? Is it experienced superficially or deep? Does it build over time and/or is there a long recovery period afterward?
      h. Use of a pain scale will be helpful, especially for reassessment after treatment.
      i. What treatment methods have been tried? What helps? What makes it worse?
   3. Gynecologic history
      a. Gravida/para, types of deliveries, breastfeeding within the last 6 months
      b. Menstrual history
      c. Contraception
      d. Menopausal symptoms
      e. History of abnormal Pap test
      f. History of sexually transmitted infections (STIs)
      g. Sexual history, current partner, duration of time with current partner

---

BOX 26.2 Examples of Common Complaints

"My yearly Pap smear is very painful; please use your smallest speculum."
"I can't use tampons because they hurt too much."
"I cannot have sex anymore" or "My partner is too big."
"It feels like sandpaper."
"I am always aware of my vagina or vulva."
"I have a disgruntled vagina."
"I'm scratching all night long."
"I've had yeast infections/bacterial vaginosis for years."
"It hurts to wear jeans."
Or worse, "My doctor told me to drink more wine—this is all in my head."

    h. History of yeast or bacterial vaginosis

    i. Genital injury or trauma

    j. **Orgasm:** Is the client able to achieve orgasm? Has she ever achieved an orgasm?

    k. History of gynecologic surgery, including urogynecological repairs

4. Review of systems may reveal a constellation of other related disorders or autoimmune dysfunction.

    a. Urinary symptoms, especially frequency, urgency, bladder pain

    b. Gastrointestinal symptoms, especially constipation

    c. Dermatologic symptoms, including oral mucosa

    d. Musculoskeletal symptoms, including back pain

    e. Psychological symptoms, including anxiety related to vulvar symptoms, depression, or loss of sleep

    f. Family history of vulvovaginal symptoms or disorders

5. **Medications:** There are numerous medications that may be associated with lichen planus or lichenoid-like vulvar eruptions; most common are nonsteroidal anti-inflammatory drugs (NSAIDs), beta blockers, and hydrochlorothiazide

6. Allergies

7. Past medical and surgical histories

B. Examination

1. **Nongenital examination:** Check general appearance, stature, weight, posture, mouth (looking for ulcers, Wickham's striae, cold sores), skin, nails, thyroid, abdomen, groin, and thighs.

2. Examination of the external pelvic and vulvar structures, beginning anteriorly (closest to abdomen) and progressing posteriorly (toward the anus). *Proceed with gentleness, respect, and caution.* If the patient is unable to tolerate any portion of the examination, consider relaxation techniques, pelvic floor therapy, psychopharmacology consult, or cognitive behavioral therapy.

    a. **Mons pubis:** Note hair distribution and any fissuring or cracking of the skin, especially at the natal cleft.

    b. **Labia majora:** Note hair distribution, skin changes.

        (1) **Skin pigmentation:** Observe for whitening, darkening, erythema.

        (2) **Lesions:** Note any ulcers, fissures, elevated dark lesions, excoriation, thickened areas (lichenification).

    c. Labia minora

        (1) **Architectural changes:** Note any agglutination or scarring. Do the labia minora extend fully to the perineum or are they flattened posteriorly? Vulvar dermatoses, such as lichen planus and lichen sclerosus, may cause scarring and/or resorption of the labia minora.

        (2) **Pigmentation:** Observe for whitening, darkening, erythema.

        (3) **Lesions:** Note ulcers, fissures, elevated dark lesions, excoriation, thickened areas (lichenification).

    d. **Clitoris:** Does the clitoral hood retract easily over the clitoris? Are the clitoral hood and clitoris scarred? Are they obliterated? Lichen planus and lichen sclerosus can both cause scarring and resorption.

    e. Vestibule

        (1) Pigmentation

        (2) **Texture:** Is the skin supple, smooth, shiny, or tissue-papery?

        (3) **Tenderness:** Cotton swab examination may produce allodynia, pain elicited by a stimulus that is not normally painful, and/or hyperpathia, when a stimulus causes greater pain than is expected.

(4) Scarring, or changes in architecture
- f. **Perineum:** As described previously, examine for color, texture, and lesions.
- g. **Anus:** As described previously, examine for color, texture, and lesions.
3. **Examination of the vagina:** Use of a virginal speculum is preferred.
   - a. Assess discharge color, consistency, and odor.
      (1) Yeast may present as white, thick discharge.
      (2) Bacterial vaginosis discharge may be off-white or grey with a fishy odor. It never causes vaginal mucosal inflammation.
      (3) Inflammatory conditions of the vagina may cause yellow discharge with a sour odor.
   - b. Vaginal walls may be a normal pink, pale, or may be inflamed. There may be telescoping (narrowing of the vaginal fornix) or strictures noted during bimanual examination.
   - c. **Texture of vaginal walls:** Supple versus smooth.
   - d. Note unusual fissures, lacy patterns, or lesions.
   - e. **Vaginal tone:** Generalized hypertonicity can be noted during speculum and manual examination; however, during manual examination, the clinician may be able to identify highly localized areas.
      (1) It may also be possible to assess involuntary pelvic floor spasms.
      (2) Use caution with evaluation of Kegel; women with PFD may have difficulty returning to resting tone, resulting in increased pain.
   - f. Perform wet mount, KOH, and pH evaluation.
      (1) Inflammatory conditions may present with elevated pH, an increased number of white blood cells, and presence of immature epithelial cells.
      (2) These conditions include vaginal atrophy, desquamative inflammatory vaginitis (DIV), lichen planus, and trichomoniasis. Yeast typically presents with a normal pH; however, yeast is often *not* observed by microscopy. Bacterial vaginosis will present with elevated pH and clue cells will be noted by microscope.
   - g. **Yeast culture:** Yeast is only observed 30% to 40% of the time by wet mount; therefore, a culture is imperative. Eighty percent to 90% of yeast is caused by *Candida albicans*. If speciation is not done automatically, it should be requested. Non-albicans yeast may require different treatment regimens.
   - h. **Vulvar biopsy:** A biopsy used to confirm dermatoses diagnosis and rule out vulvar cancer.

DIFFERENTIAL DIAGNOSES

- A. The following list is by no means complete. These are some of the more common disorders. Referral to a vulvovaginal specialist may be necessary.
- B. **Vulvodynia:** A spontaneous, generalized vulvar pain disorder, which may or may not involve dyspareunia. The pain has no known cause and has lasted for more than 3 months.
   1. Pain may be generalized and provoked, unprovoked, or mixed.
   2. Pain may be localized (e.g., the vestibule or clitoris) and provoked, unprovoked, or mixed.
- C. Yeast
- D. Herpes
- E. *Trichomonas*
- F. Inflammatory conditions
   1. **Lichen sclerosus:** This condition is 10 times more prevalent in women than in men, is often associated with other autoimmune disorders, runs in families, and can occur any time in life.
      - a. Lesions can be present on back/shoulders/wrists.
      - b. There is a 4% to 5% associated risk for squamous cell carcinoma.

    c. Typical presentation includes itching and, classically, whitening (often presents in a "keyhole pattern," surrounding the vulva and anus), dry, tissue-paper appearance; however, it can be more subtle. Excoriations, fissures, and lichenification can be observed in women who have been scratching.

    d. Agglutination, a type of scarring, can occur and will present as flattening of labia minora, appearance of synechiae or fusion of minora, clitoris, or other structures.

    e. Diagnosis can be confirmed by biopsy.

  2. **Lichen planus:** Vulvar appearance can be reticular or lacy, with Wickham's striae (a reticular, lacy pattern) or erosive (intensely bright red, exquisitely tender mucosa, typically well demarcated). Erosions may appear smooth and shiny. There may be resorption or scarring of normal architecture.

    a. Similar to lichen sclerosus, this condition is also present elsewhere on the body.

    b. Diagnosis may be confirmed by biopsy.

  3. **Lichen simplex chronicus:** Known as the "itch that rashes" with worsening symptoms resulting from "itch–scratch–itch" cycling.

    a. Skin may appear thickened, but there may also be excoriations and/or fissuring.

    b. Watch for superimposed infection.

    c. Patients may report worsening symptoms with heat, humidity, and irritants.

  4. **DIV, also known as *lichenoid vaginitis*:** This is a vaginal inflammatory condition presenting with profuse, yellow, vaginal discharge.

    a. Wet mount will reveal many white blood cells and parabasal cells.

    b. Discharge may or may not be irritating.

    c. Because DIV is very similar in presentation to vaginal lichen planus, there are some vulvar experts who believe that they are strongly associated with each other.

  5. **Atrophic vaginitis** (also known as *genitourinary syndrome of menopause [GSM]*, the preferred new term of the ISSWSH and the North American Menopause Society [NAMS]): Lack of estrogen may cause inflammation of the vulva and vaginal walls.

    a. Presentation may include elevated pH and profuse, yellow discharge; wet mount may reveal many white blood cells and parabasal cells.

    b. This condition is seen not only in postmenopausal women but also in women using medroxyprogesterone (Depo-Provera), breastfeeding mothers, women being treated with gonadotropin-releasing hormone agonists, and, occasionally, oral contraceptive users.

    c. Atrophic vaginitis cannot be distinguished from DIV or inflammatory vaginal conditions either clinically or microscopically.

  6. Irritant/contact dermatitis is a response to any exogenous substance.

    a. Affected area may appear erythematous with poorly demarcated slightly elevated plaques.

    b. Evaluate to determine whether chronic or acute; many long-used personal hygiene products may be responsible.

  7. Psoriasis

    a. Characterized by well-demarcated, thickened red plaques with silvery scaling, common on elbows, knees, scalp, and vulva.

    b. Itching is reported, often severe.

G. Neoplastic conditions

  1. **Paget's disease:** Presents with pruritus as primary symptom; may be eczematous with well-demarcated raised edges.

  2. **Squamous cell carcinoma:** Presents with pruritus as primary symptom; may appear as vulvar plaque, ulcer, or fleshy, nodular, or warty mass.

   3. **Vulvar intraepithelial neoplasia (VIN):** Like cervical intraepithelial neoplasia, VIN is strongly associated with human papillomavirus (HPV). Symptoms may be milder than other neoplastic conditions. Appearance is typically condyloma-like.

H. Neurologic conditions
   1. **Postherpetic neuralgia:** Onset of pain, tingling, or burning more than 4 months after the onset of herpetic lesions
   2. **Spinal nerve compression:** Symptoms may include sharp pain or burning.
   3. **Pudendal neuralgia:** Burning, constant pain, often relieved only while sitting on a toilet

I. Anatomic/structural conditions
   1. **Bartholin's gland:** Glands located bilaterally just inside the vaginal opening at the 4 o'clock and 8 o'clock positions. Pain associated with Bartholin's glands is typically caused by cyst or abscess.
   2. **Unruptured or tight hymen:** Condition is caused by incomplete degeneration of the central portion of the hymen.
   3. **Post-episiotomy:** Disruption of the nerve pathways may result in pain.
   4. **Post-surgery:** Disruption of the nerve pathways may result in pain.

J. Table 26.1 summarizes the assessment of the vaginal environment.

TABLE 26.1 Assessment of Vaginal Environment

CONDITION	CONDITION OF VAGINAL WALLS	ODOR	DISCHARGE COLOR	EPITHELIAL CELLS	WBC/ EPITHELIAL CELL RATIO	PH	CLUE CELLS OR OTHER
Normal	Normal, supple, pink	None	White	Mature appearance	01:01	3.8–4.6	None
Atrophic vaginitis	Smooth, pale, or inflamed	May be strong/ sour	May be scant or yellow	Immature cells are typically present	>1:1	Elevated ——— >4.6	None
DIV/lichenoid vaginitis	Inflamed	May be strong/ sour	Yellow	Immature cells are typically present	>1:1	Elevated ——— >4.6	None
Lichen planus	Inflamed, erosions may be noted	May be strong	Yellow	Immature cells are typically present	>1:1	Elevated ——— >4.6	None
Bacterial vaginosis	Normal	Fishy	Off-white, grey	Mature appearance	01:01	Elevated ——— >4.6	Clue cells present
Yeast	May be inflamed	Yeast-like	White/clumpy	Immature cells may be present	Often >1:1	3.8–4.6	None
Trichomonas	May be inflamed	May be strong	Yellow/green, frothy	Immature cells may be present	Often >1:1	Elevated ——— >4.6	Trichomonads present, no clue cells

DIV, desquamative inflammatory vaginitis; WBC, white blood cells

MANAGEMENT

A. Vulvovaginal complaints are often complex; rarely do they resolve simply. Pain management often requires a multimodal approach, which may include medication, physical therapy, lifestyle changes, and psychological support. Management of pain is complicated by treatment of underlying conditions, treatment of vaginal atrophy, and herpes suppression. Improvement is rarely quick: It can take weeks, months, or years. Women may require frequent visits with varied treatment trials before symptoms are stable and manageable. Providers may also provide much-needed psychological support that can be a cornerstone of all treatments: These women will need understanding and patience. The provider/patient relationship is often therapeutic in and of itself. Following is a list of possible options for treatment of vulvodynia and vulvar pain, along with treatment for some of the many possible conditions that cause it. This list is, by no means, exhaustive. Many treatments are off label.

B. **Lifestyle comfort measures:** Gentle care is advised.
   1. Sitz bath/cool soaks and then "seal" area with petrolatum or vegetable oil to keep in moisture and improve barrier function.
   2. Administer cool packs, refrigerated (freezing can burn the skin).
   3. Avoid and eliminate irritants (soaps, perfumed soaps/shampoos, perfumed laundry detergent, douching).
   4. Use cotton underwear during the day, no underwear at night.

C. Topical treatments for pain (Table 26.2)
   1. Five percent lidocaine may be applied up to five times daily. Useful for generalized, localized, provoked, or unprovoked pain. Instruct women to use a very small "test spot" first, as the initial sensations can be surprising (burning, stinging) but typically resolve within 5 to 10 minutes. If this occurs for more than 15 minutes, it should be compounded in a neutral base. *Avoid benzocaine, the active ingredient in Vagisil brand, which has been shown to be a contact irritant.*
   2. **EMLA cream:** Lidocaine 2.5%/prilocaine 2.5% combination cream. Prilocaine enhances the effect of lidocaine, but it can cause more burning/irritation initially. Follow instructions described previously.
   3. **Compounding:** It is very helpful to have a good working relationship with a local compounding pharmacist.
      a. Commercially prepared lidocaine or EMLA cream may be very irritating. These can be prepared in a neutral, nonirritating base.
      b. Numerous topical compounds have been used, including tricyclic antidepressant medication, gabapentin, baclofen (skeletal muscle relaxant), and ibuprofen. Typically, topical applications of these medications have fewer side effects. These should always be compounded in a neutral, nonirritating base.

D. **Dietary treatments:** A small number of women have found it helpful to lessen or eliminate high-oxalate foods from their diet. These diets can be restricting, and it may be enough to add calcium citrate to bind oxalates and avoid the worst triggers. High-oxalate foods include, but are not limited to, berries, nuts, legumes (including soy), grains, chocolate, and various vegetables.

E. Treatment for yeast
   1. Most patients tolerate fluconazole 150 mg. Topical azoles have the potential to irritate, especially with 1- or 3-day regimens.
   2. Treat the itch. Add an over-the-counter hydrocortisone ointment to quiet symptoms. Patients may need oral diphenhydramine or hydroxyzine to reduce nighttime itching.
   3. After treatment of active infection, long-term weekly suppression with one dose of 150 mg of fluconazole may be necessary.

TABLE 26.2 Pharmacologic Management of Vulvar Pain				
CLASS	**GENERIC NAME**	**BRAND NAME**	**DOSE/FREQUENCY/ ROUTE**	**CONSIDERATIONS**
Topical analgesic/ anesthetics	Lidocaine 5% ointment		Apply ½- to 1-inch ribbon (½–1 g), 3x to 5x per day	Ointment is preferable, as it tends to be less irritating. Instruct women to use a small "test spot" first. Lidocaine can be compounded in a neutral/ nonirritating base
Topical analgesic/ anesthetics	Lidocaine 2.5% with prilocaine 2.5%	EMLA	Apply ½- to 1- inch ribbon, 3x to 5x per day	See lidocaine considerations. Prilocaine enhances the effectiveness of lidocaine, but may increase initial burning sensations. A test spot prior to use is indicated.
Tricyclic antidepressants	Amitriptyline, nortriptyline, desipramine, and others	Elavil, Pamelor, Norpramin, and others	Start at 10 mg PO, qhs. Slowly titrate up by 10-mg increments q 3–5 days as tolerated	Maximum dose is 150 mg, but many women experience improvement at lower doses. Educate patients about anticholinergic side effects. Monitor for signs/ symptoms of serotonin syndrome. Tricyclics may be contraindicated with other medications
Anticonvulsants	Gabapentin or pregabalin	a. Neurontin or b. Lyrica	a. Start at 100 mg, PO, qhs. Slowly titrate up by 100 mg, q 3–5 days b. Start at 50 mg, slowly titrate up by 50-mg increments q 3–5 days as tolerated	Both are off-label for vulvar pain/vulvodynia, but are effective for neuropathic pain. Gapapentin maximum dose is 3,600 mg and should be divided into a TID regimen. Educate patients about sedation. There are very few medication interactions. Pregabalin should be divided as a TID regimen. Maximum dosing is 300 mg/ day
Selective norepinephrine reuptake inhibitors	Venlafaxine or duloxetine	a. Effexor or b. Cymbalta	a. Start at 37.5 mg, slowly titrate up by 37.5-mg increments b. Start at 20 mg, slowly titrated up by 20-mg increments	Both are off-label for vulvar pain/vulvodynia but have been studied for neuropathic pain. Venlafaxine maximum dose is 375 mg. Duloxetine maximum dose is 60 mg

PO, by mouth; q, every; qhs, every night at bedtime, TID, three times a day.

Source: Deborah A. Lipkin, NP (2017).

4. Non-albicans yeast may *not* be responsive to fluconazole. Boric acid suppositories or capsules of 600 mg can be inserted vaginally at night for 2 weeks but should not be used in pregnancy, or for more than 6 months. Single-dose intravaginal butoconazole vaginal (Gynazole) is also effective against non-albicans yeast and may be used in pregnancy if the benefits outweigh the risks (Category C).

F. **Treatment for herpes:** Long-term suppression may be achieved with antiviral agents.

G. **Treatment for *Trichomonas*:** Metronidazole 2 g, PO, once; tinidazole 2 g PO, once; or metronidazole 500 mg, BID for 7 days.

H. Systemic treatment for pain (see Table 26.2 for specific regimens)

1. **Tricyclic antidepressants:** Start at 10 mg, increase by 10 mg every 3 to 5 days as tolerated; maximum dose is 150 mg. These medications can be remarkably helpful in reducing pain, but may have significant side effects.

2. **Anticonvulsant medications:** Gabapentin—start at 100 mg, increase by 100 mg every 3 to 5 days, as tolerated; with maximum dose of 3,600 mg. Gabapentin may cause sedation. A newer option is pregabalin, or Lyrica (Pfizer Inc.), which may be taken as 100 mg dosages three times a day, with potential for a higher dose.

3. **Selective norepinephrine reuptake inhibitors (SNRI):** Venlafaxine HCl and duloxetine HCl. Both have shown some ability to treat neuropathic pain.

4. Opioid medication should be used judiciously, for short-term use, if at all. Medication contracts are strongly recommended for any patients requiring opioids longer term.

I. Treatment for inflammatory conditions

1. **Superpotent steroid:** Clobetasol, halobetasol, or betamethasone dipropionate are the cornerstones of treatment for vulvar inflammation. They can be tolerated for long-term treatment because of the high mitotic rate of the vulvar skin. Still, the skin should be evaluated regularly for signs of steroid rosacea or thinning. These medications are sometimes irritating and can be compounded in a nonirritating base. Ointments tend to be less irritating than creams.

2. **Topical calcineurin inhibitors:** Tacrolimus or other immunomodulatory medications are nearly always irritating, and so are not first-line treatments. This treatment is very effective for long-term treatment but is not well tolerated by patients. They should be used in minuscule amounts until the patient becomes less sensitive. Tiny amounts can be mixed with petrolatum. Tacrolimus can be very effective in treating otherwise unresponsive lichen planus.

3. Intralesional triamcinolone can be used for treatment of localized, unremitting lesions.

4. **Systemic triamcinolone injections for unrelenting disease:** Intramuscular triamcinolone has few side effects and is a reasonable treatment for those patients whose conditions are unresponsive to topicals or for those who cannot tolerate topicals. Referral to a vulvovaginal specialist is recommended.

5. **Vaginal estrogen can be used for atrophic conditions:** Estring, Vagifem tablets, Estrace cream, or Premarin cream. Premarin can be more irritating. Estrogen can be compounded in a non-irritating base as needed for patients who are unable to tolerate commercial preparations. Non-estrogen options include oral ospemifene (Osphena), a selective estrogen receptor modulator (SERM), and recently Food and Drug Administration (FDA)-approved dehydroepiandrosterone (DHEA; Intrarosa) vaginal suppositories. An option for women with a history of breast cancer or current breast cancer, DHEA is metabolized as estrogen intracellularly but not in the systemic circulation.

6. **Vaginal steroid suppository for DIV/lichenoid vaginitis:** May begin with commercially prepared 25 mg suppositories (prepared for rectal use) inserted in vagina. If this is ineffective, may try 100 mg compounded hydrocortisone suppositories. Regimen will vary depending on severity. Regular reevaluation for response to treatment will guide adjustment of the regimen.

7. Elimination of medications that may contribute to lichenoid conditions (most commonly NSAIDs, beta blockers, and hydrochlorothiazide) may reduce symptoms of disease. Consultation with the patient's other prescribers may be necessary. A month-long trial off these medications is sufficient.

J. Treatment for PFD/vaginismus

1. Pelvic floor physical therapy with biofeedback has been shown to help a significant number of women. Physical therapists should be experienced in working with women who have spasm of pelvic floor muscles.

2. Vaginal diazepam: Inserted vaginally, diazepam has been shown to reduce pelvic floor muscle spasm in some women. The typical dose is 5 mg but may be altered depending on response. It may be desirable to use compounded vaginal diazepam suppositories for dose adjustments *and* for better absorption of the medication.

PATIENT EDUCATION AND CLINICIAN RESOURCES

A. **ISSVD:** www.issvd.org

B. **The National Vulvodynia Association:** www.nva.org

C. **The Vulvar Pain Society:** www.vulvarpainsociety.org/vps

D. **The University of Michigan Center for Vulvar Pain:** obgyn.med.umich.edu/patient-care/ womens-health-library/vulvar-diseases

E. **Vulvovaginal disorders:** For an algorithm for basic adult diagnosis and treatment, see vulvovaginaldisorders.com. This algorithm has been available free, with registration. This may change in the future.

BIBLIOGRAPHY

American College of Obstetricians and Gynecologists' Committee on Practice Bulletins—Gynecology. (2020). Diagnosis and management of vulvar skin disorders: ACOG practice bulletin, number 224. *Obstetrics and Gynecology, 136*(1), e1–e14. https://doi.org/10.1097/AOG.0000000000003944

Bornstein, J., Goldstein, A. T., Stockdale, C. K., Bergeron, S., Pukall, C., Zolnoun, D., & Coady, D. (2016). 2015 ISSVD, ISSWSH, and IPPS consensus terminology and classification of persistent vulvar pain and vulvodynia. *Journal of Lower Genital Tract Disease, 20*(2), 126–130. https://doi.org/10.1097/LGT.0000000000000190

De Andres, J., Sanchis-Lopez, N., Asensio-Samper, J. M., Fabregat-Cid, G., Villanueva-Perez, V. L., Monsalve Dolz, V., & Minguez, A. (2016). Vulvodynia-an evidence-based literature review and proposed treatment algorithm. *Pain Practice, 16*(2), 204–236. https://doi.org/10.1111/papr.12274

Erni, B., Navarini, A. A., Huang, D., Schoetzau, A., Kind, A., & Mueller, S. M. (2021). Proposition of a severity scale for lichen sclerosus: The "Clinical Lichen Sclerosus Score." *Dermatologic Therapy, 34*(2), e14773. https://doi.org/10.1111/dth.14773

Graziottin, A., Murina, F., Gambini, D., Taraborrelli, S., Gardella, B., & Campo, M. (2020). Vulvar pain: The revealing scenario of leading comorbidities in 1183 cases. *European Journal of Obstetrics & Gynecology and Reproductive Biology, 252*, 50–55. https://doi.org/10.1016/j.ejogrb.2020.05.052

Guerrero, A., & Venkatesan, A. (2015). Inflammatory vulvar dermatoses. *Clinical Obstetrics and Gynecology, 58*(3), 464–475. https://doi.org/10.1097/GRF.0000000000000125

Guidozzi, F., & Guidozzi, D. (2021). Vulvodynia – an evolving disease. *Climacteric: The Journal of the International Menopause Society*, 1–6. https://doi.org/10.1080/13697137.2021.1956454

Leusink, P., Teunissen, D., Lucassen, P. L. B., Laan, E. T., & Lagro-Janssen, A. L. (2018). Facilitators and barriers in the diagnostic process of vulvovaginal complaints (vulvodynia) in general practice: A qualitative study. *The European Journal of General Practice, 24*(1), 92–98. https://doi.org/10.1080/13814788.2017.1420774

Martin, C. & Holland, A. C. (2020). Desquamative inflammatory vaginitis: A closer look. *Journal for Nurse Practitioners, 16*(10), 732–734. https://doi.org/10.1016/j.nurpra.2020.08.010

Moyal-Barracco, M., & Lynch, P. J. (2004). 2003 ISSVD terminology and classification of vulvodynia: A historical perspective. *Journal of Reproductive Medicine, 49*(10), 772–777.

Reed, B. D., Harlow, S. D., Plegue, M. A., & Sen, A. (2016). Remission, relapse, and persistence of vulvodynia: A longitudinal population-based study. *Journal of Women's Health, 25*(3), 276–283. https://doi.org/10.1089/jwh.2015.5397

Ringel, N. & Iglesia, C. (2020). Common benign chronic vulvar disorders. *American Family Physician, 102*(9), 550–557.

Shallcross, R., Dickson, J. M., Nunns, D., Mackenzie, C., & Kiemle, G. (2017). Women's subjective experiences of living with vulvodynia: A systematic review and meta-ethnography. *Archives of Sexual Behavior, 47*(3), 577–595. https://doi.org/10.1007/s10508-017-1026-1

Stenson, A. L. (2017). Vulvodynia: Diagnosis and management. *Obstetrics and Gynecology Clinics of North America, 44*(3), 493–508. https://doi.org/10.1016/j.ogc.2017.05.008

Stockdale, C. K., & Boardman, L. (2018). Diagnosis and treatment of vulvar dermatoses. *Obstetrics and Gynecology, 131*(2), 371–386. https://doi.org/10.1097/AOG.0000000000002460

Stone, R. H., Abousaud, M., Abousaud, A., & Kobak, W. (2020). A Systematic review of intravaginal diazepam for the treatment of pelvic floor hypertonic disorder. *Journal of Clinical Pharmacology, 60*(Suppl 2), S110–S120. https://doi.org/10.1002/jcph.1775

27

POLYCYSTIC OVARIAN SYNDROME

YVETTE MARIE PETTI AND R. MIMI SECOR

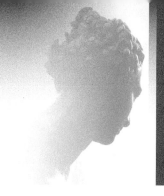

OVERVIEW AND DEFINITION OF POLYCYSTIC OVARIAN SYNDROME

A. Definition
1. Polycystic ovarian syndrome (PCOS) is the most common reproductive endocrine disorder in women.
2. PCOS is a disorder of androgen excess involving the ovaries and adrenal glands with or without insulin resistance and is associated with a complex differential.
3. PCOS affects 5% to 10% of women of reproductive age.
4. PCOS is the most common cause of female subfertility.
5. May be associated with inflammation and an increased level of oxidative stress.
6. Origins of PCOS are uncertain but emerging evidence suggests that this is:
   a. Genetic
      (1) Women with PCOS may carry a specific fragile X mental retardation 1 (FMR1) subgenotype gene.
      (2) Women with a heterozygous-normal/low FMR1 have polycystic-like symptoms of excessive follicle activity and hyperactive ovarian function.
7. Leading cause of menstrual abnormalities
B. Pathophysiology of PCOS
1. Alteration in hypothalamic–pituitary–ovarian axis due to:
   a. Elevated insulin levels, which leads to
      (1) Hyperinsulinemia associated with insulin resistance increases gonadotropin-releasing hormone (GnRH) pulse frequency.
      (2) Luteinizing hormone (LH) overrides follicle-stimulating hormone (FSH).
      (3) Increased production of ovarian androgen worsens insulin resistance.
   b. Decreased follicular maturation
   c. Decreased sex hormone-binding globulin (SHBG; inverse relationship with testosterone)
   d. Aromatase is produced by adipose tissue, which changes androstenedione to estrone and testosterone to estradiol.
   e. This creates a negative feedback loop and a paradox of excess androgens and estrogens, leading to an ineffective feedback mechanism of the effects of FSH.
   f. New research has reported elevated androgens (testosterone) may be associated with a less diverse gut microbiome.
2. The principal features are
   a. Anovulation, leading to irregular menstruation and oligomenorrhea

b. Overproduction of androgenic hormones, results in acne and hirsutism and, less common, male patterned baldness (hyperandrogenism)

c. Insulin resistance increases risk for obesity, type 2 diabetes, and elevated lipids

d. Insulin resistance is associated with normal and overweight women with PCOS.

e. Ovaries present as polycystic on ultrasound; however, this does not need to be present to meet criteria of inclusion for PCOS.

f. Symptoms and severity vary among women.

3. Ovaries become polycystic when stimulated to produce excessive androgens—namely, testosterone in one or more of the following ways:

   a. **LH and testosterone:** Thickens ovarian tissue (theca) and insulin suppresses apoptosis (programmed cell death)

   b. Hyperinsulinemia/insulin resistance

   c. Decreased levels of SHBG lead to increased free androgens (testosterone)

4. The "cysts" that develop are immature follicles; may see a "string of pearls" on ultrasound.

C. Impact of PCOS

1. Endometrial cancer

   a. Increased risk for development of uterine cancer, which is the most common gynecologic cancer in the United States (two-fold to three-fold increased risk)

   b. Overweight and obesity contribute to anovulation, irregular cycles, and/or amenorrhea.

   c. Prolonged estrogen stimulation (without ovulation) can lead to hyperplasia (thickening) of the uterine lining, atypia and type 1 endometrial/uterine cancer.

2. Infertility

   a. Inability to become pregnant after 1 year of intercourse without use of contraception

3. Psychosocial impact

   a. Emotional distress is frequently reported in women with PCOS.

   b. Higher rates of depression, anxiety, and other mental health problems have also been associated with PCOS.

   c. Risk of negative self-image, lower self-esteem, and higher rates of body dissatisfaction (associated with acne, hirsutism, and being overweight)

4. **PCOS:** Symptoms and risks

   a. **Oligomenorrhea:** Highly predictive

   b. **Hyperandrogenism:** Hirsutism, acne, and/or, less commo, male patterned baldness

   c. **Obesity:** Including central obesity (30%–70% affected)

   d. Infertility (73%–74% risk) and anovulation

   e. Abnormal uterine bleeding (AUB)

   f. **Uterine cancer:** Three-fold increased risk

   g. Breast cancer (and ovarian cancer)

   h. Insulin resistance, metabolic syndrome, type 2 diabetes

      (1) Three-fold to seven-fold increased risk for type 2 diabetes

   i. Heart disease, hypertension, dyslipidemia (70%)

   j. Mental health problems (may be linked to low allopregnanolone)

   k. Pregnancy-related risks

      (1) **Infertility:** 40% in women with PCOS

      (2) Spontaneous abortion (SAB): (25% to 73% increased risk)

      (3) **Gestational diabetes:** Three-fold increased risk

      (4) Preeclampsia/hypertension

CRITERIA FOR DIAGNOSIS OF PCOS

A. PCOS is a clinical diagnosis based on Rotterdam criteria.

B. PCOS diagnosis requires the presence of any two of the following three Rotterdam criteria:
   1. Oligomenorrhea (irregular menstrual cycles)
   2. Hyperandrogenism (acne, hirsutism, and, less common, male pattern baldness)
   3. Polycystic ovaries (noted on ultrasound; Figure 27.1)

CLINICAL SCREENING

A. Physical examination
   1. Measure blood pressure, heart rate, temperature, height, and weight (may include measure of adiposity including waist circumference and/or hip-to-waist ratio).
   2. **Hair distribution:** Assess for thinning of hair on crown of scalp, increased facial hair, hair around nipples/over chest, inner legs, and forearms. (*Note*: Ask patient if other women in the family have this hair distribution.)
   3. **Skin:** Note coarse or dry skin and/or cystic acne over face, chest, and back; examine neck for dark, velvety skin appearance (acanthosis nigricans).
   4. **Eyes:** Evaluate for exophthalmos, funduscopic–arterial venous (AV) nicking, and/or blood vessel changes.
   5. **Neck:** Evaluate for thyroid enlargement and/or nodules.
   6. **Breast examination:** Check symmetry, skin and/or hair change, nipple discharge, masses.
   7. **Cardiac:** Evaluate for tachycardia or bradycardia, rhythm abnormalities, murmurs.
   8. **Lungs:** Check breath sounds/wheezing/rhonchi.
   9. **Abdomen:** Note contour, central obesity, purple striae around anterior abdomen, organomegaly, bruits, masses.

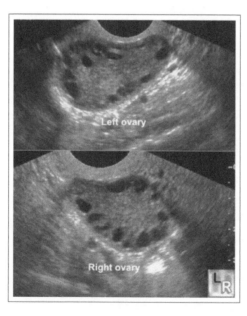

FIGURE 27.1 Classic presentation on ultrasound of the "string of pearls" presentation in PCOS.
Source: Used with permission from Learning Radiology.

10. **Peripheral exam:** Note edema, pulses, loss of vibratory and/or monofilament sensation over extremities.
11. **Genitalia:** Note virilization of labia, vaginal atrophy, use speculum examination to evaluate vaginal canal and cervix, bimanual examination to evaluate size and contour of uterus, also evaluate ovaries noting enlargement.

B. Diagnostic testing
   1. Screening labs (Table 27.1)

TABLE 27.1 Summary of Differential Laboratory Workup for PCOS

Baseline labs
- HCG—human chorionic gonadotropin (rule out pregnancy)
- CBC—complete blood count (anemia or iron overload in PCOS)
- TSH—thyroid stimulating hormone (hypothyroidism can mimic PCOS)
- CMP—comprehensive metabolic panel (older adults or if comorbid conditions like DM)

Fasting serum glucose or random glucose or HGBA1C-glycosylated hemoglobin (rule out diabetes)
- GTT—glucose tolerance testing (if fasting glucose ≥126, HBGA1C or random glucose is abnormal, confirms diabetes)
- Prolactin—(if amenorrhea, galactorrhea, vision change or headaches)
- Lipid panel—(fasting or non-fasting)
- Vitamin D—(consider if suspected or has insulin resistance)
- Testosterone (free and total)—Order if rapidly virulizing hirsutism. Modest elevations with PCOS. Done with a.m. fasting.

Additional diagnostic tests (Consider consult or referral to reproductive endocrinologist or OB/GYN)
- DHEA-S—dehydroepiandrosterone sulfate
- FSH/LH ratio: (not sensitive or specific for PCOS)
- SHBG (New)—(sex binding globulin hormone) inverse relationship with testosterone

LABORATORY TESTS	PCOS	PITUITARY DISORDERS DIABETES MELLITUS TYPE 2	NC-CAH	CUSHING'S SYNDROME	THYROID DISORDERS
HCG	Neg				
TSH with free T 4	Variable				Rule out hypothyroidism, which can mimic PCOS
Fasting glucose	>126		Check serum 17-hydroxy-progesterone level; abnormal if > 200 ng/dl		
2 hr. GTT (75 g)	≥140 and <200 mg/dL impaired fasting glucose	= 200 mg/dL diabetes mellitus			
HgBA1C	>6.5 diabetes	≥5.6 to 6.4 at risk	Variable		
Fasting or non-fasting Lipid panel	Elevated LDL Lower HDL Triglycerides may be elevated				
Total testosterone	>60 PCOS >200 Tumor				
Free testosterone	Normal range				

(continued)

TABLE 27.1 Summary of Differential Laboratory Workup for PCOS (*continued*)					
LABORATORY TESTS	**PCOS**	**PITUITARY DISORDERS DIABETES MELLITUS TYPE 2**	**NC-CAH**	**CUSHING'S SYNDROME**	**THYROID DISORDERS**
Estradiol	Decreased				
FSH/LH ratio	>3.0 or normal in PCOS Non-diagnostic		Normal FSH and LH		
Serum prolactin	Normal range (3–27) May be slightly elevated	>250 ug/dl suspect prolactinoma	If elevated workup Obtain fasting 8 a.m. to 9 a.m.		
DHEA-S	Normal range		Elevated	Elevated	
Serum fasting morning cortisol	Normal range	Variable if co-existence of other disorders	Elevated	Elevated	

NC-CAH, nonclassical-congenital adrenal hyperplasia; PCOS, polycystic ovarian syndrome.

2. **Additional labs:** Often ordered in consultation with or by referral to endocrinology/OB-GYN
   a. **Dehydroepiandrosterone sulfate (DHEA-S):** Levels of 700 to 800 mcg/dL are likely to indicate adrenal dysfunction.
   b. For hirsutism (especially rapid onset), prolactin may be ordered with androstenedione dehydroepiandrosterone sulfate (DHEA-sulfate), free and total testosterone
   c. Rule out late onset Congenital Adrenal Hyperplasia, Cushing's syndrome, Cushing's disease (consider as appropriate)
C. **Imaging:** Transvaginal ultrasound (TVUS) Refer or Order (if women's health provider)
   1. Order endometrial stripe measurement.
      a. If periods are irregular then order anytime.
      b. If periods occur at regular intervals, then ultrasound should be performed during day 6 through day 10 of menstrual cycle. This is to ensure the thickening of the endometrium is not due to premenstrual physiologic hyperplasia.
      c. For women of reproductive age an endometrial stripe greater than 10 mm is abnormal.
      d. For postmenopausal women an endometrial stripe greater than 5 mm requires an endometrial biopsy (EMB) and/or gynecologic consultation.
   2. **Evaluate ovarian status:** Note on requisition to include measurement of ovaries.
      a. **Polycystic ovaries on ultrasound:** 12 follicles 2 to 9 mm or increased volume of more than 10 mL in one or more ovaries
      b. Note cysts occur in 25% of women without PCOS
D. Referral for endometrial biopsy (EMB)
   1. Based on age, comorbidities, and TVUS endometrial stripe measurement
   2. Endometrial thickening
      a. Hyperplasia can lead to atypical cellular changes and endometrial cancer of the uterus.
      b. For women of reproductive age an endometrial stripe greater than 7 to 16 mm depending on the menstrual phase of the cycle, and for postmenopausal women an endometrial stripe greater than 5 mm requires an EMB and/or gynecologic consultation.

BOX 27.1 Patient Support Resources

- PCOS Awareness Association www.pcosaa.org
- Soul Cysters/Soul Cysters Message Board www.soulcysters.net

---

CLINICAL INTERVENTION

A. Goals of management of PCOS
   1. **Lower cardiometabolic risk:** Weight, blood pressure, insulin resistance, lipid management, lifestyle
   2. Restore/preserve fertility and establish fertility planning timeline.
   3. Treat hirsutism and/or acne.
   4. Manage oligomenorrhea/anovulation (regulate menstrual cycles), thus reducing risk of endometrial hyperplasia and endometrial cancer.
   5. The management plan is influenced by age of the woman, her symptoms, risks, and fertility planning timeline.
   6. Provide contraception that will help manage symptoms and provide contraception (if needed).
   7. Manage/promote mental health.
   8. Promote healthy lifestyle.

B. Patient education
   1. If overweight, evaluate dietary intake and physical activity and negotiate an initial weight loss goal of at least 10% of total body weight.
   2. **New research:** Moderate-intensity regular aerobic exercise over a short period of time improved menstrual irregularity and ovulation as well as reduced weight and insulin reduction.
   3. Patient support resources are listed in Box 27.1.

C. **Pharmacotherapy** (see Table 27.2)

D. Follow-up
   1. Negotiate a clinical follow-up schedule. Initially every 3 to 6 months, then if symptoms are managed and risks reduced, consider follow-up visits every 6 to 12 months.
   2. Follow-up transvaginal ultrasound (TVUS) as indicated.
   3. Encourage continued lifestyle modifications: Encourage a Mediterranean type of nutritional plan focusing on moderate amounts of lean protein, low glycemic vegetables, whole grains/beans, small quantities of fresh fruits and small quantities of healthy fats (calorically dense); daily physical activity; weight loss if possible; adequate sleep, stress reduction, and good mental health.

TABLE 27.2 Pharmacologic Management of Polycystic Ovarian Syndrome

IMPACT	GENERIC/ BRAND	DOSAGE: ADULT	SIDE EFFECTS/ MONITORING	COMMENTS
Managing irregular menses/ anovulation/AUB/ hyperandrogenism (acne, hirsutism)	Combination hormonal contraceptives (chc); typically, combination oral contraceptives	One PO daily, 21 or 28 day packets	• Nausea (take with food) • Spotting • Decreased libido • Development of elevated BP and/or headache especially with aura; discontinue and re-evaluate	Refer to CDC contraception guidelines 2016 Contraindicated if migraine with aura per CDC

(continued)

TABLE 27.2 Pharmacologic Management of Polycystic Ovarian Syndrome *(continued)*

IMPACT	GENERIC/ BRAND	DOSAGE: ADULT	SIDE EFFECTS/ MONITORING	COMMENTS
Contraception/ Prevents endometrial cancer	Levonorgestrel-releasing intrauterine systems/ devices _8 years_ Mirena IUD _5 years_ Kyleena IUD Liletta IUD _3 years_ Skyla IUD	 52 mg with release of 20 mcg/day 19.5 mg 52 mg with release of 18.6 mcg/day 13.5 mg with release of 14 mcg/day	• Risk of expulsion first 6 to 8 weeks • Cramping; may give NSAID first 30 days • Displacement • Infection • Spotting	Spotting often improves after 6 months **Pregnancy is rare, but if occurs more likely ectopic (suspect if unilateral lower abdominal pain)**
Improves insulin resistance	Metformin or Metformin ER	500 mg QD x 2 weeks and increase to BID and titrate by 500 mg up to 1,000 mg BID as indicated/tolerated Dosing: "Start low, go slow" to minimize GI side effects or consider ER	• Nausea • Diarrhea • Lactic acid ketosis in less than 10% of patients	Use ER if issues with loose stools Target over 1–2 months in patients with GI symptoms Higher dose associated with more weight loss Safe in pregnancy
Improves insulin resistance/ fasting glucose	Liraglutide (Victoza, Saxenda) Semaglutide (Ozempic, Rybelsus) Plus, CHCs, or levonorgestrel IUD if indicated	Titrate up weekly or as specified Renal dose	• Monitor renal functions • May cause nausea • Concomitant use of reliable contraception	Improves insulin resistance, facilitates modest weight loss Also cardioprotective *Do not use if history of:* Medullary thyroid cancer Multiple endocrine neoplasia syndrome type 2 Pancreatitis Primary or secondary adenoma **Safety not established, so do not use in pregnancy** Precautions: Renal disease

(continued)

TABLE 27.2 Pharmacologic Management of **POLYCYSTIC OVARIAN SYNDROME** (*continued*)

IMPACT	GENERIC/ BRAND	DOSAGE: ADULT	SIDE EFFECTS/ MONITORING	COMMENTS
				Disorders of pancreas
				May precipitate depression or suicidal ideation
Fertility preservation		Combination hormonal contraceptives		
Hirsutism	Spironolactone	25 mg to 100 mg QD to BID NOTE: 100 mg BID is very effective	• Monitor serum potassium first week, then periodically • Diuresis • Hyperkalemia • Liver dysfunction	**Do not use in pregnancy, must use effective contraception with this medication**
Hirsutism	Vaniqua (Eflornithine) Topical cream	Apply thin layer to affected areas twice daily	• Skin irritation • Discoloration	Expensive Other options: include electrocautery and laser treatment (may not be covered by insurance) **Do not use in pregnancy**
Abnormal lipids: Lower cardiovascular risk/endothelial inflammation	Atorvastatin (Lipitor) OR Simvastatin (Zocor)	20 mg to 40 mg daily by mouth usually at hs	• Monitor LFTs 4 to 6 weeks after initiation and then every 4 to 6 months • NOTE: Effective contraception is imperative • If pregnant, discontinue immediately	Benefits include reduced impact of fatty liver **Do not use in pregnancy**

CASE STUDY: Polycystic Ovarian Syndrome and Fertility Preservation

A 30-year-old female presents to your office for the first-time visit. She recently got married and is concerned about her ability to conceive as she reports that her periods have "always been irregular" and she has not used contraception the past year and has not become pregnant.

1. What questions may be helpful in understanding her "irregular periods"?
2. What information about her family history would be helpful?
3. What other clinical physical (including laboratory) measures would be needed to understand if she had polycystic ovarian syndrome versus other reasons for her irregular periods?

CASE STUDY: Polycystic Ovarian Syndrome and Fertility Preservation (*continued*)

4. How can her fertility status be determined in addition to her menstrual history?
5. If it is determined that she has polycystic ovarian syndrome, what first line pharmacotherapy could be employed?

BIBLIOGRAPHY

Abdalla, M. A., Deshmukh, H., Atkin, S., & Thozhukat, S. (2020). A review of therapeutic options for managing the metabolic aspects of polycystic ovary syndrome. *Therapeutic Advances in Endocrinology and Metabolism, 11,* https://doi .org/10.1177/2042018820938305 (retrieved 10/17/2021).

Al Khalifah, R. A., Florez, I. D., Dennis, B., Thabane, L., & Bassilious, E. (2016). Metformin or oral contraceptives for adolescents with polycystic ovarian syndrome: A meta-analysis. *Pediatrics, 137*(5), 1–12. https://doi.org/10.1542/ peds.2015-4089

Azziz, R. (2006). Diagnosis of polycystic ovarian syndrome: The Rotterdam criteria are premature. *Journal of Clinical Endocrinology & Metabolism, 91*(3), 781–785. https://doi.org/10.1210/jc2005-2153

Azziz, R., Woods, K. S., Reyna, R., Key, T. J., Knochenhauer, E. S., & Yildiz, B. O. (2004). The prevalence and features of the polycystic ovary syndrome in an unselected population. *Journal of Clinical Endocrinology and Metabolism, 89*(6), 2745–2749. https://doi.org/10.1210/jc.2003-032046

Balen, A. H., Conway, G. S., Homburg, R., & Legro R. S. (2005). *Polycystic ovary syndrome: A guide to clinical management.* Taylor & Francis.

Banaszewska, B., Spaczyński, R. Z., Pelesz, M., & Pawelczyk, L. (2003). Incidence of elevated LH/FSH ratio in polycystic ovary syndrome women with normo- and hyperinsulinemia. *Roczniki Akademii Medycznej w Bialymstoku, 48,* 131–134. Retrieved from https://pdfs.semanticscholar.org/3c6e/dbe9182dd917677372a172cde844d784f008 .pdf

Barry, J. A., Kuczmierczyk, A. R., & Hardiman, P. J. (2011). Anxiety and depression in polycystic ovary syndrome: A systematic review and meta-analysis. *Human Reproduction, 26*(9), 2442–2451. https://doi.org/10.1093/humrep/der197

Bates, G. W., & Legro, R. S. (2013). Longterm management of polycystic ovarian syndrome (PCOS). *Molecular and Cellular Endocrinology, 373*(1–2), 91–97. https://doi.org/10.1016/j.mce.2012.10.029

Batra, M., Bhatnager, R., Kumar, A., Suneja, P., & Dang, A. S. (2022). Interplay between PCOS and Microbiome: The road less travelled. *American Journal of Reproductive Immunology, 88*(2), e13580. https://doi.org/10.1111/aji.13580

Bruni, V., Capozzi, A., & Lello, S. (2022). The role of genetics, epigenetics and lifestyle in polycystic ovary syndrome development: The state of the art. *Reproductive Sciences, 29*(3), 668–679. https://doi.org/10.1007/s43032-021-00515-4

Dalibalta, S., Abukhaled, Y., & Samara, F. (2022). Factors influencing the prevalence of polycystic ovary syndrome (PCOS) in the United Arab Emirates. *Reviews on Environmental Health, 37*(3), 311–319. Advance online publication. https://doi .org/10.1515/reveh-2021-0036

de Groot, P. C., Dekkers, O. M., Romijn, J. A., Dieben, S. W., & Helmerhorst, F. M. (2011). PCOS, coronary heart disease, stroke and the influence of obesity: A systematic review and meta-analysis. *Human Reproduction Update, 17*(4), 495–500. https://doi.org/10.1093/humupd/dmr001

de Niet, J. E., de Koning, C. M., Pastoor, H., Duivenvoorden, H. J., Valkenburg, O., Ramakers, M. J., Passchier, J., de Klerk, C., & Laven, J. S. (2010). Psychological well-being and sexarche in women with polycystic ovary syndrome. *Human Reproduction, 25*(6), 1497–1503. https://doi.org/10.1093/humrep/deq068

Duleba, A. J. (2012). Medical management of metabolic dysfunction in PCOS. *Steroids, 77*(4), 306–311. https://doi .org/10.1016/j.steroids.2011.11.014

Duleba, A. J., & Dokras, A. (2012). Is PCOS an inflammatory process? *Fertility and Sterility, 97*(1), 7–12. https://doi .org/10.1016/j.fertnstert.2011.11.023

Ee, C. C., Venetis, C., & Costello, M. F. (2020). Metformin versus the combined oral contraceptive pill for hirsuitism, acne, and menstrual pattern in polycystic ovary syndrome. *The Cochrane Database of Systematic Reviews, 8*(8), CD005552. https://doi.org/10.1002/14651858.CD005552.pub3

González, F. (2012). Inflammation in polycystic ovary syndrome: Underpinning of insulin resistance and ovarian dysfunction. *Steroids, 77*(4), 300–305. https://doi.org/10.1016/j.steroids.2011.12.003

Graham, A., & Hamoda, H. (2016). Treatment of polycystic ovarian syndrome in primary care. *Prescriber, 27*(11), 36–45. https://doi.org/10.1002/psb.1515

Gu, Y., Zhou, G., Zhou, F., Li, Y., Wu, Q., He, H., Zhang, Y., Ma, C., Ding, J., & Hua, K. (2022a). Gut and vaginal microbiomes in PCOS: Implications for women's health. *Frontiers in Endocrinology, 13,* 808508. https://doi.org/10.3389/ fendo.2022.808508

Gu, Y., Zhou, G., Zhou, F., Wu, Q., Ma, C., Zhang, Y., Ding, J., & Hua, K. (2022b). Life modifications and PCOS: Old story but new tales. *Frontiers in Endocrinology, 13,* 808898. https://doi.org/10.3389/fendo.2022.808898

Guo, J., Shao, J., Yang, Y., Niu, X., Liao, J., Zhao, Q., Wang, D., Li, S., & Hu, J. (2022). Gut microbiota in patients with polycystic ovary syndrome: A systematic review. *Reproductive Sciences, 29*(1), 69–83. https://doi.org/10.1007/s43032-020-00430-0

Kite, C., Lahart, I. M., Afzal, I. Broom, D. R., Randeva, H., Kyrou, I., & Brown, J. E. (2019). Exercise, or exercise and diet for the management of polycystic ovary syndrome: A systematic review and meta-analysis. *Systematic Reviews, 8*(1), 51. https://doi.org/10.1186/s13643-019-0962-3

Leeman, L., & Acharya, U. (2009). The use of metformin in the management of polycystic ovary syndrome and associated anovulatory infertility: The current evidence. *Journal of Obstetrics and Gynaecology, 29*(6), 467–472. https://doi.org/10.1080/01443610902829414

Legro, R. S., Kunselman, A. R., & Dunaif, A. (2001). Prevalence and predictors of dyslipidemia in women with polycystic ovary syndrome. *American Journal of Medicine, 111*(8), 607–613. doi:10.1016/S0002-9343(01)00948-2

Makrantonaki, E,. & Zouboulis, C. C. (2020). Hyperandrogenismus, adrenal dysfunction und Hirsutismus [Hyperandrogenism, adrenal dysfunction, and hirsutism]. *Der Hautarst;Zeitschrift fur Dermatologie, Venerologie, und verwandte Gebiete, 71*(10), 752–761. https://doi.org/10.1007/s00105-020-04677-1

Marzouk, T., Nabil, H., & Senna, M. (2015). Impact of lifestyle modification program on menstrual irregularity among overweight or obese women with polycystic ovarian syndrome. *Korean Journal of Women Health Nursing, 21*(3), 161–170. https://doi.org/10.4069/kjwhn.2015.21.3.161

Moran, L. J., Misso, M. L., Wild, R. A., & Norman, R. J. (2010). Impaired glucose tolerance, type 2 diabetes and metabolic syndrome in polycystic ovary syndrome: A systematic review and meta-analysis. *Human Reproduction Update, 16*(4), 347–363. https://doi.org/10.1093/humupd/dmq001

Murri, M., Luque-Ramírez, M., Insenser, M., Ojeda-Ojeda, M., & Escobar-Morreale, H. F. (2013). Circulating markers of oxidative stress and polycystic ovary syndrome (PCOS): A systematic review and meta-analysis. *Human Reproduction Update, 19*(3), 268–288. https://doi.org/10.1093/humupd/dms059

Osibogun, O., Ogunmoroti, O., & Michos, E. D. (2020). Polycystic ovary syndrome and cardiometabolic risk: Opportunities for cardiovascular disease prevention. *Trends in Cardiovascular Medicine, 30*(7), 339–404. https://doi.org/10.1016/j.tcm.2019.08.010

Rashid, R., Mir, S. A., Kareem, O., Ali, T., Ara, R., Malik, A., Amin, F., & Bader, G. N. (2022). Polycystic ovarian syndrome-current pharmacotherapy and clinical implications. *Taiwanese Journal of Obstetrics & Gynecology, 61*(1), 40–50. https://doi.org/10.1016/j.tjog.2021.11.009

Sadeghi, H. M., Adeli, I., Calina, D., Docea, A. O., Mousavi, T., Daniali, M., Nikfar, S., Tsatsakis, A., & Abdollahi, M. (2022). Polycystic ovary syndrome: A comprehensive review of pathogenesis, management, and drug repurposing. *International Journal of Molecular Sciences, 23*(2), 583. https://doi.org/10.3390/ijms23020583

Sheely, D., & Pujare, D. (2022). Endocrinopathies. *The Medical Clinics of North America, 106*(3), 495–507. https://doi.org/10.1016/j.mcna.2021.12.010

Smith, H. A., Markovic, N., Matthews, A. K., Danielson, M. E., Kalro, B. N., Youk, A. O., & Talbott, E. O. (2011). A comparison of polycystic ovary syndrome and related factors between lesbian and heterosexual women. *Women's Health Issues, 21*(3), 191–198. https://doi.org/10.1016/j.whi.2010.11.001

Veltman-Verhulst, S. M., Boivin, J., Eijkemans, M. J., & Fauser, B. J. (2012). Emotional distress is a common risk in women with polycystic ovary syndrome: A systematic review and meta-analysis of 28 studies. *Human Reproduction Update, 18*(6), 638–651. https://doi.org/10.1093/humupd/dms029

Xu, Y., & Qiao, J. (2022). Association of insulin resistance and elevated androgen levels with polycystic ovarian syndrome (PCOS): A review of literature. *Journal of Healthcare Engineering, 2022*, 9240569. https://doi.org/10.1155/2022/9240569

28

ABNORMAL UTERINE BLEEDING

ANNETTE JAKUBISIN KONICKI AND IVY M. ALEXANDER

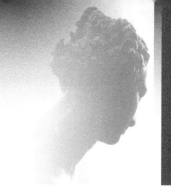

ABNORMAL UTERINE BLEEDING

A. Definition

1. Any uterine bleeding that occurs outside of the normal menstrual parameters for duration of bleeding, amount of flow, cycle length, and timing is considered abnormal uterine bleeding (AUB).
   a. Duration less than 2 days or more than 7 days
   b. Flow of more than 80 mL
   c. Cycle length of less than 21 days or more than 38 days
   d. Intermenstrual bleeding or postcoital spotting
   e. Unscheduled bleeding when using progestion+estrogen gonadal steroids (varying delivery routes)
2. Many different terms have been used historically to describe symptoms or diagnoses of AUB. Terms used to describe AUB are listed in Box 28.1.
3. Due to this lack of consistency in nomenclature used for AUB, a new classification system was adopted by the Fédération Internationale de Gynécologie et d'Obstétrique (FIGO) in November 2010 and updated in 2018.
4. The FIGO classification system was developed by an international workgroup and used an acronym to identify the possible causes for AUB: PALM–COEIN (Box 28.2).
   a. The FIGO classification system guides clinical evaluation and diagnosis for AUB (see Pathophysiology and Differential Diagnoses section).
   b. PALM etiologies are generally structural problems and the COEIN entities are nonstructural.

BOX 28.1 Terms Used to Describe Abnormal Uterine Bleeding

- Dysfunctional uterine bleeding (now called *heavy menstrual bleeding*)
- Oligomenorrhea
- Menorrhagia
- Intermenstrual bleeding
- Amenorrhea
- Polymenorrhea
- Metrorrhagia
- Menometrorrhagia
- Premenstrual spotting
- Hypermenorrhea
- Hypomenorrhea

BOX 28.2 PALM–COEIN

Polyps
Adenomyosis
Leiomyoma
Malignancy and hyperplasia
Coagulopathy
Ovulatory disorders
Endometrial disorders
Iatrogenic causes
Not classified

---

    c. The FIGO classification system recognizes that a woman may have one or more entities causing AUB and/or have entities that are symptomatic and do not contribute to the bleeding (e.g., leiomyomas, polyps, adenomyosis).

    d. The work group also recommended retiring the terms *dysfunctional uterine bleeding, menorrhagia,* and *metrorrhagia.*

B. Epidemiology

    1. Approximately 1.4 million women report AUB annually.

        a. Prevalence is difficult to estimate accurately due to the variations in nomenclature used for AUB.

    2. The incidence of abnormal bleeding increases during adolescence and perimenopause.

    3. Approximately 10% to 30% of all women report heavy bleeding.

    4. Approximately 11% of postmenopausal women have spontaneous bleeding.

    5. AUB is more common among White women, younger women (18–30 years), and women who are obese.

    6. Approximately 30% of outpatient office visits in gynecology are related to menstrual problems.

C. Health-related complications associated with AUB

    1. AUB is correlated with lower quality of physical and mental health.

    2. Persistent menstrual blood loss of more than 80 mL per cycle is associated with anemia.

    3. AUB accounts for approximately two thirds of all hysterectomies.

    4. AUB is associated with increased healthcare costs.

CLINICAL EVALUATION OF THE WOMAN WHO PRESENTS WITH ABNORMAL UTERINE BLEEDING

A. History

    1. Establish the onset, duration, severity, and course of the changes in bleeding patterns.

        a. Is this an acute change? Need to stabilize the patient due to heavy bleeding?

        b. Is this a chronic problem—persistent pattern (timing, amount, regularity) for most of a 6-month time period?

    2. Clarify the women's bleeding pattern.

        a. Are her cycles longer, shorter, or irregular?

        b. Is her flow heavier or lighter?

        c. Is she passing clots? Size of clots?

        d. Where does the blood originate (vulva, vagina, cervix, cervical os)?

        e. Are there changes in the pattern of her bleeding (spotting, midcycle bleeding, postcoital bleeding, bleeding after exercise)?

        f. Is there a change in the volume of bleeding? Quantify the number of pads/tampons used (an increase of two or more pads/tampons per day helps to quantify an increase in blood loss).

3. Has she experienced similar changes in the past?
4. Has she had previous treatment for this or a similar problem?
5. Has she tried any alternative or complementary medicine therapies or other methods for self-care?
6. Does she have symptoms of ovulation?
7. Identify whether she is experiencing any associated symptoms with a review of systems (ROS).
   a. **Constitutional:** Fatigue, malaise, myalgia, chills, fever, weight loss, anorexia
   b. **Head, eyes, ears, nose, and throat (HEENT):** Dizziness, especially with change in position; gum bleeding
   c. **Breast:** Nipple discharge, masses, pain
   d. **Respiratory:** Shortness of breath, especially with exertion
   e. **Cardiac:** Tachycardia, palpitations, chest pain, radiating pain
   f. **Gastrointestinal:** Abdominal pain, cramping, pelvic pain, bloating, elimination changes (constipation, diarrhea, bleeding), flatulence
   g. **Genitourinary:** Urinary urgency, frequency, dysuria, hematuria, odor, color changes, flank pain; genital pruritis, lesions, burning, pain, discharge, odor, dyspareunia
   h. **Neurological:** Dizziness, light-headedness, syncope
   i. **Skin:** Rash, bruising, petechiae
   j. **Extremities:** Arthralgias, joint stiffness, swelling
8. Complete a full gynecologic history.
   a. Pregnancy history summary, including gravida, parous
      (1) How many pregnancies and live births has she had?
      (2) Any problems with bleeding after delivery?
      (3) Has she had any abortions? If yes, were they spontaneous, medical, or surgical?
      (4) Any obstetric or gynecologic surgery?
         • Prior cesarean section
         • Myomectomy
         • Excisional cervical procedures like loop electrosurgical excision procedure (LEEP)
   b. Menstrual history
      (1) What was her last menstrual period like—normal, late, lighter than normal?
      (2) Age of menarche; what is her usual cycle length, days of flow, flow pattern?
      (3) Does she have any dysmenorrhea? Is it new onset or worsening?
      (4) If she has a male partner, is she using any form of contraceptive?
      (5) Any history of vaginitis? If yes, how was it treated?
   c. Sexual history
      (1) **Partner history:** How many currently and over lifetime? Does she have sex with men, women, or both?
      (2) When was her most recent sexual activity?
      (3) What is the frequency and type of sexual activity she engages in? Are there any risky behaviors or activities that correlate with her bleeding?
   d. Sexually transmitted infection (STI) history
      (1) Document any STIs: type, date, treatment
      (2) Date last tested, what tests done, and results
   e. Gynecologic surgery, procedures, problems
   f. Contraceptive history
      (1) **Type of contraception used:** Currently? In the past? Any previous changes in bleeding patterns with these? Use of TCu-380A (ParaGard) intrauterine device (IUD)?
      (2) Consistency in use of contraceptive method? Specify dates of unprotected sex, and/or non-use of contraceptive.
   g. Personal hygiene
      (1) Is she douching, using a new type of pad or tampon, or any new products?

9. Social history
   a. Does she have any history of sexual, physical, or verbal abuse?
   b. What is her lifestyle? Diet (any history of eating disorders?), exercise (excessive exercise? female athlete triad?), sleep, stressors (excessive stress?), occupation, and recreation, alcohol/drug abuse, tobacco?
   c. Increased work absence?
10. Medical history
    a. Identify current or past medical conditions; how managed?
    b. Any personal history of bleeding disorders?
    c. Any history of bleeding associated with surgeries or dental work?
    d. Any history of anemia?
11. Medications and allergies
    a. **Prescription:** Borrowed or self-medicated?
    b. Does she have any allergies to medications, environment, or animals?
    c. What over-the-counter medications does she use?
    d. Any use of complementary and alternative medication therapies?
12. Family history
    a. Has a sister or mother had similar abnormal bleeding?
    b. Any family history of bleeding disorders?
    c. Any family history of polycystic ovary syndrome?
    d. Any family history of either endometrial or colon cancer?
13. Health screenings
    a. When was her last cervical cancer screening (and results), pelvic examination, mammogram (if of age), colonoscopy (if of age), lipids and fasting glucose or hemoglobin A1C?
    b. Are her immunizations up to date?
    c. Does she need special testing, such as tuberculosis (TB) screening or screening for lung cancer?

B. Physical examination
   1. **Vital signs:** Include orthostatic blood pressures and pulses; include height and weight to calculate body mass index (BMI). Has she lost or gained weight recently?
   2. General appearance and systemic evaluation
      a. Identify level of sexual maturity
      b. Evaluate body habitus
      c. **Skin and hair:** Distribution (hirsute)? Acanthosis nigricans? Pallor, petechiae, ecchymoses?
   3. HEENT
      a. Mucosal color
      b. Thyroid examination
   4. Breast examination
      a. Evaluate for galactorrhea (bilateral, unrelated to pregnancy/breastfeeding suggests presence of hyperprolactinemia).
   5. Cardiac examination
      a. Evaluate for tachycardia, arrhythmias, murmurs.
   6. Abdominal examination
      a. Evaluate for striae, hepatosplenomegaly, tenderness, masses, ascites.
   7. Pelvic examination
      a. Identify source of bleeding; examine external genitalia, vagina, cervix.
      b. Assess for cervical motion tenderness.
      c. Cervical cancer screening test; STI testing; vaginal discharge for potassium hydroxide (KOH) test, pH test; wet mount (see Chapter 45, "Cervical Cancer Screening and Colposcopy").

    d. Perform a bimanual examination of her uterus and adnexae; assess for tenderness including rebound; uterus size, shape, firmness; adnexa palpability, firmness, fullness, or enlargement.

    e. Rectal exam

       (1) Are there any lesions, hemorrhoids?

       (2) Is there any rectal bleeding?

       (3) Test stool for occult blood.

PATHOPHYSIOLOGY AND DIFFERENTIAL DIAGNOSES

A. The FIGO PALM–COEIN acronym (see Box 28.2) provides guidance to the underlying pathophysiology and potential differential diagnoses for AUB in reproductive-aged women

B. PALM—structural disorders

   1. **Infections:** STIs, cervicitis, vaginitis, endometritis

   2. **Benign structural abnormalities:** Endocervical and endometrial polyps (AUB-P), ectropion, cysts, adenomyosis (AUB-A), leiomyomata (AUB-L)

   3. Premalignant/malignant lesions (AUB-M)

   4. **Trauma/irritation:** Intercourse, sexual assault, presence of foreign body

C. COEIN—nonstructural disorders

   1. **Endocrine disorders (AUB-O):** Hyper-/hypothyroidism, hyperprolactinemia, polycystic ovary syndrome, adrenal hyperplasia/Cushing's disease; interrupts the hypothalamic-pituitary-ovarian axis

   2. Endometrial (AUB-E)

   3. **Hematologic disorders (AUB-C):** Coagulopathy, leukemia

   4. Renal or liver disorders

   5. **Mucosal diseases:** Crohn's, Bechet's

   6. Extreme stress or extreme exercise

   7. **Medications:** Oral contraceptive pills, hormone therapy, selective serotonin reuptake inhibitors (SSRI), antipsychotics, anticoagulants, corticosteroids

   8. Herbal supplements

   9. Intrauterine devices

   10. Eating disorders

   11. Weight loss

D. AUB not specified; diagnosis of exclusion, no cause for bleeding identified (organic, structural)

   1. Periodic uterine blood loss of more than 80 mL per cycle

   2. Negatively affects woman's quality of life

E. Different diagnoses vary among different age groups. For example, bleeding (even a scant amount) in a postmenopausal woman is considered malignant until proven otherwise (Table 28.1).

DIAGNOSTIC TESTING

A. Diagnostic testing is based on the most likely differential diagnoses and the FIGO PALM–COEIN categorization.

B. PALM entities are generally structural problems that are identified with direct visualization, imaging (e.g., transvaginal ultrasound, saline infusion sonography), and/or histopathology.

C. COEIN entities are generally nonstructural problems that are not identified with imaging or direct visualization and other laboratory testing may be warranted.

D. Serology

   1. Consider testing for bleeding disorders if the patient has two or more of the following symptoms: bruising one to two times per month, frequent gum bleeding, epistaxis one to two times per month, or a family history of bleeding symptoms; or if she has a history of heavy

TABLE 28.1 Differential Diagnoses for Abnormal Uterine Bleeding Categorized by Age

AGE GROUP	POTENTIAL DIAGNOSES
Neonate	Estrogen withdrawal
Premenarche	Trauma or foreign body Infection/vulvovaginitis Urologic factors Precocious puberty (rare) Neoplasm (rare)
Early postmenarche	Anovulation/polycystic ovarian syndrome Coagulation disorder Pregnancy Stress/extreme exercise Infection Neoplasm (rare) Trauma
Reproductive years	Anovulation Pregnancy Infection Benign growths Medication Coagulation disorders Endocrine disorders Liver disease Malignancy Trauma Stress/extreme exercise
Perimenopause	Anovulation Medications Malignancy Benign growths
Postmenopause	Malignancy Medications Atrophy Benign growths

bleeding since menarche or has had a postpartum hemorrhage, bleeding related to surgery, or bleeding associated with dental work.

2. Complete blood count (CBC) with platelet count is recommended for both women and adolescent females with heavy menstrual bleeding. Adolescents with abnormalities of platelet function or count may have heavy menstruation.

3. Ferritin level to identify iron stores in those who may not currently be anemic. Test thyroid-stimulating hormone (TSH; serum) if signs or symptoms of thyroid disorders.

E. Transvaginal ultrasound is used to identify structural abnormalities and the thickness of the endometrial stripe.

1. An endometrial stripe less than or equal to 4 mm correlates with very low risk for endometrial cancer (1 in 917) and thus endometrial biopsy is not needed.

   a. Premenopause >8 mm

   b. Postmenopause >4 mm

   c. https://www.ogscience.org/m/journal/view.php?number=611

2. In adolescents, a transabdominal ultrasound may be more appropriate than transvaginal ultrasound.
3. Sonohysteroscopy may be indicated if inconclusive ultrasound findings or ultrasound identified a focal lesion.

F. Endometrial biopsy is needed for all postmenopausal women with bleeding and for women older than 40 years and for women younger than 45 years with endometrial cancer risk factors.
   1. Endometrial cancer risk increases with age.
      a. Incidence at age 13 to 18 years is approximately 0.1 out of 100,000 women.
      b. Incidence at age 19 to 34 years is approximately 2.3 out of 100,000 women.
      c. Incidence at age 35 to 39 years is approximately 6.1 out of 100,000 women.
      d. Incidence at age 40 to 49 years is approximately 36.0 out of 100,000 women.

G. Diagnostic studies to consider for women with AUB (Table 28.2).

CLINICAL MANAGEMENT OF ABNORNMAL UTERINE BLEEDING

A. Management is tailored to the cause of the bleeding if one can be identified.

TABLE 28.2 Diagnostic Studies to Consider for Women With Abnormal Uterine Bleeding

AGE (YEARS)	DIAGNOSTIC TEST
13–18	hCG to rule out pregnancy Cultures if sexually active Coagulation studies: INR or PT and PTT, fibrinogen, von Willebrand factor, ristocetin cofactor CBC with platelet count to identify coagulation defects, leukemia, anemia
19–50	hCG, cervical cancer screening, cultures TSH—to identify hypo-/hyperthyroidism, especially if untested in 5 years FSH (controversial), maybe with estradiol, progesterone, LH, FSH:LH ratio CBC with platelet count and serum iron, blood drawn early in cycle (day 3) Coagulation studies if screening questions positive Urine analysis to identify urinary tract infection, renal calculi, bladder cancer Stool guaiac test to identify colon polyps, diverticula, gastrointestinal cancers, ulcer, hemorrhoids, fissures Ultrasound (US) to identify leiomyomata, structural abnormalities; follow-up with saline infusion sonography (SIS) or hysteroscopy if structural abnormalities identified via US Endometrial biopsy if 40 years or older and in younger women if any concern for endometrial cancer Consider fasting serum prolactin test to identify pituitary adenoma if bleeding is infrequent or minimal Consider head MRI to identify pituitary adenoma Consider liver function tests and renal function studies to identify systemic illness

CBC, complete blood count; FSH, follicle-stimulating hormone; hCG, human chorionic gonadotropin; INR, international normalized ratio; LH, luteinizing hormone; PT, prothrombin time; TSH, thyroid-stimulating hormone.

Sources: American College of Obstetrics and Gynecology. (2013a). ACOG practice bulletin: Management of abnormal uterine bleeding associated with ovulatory dysfunction. *Obstetrics & Gynecology, 122*(1), 176–185; American College of Obstetrics and Gynecology. (2013b). ACOG practice bulletin: Management of acute abnormal uterine bleeding in nonpregnant reproductive-aged women. *Obstetrics & Gynecology, 122*(1), 891–896; Taylore, H. S., Pal, L., & Seli, E. (2020). *Speroff's Clinical gynecologic endocrinology and infertility* (9th ed.). Philadelphia, PA: Lippincott, Williams & Wilkins; James A. H., Kouides, P. A., Abdul-Kadir R., Edlund, M., Federici, A. B., Halimeh, S., . . . Winikoff, R. (2009). Von Willebrand disease and other bleeding disorders in women: Consensus on diagnosis and management from an international expert panel. *American Journal of Obstetrics and Gynecology, 201*, 12–18. doi:10. 1016/j. ajog. 2009. 04. 024; Munro, M. G., Critchey, H. O. D., Broder, M. S., & Fraser, I. S. (2011). FIGO classification system (PALM–COEIN) for causes of abnormal uterine bleeding in nongravid women of reproductive age. *International Journal of Gynecology and Obstetrics, 113*, 3–13. doi:10.1016/j.ijgo.2010.11.011. Munro, M. G., Critchley, H. O. D., Fraser, I.S., FIGO Menstrual Disorders Committee (2018) The two FIGO systems for normal and abnormal uterine bleeding symptoms and classification of causes of abnormal uterine bleeding in the reproductive years: 2018 revisions. International Journal of Gynaecology and Obstetrics, 143(3), 393-408. DOI: 10.1002/ijgo.12666.

B. The goal of therapy (after pregnancy and malignancy have been excluded) is to restore normal menstrual cycles and minimize blood loss and disruption to the woman's life.

C. Management options for heavy menstrual bleeding (HMB)

1. Medications (Table 28.3)

TABLE 28.3 Pharmacologic Management of Abnormal Uterine Bleeding: Heavy Menstrual Bleeding

TREATMENT OPTIONS WILL VARY BASED ON ETIOLOGY OF AUB

General Comments:
- FDA indication: Heavy menstrual bleeding
- Must be taken as directed for efficacy.

GENERIC/BRAND AVAILABILITY	DOSAGE: ADULT	DOSAGE: PEDIATRIC	SIDE EFFECTS/ MONITORING	COMMENTS
Acute: Monophasic combination oral contraceptive, multiple choices. Example: *Levonorgestrel/ethinyl estradiol (BRAND Alesse)* HMB: Cyclic monophasic or triphasic pills, extended or continuous monophasic OC, vaginal ring or transdermal patch. Example: *Levonorgestrel/ethinyl estradiol* **Availability:** Oral combination pill, estrogen/progesterone dose dependent upon brand. *(BRAND Larissia)*	Acute: 35 mcg estradiol, 3x per day for 1 week then daily dosing for 3 weeks HMB: Monophasic: Levonorgestrel / ethinyl estradiol 0.1 mg/20 mcg tab formulation once daily as either the 21- or 28-day pack option Or if continuously use the 21-day pack with no interruption	Same, no dose adjustments made	May experience spotting or breakthrough bleeding, headache, breast tenderness, nausea, VTE, MI, or CVA	If pre-diabetes or diabetes, monitor glucose; if hyperlipidemia, monitor lipid panel; if HTN, monitor BP
Vaginal ring **Availability:** (BRAND *Nuvaring*)	Vaginal ring: 0.12 mg/0.015 mg per day; insert once a month, remove on day 21		May experience bleeding irregularities, nausea, vomiting, breast tenderness, headache, abdominal distention or pain, edema, weight changes.	
Ethinyl estradiol/ norelgestromin transdermal patch **Availability:** (BRAND *Ortho Evra* or *Xulane*)	Patch: 150 mcg/ 35 mcg per day; applied once per week × 3 weeks, off × 1 week		Serious reactions include thrombosis, thromboembolism, MI, CVA, HTN. Same as for the vaginal ring and transdermal patch	

(continued)

TABLE 28.3 Pharmacological Management of Abnormal Uterine Bleeding: Heavy Menstrual Bleeding (*continued*)

GENERIC/BRAND AVAILABILITY	DOSAGE: ADULT	DOSAGE: PEDIATRIC	SIDE EFFECTS/ MONITORING	COMMENTS
Depot medroxyprogesterone acetate (DMPA) **Availability:** (Depo-Provera *CL* 150 mg pre-filled syringe or 150 mg /mL vial)	150 mg IM every 3 months	Same, no dose adjustments made	May experience headache, weight gain, menstrual irregularities, amenorrhea. Serious reactions include bone density loss, thromboembolism, osteoporosis, anaphylaxis	Monitor glucose, if diabetic; pregnancy test if >14 weeks between doses. Check bone density if treatment >2 years
Levonorgestrel intrauterine device Dose range dependent upon brand, range 13.5–52 mg per intrauterine device **Availability:** Mirena, 52 mg IUD q 8 years Kyleena, 19.5 mg IUD q 5 years Skyla, 13.5 mg IUD q 3 years	1 IUD every 8 years Start within 7 days of menses onset	Same, no dose adjustments made	May experience vulvovaginal mycotic infections, menstrual irregularities, amenorrhea, vaginitis, acne, ovarian cyst, anxiety, abdominal or pelvic pain, dysmenorrhea. Serious reactions include ectopic pregnancy, sepsis, PID, myometrial embedment	Pelvic exam performed 4–12 weeks after insertion, then annually or as needed. If diabetes, monitor glucose
Tranexamic acid 650 mg tablet **Availability:** **Oral preparation** (Lysteda, 650 mg tabs) Generic tranexamic acid 650 mg tablets	2 tabs PO TID during menses for 5 days		With oral use may experience headaches, backpain, upper respiratory infection symptoms, musculoskeletal pain, athralgia, migraines. Serious reactions include: anaphylaxis, hypersensitivity reaction, thromboembolism, retinal vascular occlusion, cerebral edema, cerebral infarction	Obtain creatine at baseline. May be treatment option for patients who are currently bleeding and decline hormonal options

a. Combined oral contraceptive pills
b. Postmenopausal hormone therapy
c. Progestin-only contraceptive pills
d. Depot medroxyprogesterone acetate (DMPA)
e. Levonorgestrel intrauterine device
f. Nonsteroidal anti-inflammatory drugs (NSAIDs)
g. Tranexamic acid

2. **Endometrial ablation:** The benefits and risks of various techniques should be considered and discussed with the patient.
3. Myomectomy
4. Uterine artery embolization
5. Hysterectomy (last resort)

D. Management options for anovulatory bleeding
  1. Medications (Table 28.4)
    a. Estrogen or progestin to stop bleeding
    b. Combined oral contraceptive pills
    c. Metformin if the woman has insulin resistance

E. Management options for structural causes of bleeding (polyps, leiomyomata)
  1. Medications (Table 28.5)
    a. Combined oral contraceptive pills
    b. Levonorgestrel intrauterine device

TABLE 28.4 Pharmacologic Management of Abnormal Uterine Bleeding: Anovulatory Bleeding

TREATMENT OPTIONS WILL VARY BASED ON ETIOLOGY OF ABNORMAL UTERINE BLEEDING

General Comments:
- FDA indication: Anovulatory bleeding
- Must be taken as directed for efficacy.

GENERIC/BRAND AVAILABILITY	DOSAGE: ADULT	DOSAGE: PEDIATRIC	SIDE EFFECTS/ MONITORING	COMMENTS
Cyclic monophasic or triphasic pills, extended or continuous monophasic OC with at least 30 mcg of estrogen to reduce risk of break through bleeding. Example: *Levonorgestrel/ethinyl estradiol* **Availability:** Oral combination pill, estrogen/progesterone dose dependent upon brand *(BRAND Levora)*	Monophasic: Levonorgestrel/ ethinyl estradiol 0.15 mg/30 mcg tab formulation once daily as either the 21- or 28-day pack option. Or if continuously, use the 21-day pack with no interruption	Same, no dose adjustments made	May experience spotting or breakthrough bleeding, headache, breast tenderness, nausea, VTE, MI or CVA.	If pre-diabetes or diabetes, monitor glucose; if hyperlipidemia, monitor lipid panel; if HTN, monitor BP
Depot medroxyprogesterone acetate (DMPA) **Availability:** *(BRAND Depo-Provera CL 150 mg pre-filled syringe or 150 mg/mL vial)*	150 mg IM every 3 months	Same, no dose adjustments made	May experience headache, weight gain, menstrual irregularities, amenorrhea. Serious reactions include bone density loss, thromboembolism, osteoporosis, anaphylaxis	Monitor glucose if pre-diabetes or diabetes, pregnancy test if >14 weeks between doses. Check bone density if treatment >2 years

(continued)

TABLE 28.4 Pharmacologic Management of Abnormal Uterine Bleeding: Anovulatory Bleeding (*continued*)

GENERIC/BRAND AVAILABILITY	DOSAGE: ADULT	DOSAGE: PEDIATRIC	SIDE EFFECTS/ MONITORING	COMMENTS
NOT ACTIVELY bleeding: Progestin/progesterone only regimens		Same, no dose adjustments made	May experience irregular bleeding, amenorrhea, nausea, breast pain/tenderness, weight changes or fluid retention	Monitor glucose if pre-diabetes or diabetes, monitor lipid panel closely if hyperlipidemia; mammography, frequency based on age, risk factors, prior results
Generic: Norethindrone acetate 5 mg tabs	5 mgs PO q HS for 10 days of each calendar month			
Micronized progesterone 200 mg tabs	200 mg PO q HS for first 12 days of calendar month			
Medroxyprogesterone acetate 10 mg tabs	10 mg PO q HS first 10 days of each calendar month			
ACTIVELY bleeding: Continuous monophasic OC with no placebo week Example: Levonorgestrel/ethinyl estradiol **Availability:** Oral combination pill, estrogen/progesterone dose dependent upon brand (*BRAND, Levora*)	Monophasic: Levonorgestrel / ethinyl estradiol 0.15 mg/30 mcg tab formulation once daily as either the 21- or 28-day pack option. Or if continuously, use the 21-day pack with no interruption		May experience spotting or breakthrough bleeding, headache, breast tenderness, nausea, VTE, MI, or CVA	
If insulin resistance: Metformin Immediate-release formulations, 500 mg tablets Extended-release formulations, 1,500 mg–2,000 mg ER	500 mg TID PO OR 1,500 mg PO at bedtime	10–16-year-olds 500–1,000 mg BID; immediate release only	May experience diarrhea, nausea, vomiting, flatulence, or indigestion. Serious reactions include lactic acidosis, megaloblastic anemia or hepatotoxicity	Will need to test eGFR at baseline, then periodically or more frequently in individuals 65 years old and older; CBC at baseline, then at least q12mo; vitamin B_{12} levels q2–3y if vitamin B_{12} deficiency risk

2. Surgical excision of polyp, leiomyomata
3. Uterine artery embolization (for leiomyomata)
4. High intensity focus ultrasound (for leiomyomata)
5. Hysterectomy (last resort)

TABLE 28.5 Pharmacologic Management of Abnormal Uterine Bleeding: Structural Causes of Bleeding

General Comments:
* Options for structural causes of bleeding (polyps, leiomyomata)

GENERIC/BRAND AVAILABILITY	DOSAGE: ADULT	DOSAGE: PEDIATRIC	SIDE EFFECTS/ MONITORING	COMMENTS
Cyclic monophasic or triphasic pills, extended or continuous monophasic OC, vaginal ring or transdermal patch Example: *Levonorgestrel/ethinyl estradiol* **Availability:** Oral combination pill, estrogen/progesterone dose dependent upon brand. (*Larissia*)	Monophasic: Levonorgestrel / ethinyl estradiol 0.1 mg/20 mcg tab formulation once daily as either the 21- or 28-day pack option. Or if continuously, use the 21-day pack with no interruption	Same, no dose adjustments made	May experience spotting or breakthrough bleeding, headache, breast tenderness, nausea, VTE, MI, or CVA	If pre-diabetes or diabetes, monitor glucose; if hyperlipidemia, monitor lipid panel; if HTN, monitor BP
Levonorgestrel intrauterine device Dose range dependent upon brand, range 13.5–52 mg per intrauterine device **Availability:** *Mirena*, 52 mg IUD q 7 years *Kyleena*, 19.5 mg IUD q 5 years *Skyla*, 13.5 mg IUD q 3 years	1 IUD every 8 years. Start within 7 days of menses onset	Same, no dose adjustments made	May experience vulvovaginal mycotic infections, menstrual irregularities, amenorrhea, vaginitis, acne, ovarian cyst, anxiety, abdominal or pelvic pain, dysmenorrhea. Serious reactions include ectopic pregnancy, sepsis, PID, myometrial embedment	Pelvic exam performed 4–12 weeks after insertion, then annually or as needed. If diabetes, monitor glucose

CASE STUDY

Patient Situation

A 46-year-old Black cis-gender female presents with complaint of irregular, heavier menses with increasing frequency.

Subjective Data

* **History of presenting issue:** Bleeding every 2 weeks for the past 4 to 6 months, usually cycle is 30 to 32 days; flow heavier (using five to six pads/day, up from usual of three/day), passing clots sized ranges from raisin to grape; unrelated to exercise, coitus, etc.; experiencing increased pelvic pressure and cramping with menses; minimal relief with over-the-counter ibuprofen (400 mg three to four times per day with food). Says her friend had a similar problem and ended up having surgery, which she wants to avoid.

(*continued*)

CASE STUDY (*continued*)

- Review of Relevant Systems:
  - ○ **Constitutional:** Feels well overall, some fatigue because of cramping at night
  - ○ **Head, Eyes, Ears, Nose, Throat:** No gum bleeding
  - ○ **Breast:** No nipple discharge
  - ○ **Cardiac:** No palpitations
  - ○ **Gastrointestinal:** No bowel changes, no bleeding with defecation, no abdominal cramping
  - ○ **Urinary:** No urinary symptoms
  - ○ **Gynecologic:** G2P2, no hemorrhaging after deliveries, no surgeries, menarche age 13, usual menses 28 to 32 days, medium flow three pads/day, lasts 4 to 5 days, some cramping that usually resolves with ibuprofen or warm bath, one male sexual partner for 18 years (exclusive, not concerned about sexually transmitted infections, has never had any STIs, no prior vaginitis), uses condoms consistently for birth control (tried oral contraceptives in the past but did not remember to take them), not interested in more pregnancies, no recent change in feminine hygiene or menstrual products, does not douche.
  - ○ **Neurologica:** No dizziness/light headedness/syncope
- **Current Medical History:** Hypertension
- **Family History:** Dad (72, hypertension, diabetes type 2), mom (74, osteoporosis, hypertension), maternal grandmother (deceased at 66, heart attack)
- **Medications:** Amlodipine (Norvasc) 5 mg daily, no vitmains/supplements/herbals
- **Allergies:** NKDA
- **Social History:** Married to male partner, two high school-aged children, works full-time as supervisor for medical billing company, enjoys her work, exercises regularly—usually walking, no injectable/recreational drugs, never smoked, social alcohol—one to two drinks weekend evenings, has never been hit/kicked/slapped or forced to do sexual things she did not want to do, feels safe in relationship and at home.

Objective Data

- **Vital signs:** BP: 124/72 P: 74 T: 98.0°F BMI: 32
- **General:** Relaxed, dressed appropriately to weather, appears stated age
- **HEENT:** Mucosal color pink, thyroid supple, midline, without palpable nodules
- **Cardiac:** RRR 74, no murmurs/rubs/gallops
- **Pulmonary:** Clear to auscultation
- **Abdominal:** Bowel sounds present, soft, non-tender, no hepatosplenomegaly
- **GYN:** External genitalia without lesions, vaginal mucosa pink, moist with rugae, scant blood present at cervical os, no cervical motion tenderness, mild uterine tenderness, and no adnexal tenderness on bimanual exam

Clinical Analysis

1. Which characteristics of the patient's current menstrual pattern align with a diagnosis of abnormal bleeding and why?
   a. Interval—short; approximately 14 days (about 2 weeks) [normal is 28–30 days (range 24–35 days)]
   b. Duration—no change
   c. Flow amount—heavy, increased number of pads needed per day (up to 5–6/day from 3/day), passing clots [normal is 30–40 mL (range 20–80)]

(*continued*)

CASE STUDY (*continued*)

    d. Interval and flow amount have changed significantly from her usual pattern and are above both average and range.

2. What are the top seven differential diagnoses that need to be considered for the patient? Provide subjective and objective data that support and refute each potential differential diagnosis.

    a. Structural – Leiomyomata
       i. Supporting: irregular bleeding, heavier menses, passing clots, dysmenorrhea, midlife age, race
       ii. Refuting: (none)

    b. Anovulatory cycles
       i. Supporting: irregular bleeding, heavier menses, midlife age
       ii. Refuting: dysmenorrhea

    c. Infection
       i. Supporting: irregular menses, dysmenorrhea
       ii. Refuting: one partner

    d. Premalignant/malignant lesions
       i. Supporting: irregular bleeding
       ii. Refuting: normal examination

    e. Hypothalamic-Pituitary-Ovarian (HPO) Axis Disruption Endocrine Disorders – Thyroid, ex
       i. Supporting: irregular bleeding, heavier menses, passing clots
       ii. Refuting: midlife age, no weight changes or other physical exam findings

    f. Bleeding disorder
       i. Supporting: increased bleeding, passing clots
       ii. Refuting: midlife age, no family history

    g. Pregnancy/Incomplete spontaneous abortion
       i. Supporting: heavy bleeding, passing clots
       ii. Refuting: occurring for multiple months, using birth control method regularly

3. What diagnostic testing will you order for the patient? Provide rationale for each test.

    a. Urine human chorionic gonadotropin (HCG)—rule-out pregnancy
    b. Cervical cytology—evaluate for malignant/premalignant lesion
    c. Complete blood count and ferritin—evaluate for anemia, ferritin stores
    d. Chlamydia and gonorrhea cultures or urine testing—evaluate for sexually transmitted infection
    e. Thyroid stimulating hormone—evaluate for hypo- or hyperthyroidism
    f. Liver function tests —evaluate for liver disease affecting clotting
    g. Pelvic and vaginal ultrasound—evaluate for structural abnormalities

4. What will your management plan recommendations be for the patient if she has an ultrasound that shows a small leiomyoma located in the uterine wall and all other diagnostic testing results are normal/negative? Include short- and long-term goals, any prescriptions, patient education, and follow-up plans.

    a. Short-term goals
       i. Reduce dysmenorrhea
       ii. Decrease frequency and quantity of bleeding

    b. Long-term goals
       i. Return to usual menstrual pattern
       ii. Pregnancy prevention
       iii. Avoid surgery

(*continued*)

CASE STUDY (*continued*)

    c. Medications

      i. Naproxen sodium for dysmenorrhea, start 2 to 3 days prior to menses, take with food

      ii. Levonorgestrel IUD to reduce heavy bleeding and prevent pregnancy

    d. Patient education

      i. Discuss nature of leiomyoma

      ii. Review how to take medications, risks/benefits, potential adverse effects

      iii. When to call

    e. Follow-up

      i. Phone or in-person in 2 to 3 months, re-evaluate bleeding frequency and amount, re-evaluate dysmenorrhea

BIBLIOGRAPHY

Abou-Salem, N., Elmazny, A., & El-Sherbiny, W. (2010). Value of 3-dimensional sonohysterography for detection of intrauterine lesions in women with abnormal uterine bleeding. *Journal of Minimally Invasive Gynecology, 17*(2), 200–204. https://doi.org/10.1016/j.jmig. 2009. 12. 010

American College of Obstetricians and Gynecologists. (2012). Practice bulletin no. 128: Diagnosis of abnormal uterine bleeding in reproductive-aged women. *Obstetrics & Gynecology, 120*(1), 197–206. https://doi.org/10.1097/AOG. 0b013e318262e320

American College of Obstetrics and Gynecology. (2013a). ACOG practice bulletin: Management of abnormal uterine bleeding associated with ovulatory dysfunction. *Obstetrics & Gynecology, 122*(1), 176–185. https://doi.org/10.1097/01. AOG. 0000431815. 52679. bb

American College of Obstetrics and Gynecology. (2013b). ACOG practice bulletin: Management of acute abnormal uterine bleeding in nonpregnant reproductive-aged women. *Obstetrics & Gynecology, 122*(1), 891–896. https://doi.org/10. 1097/01. AOG. 0000428646. 67925. 9a

Attia, A. H., Youssef, D., Hassan, N., El-Meligui, M., Kamal, M., & Al-Inany, H. (2007). Subclinical hyperthyroidism as a potential factor for dysfunctional uterine bleeding. *Gynecological Endocrinology, 23*(2), 65–68. https://doi.org/10. 1080/09513590601095061

Bevan, J. A., Maloney, K. W., Hillery, C. A., Gill, J. C., Montgomery, R. R., & Scott, J. P. (2001). Bleeding disorders: A common cause of menorrhagia in adolescents. *Journal of Pediatrics, 138*(6), 856–861. https://doi.org/10. 1067/mpd.2001. 113042

Côté, I., Jacobs, P., & Cumming, D. (2002). Work loss associated with increased menstrual loss in the United States. *Obstetrics and Gynecology, 100*(4), 683–687. https://doi.org/ 10.1016/s0029-7844(02)020943-x.

Davidson, B. R., Dipiero, C. M., Govoni, K. D., Littleton, S. S., & Neal, J. L. (2012). Abnormal uterine bleeding during the reproductive years. *Journal of Midwifery & Women's Health, 57*(3), 248–254. https://doi.org/10.1111/j.1542-2011. 2012. 00178. x

De Souza, M. J., Nattiv, A., Joy, E., Misra, M., Williams, N. I., Mallinson, R. J., Gibbs, J. C., Olmsted, M., Goolsby, M., Matheson, G., & Panel, E. (2014). 2014 Female athlete triad coalition consensus statement on treatment and return to play of the female athlete triad: 1st International conference held in San Francisco, CA, May 2012, and 2nd International Conference held in Indianapolis, IN, May 2013. *Clinical Journal of Sport Medicine, 24*(2), 96–119. https://doi.org/10.1097/JSM. 0000000000000085

Hobby, J. H., Zhao, Q., & Peipert, J. F. (2018). Effect of baseline menstrual bleeding pattern on copper intrauterine device continuation. *American Journal of Obstetrics and Gynecology, 219*(5), 465.e1–465. e5. https://doi.org/10-1016/j. ajog.2018.08.028

James, A. H., Kouides, P. A., Abdul-Kadir, R., Edlund, M., Federici, A. B., Halimeh, S., Kamphuisen, P. W., Konkle, B. A., Martínez-Perez, O., McLintock, C., & Peyvandi, F. (2009). Von Willebrand disease and other bleeding disorders in women: Consensus on diagnosis and management from an international expert panel. *American Journal of Obstetrics and Gynecology, 201*(1), 12. e1–12. e8. https://doi.org/10.1016/j. ajog. 2009. 04. 024

Kaunitz, A. M. (2021). Abnormal uterine bleeding in nonpregnant reproductive-age patients: Evaluation and approach to diagnosis. Up-To-Date Topic 3263. Available with subscription at: https://www.uptodate.com/contents/abnormal-uterine-bleeding-in-nonpregnant-reproductive-age-patients-evaluation-and-approach-to-diagnosis

Khan, F., Jamaat, S., & Al-Jaroudi, D. (2011). Saline infusion sonohysterography versus hysteroscopy for uterine cavity evaluation. *Annals of Saudi Medicine, 31*(4), 387–392. https://doi.org/10.4103/0256-4947.83213

Matteson, K. A., Raker, C. A., Clark, M. A., & Frick, K. D. (2013). Abnormal uterine bleeding, health status, and usual source of medical care: Analyses using the medical expenditures panel survey. *Journal of Women's Health (2002), 22*(11), 959–965. https://doi.org/10. 1089/jwh. 2013. 4288

Mishell Jr., D. R., Guillebaud, J., Westhoff, C., Nelson, A. L., Kaunitz, A. M., Trussell, J., & Davis, A. J. (2007). Recommendations for standardization of data collection and analysis of bleeding in combined hormone contraceptive trials. *Contraception, 75*(1), 11–15. https://doi.org/10.1016/j.contraception.2006.08.012

Munro, M. G., Critchley, H. O., Broder, M. S., & Fraser, I. S. (2011). FIGO classification system (PALM-COEIN) for causes of abnormal uterine bleeding in nongravid women of reproductive age. *International Journal of Gynaecology and Obstetrics, 113*(1), 3–13. https://doi.org/10. 1016/j. ijgo. 2010. 11. 011

Munro, M. G., Critchley, H. O., & Fraser, I. S. (2011). The FIGO classification of causes of abnormal uterine bleeding in the reproductive years. *Fertility and Sterility, 95*(7), 2204–8, 2208. e1. https://doi.org/10. 1016/j. fertnstert. 2011. 03. 079

Munro, M. G., Critchley, H. O. D., Fraser, I. S., & FIGO Menstrual Disorders Committee. (2018). The two FIGO systems for normal and abnormal uterine bleeding symptoms and classification of causes of abnormal uterine bleeding in the reproductive years: 2018 revisions. *International Journal of Gynaecology and Obstetrics, 143*(3), 393–408. https://doi.org/ 10.1002/ijgo.12666.

Singh, S., Best, C., Dunn, S., Leyland, N., & Wolfman, W. L. & Clinical Practice– Gynaecology Committee. (2013). Abnormal uterine bleeding in pre-menopausal women. *Journal of Obstetrics and Gynaecology Canada, 35*(5), 473–475. https://doi.org/10. 1016/S1701-2163(15)30939-7

Sweet, M. G., Schmidt-Dalton, T. A., Weiss, P. M., & Madsen, K. P. (2012). Evaluation and management of abnormal uterine bleeding in premenopausal women. *American Family Physician, 85*(1), 35–43. https://www. aafp. org/afp/2012/0101/ p35. html

Taylor, H. S., Pal, L., & Seli, E. (2020). *Spiroff's clinical gynecologic endocrinology and infertility* (9th ed.). Lippincott Williams & Wilkins. ISBN: 978-1-4511-8976-6

Tower, A. M., & Frishman, G. N. (2013). Cesarean scar defects: An underrecognized cause of abnormal uterine bleeding and other gynecologic complications. *Journal of Minimally Invasive Gynecology, 20*(5), 562–572. https://doi.org/10.1016/j. jmig.2013.03.008

Tsai, M. C., & Goldstein, S. R. (2012). Office diagnosis and management of abnormal uterine bleeding. *Clinical Obstetrics and Gynecology, 55*(3), 635–650. https://doi.org/10. 1097/GRF. 0b013e31825d3cec

29

AMENORRHEA

SHELAGH B. LARSON

AMENORRHEA

A. Definition
1. Amenorrhea is the absence of a menstrual period when not caused by pregnancy, breastfeeding, or menopause.
2. Oligomenorrhea is going longer than 35 days without a period.
3. It is not a disease process, but it can be a sign of other health problems.
4. Menstruation usually begins with menarche at age 12.8 and ceases at age 51 with menopause.
5. About one in 25 women who are not pregnant, breastfeeding, or going through menopause experience amenorrhea at some point in their lives.

B. Types of amenorrhea
1. **Primary:** Primary amenorrhea is defined as no menstruation by age 15.
   a. Cause
      (1) Chromosomal or genetic problem with the ovaries
         - Vaginal agenesis is a rare disorder that occurs when the vagina does not develop, and the uterus may only develop partially or not at all.
         - **Turner syndrome**: A condition caused by a partially or completely missing X chromosome that can cause a variety of developmental and physical issues such as short in stature, failure of the ovaries to fully develop, hearing and vision problems, kidney problems, and cardiac problems including high blood pressure. Women with Turner syndrome usually have webbed folds of skin that stretch from about the ears to shoulders and lower hairline in the back of the head.
         - **Androgen Insensitivity Syndrome, or Reifenstein syndrome:** Occurs when a person is genetically a male with XY chromosomes however, the body does not respond to the androgen hormone. The body forms external female sex characteristics. Internally, they are male with undescended testes and no uterus.
      (2) Structural problem with the reproductive organs, such as missing parts of the reproductive system.
2. **Secondary**: Secondary amenorrhea is defined as the absence of menses for 6 or more months or the length of three cycles after the establishment of regular menstrual cycles
   a. Causes (Table 29.1)
      (1) Functional hypothalamic amenorrhea (FHA) is the most common cause of secondary amenorrhea. It is defined as the absence of menses, caused by a suppression of the hypothalamic-pituitary-ovarian (HPO) axis, in which no anatomic or organic cause is found. Stress related to insufficient nutrition, excessive physical effort, and psychological trauma can cause the body to become hormonally imbalanced. FHA is the most common cause of missed periods in dancers and athletes. If left untreated, FHA can have a detrimental impact on bone, cardiovascular, mental, metabolic, and reproductive health.
      (2) Polycystic ovarian syndrome (PCOS) occurs when an ovarian follicle does not mature enough to release an egg. These women usually have insulin insensitivity wherein the

TABLE 29.1 Causes of Secondary Amenorrhea	
Physiological	Breastfeeding Contraception Exogenous androgens Menopause Pregnancy
Intrauterine adhesions	Asherman syndrome

Ovarian	Polycystic ovarian syndrome
	Premature ovarian insufficiency:
	    Acquired
	        Autoimmune
	        Chemotherapy or radiation
	    Congenital
	        Gonadal dysgenesis (other than Turner syndrome)
	        Turner syndrome or variant
	Ovarian tumors

Brain:
Hypothalamic,
pituitary
	Autoimmune disease
	Brain radiation
	Constitutional delay of puberty
	Cushing's syndrome
	Empty sella syndrome
	Functional
	    Eating disorder
	    Stress
	    Vigorous exercise
	    Weight loss
	Gonadotropin deficiency (e.g., Kallmann syndrome)
	Hyperprolactinemia
	    Adenoma (prolactinoma)
	    Chronic kidney disease
	    Medications or illicit drugs (e.g., antipsychotics, opiates)
	Sheehan syndrome

Other	Adrenal insufficiency Androgen-secreting tumor (e.g., ovarian or adrenal) Celiac disease Congenital adrenal hyperplasia Diabetes mellitus, uncontrolled Hypothyroidism Inflammatory bowel disease Late-onset congenital adrenal hyperplasia
Medications	Certain medications that treat cancer, seizures, psychosis, or schizophrenia
Illegal drugs	Cocaine, heroin, methadone, and marijuana

body is not reacting to its insulin or an overproduction of testosterone. It can also be both conditions. Individuals present with acne, excessive facial and body hair, and/or obesity. A diverse endocrine condition in reproductive aged women commonly associated with menstrual irregularities or absence, physical or biochemical evidence of androgen excess, and an increased number of immature ovarian follicles. This diagnosis can only be made after excluding other pathologic conditions.

(3) Hypothyroidism can cause missed periods.

(4) Premature ovarian insufficiency (POI), also known as premature ovarian failure, is a condition characterized by hypergonadotropic hypogonadism, a disorder of abnormal

function of gonads with a deficiency of testosterone in males and estradiol in females. This results in the development of menopause before the age of 40. It affects approximately 1 in 100 females and is defined by ovarian follicle dysfunction or depletion. It is usually diagnosed with two serum follicle-stimulating hormone levels in the menopausal range obtained at least 1 month apart.

C. Pathophysiology of amenorrhea
  1. No uterus
  2. Lack of endometrium
  3. Genetic disorder
  4. Hormone imbalance

D. Impact of amenorrhea
  1. Infertility
  2. Low bone density, osteoporosis
  3. Polycystic ovarian syndrome/metabolic disorder
  4. **Emotional health:** Stress, eating disorders
  5. Depression

E. Evaluation of amenorrhea (Figures 29.1 and 29.2)
  1. Blood work can further help determine the source of the amenorrhea (Table 29.2).
     a. If gonadotropins are elevated and POI is diagnosed, other testing would be required including autoimmune antibodies and fragile X testing. An abnormal karyotype is apparent in approximately one third of patients with primary amenorrhea, and it should be offered to all patients with a diagnosis of POI.
  2. Imaging studies
     a. Pelvis ultrasonography can identify any congenital abnormalities of the uterus, fallopian tubes, or ovaries.
     b. MRI of the sella turcica can rule out a pituitary tumor. Normal MRI indicates a hypothalamic cause of amenorrhea.
     c. Abdominal ultrasound can assess adrenal tumors.
  3. Hormone challenge
     a. Progesterone challenge begins by giving medroxyprogesterone 5 to 10 mg or norethindrone 2.5 to 10 mg orally daily for 7 to 10 days to produce secretory transformation of an endometrium that has been adequately primed with either endogenous or exogenous estrogen.
        (1) If bleeding occurs, amenorrhea is most likely not caused by an endometrial issue (e.g., Asherman syndrome) or outflow tract obstruction, and the cause is probably hypothalamic–pituitary dysfunction, ovarian insufficiency, or estrogen excess.
        (2) If bleeding does not occur, this may suggest an outflow tract abnormality or a hypoestrogenic state, as estrogen is responsible for thickening the endometrial lining. Evaluate with an estrogen challenge; e.g., conjugated equine estrogen 1.25 mg, estradiol 2 mg orally once a day is given for 21 days, followed by daily medroxyprogesterone 10 mg or norethindrone 10 mg orally for 7 to 10 days. If bleeding does not occur after estrogen is added, patients may have an endometrial issue or outflow tract obstruction. However, bleeding may not occur in patients who do not have these abnormalities (e.g., because the uterus is insensitive to estrogen); thus, the trial using estrogen and progestin may be repeated for confirmation.

F. Treatment
  1. Lifestyle changes
     a. Healthy weight, too little or too much weight can impact hormone balance
     b. Reduce stress
     c. **Physical activity:** may need to reduce or increase physical activity

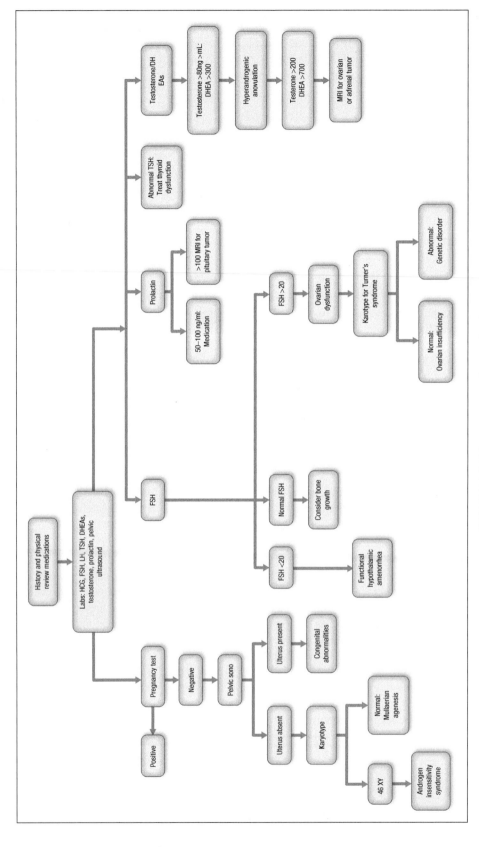

FIGURE 29.1 Primary amenorrhea evaluation.

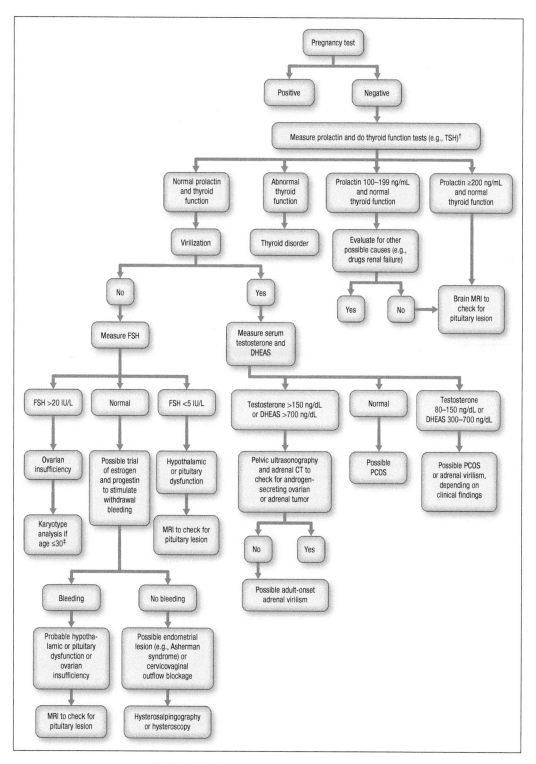

FIGURE 29.2 Secondary amenorrhea evaluation.

TABLE 29.2 Normal Lab Values

ANTI-MULLERIAN HORMONE		LOW DECREASE OVARIAN RESERVE HIGH: MAY BE INDICATIVE OF POLYCYSTIC OVARIAN SYNDROME (PCOS)
Estradiol	30 to 400 pg/mL	<50 pg/mL indicate hypoestrogenism
Dehydroepiandrosterone sulfate	250–300 ng/dL	Elevated may indicate hyperandrogenism
Follicle stimulating hormone	5–20 IU/L	Elevated suggests an ovarian anomaly (hypergonadotropic hypogonadism, menopause) Normal or low levels suggest a pituitary or hypothalamic abnormality (hypogonadotropic hypogonadism)
Luteinizing hormone	5–40 IU/L	
Progesterone	Pre-ovulation: <1 ng/mL or 3.18 nmol/L Mid-cycle: 5–20 ng/mL or 15.90–63.60 nmol/L	<1 ng.nL no ovulation
Prolactin	2 to 29 ng/mL	50–100 ng/mL mildly elevated and may be due to use of medication (oral contraceptive pills, antipsychotics, antidepressants, antihypertensives, histamine H_2 blockers, opiates) >100 ng/mL usually corresponds to a pituitary tumor.
Testosterone (total and free)	20–80 ng/dL	High: Hyperandrogenism, PCOS, ovarian or adrenal tumor, congenital adrenal hyperplasia, Cushing syndrome
Thyroid stimulating hormone	0.5 to 5.0 mIU/L	

2. Medical interventions
   a. For primary amenorrhea, hormone therapy consisting of an estrogen and a progestin (combination birth control) is recommended first line for women with estrogen deficiency.
   b. Hormone therapy with primary ovarian insufficiency or fragile X-associated primary ovarian insufficiency
   c. For secondary amenorrhea, dopamine agonists are the only medical therapy specifically approved to reverse an underlying pathology that leads to amenorrhea. In most cases, dopamine agonists effectively reduce hyperprolactinemia.
   d. Balance thyroid levels
   e. Insulin-sensitizing agents such as metformin (Glucophage) can reduce insulin resistance and improve ovulatory function.
   f. **Medication-induced amenorrhea:** Adjust dose or duration.
3. Surgical intervention
   a. **Uterine scarring:** Removal of scar tissue resulting from a cesarean section, prior medical procedure, endometriosis, or other condition may be helpful in treating amenorrhea.
   b. Pituitary tumor removal if medication has not been successful

BIBLIOGRAPHY

American College of Obstetricians and Gynecologist. (2020). *Amenorrhea: Absences of Periods. FAQ513*. https://www. acog.org/womens-health/faqs/amenorrhea-absence-of-periods (ACOG) 2020. Revitalize: Gynecology Data Definitions

Gordon, C. M. (2010). Clinical practice. Functional hypothalamic amenorrhea. *New England Journal of Medicine, 363*(4), 365–371. https://doi.org/10.1056/NEJMcp0912024

Klein, D., Paradise, S. L., & Reeder, R. M. (2019). Amenorrhea: A systematic approach to diagnosis and management. *American Family Physician, 100*(1), 40–48.

Landau, M. D. (2020). What is amenorrhea? Symptoms, causes, diagnosis, treatment, and prevention. *Everyday Health Newsletter*. https://www.everydayhealth.com/amenorrhea/guide/#diagnosis

Lawson, E. A., Donoho, D., Miller, K. K., Misra, M., Meenaghan, E., Lydecker, J., Wexler, T., Herzog, D. B., & Klibanski, A. (2009). Hypercortisolemia is associated with severity of bone loss and depression in hypothalamic amenorrhea and anorexia nervosa. *The Journal of Clinical Endocrinology & Metabolism, 94*(12), 4710–4716. https://doi.org/10.1210/jc.2009-1046

Pereira, K., & Brown, A. J. (2017). Secondary amenorrhea: Diagnostic approach and treatment considerations. *The Nurse Practitioner, 42*(9), 34–41. https://doi.org/10.1097/01.NPR.0000520832.14406.76. PMID: 28832422.

Pinkerton, J. (2020). *Amenorrhea. Merck Manuals*. https://www.merckmanuals.com/en-ca/professional/gynecology-and -obstetrics/menstrual-abnormalities/amenorrhea

Pletcher, J. R., & Slap, G. B. (1999). Menstrual disorders: amenorrhea. *Pediatric Clinics of North America, 46*(3), 505–518. https://doi.org/10.1016/s0031-3955(05)70134-6

Podfigurna, A., & Meczekalski, B. (2021). Functional hypothalamic amenorrhea: A stress-based disease. *Endocrines, 2*(3), 203–211. https://doi.org/10.3390/endocrines2030020

Sophie Gibson, M. E., Fleming, N., Zuijdwijk, C., & Dumont, T. (2020). Where have the periods gone? The evaluation and management of functional hypothalamic amenorrhea. *Journal of Clinical Research in Pediatric Endocrinology, 12*(Suppl 1), 18–27. https://doi.org/10.4274/jcrpe.galenos.2019.2019.S0178

The Practice Committee of the American Society for Reproductive Medicine: Current evaluation of amenorrhea. *Fertility and Sterility, 90*(5 Suppl), S219–S225, 2008. https://doi.org/10.1016/j.fertnstert.2008.08.038

30

PREMENSTRUAL SYNDROME AND PREMENSTRUAL DYSPHORIC DISORDER

SHELAGH B. LARSON

DEFINITIONS

A. Premenstrual yndrome
   1. Premenstrual syndrome (PMS) is a combination of physical and emotional symptoms that many women get after ovulation and before the start of their menstrual period.
   2. It is thought to be caused by a dramatic drop in estrogen and progesterone levels if the woman is not pregnant.
   3. PMS usually starts 5 days before the period starts until 4 days into the cycle.
   4. Over 90% of women verbalize having some degree of PMS, such as bloating, headaches, and moodiness.
   5. It is estimated that up to 12% of women suffer with PMS, and in most of those cases, the symptoms are moderate. It is believed that about 1% to 5% of women have premenstrual dysphoric disorder (PMDD).
   6. PMS is more common from the late 20s to the 40s with the most intense symptoms often arising in the late 30s into the 40s.
   7. Women may have PMS during some menstrual cycles but not with every cycle. It estimated that, at some point during a woman's life, nearly 75% will experience PMS-like symptoms.
B. Premenstrual dysphoric disorder
   1. Premenstrual dysphoric disorder (PMDD) is a condition much like PMS in that it happens in the week 1 or 2 prior to the onset of the period when hormone levels begin to plunge after ovulation.
   2. PMDD causes more severe symptoms than PMS, including severe depression, irritability, and tension that can trigger problems with work or personal relationships.
   3. PMDD affects up to 5% of women of childbearing age.
   4. Many women with PMDD may also have underlying anxiety or depression.
   5. PMDD can disrupt a woman's life and relationships so completely, the woman may despair that life itself is not worth living. About 15% of women with PMDD attempt suicide.

ETIOLOGY

A. Cause is not fully understood.
B. Fluctuations in hormones estradiol and progesterone appear to be involved; a person's sensitivity to these hormones may have links to PMDD and PMS.
C. Chemical change in the brain and fluctuation in serotonin also appear to have an impact.
   1. Alterations in temperament may be attributable to the effect that estrogen and progesterone have on the serotonin, γ-aminobutyric acid, and dopamine systems.

2. Serotonergic function seems to be altered in the luteal phase of the menstrual cycle in women with PMS/PMDD.
3. Insufficient amounts of serotonin cause depression, fatigue, food cravings, and sleep problems.
4. Studies found 60% to 90% of women with PMDD respond to treatment with drugs that block reuptake of serotonin, compared with 30% to 40% on placebos.

D. Several vitamins and minerals including vitamin B, vitamin D, calcium, and magnesium are essential for neurotransmitter synthesis and hormonal balance, both of which are potentially involved in the underlying pathogenesis of PMS.
   1. Magnesium is essential for the brain's dopaminergic synthesis. Dopamine imbalance can affect mood and can lead to overwhelming anxiety. Magnesium is also noted in reducing bloating, fluid retention, and breast tenderness.
   2. Decreased circulating magnesium concentrations during the luteal phase suggest that magnesium deficiency may be a key factor in PMS.
   3. Vitamin B is involved in various steps of serotonin metabolism including converting the amino acid tryptophan to serotonin and generating the active substances required for metabolism of serotonin.
   4. Vitamin B_6 (pyridoxine) deficiency can deter serotonin production, which can result in mood disorders.
   5. Nurses' Health Study found that women with high intake of vitamin D and calcium carried lower risk of developing PMS compared with those in the group with low intake

E. Supplements: Chasteberry Extract (Vitex agnus-castus) is known traditionally for balancing the female sex hormones estrogen and progesterone and their interaction with the pituitary gland, which is responsible for releasing follicular stimulating hormone (FSH) and luteinizing hormone (LH). Several studies support the use of chasteberry to modulate hormones that can contribute to PMS/PMDD and other reproductive conditions like polycystic ovarian syndrome (PCOS), mild hyperprolactinemia, mastalgia/mastodynia, amenorrhea, and oligomenorrhea.
   1. In a meta-analysis review comparing Vitex to vitamin B_6 and the SSRI, fluoxetine, the author found Vitex to be superior to B_6 in alleviating PMS symptoms but found that fluoxetine was more effective in alleviating psychological symptoms. Vitex did better than magnesium, pyridoxine, St. John's wort, and vitamin E, and significantly improved all PMS-related symptoms. Reviews concluded that Vitex could be offered to people with PMS or PMDD who either do not want or cannot use prescription medications.

SYMPTOMS

A. Diagnosis of PMS
   1. Symptoms for both PMS and PMDD are similar, the difference is the severity (Table 30.1).
   2. With PMS, a woman experiences at least one affective symptom and one somatic symptom that cause dysfunction in social, academic, or work performance.
   3. Symptom resolution after day 4 on menses without recurrence until at least day 13 of the cycle and occur without any pharmacologic therapy, hormone ingestion, or drug or alcohol use.
   4. The symptoms must occur reproducibly during two cycles of prospective recording. The patient must exhibit identifiable dysfunction in social, academic, or work performance.
   5. Women with PMS are at least twice as likely to experience insomnia before and during their period. Poor sleep may cause excessive daytime sleepiness and feeling tired or drowsy around their period.

B. Diagnosis of PMDD: For a diagnosis of PMDD, a patient must experience at least *five PMS* symptoms during the week before menses that improve within a few days after the onset of menses.

TABLE 30.1 Premenstrual Syndrome Symptoms	
EMOTIONAL	**PHYSICAL**
• Fatigue or feeling tired • Irritability • Problems with sleeping too much or too little • Changes in appetite • Mood swings • Issues with memory or concentration • Anxiety, tension • Decreased sex drive • Loss of interest in daily activities • Feeling sad, frequent crying, or depression	• Acne flares • Abdomen bloated or gassy • Breast tenderness/swelling • Diarrhea or constipation • Cramping • Lower tolerance for light or noise • Clumsiness • Headaches or backaches • Joint pain • Weight gain/fluid retention

C. Symptoms
 1. Marked anxiety, restlessness, or feeling on edge
 2. Marked depression, despondency, or self-depreciation
 3. Marked irritability, anger, or social tensions
 4. Marked emotional signs; feelings of unexplained sadness, dread, or tearful, mood swings, insensitivity to negativity/rejection
 5. Lack of energy, fatigue, weary, sluggish
 6. Lack of interest in normal activities (friends, work, school, interests)
 7. Noticeable difficulty concentrating and staying focused
 8. Marked change in appetite; overeating, binging, cravings (especially sweets)
 9. Extreme insomnia or sleeplessness
 10. Sense of being out of control, "out of body," not coping well
 11. Physical symptoms (i.e., abdominal bloating, breast tenderness/swelling, muscle/joint pain, weight gain)

D. The symptoms are associated with clinically significant distress and interferences with work, school, usual social activities, or relationships with others including avoiding social activities, decreased productivity and efficiency at home, school, and work.

E. The episodes are not just an exacerbation of the symptoms of another disorder, major/persistent depressive disorder, panic disorder, or a personality disorder; however, these disorders may co-exist with PMDD.

F. Criteria should be confirmed by prospective daily ratings during at least two symptomatic cycles.

G. The symptoms are not attributed to any physiological side effects of medication, substance abuse, other treatment, or medical conditions.

PHARMACOLOGIC MANAGEMENT (TABLE 30.2)

Non-Pharmaceutical Treatments

A. Diet
 1. Women with PMS typically consume more dairy products, high-sodium foods, and refined sugar than women without PMS. Therefore, limiting these foods as well as salt, caffeine, alcohol, chocolate, or simple carbohydrates may alleviate symptoms.
 2. Eating smaller meals yet more frequently (i.e., four to six times a day) during the premenstrual period may help reduce symptoms or food cravings that can contribute to bloating, changes in bowel habits, and weight gain.

TABLE 30.2 Pharmacologic Management of Premenstrual Syndrome/Premenstrual Dysphoric Disorder

General Comments:
- Selective serotonin reuptake inhibitors (SSRIs) are first line for PMD/PMDD and may be taking only from ovulation to menstruation or continuously
- Oral contraceptive pills (OCP) therapy balances estradiol and progesterone and is FDA approved for treatment in women who also desire contraception.

GENERIC/BRAND AVAILABILITY	CONTINUOUS DOSING	LUTEAL-PHASE DAILY DOSE	SIDE EFFECTS/ MONITORING	COMMENTS
Selective serotonin reuptake inhibitors (SSRIs) Escitalopram Fluoxetine* Paroxetine* Paroxetine CR Sertraline*	5–20 mg 10–30 mg 10–30 mg 12.5–37.5 mg 25–150 mg	5–20 mg 10–30 mg 10–40 mg 12.5–50 mg 25–200 mg	Nausea, vomiting, diarrhea, fatigue, headaches, insomnia, jittery, sexual dysfunction, weight gain, serotonin syndrome	Intermittent dosing is sufficient for treating irritability or mood, but daily medication may be necessary to control somatic symptoms such as fatigue and physical discomfort
Serotonin and norepinephrine reuptake inhibitors (SNRIs) Venlafaxine	37.5–112 mg	20–200 mg	Nausea, anorexia, anxiety, constipation diaphoresis, dry mouth sexual dysfunction, serotonin syndrome	
Oral contrceptive pills (OCPs) Drospirenone/ethinyl estradiol*	3 mg/20 mcg for 24 active pills, 4 placebos		Nausea, vomiting, abdominal cramping, breast pain, headaches, moodiness, sexual dysfunction	
Benzodiazepines Alprazolam is considered a second-line treatment option	None	0.25 mg 0.50 mg 0.75 mg	Drowsiness, weakness, fatigue, impaired coordination, and dizziness	Habit forming
Gonadotropin-releasing hormone (GnRH) agonists	No longer a treatment suggestion due to side effects		May cause hypoestrogen adverse effects including hot flashes, night sweats, and decreased bone density	Not practical for long-term use because of the increased cardiovascular and osteoporosis risks associated with extended use
Vitamins Calcium carbonate Vitamin B$_6$ Vitamin D Magnesium	1,000–1,300 mg 80 mg/day 360 mg/day			
Chasteberry extract	20 mg			

*FDA-approved treatment for PMS/PMDD.

B. Exercise
   1. Exercise is known to increase endorphin levels, to help regulate progesterone and estrogen synthesis, and to encourage the production of endogenous anti-inflammatory chemicals.

2. Exercising improves overall fitness, opportunities to socialize, and the potential for reduction in feelings of depression, all of which may help to moderate the symptom profile in PMS.

C. Sleep

1. Having a consistent sleep schedule, avoiding excess caffeine, getting exposure to daylight, and developing a relaxing bedtime routine are all examples of strategies that can strengthen sleep hygiene.

2. Avoid any bedroom light at night before bed from TV, phones, computers, and/or tablets.

CASE STUDY

Patient Situation

A 21-year-old G2P2 female presents to your clinic complaining of depression, diarrhea, fatigue, and severe mood swings the week before her period. She also has acne and dysmenorrhea. Her headaches are so bad she cannot get out of bed to help with her children. It has gotten so bad she has called in sick to work the past 3 months. This started about 6 months ago after she stopped nursing her baby. But the last 4 months the symptoms have become unbearable. "The symptoms start to go away by the time my period is over. I cannot do this anymore. This is starting to affect my relationships with my parents, kids, and now my job. When I am like this, I don't care about anyone or anything. I cannot focus on work or at home. I am afraid I will get fired."

Subjective Data

- Rates headaches, cramping pain as 8/10 (with 10 being the worst pain possible) that slowly builds the week before her period.
- The depression she ranks as severe, PHQ9: 7 during this period, otherwise not emotional, not sad.
- Current medical history: None
- Not sexually active, so not interested in birth control.
- Home medications: Excedrin for the headaches, Motrin for the cramping, and Tums as needed for the bloating
- Denies history of sexually transmitted infections or UTIs.
- Non-smoker
- Denies physical activity
- Normally sleeps 7 hours a night; however, during this 2-week period she finds she is very tired and just wants to stay in bed and sleep. Her sleep is restless.

Objective Data

- No abdominal tenderness
- Alert and oriented to person, place, time
- Vital signs: Blood pressure 115/65, pulse 78/min, respiration 18/min
- Height: 5'4" Weight 204 lbs. but will go down to 196 after period

Clinical Analysis

What diagnostics do you anticipate that will be ordered, and why?

- Urine drug screen to rule out drugs
- Urine analysis to rule out UTI
- Laboratory tests: pregnancy test, thyroid stimulating hormones, estradiol, progesterone, complete metabolic panel (magnesium, calcium), vitamin D and pyridoxine (B_6) levels

(continued)

CASE STUDY (*continued*)

Identify this patient's modifiable and non-modifiable risk factors.
- Modifiable: Weight, exercise, sleep, diet
- Non-modifiable: Race, age, female

Diagnosis: *PMDD*

What is the priority intervention based on the patient's clinical presentation?

The symptoms are interfering with her ability to care for herself, her children, and now her job performance. The symptoms are becoming worse over time. Balancing hormones and neurotransmitters will enable her to gain control over her body and emotions. **After receiving the results of the diagnostics, the patient is scheduled to begin Plan of Care.**

What should be included in this patient's plan of care?

- Start on daily SSRI.
- Discuss the need and benefits of starting birth control pills versus chasteberry extract to stabilize hormones.
- Start daily exercise program.
- Begin taking a multivitamin.
- Establish a bedtime routine.
- Follow up in 3 months to assess treatment.

BIBLIOGRAPHY

Burnett, T. (2021, March 11). *Premenstrual dysphoric disorder: Different from PMS?* Mayo Clinic. Retrieved November 14, 2021, from https://www.mayoclinic.org/diseases-conditions/premenstrual-syndrome/expert-answers/pmdd/fahttps://www.mayoclinic.org/diseases-conditions/premenstrual-syndrome/expert-answers/pmdd/faq-20058315q-20058315

Fletcher, J. (2021, March 17). *Pmdd vs. pms: What are the differences? how are they treated?* Retrieved November 14, 2021, from https://www.medicalnewstoday.com/articles/pmdd-vs-pms

Kaewrudee, S., Kietpeerakool, C., Pattanittum, P., & Lumbiganon, P. (2018). Vitamin or mineral supplements for premenstrual syndrome. *Cochrane Database of Systematic Reviews.* https://doi.org/10.1002/14651858.cd012933

Lete, I., & Lapuente, O. (2016). Contraceptive options for women with premenstrual dysphoric disorder: Current insights and a narrative review. *Open Access Journal of Contraception, 7,* 117–125. https://doi.org/10.2147/oajc.s97013

National Universilty of Natural Medicine. (2019, May 30). *Vitex for pms and pmdd - national university of natural medicine.* National University of Natural Medicine. https://nunm.edu/2019/05/chaste-tree-berry-pms

Office on Women's Health. (2018, March 16). *Premenstrual dysphoric disorder (pmdd) | office on women's health.* https://www.womenshealth.gov/menstrual-cycle/premenstrual-syndrome/premenstrual-dysphoric-disorder-pmdd

Pearce, E., Jolly, K., Jones, L. L., Matthewman, G., Zanganeh, M., & Daley, A. (2020). Exercise for premenstrual syndrome: A systematic review and meta-analysis of randomized controlled trials. *British Journal of General Practice, 4*(3), https://doi.org/10.3399/bjgpopen20X101032

Shaw, S., Wyatt, K., Campbell, J., Ernst, E., & Thompson-Coon, J. (2018). Vitex agnus castus for premenstrual syndrome. *The Cochrane Database of Systematic Reviews, 2018*(3), CD004632. https://doi.org/10.1002/14651858.CD004632.pub2

Vyas, N. (2021, November 17). *PMSand insomnia.* Sleep Foundation. https://www.sleepfoundation.org/insomnia/pms-and-insomnia

Unit V

EVALUATION OF THE PELVIC FLOOR

31
PELVIC ORGAN PROLAPSE

LISA S. PAIR AND HELEN A. CARCIO

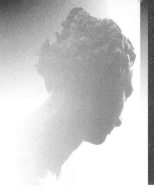

PELVIC ORGAN PROLAPSE EXPLAINED

A. Pelvic organ prolapse is defined as a downward descent of the anterior vaginal wall, posterior vaginal wall, uterus, or vaginal apex (female pelvic organs) into or through the vagina. Descent against the vaginal wall or actual protrusion through the vaginal outlet may occur in one or more of these structures. Prolapse of pelvic structures can cause a sensation of pelvic pressure or bulging through the vaginal opening and may be associated with urinary incontinence, voiding dysfunction, fecal incontinence, incomplete defecation, and sexual dysfunction.

B. Pelvic organ prolapse is caused by the failure of both the pelvic floor muscles and connective tissue. The muscles of the pelvic floor lie at the bottom of the abdominopelvic cavity.
   1. The levator ani muscles form a supportive layer that prevents the pelvic organs (uterus, rectum, or bladder) from descending through the bony pelvis.
   2. When these muscles become weakened, torn, or stretched, the vaginal outlet enlarges, allowing for easier descent of the uterus, rectum, or bladder to or through the vaginal opening (Figure 31.1).
   3. It supports conception and parturition.
   4. It controls storage and evacuation of feces and urine.
   5. A network of connective tissue, the endopelvic fascia, surrounds the muscles and functions to attach the muscles to the bony pelvic sidewalls.
   6. Provides a loose support allowing movement of the uterus, vagina, bladder, and rectum.
   7. Divided into three levels of support (Delancey's):
      a. Support focus is the cervix and upper third of the vagina. The cardinal and uterosacral ligaments attach the uterus and vaginal vault apically to the bony sacrum.
      b. Support focus is the middle third of the vagina. The connective tissue support arcus tendinous fascia pelvic (ATFP), and the fascia overlie the levator ani muscles and provide support to the middle section of the vagina including supporting the bladder and rectum.
      c. Support focus is the lower section of the vagina. In the perineal body, perineal muscles support the distal one third of the vagina and the introitus.

C. Mechanical principles in relation to prolapse of pelvic organs:
   1. The uterus and vagina lie suspended in a sling-like network of ligaments and fascial structures attached to the side walls of the pelvis.
   2. Levator ani muscles constrict, forming an occlusive layer on which the pelvic organs may rest.
      a. They consist of strong striated muscle tissue, comprising the iliococcygeus, the pubococcygeus, and the puborectalis (Figure 31.2).
      b. They compress the rectum, vagina, and urethra against the pubic bone, holding them in position.
   3. If the pelvic floor musculature functions normally, the pelvic floor is closed, and the ligaments and fascia (connective tissue) are under no tension.
   4. Problems exist when the pelvic floor muscles (PFMs) relax or are damaged. Risk factors are listed in Box 31.1.

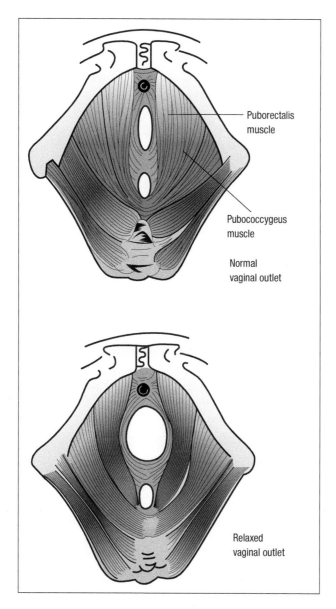

Puborectalis muscle

Pubococcygeus muscle

Normal vaginal outlet

Relaxed vaginal outlet

FIGURE 31.1 Graphical pictures of the widened vaginal outlet that puts the woman at risk for prolapse.

    a. The pelvic floor opens, and the vagina lies between the high intra-abdominal pressure and the low atmospheric pressure, where it must be held in place by ligaments.

    b. Eventually, connective tissue will become damaged and fail to hold the vagina in place.

  5. The increase in intra-abdominal pressure placed on the PFMs and ligaments causes the development of a prolapse, rather than problems with the organs themselves.

D. Urinary continence

  1. Depends on urethral support

    a. Failure of level III support. Weakness of the structures supporting the urethra at the vesical neck

    b. Active muscle contraction

    c. Intact neuromuscular mechanisms

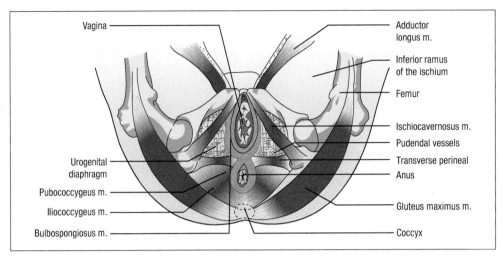

FIGURE 31.2 Muscles of the pelvic floor. The pubococcygeus muscle provides the main support for the pelvic floor.

   2. Ability of the urethra to remain closed
   3. Note: Closure pressure of the urethra must be equal to or exceed intravesical pressure.

ASSESSMENT

A. History
   1. Obtain a history of present illness concerning pelvic prolapse symptoms using OLDCARTS (Onset, Location/radiation, Duration, Character, Aggravating factors, Relieving factors, Timing and Severity).
   2. The degree of bother is important to ascertain for management purposes.
   3. Does prolapse limit sexual function or physical activity?
   4. Assess for urinary storage and emptying symptoms.
   5. Assess for bowel elimination symptoms such as splinting, straining to eliminate, or accidental bowel leakage.
B. Physical examination
   1. Perform an abdominal, pelvic, and neurologic assessment.

BOX 31.1 Risk Factors for the Development of Pelvic Floor Relaxation

- Chronic cough (due to asthma or chronic bronchitis)
- Heavy lifting (prolonged)
- High-impact sports
- Obesity
- High parity
- Caucasian (higher incidence in this population)
- Advancing age (estrogen deficiency)
- Vaginal delivery
- Previous hysterectomy
- Genetic predisposition (connective tissue disorders, family history of pelvic organ prolapse)
- Previous pelvic or vaginal irradiation
- Decreased pelvic muscle strength

2. Patient should void prior to the exam.
   a. Abdomen is assessed for gross masses, scars, tenderness, and herniation
   b. Neurologic assessment of sacral nerve roots (S2–S4) focusing on perineal sensation and anal and bulbocavernosus reflexes. If neurologically intact, one will see contraction of the external anal sphincter.
      (1) Anal wink is demonstrated when cotton tip applicator is stroked adjacent to the anus.
      (2) Bulbocavernosus reflex is demonstrated when the clitoris is lightly squeezed.
   c. Pelvic assessment
      (1) Inspection of external vaginal area and vagina for evidence of contact dermatitis from urine leakage, genitourinary syndrome of menopause, or vaginal discharge. The vagina is further assessed for prolapse with Valsalva; any prolapse should be identified and quantified. For optimal prolapse evaluation, the patient may need to stand. The clinician may use a handheld mirror to explain pelvic findings.
      (2) Perform bimanual exam. Assess for uterine size if application, any tenderness, or adnexal masses.
      (3) Assess for pelvic floor muscle strength. Place two fingers (index and middle fingers) into the vagina and have the patient squeeze around your fingers. Instruct the patient to avoid tightening the abdomen and gluteal regions and the legs. Explain to the patient to squeeze like trying to inhibit passage of flatus. The strength of the pelvic floor contraction is described as absent, weak, normal, or strong. Note the patient's ability to sustain a constriction and palpate for any deflection of finger or fingers upward with a good squeeze. No deflection indicates weaker muscles (see Table 31.1). As described previously, a rectal squeeze draws the rectum and vagina upward and forward toward the symphysis pubis to tighten and close the vagina.
      (4) **Digital rectal examination:** Assess for any fecal impaction. Note sphincter muscle tone.
      (5) **Assess urethral mobility:** This can be through visual inspection of urethral mobility with Valsalva.
      (6) **Or perform the Q-tip test:** A sterile Q-tip with lidocaine jelly is inserted into the urethra to the urethrovesical junction (level of the bladder neck) and the angle of the Q-tip change with Valsalva is measured from a horizontal plane. An axis change with Valsalva of $\geq 30°$ is defined as urethral hypermobility.
      (7) Assess post-void residual (PVR) either via ultrasound or catherization.
         • High residual may indicate obstructive voiding due to prolapse
         • High residual may indicate neurologic disorder
         • Normal PVR <200 mL
         • PVR should be assessed within 20 minutes of voiding

TABLE 31.1 Assessment of Pelvic Muscle Strength				
PARAMETERS	0	1	2	3
Pressure	None	Weak	Moderate	Strong; fingers compressed
Duration	None	Less than 1 sec	1–3 sec	More than 3 sec
Displacement	None	Slight incline	Noticeable incline	Fingers drawn in

STEP-BY-STEP ASSESSMENT OF PELVIC ORGAN PROLAPSE

A. Once the prolapse is visible, other structures need to be systematically assessed.
  1. Focus on the specific defects.
  2. Note the severity of the prolapse (i.e., prolapse in relation to hymenal ring).
  3. Stage the prolapse.
B. Identify the extent of descent of the anterior vagina, cervix or apex of the vagina, and posterior vagina.
  1. Examine the anterior and posterior vagina by retracting the opposite wall with the posterior half of a vaginal speculum so that a larger anterior vaginal prolapse does not obscure a smaller posterior vaginal prolapse.
C. Staging the prolapse
  1. Prolapse staging systems are varied and can be subjective. Table 31.2 lists one form of classification. The best grading system for prolapse is the Pelvic Organ Prolapse Quantification (POP-Q) system. The POP-Q system is a validated method for objective prolapse measurement. It is more precise and reproducible. (Explaining this system is beyond the scope of this chapter.)
  2. It is best to describe the size of a prolapse in terms of the distance the prolapse descends below or rises above the hymenal ring with the prolapse extended to its fullest (e.g., "The cervix lies 2 cm below the hymenal ring." "The anterior wall extends 3 cm beyond the hymenal opening.").
D. Evaluate the anterior vaginal wall support.
  1. Establish status of urethral and bladder support.
  2. Urethra is fused with the lower 3 to 4 cm of the vaginal wall.
  3. Urethrocele
    a. Diagnosed by descent of the lower anterior vaginal wall to the level of the hymenal ring during straining.
    b. Seen as a herniation between the urethra and vagina, as the urethra prolapses into the anterior vaginal vault, out of the correct angle with the bladder.
    c. Can be associated with stress incontinence and loss of urethral support.
  4. Anterior vaginal wall prolapse (formerly called a cystocele)
    a. Loss of support of the anterior vaginal wall (Figure 31.3)
    b. Descent of the bladder into a portion of the common wall between the bladder and vagina. The vaginal wall descends from the pressure of the bladder pushing against the vaginal wall.
    c. Measure the prolapse of the anterior vaginal wall in relation to the hymenal plane.
E. Evaluate position of the apex (most distal) of the vagina (also known as uterine or vaginal vault prolapse).
  1. Insert a normal speculum and locate the apex of the vagina or the cervix. Have the patient Valsalva and note the descent of the cervix or the apex of the vagina.

TABLE 31.2 Staging of Pelvic Organ Prolapse (Baden-Walker Staging System)	
STAGE	**DESCRIPTION**
Stage 0	No prolapse
Stage 1	Descent halfway to the hymen >1 cm above the hymen
Stage 2	Descent to the hymen ≤1 cm proximal or distal to the hymenal plan
Stage 3	Descent halfway past the hymen >1 cm below the hymenal plane but protrudes <2 cm of the total vaginal length
Stage 4	Total vaginal or uterine eversion

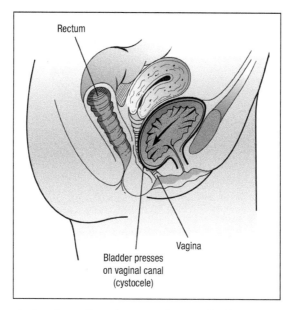

Rectum

Vagina

Bladder presses
on vaginal canal
(cystocele)

FIGURE 31.3 Anterior vaginal prolapse. Note the arrow showing the downward descent of the bladder into the vaginal canal and through the vaginal outlet.

2. Normal total vaginal length (TVL) in a person who has not had a hysterectomy is 10 to 12 cm to the hymen with no Valsalva.
3. Measure the TVL (length of the vagina with no Valsalva in centimeters)
4. Measure the loc.ation of the cervix or the apex of the vagina with Valsalva to the hymenal opening.
5. If the cervix or apex descends to within 1 cm of the hymenal ring, there is considerable loss of support. Note the location in relation to the hymenal ring for staging purposes. See Figure 31.4.
6. Complete uterine eversion outside the vagina (Stage 4) is called procidentia.

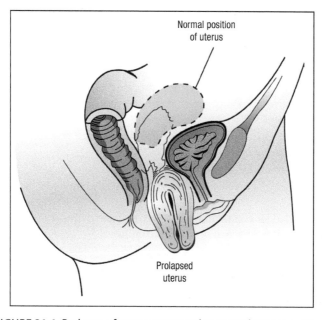

Normal position
of uterus

Prolapsed
uterus

FIGURE 31.4 Prolapse of uterus compared to normal uterus position.

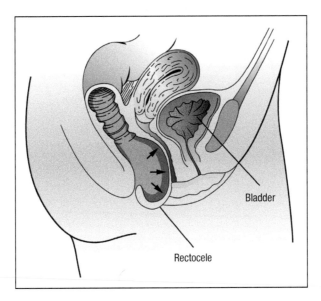

FIGURE 31.5 Posterior vaginal prolapse (sagittal section showing relative position of uterus and bladder). The arrows demonstrate the downward forces of the rectum against the wall of the vagina.

F. Evaluate the posterior vaginal wall support:
  1. Posterior vaginal prolapse (formerly referred to as a rectocele; see Figure 31.5):
     a. Protrusion of the anterior rectal wall and posterior wall of the overlying vagina
     b. Posterior vaginal wall protrudes below the hymenal ring to form a bulging mass, from the anterior rectal wall ballooning down and pushing the posterior vaginal tissue.
     c. Measure the posterior vaginal wall with Valsalva in relation to the hymenal plane.
  2. Enterocele
     a. The cul-de-sac becomes distended with intestine and bulges the posterior vaginal wall outward or the apex of the vagina downward.
     b. Hernia of the connective tissue of the apex or posterior vagina above the rectovaginal septum
     c. Sometimes mistaken for a posterior vaginal wall prolapse (rectocele).
     d. Measure with Valsalva to the hymenal plane as you would an apical or posterior prolapse.

MANAGEMENT OF PELVIC ORGAN PROLAPSE

A. Conservative management
  1. **Expectant management:** If the patient has less than stage 3 prolapse, and has no bothersome bladder or bowel symptoms
  2. Pessary
B. May refer the patient for a simple cystometrogram or urodynamic techniques if bladder symptoms.
  1. To assess for any bladder contractions that may indicate detrusor instability before surgery
  2. To evaluate for urge incontinence or stress incontinence
C. Refer for surgical consultation
  1. Based on the situation and symptoms of the woman depending on:
     a. Stage of prolapse
     b. Degree of symptoms and bother
     c. Patient's desire for surgical intervention

BIBLIOGRAPHY

Abrams, P., Andersson, K. E., Apostolidis, A., Birder, L., Bliss, D., Brubaker, L., Cardozo, L., Castro-Diaz, D., O'Connell, P. R., Cottenden, A., Cotterill, N., de Ridder, D., Dmochowski, R., Dumoulin, C., Fader, M., Fry, C., Goldman, H., Hanno, P., . . . Khullar, V.; members of the committees (2018). 6th International Consultation on Incontinence. Recommendations of the International Scientific Committee: Evaluation and treatment of urinary incontinence, pelvic organ prolapse and faecal incontinence. *Neurourology and Urodynamics, 37*(7), 2271–2272. https://doi.org/10.1002/nau.23551

ACOG Practice Bulletin, Number 214. (2019). Pelvic Organ Prolapse: *Obstetrics and Gynecology, 134*(5), e126–e142. https://doi.org/10.1097/AOG.0000000000003519

Barber M. D. (2016). Pelvic organ prolapse. *BMJ (Clinical Research ed.), 354*, i3853. https://doi.org/10.1136/bmj.i3853

DeLancey J. O. (2016). What's new in the functional anatomy of pelvic organ prolapse? *Current Opinion in Obstetrics & Gynecology, 28*(5), 420–429. https://doi.org/10.1097/GCO.0000000000000312

Hoffman, B. L., Schorge, J. O., Halvorson, L. M., Hamid, C. A., Corton, M. M., & Schaffer, J. I. (Eds.), (2020). Pelvic organ prolapse. *Williams Gynecology*, (4th ed.). McGraw Hill. https://accessmedicine-mhmedical-com.ezproxy3.lhl.uab.edu/content.aspx?bookid=2658&sectionid=241011397

Iglesia, C. B., & Smithling, K. R. (2017). Pelvic organ prolapse. *American Family Physician, 96*(3), 179–185.

Kegel A. H. (1948). Progressive resistance exercise in the functional restoration of the perineal muscles. *American Journal of Obstetrics and Gynecology, 56*(2), 238–248. https://doi.org/10.1016/0002-9378(48)90266-x

Somerall, Jr. W. E., & Pair, L. S. (2020). Importance of urologic assessment for pelvic organ prolapse with occult incontinence: A case study. *Urologic Nursing, 40*(5), 245–257. https://doi.org/10.7257/1053-816X.2020.40.5.245

Vergeldt, T. F., Weemhoff, M., IntHout, J., & Kluivers, K. B. (2015). Risk factors for pelvic organ prolapse and its recurrence: A systematic review. *International Urogynecology Journal, 26*(11), 1559–1573. https://doi.org/10.1007/s00192-015-2695-8

Wang, M., & Smith, A. L. (2017). Pelvic organ prolapse. In D.K. Newman, J.F. Wyman, & V.W Welch (Eds.), *Core curriculum for urologic nursing* (1st ed., pp. 539–543). Society of Urologic Nurses and Associates.

32

URINARY INCONTINENCE

LISA S. PAIR AND HELEN A. CARCIO

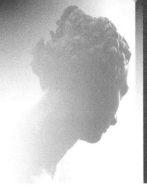

BLADDER DYSFUNCTION EXPLAINED

A. Statistics for urinary incontinence (UI)
1. Epidemiological studies suggest that 30% to 40% of all adults in the United States have some degree of incontinence.
2. The actual frequency is probably much higher considering the significant underreporting of the problem because of patients' reluctance (Box 32.1).
3. An estimated 50% of people affected are women, with this percentage increasing as women age.
4. Demographic trends are changing the nature of the country and the healthcare landscape.
   a. The fastest growing segment of the population is the aging baby boomers; those between the ages of 45 and 65 years have dramatically increased over the past 10 years.
   b. As the number of elderly increases, so will the need for incontinence services.
5. Approximately 50% of women affected never bring up the subject to their healthcare provider.
6. Conversely, very few healthcare providers inquire about symptoms of UI.
7. The economic burden of UI is approximately $65 billion annually.

B. Some thoughts
1. Aging does not cause incontinence, but the lower urinary tract does undergo some changes with age including:
   a. Diminished muscle tone, bladder capacity, and voided volume
   b. The bladder is less compliant and less able to easily stretch with filling.
   c. Uninhibited bladder contractions and postvoid residual volumes increase.
   d. The functioning of the main pelvic floor muscle, the levator ani, deteriorates.
   e. These changes are thought to be related to loss of estrogen to the cells and vascular insufficiency.

BOX 32.1 Common Reasons Why Women May Be Reluctant to Discuss Incontinence

- They believe incontinence is a normal part of aging.
- They are unaware there are conservative methods of treatment.
- They erroneously think that surgery is the only treatment option.
- They do not realize that they are not alone.
- They are afraid they will be put in a nursing home.
- They fear it is some form of cancer.
- They can rely on incontinence products.
- They are not able to find resources to help with their problems.
- They are ashamed and embarrassed.
- They feel powerless and are resigned to their situation.

(1) Symptoms include urgency, dysuria, incontinence, and urinary frequency.
(2) There is an increased risk of urinary tract infections (UTIs).
(3) These symptoms and signs of genitourinary syndrome of menopause usually develop slowly over several months or years.
(4) Urogenital atrophy is the most likely consequence of menopause.
  f. The lower urinary tract and pelvic musculature are under the influence of estrogen and share a common embryologic origin with the vagina.
  g. The squamous epithelium of the trigone and urethra thins and blood flow decreases.

PATHOPHYSIOLOGY OF THE LOWER URINARY TRACT SYSTEM

A. The bladder and the urethra make up the lower urinary tract (LUTS) (Figure 32.1).
  1. The bladder is both a holding tank and a pump.
    a. Stores urine
    b. Empties when full
  2. The dome is the top of the bladder and is thin, stretchy, and collapsible.
    a. Extends as the bladder fills, much like a balloon
    b. Collapses when empty
  3. The base of the bladder is the thicker and less distensible portion.
    a. The trigone is the lower portion where the ureters enter the bladder.
    b. The bladder fills from the bottom and rises above the pubic bone when full.
    c. Bladder fills at a rate of 1 mL/min.
    d. The bladder has an average capacity of 400 to 600 mL.
B. The bladder wall consists of three layers.
  1. Smooth involuntary detrusor muscle of the bladder

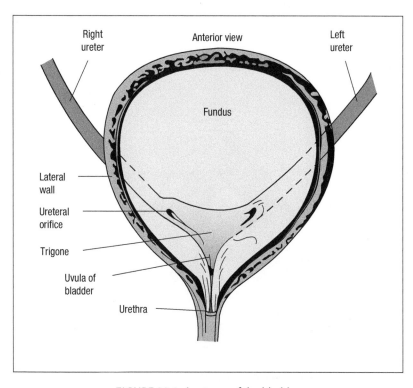

FIGURE 32.1 Anatomy of the bladder.

2. Lamina propria found deep in the urothelium; composed of thick fibroelastic connective tissue; allows for bladder distention
3. Urothelium, which is 6 cell layers thick

C. Urethral sphincter
1. Passes through the urogenital diaphragm and acts as a purse string to tighten the sphincter
2. Muscles provide passive compression to keep the urethra closed during filling.
3. Less adrenergic innervation of nerves than in males

D. **Pelvic floor muscle:** The levator ani is an internal diaphragm, which supports and stabilizes the pelvic organs.
1. It acts as a voluntary sphincter for the urethra.
2. It forms an occlusive layer that closes the lower pelvic floor to resist the downward thrust of an increase in intra-abdominal pressure.
3. It consists of a strong striated long muscle.
4. Figure 32.2 clearly demonstrates a normal and relaxed pelvic floor outlet.

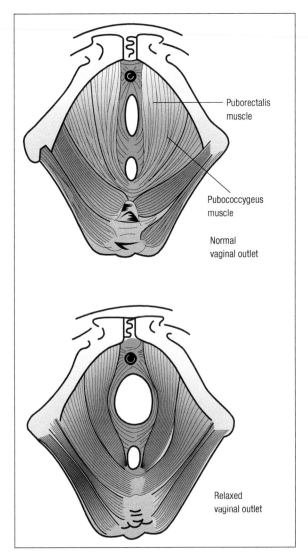

FIGURE 32.2 The dramatic difference between a normal vaginal outlet and a relaxed pelvic outlet due to weakened pelvic floor muscles.

E. Neurophysiology
   1. Distention of the bladder activates stretch receptors at approximately 200 mL of urine.
   2. Sympathetic response facilitates urine storage by inhibiting the bladder contractions and stimulating the urethra to contract.
   3. Afferent impulses travel to the sacral spinal cord and to the brain and the urge to urinate is felt.
   4. Efferent impulses return via the parasympathetic system.
      a. Detrusor muscle of the bladder contracts and the bladder empties.
      b. The urethral sphincter at the bladder neck simultaneously relaxes to allow the urine to escape.
   5. Pudendal nerve causes voluntary relaxation of the external sphincter and the levator ani.
   6. Figure 32.3 provides a schematic diagram of the neurologic innervation of the bladder.

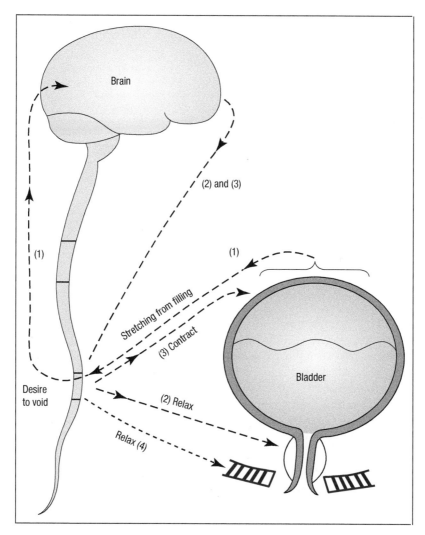

FIGURE 32.3 Schematic of neurologic innervation of the bladder. Arrows pointing upward show the afferent sensory nerves' pathway, caused by the stretching of a full bladder, to the spinal column to the brain. The downward arrows represent the efferent motor pathways from the brain to the bladder, causing it to relax and empty.

URINARY INCONTINENCE EXPLAINED

A. Functional classification
1. Failure to store
   a. Bladder
      (1) Involuntary muscle contractions
      (2) Low compliance or stretchability
      (3) Hypersensitivity to filling pressures
2. Failure to empty
   a. Bladder does not contract efficiently
   b. Outlet obstruction due to a stricture or kink in the urethra (cystocele) or the pressure of an enlarged prostate
3. Incontinence can be a sign of storage failure.
B. Requirements for urinary continence
1. Intact intrinsic urethral sphincteric mechanism
2. Well-supported bladder neck and urethra
3. Normal bladder storage capacity at low pressure
4. Good compliance
5. Competent pelvic floor muscle
6. Intact autonomic and somatic nervous system

TYPES OF URINARY INCONTINENCE

A. Stress UI (SUI)
1. Involuntary loss of urine due to increased abdominal pressure on the bladder that exceeds maximal urethral pressure (the ability of the urethra to hold the urine in).
2. Symptoms
   a. Urine loss, usually occurring at unexpected or inappropriate times
   b. Volume varies and is often described as occurring in spurts or drops
   c. Precipitated by cough, sneeze, change in position, or other types of impact or exertional activities
   d. Rare nighttime occurrence
3. Cause
   a. Pelvic muscles act as a backboard or spring to absorb any increases in abdominal pressure and prevent overwhelming the urethral sphincter.
   b. When this backboard becomes weakened or damaged, the bladder neck becomes displaced and opens the urethra to allow leaking.
   c. Abdominal forces generated to the bladder overcome the closing ability of the urethra and leaking occurs.
   d. Urethral sphincter is weak.
B. Overactive bladder
1. Symptom
   a. Symptom complex consists of urgency, frequency, and urge incontinence; may not always be incontinent.
   b. Is characterized by sudden, strong feeling of urgency caused by uncontrolled (overactive) contractions of the detrusor during filling.
   c. The urgency may be very strong or very subtle.

    d. The urge a woman experiences is a bladder contraction that creates a false need to empty the bladder before it is full.

    e. If the force of the contractions is too strong and overcomes the urethral closing pressure, uncontrollable urine leakage can occur.

C. Urge incontinence

    1. The involuntary leakage of urine that is often immediately preceded by an urge to urinate in the absence of physical activity

    2. Frequency associated with "triggers," such as running water or placing the house key in the front door

    3. Urine loss may be substantial since contractions may continue until the bladder is empty

    4. Must distinguish from a normal strong urge to void, which can be controlled

D. Mixed incontinence

    1. A combination of stress and urge incontinence (Table 32.1)

    2. Probability increases with age

    3. Usually described as being "stress dominant" or "urge dominant" depending on which type of symptoms are more prevalent

    4. It is a combination of symptoms in which each requires special consideration.

    5. Table 32.2 compares the causes of stress and urge incontinence.

E. Transient incontinence: Causes of incontinence that are usually caused by outside forces, which can be controlled or reversed (Box 32.2)

F. Bladder pain syndrome, formerly interstitial cystitis (IC)

    1. Symptoms

        a. Complex of symptoms characterized by urinary urgency and frequency, pelvic pain, pressure, discomfort, dysuria, dyspareunia, and nocturia

        b. Bladder is tender, and pain increases with filling and is relieved with emptying.

        c. Is often misdiagnosed in the early phases of the condition as overactive bladder or recurrent urinary tract infections

        d. Pelvic pain increases over the years and is often diagnosed as endometriosis.

        e. Symptoms worsen with intercourse (12–24 hours), menstrual cycle changes, seasonal allergies, and stress.

        f. No underlying cause has been identified.

        g. Diagnosis is difficult and may take up to 7 years of seeing various providers; diagnosis is usually made by exclusion.

TABLE 32.1 Comparison of Presenting Symptoms

SYMPTOM	OVERACIVE BLADDER	STRESS INCONTINENCE
Urgency	X	
Frequency	X	
Leaking with physical activity		X
Leakage volume	Large	Drops to small amounts
Nighttime urination	X	Rare
Inability to reach toilet in time with urgency	X	

Note: Mixed incontinence is a combination of the symptoms of urge and stress incontinence.

TABLE 32.2 Comparison of the Risk Factors and Possible Causes of Incontinence

CAUSES OF STRESS INCONTINENCE	CAUSES OF URGE INCONTINENCE/OVERACTIVE BLADDER
Pregnancy	Urinary tract infection
Genetic factors	Bladder stones or tumor
Vaginal delivery, particularly if multiple	Bladder stones or tumor
Pelvic organ prolapse	Lack of vaginal estrogen
Genitourinary syndrome of menopause	Urethritis/urethral diverticulum
Previous pelvic surgeries/radiation	Cystocele
Obesity, particularly a high waist-to-hip ratio	Neurologic problems associated with stroke, Parkinson's disease, multiple sclerosis, or spinal cord problems
High-impact sports	Habitual frequent voiding
Medications (ACE inhibitors, alpha-adrenergic blockers, diuretics)	Systemic disorders such as diabetes
Long-term heavy lifting	Incomplete emptying of the bladder
Chronic constipation	Smoking
Elevated BMI	
Chronic cough, often related to smoking	
Systemic disorders such as diabetes	

ACE, angiotensin-converting enzyme; BMI, body mass indexr.

DIAGNOSTIC TESTING AND DIFFERENTIAL DIAGNOSIS

A. Health history
   1. Because most women do not report symptoms of UI, the Women's Preventive Services Initiative (WPSI) recommends screening women annually over the age of 25 for UI and its effect on their quality of life.
   2. Begin by reassuring the woman that incontinence is a relatively common problem and that effective treatment is available.
   3. History includes the patient's perception of her symptoms, which helps determine the type and extent of UI.

BOX 32.2 Causes of Transient Incontinence

- Delirium/dementia
- Bladder infection
- Atrophic vaginitis/urethritis
- Medications
- Endocrine causes
- Restricted mobility
- Stool impaction/constipation
- Polyuria

4. Urinary symptoms of frequency, urgency, and incontinence mimic other bladder disorders and require special evaluation.
5. Assess bowel function and type.
6. Address the impact that incontinence has on the patient's life, self-esteem, and activities of daily living.
7. Inquire about medical history, prior pelvic surgeries, obstetrical and gynecologic history, patient motility, current medications, and history of UTI.
8. Review use and extent of "self-help" measures, such as pad use and fluid reduction.
9. See Box 32.3 for a sample of a tool used to assess the severity of UI.

B. Bladder voiding diary
1. Obtain a 3-day recorded history of the woman's day-to-day bladder habits and patterns.
2. Objectively document intake and output and extent of the problem.
3. The diary allows the woman to focus on her behavior and how it relates to symptoms.

BOX 32.3 Urinary Incontinence Assessment Tool

Do you experience and, if so, how much are you bothered by:
1. Urine leakage related to the feeling of urgency
   - Not at all 0
   - Slightly 1
   - Moderately 2
   - Greatly 3
2. Urine leakage related to physical activity, coughing, or sneezing
   - Not at all 0
   - Slightly 1
   - Moderately 2
   - Greatly 3
3. Small amounts of urine leakage (drops)
   - Not at all 0
   - Slightly 1
   - Moderately 2
   - Greatly 3
4. How often do you experience urine leakage?
   - Never 0
   - Less than once a month 1
   - A few times a month 2
   - A few times a week 3
   - Every day and/or night 4
5. How much urine do you lose each time?
   - None 0
   - Drops 1
   - Small splashes 2
   - More 3

The Results
0–3: No urinary incontinence or extremely mild ("slight") or occasional ("rare") incontinence
4–9: Mild urinary incontinence
9–12: Moderate urinary incontinence
13–16: Severe urinary incontinence (scores of 15–16 could be considered very severe)
Finally, users should check that each question has a response option selected to avoid any missing data.

4. The mere keeping of the diary can be therapeutic, and continence may improve once a causal relationship is established and documented.

5. Download an example of a bladder diary at https://www.niddk.nih.gov/-/media/Files/Urologic-Diseases/diary_508.pdf

6. Review the use of any bladder irritants.
   a. The lining of the bladder is sensitive to certain types of foods and fluids, particularly those with high caffeine and acid content.
   b. These irritants can cause "irritative symptoms" such as urgency and frequency.
   c. See Box 32.4 for common bladder irritants.

C. The physical examination is outlined in Table 32.3.

1. Urinalysis
   a. Rule out infection. Geriatric women may not have the characteristic symptoms of a UTI, such as burning urination, and may only have frequency and incontinence.
   b. The presence of leukocytes and nitrates on a Multstix reagent strip is a sensitive and inexpensive indicator.
   c. The presence of glucosuria or proteinuria requires further investigation.
   d. Hematuria may be indicative of bladder cancer and may require referral for cystoscopy. Microscopic hematuria is defined as three or more red blood cells per high-power field on examination under a microscope of urinary sediment and not on a Multistrip reading. If the urine multistep strip is positive for hematuria, a laboratory urinalysis should be performed.

2. Postvoid residual
   a. This is the integral result of bladder contractility and urethral resistance.
   b. It measures the amount of urine left in the bladder after an attempt to empty it completely.
   c. A high residual may indicate
      (1) An inability of the bladder to contract against an increase in urethral pressure, often due to bladder outlet obstruction
      (2) A hypotonic bladder as seen with diabetic neurogenic lower urinary tract dysfunction
      (3) Detrusor sphincter dyssynergia, which is lack of coordination between contraction of the bladder and urethral sphincter relaxation
   d. It should be done within 10 minutes of bladder emptying.

BOX 32.4 Common Bladder Irritants

- Coffee and tea (sometimes even decaffeinated)
- Chocolate
- Carbonated beverages
- Citrus (whether juice or fresh)
- Cranberry juice or pills
- Vitamin C
- Cocktails (beer and wine)
- Crystal Light
- Candy and other sugars
- Chili and other tomato-based products
- Chinese food (spicy or with monosodium glutamate)
- Cigarette smoking
- Condiments such as honey and artificial sweeteners—aspartame (NutraSweet, Equal)
- Cold remedies

TABLE 32.3 The Focused Physical Examination in the Evaluation of Incontinence	
Abdominal examination	Abdominal skin condition Bowel sounds Masses Suprapubic tenderness Bladder distention
Pelvic examination	Vulva/perineal skin condition Urethral characteristics Genitourinary syndrome of menopause Vaginal discharge Pelvic organ prolapse such as cystocele or rectocele Palpation of the strength and symmetry of the levator ani muscle Bladder base tenderness in the anterior vagina Pelvic mass Provocative stress test with direct observation of urine loss
Rectal examination	Skin irritation Perineal sensation Sphincter tone Presence and consistency of stool Masses or fecal impaction
Neurologic examination	Gait Mental status Knee and ankle reflexes Perineal sensation of S2–S4 dermatomes Anal reflex or "wink" (S2–S5) Bulbocavernosus reflex (S2–S4)
Laboratory assessment	Urinalysis for infection, blood, glucose, protein Urine culture for infection if point of care testing is positive

    e. There is no consensus on normal post-void residual (PVR) amount. However, most urologists and urogynecologists agree that a PVR of less than 150 mL is normal.

    f. Prior to assessing the PVR, if the patient has symptoms of UI, have the patient Valsalva and cough to assess for leakage. If she leaks with her PVR and the PVR is within normal limits, she is noted to have a positive empty bladder stress test for UI.

  3. Assess for vaginal discharge as this can be mistaken for UI.

  4. Assess for STIs as indicated from sexual history.

  5. Assess for genitourinary syndrome of menopause

    a. The presence of any parabasal cells on a wet mount may be considered documentation of genitourinary syndrome of menopause.

    b. Observe for the presence of a urinary caruncle, which can cause symptoms of urgency, frequency, and bleeding.

D. Assess for pelvic floor muscle tone.

  1. Ask patient to squeeze around your two examining fingers while palpating the levator ani muscle. Tell the patient to squeeze like she is trying to prevent the passage of flatus or to squeeze as she would if she was trying to pull up tight pants over her hips.

  2. Note the patient's ability to sustain constriction and deflection of finger or fingers upward with a good squeeze. No deflection indicates weaker muscles.

  3. Constriction lasting a few seconds indicates weakening.

  4. A weakness may be indicative as the cause of SUI.

E. Provocative stress test
   1. Stress testing has a sensitivity and specificity of more than 90%.
   2. See the preceding PVR section for provocative stress test: empty bladder stress test.
   3. Delayed or persistent leakage suggests detrusor overactivity (triggered by coughing) rather than outlet incompetence.
F. Assess the neuronal support to the sacral dermatome, S2, S3, and S4; these dermatomes innervate the micturition reflex (Figure 32.4).
   1. Lightly stroke the skin area innervated by the dermatomes in the inner thighs; note response to light touch; compare contralateral sides.
   2. Bulbocavernosus reflex
      a. Stroke or gently squeeze the clitoris.
      b. Note contraction of the bulbocavernosus muscle around the clitoris.
   3. Anal reflex (so-called anal wink)
      a. Lightly stroke the skin lateral to the anus.
      b. Note contraction of the anal sphincter.
G. The cotton-tipped swab (Q-tip) test or visual exam of urethra during Valsalva
   1. This determines the degree of proximal urethra compromise (Figure 32.5).
   2. Place the cotton-tipped swab through the urethra to the midurethral area.
   3. Ask patient to perform a Valsalva maneuver (hold breath while bearing down).
   4. Note change in the angle of the cotton-tipped swab.
      a. Normally, 10° to 15° from the horizontal position.
      b. If there is significant urethral support compromise, the angle will exceed 30° (Figure 32.5).
H. Perform a simple cystometrogram (CMG) to determine the presence of stress incontinence, urge incontinence, or mixed incontinence.

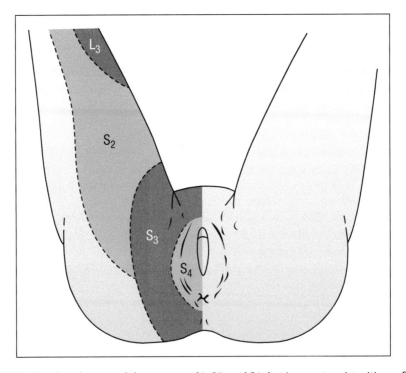

FIGURE 32.4 Sacral neuronal dermatomes S2, S3, and S4 that innervate micturition reflex.

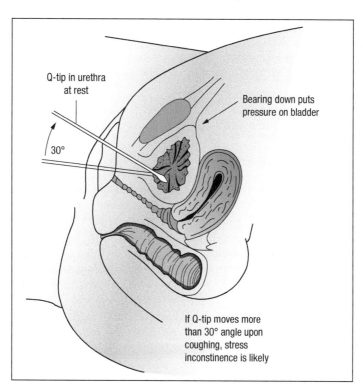

FIGURE 32.5 Cotton-tipped (Q-tip) swab test is used to determine the degree of detachment of the proximal urethra.

FOLLOW-UP

A. Follow-up visits may range from 2 weeks to 3 months based on the patient's problems, response to therapy, and clinician/patient preference.

B. Once the diagnosis is established, an individualized plan of care is developed with the patient. Options include:

1. Pelvic floor muscle strengthening
   a. Kegel exercises, which include a vaginal/rectal tightening and hold for 10 seconds followed by an equal period of relaxation
   b. The patient should perform three sets a day of 10 contractions of the pelvic floor muscles holding each contraction for 10 seconds.

2. Biofeedback training
   a. Uses computerized technology to isolate the pelvic floor muscles
   b. Monitors the electrical activity of the muscles through a vaginal or anal sensor and records any unwanted contraction of the accessory muscles using a sensor

3. Vaginal support pessary
   a. Continence pessary is a type of vaginal device that elevates and stabilizes the bladder neck and increases urethral resistance.
   b. Provides a backstop of support for the urethra preventing leakage with increased abdominal pressure

4. Electrical stimulation
   a. Non-implantable electrical stimulation (E-stim) delivers a weak, painless electrical current to the pelvic floor muscles.

    b. Inhibits bladder spasms by affecting the neural pathways between the pudendal nerve and the bladder.

  5. Percutaneous tibial nerve stimulation (PTNS)

    a. Delivers a pulsed electrical current through a fine needle electrode placed externally close to the posterior tibial nerve.

  6. Urge suppression

    a. Contracting the muscle of the pelvic floor reflexively causes the muscles of the bladder to relax.

    b. Box 32.5 lists the steps to use when teaching urge suppression.

  7. Bladder training

    a. Bladder training is an important form of behavior therapy that can be effective in treating UI.

    b. The goals are to increase the amount of time between emptying your bladder and the amount of urine your bladder can hold. It also can diminish leakage and the sense of urgency associated with the problem.

    c. Bladder training requires following a fixed voiding schedule, whether you feel the urge to urinate or not.

    d. If you feel an urge to urinate before the assigned interval, you should use urge suppression strategies and attempt to hold off voiding until the scheduled time.

    e. As success is achieved, the interval is lengthened in 15- to 30-minute increments until it is possible to hold your urine for 3 hours.

  8. Table 32.4 summarizes the UI treatment options.

  9. Table 32.5 lists pharmacologic management options for UI.

C. Certain clinical conditions should be referred to a specialist.

  1. Uncertain diagnosis

  2. Hematuria without UTI

  3. Urinary retention with persistent symptoms of inadequate bladder emptying

  4. History of incontinence surgery, radical pelvic surgery, or pelvic irradiation

---

BOX 32.5 Urge Suppression

Patient Education: Urge Suppression

In the following exercises, you will learn to decrease frequency and urgency by calming the bladder. The urgency curve is like a labor contraction; you simply must mentally and physically suppress the urge and ride through the contraction. It is a matter of "mind over bladder." Follow these simple steps. (You may leak a little during this training period.)

The Urge Strikes!

- Avoid rushing to the toilet. It will make matters worse.
- Sit down and try to relax.
- Do five "quick flicks." This is done by tightening your vaginal muscles for a couple of seconds and releasing for another few seconds. Quickly repeat this sequence five times in a row.
- Next, relax your body totally—and perform mental distraction: counting to 10 slowly, making a to-do list, or anything that will demand your focus. The urge should be decreasing by now.
- Do another set of five "quick flicks."
- This may completely make the urge go away, or at least suppress the urge long enough to allow you to squeeze and calmly walk to the bathroom.

TABLE 32.4 Options in the Treatment of Urinary Incontinence

URINARY INCONTINENCE TREATMENT OPTIONS	STRESS	URGE	MIXED
Pelvic muscle exercises	X	X	X
Biofeedback/EMG	X	X	X
Reduction in use of bladder irritants		X	X
Treatment of genitourinary syndrome of menopause	X	X	X
Pessary use	X		
Anticholinergics		X	X
Bladder training		X	X
Urge suppression		X	X
Weight reduction (8%)	X	X	X
Vaginal weights	X		X
Smoking cessation	X	X	X

Note: Mixed incontinence requires a combination of treatment options for stress and urge incontinence.

EMG, electromyography.

TABLE 32.5 Pharmacologic Management of Urinary Incontinence

MEDICATION	MECHANISM OF ACTION	RECEPTOR SELECTIVE	DOSING	PRECAUTIONS
Oxybutynin	Antimuscarinic: Blocks action of acetylcholine > smooth muscle relaxation > increased bladder capacity and decreased urgency	Primarily M_3 with some M_2	Oral: 5–15 mg 3x daily Oral extended release: 5–15 mg daily Transdermal patch: 3.9 mg/patch 2x per week	Use with care in older adults. With transdermal patch, do not exceed initial dosing of 3.9 mg 2x/ week. See contraindications.
Darifenacin		Highly selective M_3	7.5–15 mg daily	Use with care in renal or hepatic dysfunction. See contraindications
Fesoterodine		Nonselective	Oral: 4–8 mg daily	Use with care in renal or hepatic dysfunction. See contraindications
Solifenacin		Primarily M_3	Oral: 5–10 mg daily	Use with care in severe renal or moderate hepatic dysfunction. Do not use with severe hepatic dysfunction. Can be used with combination therapy with mirabegron. See contraindications

(continued)

MEDICATION	MECHANISM OF ACTION	RECEPTOR SELECTIVE	DOSING	PRECAUTIONS
				TABLE 32.5 Pharmacologic Management of Urinary Incontinence (*continued*)

MEDICATION	MECHANISM OF ACTION	RECEPTOR SELECTIVE	DOSING	PRECAUTIONS
Tolterodine		Nonselective	Oral: 2–4 mg 2x daily Oral extended release: 2–4 mg daily	Use with care in severe renal or moderate hepatic dysfunction. Do not use with severe hepatic dysfunction. Use with care in individuals with QTc prolongation. See contraindications
Trospium		Nonselective	Oral: 20 mg 1–2x daily Oral extended release: 60 mg daily	Use with care in severe renal or moderate hepatic dysfunction. Do not use with severe hepatic dysfunction. See contraindications
Mirabegron	Stimulates receptors in bladder > smooth muscle relaxation > increased bladder capacity	Beta-3 adrenergic agonist	Oral: 25–50 mg daily	Can be used with combination therapy with solifenacin. May cause elevation of blood pressure Monitor blood pressure frequently with initiation of drug. Do not use if blood pressure 160/100 mmHg. Not recommended with severe renal or hepatic disease.
Vibegron		Beta-3 adrenergic agonist	Oral: 75 mg daily Can be crushed and taken with food	Less risk of hypertension than mirabegron Not recommended with severe hepatic disease.

Note: Antimuscarinics are contraindicated in individuals with uncontrolled tachyarrhythmia, myasthenia gravis, gastric retention, narrow angle-closure glaucoma, and in older adults with cognitive impairment. Use with caution with other drugs that have anticholinergic effects.

Source: Pair LS, Somerall WE Jr. Evaluation and conservative management of urinary incontinence in women. (2022). *Women's Healthcare*. *10*(3), 10–17. Reprinted from *Women's Healthcare*. 2022 HealthCom Media. Used with permission. All rights reserved. Npwomenshealthcare .com

5. Neurologic conditions such as multiple sclerosis (MS), spinal cord injury, or neuropathy
6. Suspicion of fistula or suburethral diverticula

NATIONAL ORGANIZATIONS THAT PROVIDE VALUABLE URINARY INCONTINENCE RESOURCES

A. National Association for Continence (NAFC)
B. Society for Urologic Nurses and Associates (SUNA)
C. American College of Obstetricians and Gynecologist (ACOG)
D. American Urogynecologic Society (AUGS)

BIBLIOGRAPHY

Abrams, P., Cardozo, L., Fall, M., Griffiths, D., Rosier, P., Ulmsten, U., Kerrebroeck, P. V., Victor, A., & Wein, A.; Standardisation Sub-Committee of the International Continence Society. (2003). The standardisation of terminology in lower urinary tract function: Report from the standardisation sub-committee of the International Continence Society. *Urology, 61*(1), 37–49. https://doi.org/10.1016/s0090-4295(02)02243-4

ACOG Practice Bulletin No. 155: Urinary Incontinence in Women. (2015). *Obstetrics and Gynecology, 126*(5), e66–e81. https://doi-org.ezproxy3.lhl.uab.edu/10.1097/AOG.0000000000001148

ACOG WPSI Screening for Urinary Incontinence. (2018). https://www.womenspreventivehealth.org/recommendations/screening-for-urinary-incontinence. Accessed October 9, 2021.

American Urogynecologic Society and American College of Obstetricians and Gynecologists. (2014). Committee opinion: Evaluation of uncomplicated stress urinary incontinence in women before surgical treatment. *Female Pelvic Medicine & Reconstructive Surgery, 20*(5), 248–251. https://doi.org.ezproxy3.lhl.uab.edu/10.1097/SPV.0000000000000113

Castillo, P. A., Espaillat-Rijo, L. M., & Davila, G. W. (2010). Outcome measures and definition of cure in female stress urinary incontinence surgery: A survey of recent publications. *International Urogynecology Journal, 21*(3), 343–348. https://doi.org/10.1007/s00192-009-1032-5

Coyne, K. S., Wein, A., Nicholson, S., Kvasz, M., Chen, C. I., & Milsom, I. (2014). Economic burden of urgency urinary incontinence in the United States: A systematic review. *Journal of Managed Care Pharmacy, 20*(2), 130–140. https://doi.org/10.18553/jmcp.2014.20.2.130

Dennis, J. (2016). Changing our view of older people's continence care. *Nursing Times, 112*(20), 12–14.

Handler, S. J., & Rosenman, A. E. (2019). Urinary incontinence: Evaluation and management. *Clinical Obstetrics and Gynecology, 62*(4), 700–711. https://doi-org.ezproxy3.lhl.uab.edu/10.1097/GRF.0000000000000488

Hannestad, Y. S., Rortveit, G., Daltveit, A. K., & Hunskaar, S. (2003). Are smoking and other lifestyle factors associated with female urinary incontinence? The Norwegian EPINCONT Study. 2003. *BJOG, 110*, 247–54.

Hu, J. S., & Pierre, E. F. (2019). Urinary incontinence in women: Evaluation and management. *American Family Physician, 100*(6), 339–348.

Kegel, A. H. (1949). Progressive resistance exercise in the functional restoration of the perineal muscle. *American Journal of Obstetrics and Gynecology, 56*(2), 239–249. https://doi.org/10.1016/0002-9378(48)90266-x

Lightner, D. J., Gomelsky, A., Souter, L., & Vasavada, S. P. (2019). Diagnosis and treatment of overactive bladder (Non-Neurogenic) in adults: AUA/SUFU guideline amendment 2019. *The Journal of Urology, 202*(3), 558–563. https://doi-org.ezproxy3.lhl.uab.edu/10.1097/JU.0000000000000309

Lukacz, E. S., Santiago-Lastra, Y., Albo, M. E., & Brubaker, L. (2017). Urinary incontinence in women: A review. *Journal of the American Medical Association, 318*(16), 1592–1604. https://doi.org.ezproxy3.lhl.uab.edu/10.1001/jama.2017.12137

Newman, D. K., Wyman, J. F. & Welch, V. W. (Eds.). (2017). *Society of urologic nurses and associates core curriculum for urologic nursing* (1st ed.). Anthony J. Jannetti, Inc.

Pair, L S., & Somerall, Jr. W. E. (2018). Urinary incontinence: Pelvic floor muscle and behavioral training for women. *Nurse Practitioner, 43*(1), 21–25. https://doi.org/10.1097/01.NPR.0000527571.66854.0d

Qaseem, A., Dallas, P., Forciea, M. A., Starkey, M., Denberg, T. D., & Shekelle, P.; Clinical Guidelines Committee of the American College of Physicians. (2014). Nonsurgical management of urinary incontinence in women: A clinical practice guideline from the American College of Physicians. *Annals of Internal Medicine, 161*(6), 429–440. https://doi.org/10.7326/M13-2410

Subak, L. L., Wing, R., West, D. S., Franklin, F., Vittinghoff, E., Creasman, J. M., Richter, H. E., Myers, D., Burgio, K. L., Gorin, A. A., Macer, J., Kusek, J. W., & Deborah Grady, D.; PRIDE Investigators. (2009). Weight loss to treat urinary incontinence in overweight and obese women. *New England Journal of Medicine, 360*(5), 481–90. https://doi.org/10.1056/NEJMoa0806375

Sussman, R. D., Syan, R., & Brucker, B. M. (2020). Guideline of guidelines: Urinary incontinence in women. *BJU International, 125*(5),638–655. https://doi.org/10.1111/bju.14927

Vaughan, C. P., & Markland, A. D. (2020). Urinary Incontinence in Women. *Annals of Internal Medicine, 172*(3), ITC17–ITC32. https://doi-org.ezproxy3.lhl.uab.edu/10.7326/AITC202002040

APPENDIX 32.1: HOW TO RECORD A BLADDER (VOIDING) DIARY

Voiding diaries are important to help you understand the functioning of your bladder. It helps you track and know how much and when you drink liquids, how much and when you urinate, when you have that "gotta go" feeling, and how much and when you leak urine. It describes your day-to-day bladder habits and patterns related to urination. It typically documents the time and amount of fluid intake (great way to look for bladder irritants), the time of each void, each accidental leaking, and a notation of the volume of urine loss. It is an accurate measure of the urinary frequency, volume, and circumstance surrounding urinary accidents. If you leak stool, put a square around the amount; if you leak urine, put a circle around the amount leaked.

How to Complete the Diary

1. Begin your diary when you wake up each day. Take notes throughout the day and continue until you complete 24 hours. For example, if you wake up at 7 a.m. on the first day of your diary, take notes until 7 a.m. the next day.
2. During the day, write down how much liquid you drink. If you do not know exactly how much liquid you are drinking, it is important to take a good guess about the number of ounces every time. Most containers will list the number of ounces they contain. Use these listings to help you make an estimate—for example, a 5-ounce cup of coffee, 8-ounce cup of juice, 12-ounce can of soda, or a 16-ounce bottle of water.
3. Take note of how much urine you produce during the day. If your healthcare professional asks you to keep a bladder diary, you will probably get a special collection device to use. It sits under your toilet seat. It is marked with measurements to let you know how much urine you void. Otherwise, you can record the amounts in subjective terms of large (more than one-quarter cup), medium (less than one-quarter cup), or small (dribbles).
4. It is best to keep a bladder diary for 3 days to get the most accurate picture of your voiding patterns.

The diary is also a method for you to use to focus on your behavior related to overactive bladder and incontinence. Sometimes the mere fact of keeping the diary is therapeutic in and of itself, and the continence improves once a causal relationship with what you eat,and drink and related activities has been established.

33
SEXUAL HEALTH AND RELATED PROBLEMS

SHELAGH B. LARSON

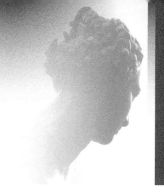

DEFINITION OF SEXUAL HEALTH AND RELATED PROBLEMS

A. Sexual health is a state of physical, emotional, mental, and social well-being in relation to sexuality and not merely the absence of disease, dysfunction, or infirmity.
   1. It requires a positive and respectful approach to sexuality and sexual relationships with the possibility of enjoying pleasurable and safe sexual experiences, free of coercion, judgment, and violence.
B. Sexual response cycle
   1. Libido (sex drive) is the desire to have sexual activity, and often involves sexual thoughts, images, and wishes.
   2. Arousal (excitement) is a sense of tangible sexual pleasure, often accompanied by an increase in physiological changes; blood flow to the genitals; increased lubrication; and an intensified heart rate, blood pressure, and rate of breathing.
   3. Orgasm is defined as a peaking of sexual pleasure and release of sexual tension, usually with contractions of the muscles in the genital area and reproductive organs. It is possible to experience sexual pleasure without orgasm; absence of orgasm does not necessarily mean there is a problem unless the woman is bothered by this.
   4. Resolution is the time after orgasm when the body slowly returns to its normal level of functioning and swelling and erect body parts return to their previous size and color.
C. Sexual response theories (Figure 33.1)
   1. Masters and Johnson (1966) proposed a four-stage "linear" model of human sexual response: (a) excitement, (b) plateau, (c) orgasm, and (d) resolution.
      a. Limited by the assumption that sexual desire is spontaneous, automatic, and unprompted, and focus is on the physiological components, yet this conceptualization does not fit with many women's experiences of sexual response.
   2. Rosemary Basson proposed a "circular" model for human sexual response, noting that many women do not experience sexual desire spontaneously. Rather, desire is a response to sexual stimuli, creating arousal and then desire to circle back to arousal.
      a. The circular model is not so much a rejection of the linear model as it is a combination of an elaborated traditional model with greater recognition of the importance of the emotional and relational qualities integral in partnered sexual response.
      b. The final aspect of the circular model is the psychological and physical satisfaction leading to emotional intimacy as opposed to achieving an orgasm as an end point.

SEXUAL HISTORY

A. A sexual history (SH) allows you to provide high-quality patient care by appropriately assessing and screening individuals for a broad range of sexual health concerns.

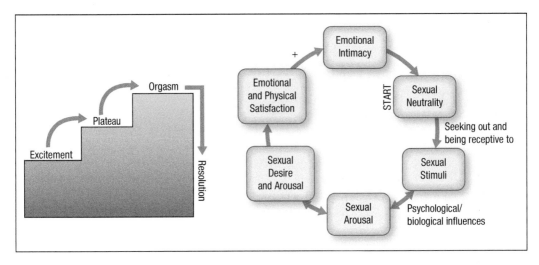

FIGURE 33.1 Sexual response cycle linear versus circular theories.

Source: Adapted from Pines, M. Human sexual response—A discussion of the work of Masters and Johnson, *Journal of Psychosomatic Research, 12*(1), 1968, 39–49, https://doi.org/10.1016/0022-3999(68)90007-X; and Basson R, Chapter 2, Human sexual response, Editor(s): D. B. Vodušek, F. Boller, *Handbook of clinicnal eurology*, Elsevier, Volume 130, 2015, Pages 11–18, https://doi.org/10.1016/B978-0-444-63247-0.00002-X)

B. A SH should be tailored to each person based on their preferences and the clinical situation. Providers may need to modify questions to accommodate a person's gender identity, race/ethnicity, culture, or other important considerations.

C. Open the dialogue by asking permission to discuss the patient's sexual health and practices as you understand that these questions are personal, but they are important for her overall health.

D. Inform the patient that this information is kept in strict confidence unless she or someone else is being hurt or is in danger.

E. Using the 5 Ps may help organize the providers thoughts and flow: Partner, Practice, Protection for STI, Past history of STIs, and Pregnancy intention.

  1. **Partner:** Ask if she has sex with men, women, or both; how many partners in the past 12 months and does the partner have risk factors such as multiple partners or drug use. Ask your patient about a history of trauma, sexual abuse, or violence, as these are common, and patients may benefit from additional care.

  2. **Practice:** Asking about sex practices will guide the assessment of patient risk, risk-reduction strategies, the determination of necessary testing, and the identification of anatomical sites from which to collect specimens for STI testing. Ask open-ended questions that are focused on the information you need to know based on what you have already learned about the patient.

  3. **Protection for STIs:** You may need to explore the subjects of abstinence, number of sex partners, condom use, the patient's perception of her own risk and her partner's risk, and STI testing while not assuming risk or lack of risk for any patient.

  4. **Past history of STIs:** Question if she has had a STI ever in the past, was she treated, and was her partner treated. Question if she is having any symptoms or concerns about an STI and whether or not she want to be tested.

  5. **Pregnancy intention:** Questions should be focused on determining pregnancy intention and what information the patient needs. This could be best assessed using the One Key Question format.

  6. **Conclusion:** What other concerns or questions regarding your sexual health or sexual practices would you like to discuss? Thank her for being candid and honest.

SEXUAL DYSFUNCTION

A. Difficulties with libido (sex drive), arousal, orgasm, or pain with sex that are bothersome to an individual and may be a lifelong problem or acquired later in life after a period of having no difficulties with sex
   1. Dyspareunia
      a. Pain from initial vaginal penetration throughout the entire experience
      b. Can arise from vulvodynia, recurrent vaginal infections, birth control pills (BCPs), breastfeeding, menopause, vulvar dermatoses, pelvic floor dysfunction, pudendal neuralgia, sexual abuse or trauma, and sexual transmitted infections
   2. Vaginismus
      a. The involuntary muscle spasms when something—a penis, finger, tampon, or medical instrument—attempts to penetrate the vagina
      b. Bladder infections, STIs, bacterial vaginosis, and yeast infections can worsen vaginismus pain.
      c. Contributing factors
         (1) Anxiety disorders
         (2) Childbirth injuries, such as vaginal tears
         (3) Prior surgery
         (4) Fear of sex or negative feelings about sex, perhaps due to past sexual abuse, rape, or trauma
      d. Treatments
         (1) Topical lidocaine or compounded creams may help with the pain.
         (2) Pelvic floor physical therapy
         (3) Vaginal dilator therapy
         (4) **Counseling:** behavior cognitive, sex therapy
   3. Female sexual arousal disorder
      a. Described by the distressing difficulty or inability to attain or maintain adequate mental excitement associated with sexual activity as manifested by problems with feeling engaged or mentally turned on or sexually aroused, for a minimum of 6 months.
   4. Female genital arousal disorder
      a. Distinguished by the distressing difficulty or inability to attain or maintain adequate genital response, including vulvovaginal lubrication, engorgement of the genitalia, and sensitivity of the genitalia associated with sexual activity, for a minimum of 6 months.
   5. Persistent genital arousal disorder
      a. Characterized by the persistent or recurrent, unwanted or intrusive, distressing feelings of genital arousal or being on the verge of orgasm (genital dysesthesia), not associated with concomitant sexual interest, thoughts, or fantasies for a minimum of 6 months.
   6. May be associated with:
      a. Limited resolution, no resolution, or aggravation of symptoms by sexual activity with or without aversive or compromised orgasm
      b. Aggravation of genital symptoms by certain circumstances
      c. Despair, emotional lability, histrionic, or suicidality
      d. Inconsistent evidence of genital arousal during symptoms
   7. Female orgasm disorder
      a. Indicated by the persistent or recurrent, distressing compromise of orgasm frequency, intensity, timing, or pleasure associated with sexual activity for a minimum of 6 months.
         (1) **Frequency:** Orgasm occurs with reduced frequency (diminished frequency of orgasm) or is absent (anorgasmia).
         (2) **Intensity:** Orgasm occurs with reduced intensity (muted orgasm).

      (3) **Timing:** Orgasm occurs either too late (delayed orgasm) or too early (spontaneous or premature orgasm) than desired by the woman.

      (4) **Pleasure:** Orgasm occurs with absent or reduced pleasure (anhedonic orgasm, pleasure dissociative orgasm disorder).

  8. Female orgasmic illness syndrome

    a. Illustrated by the peripheral or central aversive symptoms that occur before, during, or after orgasm not necessarily related to a compromise of orgasm quality.

  9. Genitopelvic pain penetration dysfunction

    a. Persistent or recurrent difficulties with one or more of the following:

      (1) Vaginal penetration during intercourse

      (2) Marked vulvovaginal or pelvic pain during genital contact

      (3) Marked fear or anxiety about vulvovaginal or pelvic pain in anticipation of, during, or as a result of genital contact

      (4) Marked hypertonicity or overactivity of pelvic floor muscles with or without genital contact

10. Hypoactive sexual desire disorder (HSDD)

    a. Affecting 10% of adult females and is associated with negative emotional and psychological states and medical conditions including depression; may be lifelong or acquired and generalized or situational

    b. **Symptoms:** Lack of motivation for sexual activity as manifested by:

      (1) Decreased or absent spontaneous desire (sexual thoughts or fantasies)

      (2) Decreased or absent responsive desire to erotic cues and stimulation or inability to maintain desire or interest through sexual activity

      (3) Loss of desire to initiate or engage in sexual activity, including social reactions such as avoidance of situations that could lead to sexual activity, that is not secondary to sexual pain disorders

      (4) Also combined with clinically significant personal distress that includes frustration, grief, guilt, incompetence, loss, sadness, sorrow, or worry

B. Etiology

  1. Factors include conditions or drugs that decrease brain dopamine, melanocortin, oxytocin, and norepinephrine levels and augment brain serotonin, endocannabinoid, prolactin, and opioid levels.

C. Decreased Sexual Desire Screener (DSDS) Tool (Table 33.1)

  1. DSDS results

    a. Answers any question 1 to 4 *no*, then she does not qualify for diagnosis of generalized acquired HSDD.

    b. If she answers *yes* to all questions 1 to 4 and no to all factors in #5, she qualifies for diagnosis of HSDD

    c. If she answers *yes* to any of the question 1 to 4 and *yes* to any of the factors in #5, determine if #5 may be due to something other than HSDD as this may be a concurrent diagnosis.

HORMONES AND SEXUALITY

A. Estradiol

  1. Estradiol and testosterone are the hormones closely linked to sexual desire in women, although, estradiol seems at first glance to be the more likely candidate for this role.

  2. Estradiol influences sexual function in women by working on the central nervous system to increase sexual desire; however, this outcome is likely facilitated by effects of estradiol acting directly on the genitals.

TABLE 33.1 Decreased Sexual Desire Screener Tool	Yes	No
1. In the past, was your level of sexual desire or interest good and satisfying to you?	☐	☐
2. Has there been a decrease in your level of sexual desire or interest?	☐	☐
3. Are you bothered by your decreased level of sexual desire or interest?	☐	☐
4. Would you like for your level of sexual desire or interest to increase?	☐	☐
5. Please all factors that you feel might be contributing to your current decrease in sexual desire or interest: a) An operation, depression, injuries, or other medical conditions b) Medications, drugs, or alcohol you are currently taking c) Pregnancy, recent childbirth, menopausal symptoms d) Other sexual issues you may be having (pain, decreased arousal, or orgasms) e) Your partner's sexual problems f) Dissatisfaction with your relationship or partner g) Stress or fatigue		

Source: Clayton, A. H., Goldfischer, E. R., Goldstein, I., DeRogatis, L., Lewis-D'Agostino, D. J., & Pyke, R. (2009). Validation of the Decreased Sexual Desire Screener (DSDS): A brief diagnostic instrument for generalized acquired female Hypoactive Sexual Desire Disorder (HSDD). *Journal of Sexual Medicine*, 6, 730–738.

3. Estradiol alone (at periovulatory levels) increases sexual desire in naturally and surgically postmenopausal women.
4. Estradiol acts on the walls of the vagina to increase lubrication.
5. Increasing vaginal lubrication increases women's sexual desire by making sexual intercourse more pleasurable.

B. Progesterone
   1. Increases in progesterone can reduce sexual desire

C. Prolactin
   1. The higher the level of prolactin inversely impacts female sexual arousal, lubrication, orgasm, sexual satisfaction, and dyspareunia.

D. Testosterone
   1. May work secondarily to regulate levels of free estradiol by its preferential attachment to Sex hormone-binding globulin (SHBG) or work centrally to increase estradiol levels in the brain through its aromatization to estradiol, or both.
   2. Testosterone can be directly metabolized to estradiol in breast, bone, adipose, and brain tissue which may account for increasing women's sexual desire.

E. Sex hormone-binding globulin
   1. SHBG preferentially binds testosterone; an increase in circulating testosterone increases the amount of SHBG bound to testosterone, which frees previously SHBG-bound estradiol.
   2. Binds both estradiol and testosterone, although it binds testosterone with twice the affinity that it binds estradiol.

F. Thyroid
   1. Low thyroid hormone levels, increasing thyrotropin-releasing hormone secretion, stimulates lactotrophs which increases prolactin production.
   2. Low thyroid levels were found to induce sexual dysfunction.

MEDICATIONS THAT IMPACT SEXUALITY (TABLE 33.2)

Contributing Factors of Other Comorbidities

A. Treating hyperprolactinemia might lessen female sexual dysfunction (FSD).

B. Polycystic ovary syndrome, obesity, and metabolic syndrome could be associated with FSD, but data are limited.

C. There is a strong association between diabetes mellitus and FSD.

TABLE 33.2 Sexual Response Dysfunction by Medication

GENERIC NAME	SEXUAL DESIRE	SEXUAL AROUSAL	ORGASM	COMMENTS
Anti-epilepsy	+	+	+	Oxcarbazepine, and lamotrigine; have less impact on SRD
Antidepressants SSRIs: citalopram, duloxetine, escitalopram, fluoxetine, paroxetine, sertraline, venlafaxine	+++	+++	+++	Block the action of three brain chemicals that relay signals between nerve cells: acetylcholine, norepinephrine, and serotonin
Bupropion SR, buspirone	+	+	+	Used as add-on lower SRD with SSRIs
Antipsychotic	+	+	+	All antipsychotic drugs block dopamine, that helps regulate emotional responses and control the brain's reward and pleasure centers. They also increase levels of prolactin, which can lead to reduced libido, dryness, and difficulties achieving orgasm
Chemotherapy and hormonal medicines" antiandrogens (flutamide, spironolactone), gonadotropin-releasing hormone agonists, combined hormonal contraceptives, tamoxifen, aromatase inhibitors	++	++	+	Alter hormone levels throughout the body by increase in SHBG. Contraceptives: switching to a low-dose or nonhormonal contraceptive method
H2 blockers/ H2-receptor antagonists	+	+	+	Affect histamines and can cause, vaginal dryness, painful sex
Hypertensives	+	+	+	Diuretics, beta-blockers, and alpha-blockers have been found to have the highest incidence of SD. Calcium channel blocker is often the best choice, have been shown to cause fewer SRD
Pain medication: NSAIDs, opioids	++/+++	++/++	+++	
Statins	+	+	+	Interfere with the production of testosterone, estrogen, and other sex hormones. Levels of sexual pleasure drop proportionately with levels of LDL

LDL, low-density lipoprotein; SHBG, sex hormone binding globulin; SD, sexual dysfunction; SRD, sexual response dysfunction.

TREATMENT (TABLE 33.3)

TABLE 33.3 Pharmacologic Management of Female Sexual Health

GENERIC/BRAND AVAILABILITY	DOSAGE: ADULT	ACTION	SIDE EFFECTS/ MONITORING	COMMENTS
VULVOVAGINAL ATROPHY, VAGINAL DRYNESS, DYSPAREUNIA				
Estradiol: Systemic FemRing (estradiol acetate)	0.05 mg, 0.1 mg ring inserted vaginally for 90 days, then replace			
Vaginal Estradiol cream (Estrace, CEE: Premarin (0.625 mg) Estradiol vaginal tablet (Vagifem)	Estradiol: 2–4 g vaginally HS x14, then reduce to 1 g BIW–TIW Premarin cream: 0.5 g vaginally BIW One tablet (10 mcg) vaginally HS x14, then one tablet BIW	Vaginal estradiol therapy benefits sexual function by improving vaginal tone and elasticity, increasing vaginal blood flow, and enhancing lubrication	No need to add progesterone if only using local estradiol	Vaginal: shown to increase sexual desire and arousal and is consider first-line treatment in patients with genitourinary syndrome of menopause
Estradiol vaginal gel cap (Imvexxy) 4 mcg, 10 mcg capsules Estradiol vaginal ring (Estring)	Insert one capsule vaginally daily x14 days, then reduce to one capsule BIW 2 mg; insert ring vaginally for 90 days, then replace			Imvexxy has a starter pack (22 capsules) and a maintenance pack (8 capsules)
DHEA prastone (Intrarosa)	6.5 mg vaginal insert Q HS	An inactive endogenous steroid and is converted into active androgens and/or estrogens		
Ospemifene (Osphena) selective estrogen receptor modulator	60 mg tablet daily with food	Helps reduce pain during sex for women with vulvovaginal atrophy	Do not use with fluconazole as it increases the concentration of ospemifene	If used as a single-agent therapy, there is no need for a progestogen
TREATMENT FOR LOW SEXUAL DESIRE IN PREMENOPAUSAL WOMEN				
Flibanserin (Addyi)	100 mg at Q HS,		Side effects: low blood pressure, sleepiness, nausea, fatigue, dizziness, and fainting, particularly if the drug is mixed with alcohol. Discontinue if no improvement in sex drive after 8 weeks	Only FDA-approved oral treatment for generalized acquired HSDD in premenopausal women in the United States

(continued)

TABLE 33.3 Pharmacologic Management of Female Sexual Health (*continued*)

GENERIC/BRAND AVAILABILITY	DOSAGE: ADULT	ACTION	SIDE EFFECTS/ MONITORING	COMMENTS
Bremelanotide (Vyleesi)	1.75 mg/0.3 mL syringe Self-injection subcutaneous in the belly or thigh 45 minutes prior to anticipated sexual activity. One injection per 24 hours		Side effects: nausea, which is more common after the first injection but tends to improve with the second injection. Other side effects include vomiting, flushing, headache and a skin reaction at the site of the injection	Only FDA-approved on-demand treatment for generalized acquired HSDD in premenopausal women in the United States
		NON-PHARMACEUTICAL		
Therapy based	Helpful for all FSD diagnoses			
Lubricants	Water based Silicone based Oil based and hybrids	Used as needed to reduce friction and enhance comfort with sexual activity		Coconut oil is high recommended
Pelvic floor physical therapy	For treatment of pelvic floor dysfunction			
		OFF LABEL, NO FDA APPROVAL		
Transdermal testosterone	300 mcg/day patch		Can increase hair growth on the body and face and cause scalp hair loss, oily skin, acne, irreversible deepening of the voice, liver problems, and high cholesterol levels	Currently, there are no FDA-approved testosterone therapies for FSD; can be effective for the treatment of HSDD
Bupropion	150 mg SR BID to 400 mg daily	Thought to facilitate dopamine and norepinephrine neurotransmission, possibly by inhibiting the reuptake of neurotransmitters		
Buspirone	20 mg daily	Result of a reversal of SSRI-induced sexual side effects		

(*continued*)

TABLE 33.3 Pharmacologica Management of Female Sexual Health (*continued*)

GENERIC/BRAND AVAILABILITY	DOSAGE: ADULT	ACTION	SIDE EFFECTS/ MONITORING	COMMENTS
CO_2 fractional laser	May be more effective than hormonal therapy in improving sexual function in postmenopausal women		Vaginal laser treatments are very expensive and not covered by health insurance. Injuries and scarring may occur, resulting in increased pain with sex	FDA cleared, but no specific indication for genitourinary syndrome of menopause

CEE, conjugated equine estrogens; HSDD, hypoactive sexual desire disorder.

BIBLIOGRAPHY

Cappelletti, M., & Wallen, K. (2016). Increasing women's sexual desire: The comparative effectiveness of estrogens and androgens. *Hormones and Behavior, 78*, 178–193. https://doi.org/10.1016/j.yhbeh.2015.11.003

Clayton, A. H., Goldfischer, E. R., Goldstein, I., Derogatis, L., Lewis-D'Agostino, D. J., & Pike, R. (2009, March 1, 2009). Validation of the Decreased Sexual Desire Screener (DSDS): A brief diagnostic instrument for generalized acquired female Hypoactive Sexual Desire Disorder (HSDD). *Journal of Sexual Health, 6*(3), 730–738. https://doi.org/10.1111/j.1743-6109.2008.01153.x

Clayton, A. H., Goldstein, I., Kim, N. N., Larkin, L., McCabe, M., & Sadovsky, R. (2018). The International society for the study of women's sexual health process of care for management of hypoactive sexual desire disorder in women. *Mayo Clinic Proceedings, 93*(4), 267–287. https://doi.org/10.1016/j.mayocp.2017.11.002

Eftekhar, T., Forooghifar, T., Khalili, T., Shariat, M., & Haghollahi, F. (2020). The effect of the CO_2 fractional laser or premarin vaginal cream on improving sexual function in menopausal women: A randomized controlled trial. *Journal of Lasers in Medical Sciences, 11*(3), 292–298. https://doi.org/10.34172/jlms.2020.49

Goldstein, I., Kim, N. N., Clayton, A. I., DeRogatis, L. R, Giraldi, A., Parish, S. J., Simon, J. A., Kingsberg, S. A., Cindy Meston, C., Stahl, S. M., Wallen, K., & Worsley, R. (2017). Hypoactive sexual desire disorder: International Society for the Study of Women's Sexual Health (ISSWSH) expert consensus panel review. *Mayo Clinical Proceedings. 92*(1), 114–128. https://doi.org/10.1016/j.mayocp.2016.09.018

Krysiak, R., Szkróbka, W., & Okopień, B. (2018). The effect of bromocriptine treatment on sexual functioning and depressive symptoms in women with mild hyperprolactinemia. *Pharmacological Reports: PR, 70*(2), 227–232. https://doi.org/10.1016/j.pharep.2017.10.008

Parish, S., Hahn, S., Goldstein, S. W., Giraldi, A., Kingsberg, S. A., Larkin, L., Minkin, M. J., Brown, V., Christiansen, K., Hartzell-Cushanick, R., Kelly-Jones, A., Rullo, J., Sadovsky, R., & Faubion, S. S. (2019). The international society for the study of women's sexual health process of care for the identification of sexual concerns and problems in women. *Mayo Clinic Proceedings. 94*(5), 842–856. https://doi.org/10.1016/j.mayocp.2019.01.009

Rowland, D., & Gutierrez, B. R. (2017). *Phases of the sexual response cycle. The SAGE encyclopedia of abnormal and clinical psychology*: Psychology Faculty Publications. 62. https://scholar.valpo.edu/psych_fac_pub/62

Workowsky, K. A., Bolan, G. A., & Centers for Disease and Prevention. (2015). Morbidity and Mortality Weekly Report. (MMWR). *Morbidity and Mortality Weekly Report: Recommendations and Reports 64(*RR-03). 1–137. Retrieved from https://www.ncbi.nlm.nih.gov/pmc/articles/PMC5885289/

Worsley, R., Santoro, N., Miller, K., Parish, S., & Davis, S. (2016). Hormones and female sexual dysfunction: Beyond estrogens and androgens—findings from the fourth international consultation on sexual medicine. *Journal of Sexual Health, 13*(3), 283–290. https://doi.org/10.1016/j.jsxm.2015.12.014

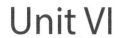Unit VI

ASSESSMENT OF WOMEN AT RISK

34

THE SEXUAL ASSAULT VICTIM

KAREN A. KALMAKIS

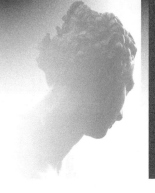

INTRODUCTION

A. Victims of sexual assault need healthcare from a practitioner who is sensitive to their circumstance, knowledgeable about prevention of sexually transmitted infections (STIs) and pregnancy, and aware of the heightened need for safety and privacy.

SEXUAL ASSAULT EXPLAINED

A. Sexual assault is an invasive, traumatic, and often violent crime that is accompanied by both legal and health concerns. All women are at risk regardless of age, socioeconomic status, ethnic background, or race.
   1. Approximately one in five women will experience sexual assault during their lifetime (Smith et al., 2018). In 51% of sexual assaults against women, the perpetrators were intimate partners, and in 41% of cases the perpetrators were acquaintances (Black et al., 2011).
   2. Men perpetrate nearly all sexual assaults against women.
   3. Of the women who report rape, 43% also reported sexual assault before the age of 18 years (Smith et al., 2018).
   4. Women who have suffered a sexual assault by a stranger are more likely to seek healthcare.
   5. Only 34% of victims report the sexual assault to police (U.S. Department of Justice, 2020).
B. Many emergency departments are well equipped with a rape crisis team, which often includes sexual-assault nurse examiners (SANEs). SANEs are specially educated registered nurses who provide comprehensive care to victims of sexual assault, including physical examination, emotional support, forensic evidence collection, and victim education.
C. The legal definition of rape varies from state to state, but all definitions share similar components.
   1. **Sexual penetration:** Invasion of the vulva, vagina, mouth, or anus
   2. **Lack of consent:** Lack of consent is assumed when:
      a. A weapon or force is used.
      b. The victim is a minor.
      c. The victim has physical or mental limitations, is under the influence of alcohol or other substances, or is unconscious.
D. Certain populations are at higher risk for sexual assault, including the homeless, people who are disabled, and young women.
E. Alcohol and drugs may be used to facilitate sexual assault. Young college women under the influence of alcohol are more likely to suffer sexual assault, particularly penetrative assault (Mellins et al., 2017). Indeed, the majority of sexual assaults among college students involve alcohol consumption by the victim, the assailant, or both.
F. Table 34.1 lists the definition of terms often used with a sexual assault.

TABLE 34.1 Explanation of Terms Used in Sexual Assault	
TERM	**DEFINITION**
Sexual assault	Unconsented sexual contact, including grabbing and fondling; includes verbal threats
Rape	Unconsented sexual contact with penetration
Stranger rape	Victim is assaulted by an unknown assailant for unknown purpose
Acquaintance rape	Assaulted by an acquaintance whom the victim has met previously during a nonthreatening social encounter—not considered a friend
Date rape	Occurred during a date or encounter in which the victim agreed to accompany the assailant; may occur after an initial encounter or after many dates of a nonthreatening nature
Intimate or partner rape or marital rape	Sexual assault perpetrated by an intimate partner
Aggravated assault	Sexual assault of a victim who is disabled (mentally or physically) or elderly; associated with excessive force to cause physical injury
Incest	Sexual assault by a blood relative who is a close family member
Statutory rape	Sexual intercourse with a minor, defined by the state in which the incident occurs; it may be with or without consent

SOME REASONS WHY WOMEN MAY NOT REPORT SEXUAL ASSAULT

A. Embarrassment
B. Feelings of self-blame that they are somehow at fault
C. Fear of retribution, especially if assailant is a known or close acquaintance
D. Lack of faith in the medical or legal system
E. Lack of knowledge concerning their legal rights
F. Lack of access to healthcare
G. Concerns about confidentiality
H. The victim may not believe that date rape constitutes true sexual assault.
I. The person may have financial constraints.
J. The person may be unsure where to go for help.

THE FORENSIC EXAMINATION

A. Best performed by a specially trained SANE or emergency department physician
B. Examinations must be done within 5 days (120 hours) of the sexual assault. This time may vary according to the jurisdiction in which the sexual assault occurred. However, victims may seek healthcare weeks or months after the assault.
C. Once a history of a sexual assault has been identified, the practitioner should follow recommended guidelines.

GUIDELINES FOR THE PRIMARY CARE PROVIDER FOLLOWING SEXUAL ASSAULT

A. Facilitate emotional stability and safety of the victim.

B. Determine time elapsed since the sexual assault; if fewer than 5 days and patient consents to forensic evidence collection, refer to the emergency department for a forensic sexual assault examination.

C. If greater than 5 days since sexual assault, or patient declines forensic examination:
   1. Obtain and document history of the assault using patient's own words when possible.
   2. Gather information about the victim's prior medical history, particularly her gynecologic history and risk for, or presence of, pregnancy.
   3. Document any injuries.
   4. If 5 days or less since assault, offer prophylaxis against STIs and pregnancy (Table 34.2). If 5 days or more since the assault, offer testing for STIs and pregnancy as indicated.

TABLE 34.2 Recommended Prophylactic Medication Regimen Following Sexual Assault for Adolescents and Adults

INFECTION/ CONDITION	TREATMENT
Gonorrhea	Ceftriaxone 500 mg IM in a single dose; for persons weighing ≥150 kg, 1 g of ceftriaxone should be administered (CDC, 2021)
Chlamydia	Doxycycline 100 mg orally 2x/day for 7 days
Trichomoniasis	Metronidazole 500 mg orally twice daily for 7 days (CDC, 2021) https://www.cdc.gov/std/treatment-guidelines/trichomoniasis.htm
Hepatitis B	Hepatitis B vaccination needed if the woman has not already been immunized and the assailant's hepatitis status is unknown. If the perpetrator is known to be HBsAg positive, unvaccinated survivors should receive both hepatitis B vaccine and HBIG. If administered at the initial visit, the vaccine (and HBIG if indicated) should be administered again 1–2 and 4–6 months after the first dose. Hepatitis B booster vaccines should be administered if the woman is unsure of her hepatitis B serology status after vaccinations.
HPV	HPV vaccination should be offered to women up to age 45 years who have not been immunized. The vaccine should be administered at the time of the initial examination, and the follow-up dose administered at 1–2 months and again 6 months after the first dose.
HIV	Recommendations for HIV PEP are made on a case-by-case basis, based on complete assessment of history, injuries, and risk (See Workowski et al., 2021, pp. 130–131).
Pregnancy	Administer ulipristal acetate (ella) 30 mg, or levonorgestrel (Plan B) 1.5 mg, orally in a single dose as indicated by history and negative hCG test. Alternatively, consider using copper-T IUC if access to insertion within 5 days of sexual assault.

HBIG, hepatitis B immunoglobulin; HBsAg, hepatitis B surface antigen; hCG, human chorionic gonadotropin; HPV, human papillomavirus; IM, intramuscularly; IUC, intrauterine contraception; nPEP, nonoccupational postexposure prophylaxis.

Note: These medical regimens are standard choices, but do not take into consideration allergies, pregnancy, or ages other than adolescents/adults. See CDC guidelines for treatment of STIs: https://www.cdc.gov/std/treatment-guidelines/sexual-assault.htm

Source: Workowski, K. A., Bachmann, L. H., Chan, P. A., Johnston, C. M., Muzny, C. A., Park, I., Reno, H., Zenilman, J. M., & Bolan, G. A. (2021). Sexually transmitted infections treatment guidelines, 2021. *Morbidity and Mortality Weekly Report Recommendations and Reports, 70*(4), 1–187.

5. Recommendations for HIV assessment of adolescent and adult patients 72 hours postsexual assault:
   a. Assess risk for HIV infection.
      (1) Increased risk of contracting HIV is associated with lack of condom use, genital and/or anal trauma, concurrent STIs, and HIV positive or unknown HIV status of assailant(s).
   b. If the patient is at risk for HIV transmission from the assault, discuss antiretroviral prophylaxis options.
   c. Consult with a specialist as needed to discuss nonoccupational postexposure prophylaxis (nPEP) for HIV.
   d. If the patient chooses to start antiretroviral nPEP, give enough medication to last until the next visit, reevaluate 3 to 7 days after initial assessment, and assess tolerance of medications.
   e. If nPEP is started, perform HIV, complete blood count (CBC), and serum chemistry laboratory testing at baseline (initiation of nPEP should not be delayed, pending results).
   f. Repeat HIV test at 6 weeks, 3 months, and 6 months.
6. Arrange mental health counseling as well as physical health follow-up examination.
7. Complete mandatory report forms as appropriate; for example, provider crime report, weapons report, elder or disabled persons' report.
8. Discuss with the patient the possibility of reporting the assault to police.
9. Send the woman home with written instructions to increase adherence to plan of care, including medication regimens.
10. Provide a list of community resources for victim support; for example, sexual assault support centers, women's centers, and 24-hour rape crisis contact information.
11. Send the victim home in the care of family or friends.

MANAGEMENT

A. Follow-up physical health examinations with a healthcare provider are recommended at 4 to 6 weeks postsexual assault in cases in which the patient received prophylactic medications immediately after the sexual assault. This follow-up examination should take place in 1 to 2 weeks if no prophylaxis was provided. The follow-up examination should include:
   1. Vaginal wet mount for microscopy examination or commercial lab tests
      a. Trichomoniasis
      b. Bacterial vaginosis
   2. Gonorrhea culture from throat, cervix, and rectum as deemed appropriate from patient report of the assault
   3. Chlamydia culture
   4. HIV antibody screening (complete at 6 weeks, 3 months, and 6 months)
   5. Hepatitis B surface antigen with hepatitis B immunizations as needed
   6. Other interventions and care as clinically indicated (e.g., herpes lesions)
   7. Provide ongoing counseling and support; determine the need for additional mental health counseling and referrals.
   8. Obtain pregnancy test ≥14 days or more post assault if no menses since the sexual assault; if pregnancy test is positive, provide pregnancy-option counseling.
B. Additional follow-up should be scheduled for testing of infections that have a long incubation period before they are discernible in the serum.
   1. Test for syphilis at 12 weeks.
   2. Test for HIV at 3 and 6 months.
C. Continue mental health counseling as needed.

BIBLIOGRAPHY

Black, M. C., Basile, K. C., Breiding, M. J., Smith, S. G., Walters, M. L., Merrick, M. T., Chen, J., & Stevens, M. R. (2011). *The National Intimate Partner and Sexual Violence Survey (NISVS): 2010 summary report.* National Center for Injury Prevention and Control, Centers for Disease Control and Prevention.

Brache, V., Cochon, L., Deniaud, M., & Croxatto, H. B. (2013). Ulipristal acetate prevents ovulation more effectively than levonorgestrel: Analysis of pooled data from three randomized trials of emergency contraception regimens. *Contraception, 88*(5), 611–618. https://doi.org/10.1016/j.contraception.2013.05.010

Centers for Disease Control and Prevention. (2021). Violence prevention. https://www.cdc.gov/violenceprevention/sexualviolence/fastfact.html

Mellins, C. A., Walsh, K., Sarvet, A. L., Wall, M., Gilbert, L., Santelli, J. S., Thompson, M., Wilson, P. A., Khan, S., Benson, S., Bah, K., Kaufman, K. A., Reardon, L., & Hirsch, J. S. (2017) Sexual assault incidents among college undergraduates: Prevalence and factors associated with risk. *PLoS ONE, 12*(11), e0186471. https://doi.org/10.1371/journal.pone.0186471

Smith, S. G., Zhang, X., Basile, K. C., Merrick, M. T., Wang, J., Kresnow, M., & Chen, J. (2018). *The National Intimate Partner and Sexual Violence Survey (NISVS): 2015 Data Brief – Updated Release.* National Center for Injury Prevention and Control, Centers for Disease Control and Prevention.

U.S. Department of Justice, Office of Justice Programs, Bureau of Justice Statistics (2020). *Criminal Victimization, 2019 Report NCJ 255113.* https://bjs.ojp.gov/content/pub/pdf/cv19.pdf

Workowski, K. A., Bachmann, L. H., Chan, P. A., Johnston, C. M., Muzny, C. A., Park, I., Reno, H., Zenilman, J. M., & Bolan, G. A. (2021). Sexually transmitted infections treatment guidelines, 2021. *Morbidity and Mortality Weekly Report Recommendations and Reports, 70*(4), 1–187. https://doi.org/10.15585/mmwr.rr7004a1

35

INTIMATE PARTNER VIOLENCE

KAREN A. KALMAKIS

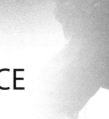

INTRODUCTION

A. Intimate partner violence (IPV) is a global public health problem, linked to long-term health, social, and economic consequences.

VIOLENCE AND ABUSE EXPLAINED

A. *IPV, domestic violence,* and *family violence* are terms that have been used to refer to physical, sexual, and psychological violence and stalking, within intimate partner relationships. The overwhelming majority of violence and abuse is perpetrated by men against women; however, IPV does occur in same-sex relationships.

B. In the United States, one third of adult females (36.4%) have experienced physical violence, sexual violence, and/or stalking perpetrated by a romantic or sexual partner in their lifetime, with sexual and gender minorities having higher rates (Smith et al., 2018).

C. IPV is a preventable public health problem.

D. Research provides evidence for a relationship with numerous adverse mental, behavioral, and physical health outcomes as well as higher healthcare utilization, often continuing after the abuse has ended (Clark et al., 2021).

E. There are four main forms of IPV.
  1. Physical violence
     a. Slapping, pushing, punching, biting, burning, kicking, and choking
     b. Use of weapons; stabbing and shooting
  2. Sexual violence
     a. Forced sexual acts
     b. Sexual contact without consent; for example, while intoxicated, ill, or disabled
     c. Use of coercion or intimidation for sexual contact
  3. Stalking
     a. Repeated, unwanted contact that causes fear or concern for the woman's safety
  4. Psychological aggression
     a. Threats of harm to the woman, her family, and/or pets
     b. Humiliation
     c. Economic control
     d. Isolation and control over activities
     e. Reproductive coercion; controlling reproductive or sexual health

F. Violence against women affects women's health.
  1. Failure to seek routine healthcare
  2. Delayed healthcare for injury or illness
  3. Delayed prenatal care

G. IPV affects
   1. Women of every age, race, religion, and sexual orientation
   2. People of all socioeconomic backgrounds and educational levels
   3. Family members, friends, coworkers, and communities
H. IPV influences the relationship between women and their healthcare provider.
   1. Most women in practice settings are not routinely assessed for IPV.
   2. Healthcare providers are underprepared to identify and respond to IPV, and often do not follow recommendations for IPV screening (Alvarez et al., 2017; Renner et al., 2021).

ASSESSMENT OF INTIMATE PARTNER VIOLENCE

A. The U.S. Preventive Services Task Force (USPSTF) recommends IPV screening for all women of reproductive age (USPSTF, 2018). There are insufficient data to support screening for women beyond reproductive age (>50; USPSTF, 2018); however, IPV has been reported among older women. Considering the current recommendations, it would be prudent to screen all women between the ages of 18 and 50 years *and* any woman who presents with vague or somatic complaints, or injuries that are unexplained or inconsistent with the history provided.
B. Many women attempt to conceal the abuse, and any clues to the abuse may be subtle or absent.
C. Some principles of assessment for abuse include the following:
   1. Because abuse may be physical, sexual, or psychological, merely observing for signs of physical abuse during a routine visit may not be sufficient to rule out abuse. If there are obvious signs of what might be physical abuse, the provider should address the signs; for example, "Often when I see marks like this on women, it is because someone is hurting them. Is anyone hurting you?"
   2. Always screen for IPV when the woman is alone. She should never be asked questions about IPV in front of anyone else. A partner who will not leave the patient alone with the provider may be attempting to control her and influence her responses.

BOX 35.1 Intimate Partner Violence Assessment Screening Intervention/Suggested Dialogue

1. Interpersonal violence is a serious health problem that affects many women. Routine screening is necessary to identify and care for women who have suffered IPV. Therefore, I would like to take this opportunity to ask you about your experiences.
2. Ask direct questions about IPV:
   a. Has your partner/boyfriend/husband (*use the term the woman has used when possible*) ever physically hurt you, or threatened to hurt you, or your family?
   b. Are you afraid of your partner?
   c. Do you feel that your partner tries to control you?
   d. Has your partner ever forced you to have sex?
   e. Do you feel safe in your home?
3. Respond with compassion.
   a. If the woman reports IPV experiences: *I am sorry/sad this is happening to you. What can I do to help?* (e.g., referral to women's support centers, shelters, counseling). If you believe children are at risk for harm, follow mandatory reporting procedures.
   b. If the woman reports that there is no IPV, respond: *Thank you for answering.*

IPV, intimate partner violence.

3. Screening questions should be direct and oral (see Box 35.1 for a suggested dialogue for screening).
4. The healthcare provider should be the one to screen for abuse. Do not delegate this task to support staff.
5. If you do not speak the same language as the woman, you must obtain a professional interpreter to screen for violence and abuse; never use a family member or friend.
6. Clinical screening tools may be used to screen women for IPV. The three-item Abuse Assessment Screen (AAS), the four-item Humiliation, Afraid, Rape and Kick (HARK), and the 10-item Women Abuse Screen Tool (WAST; also available as short form two-item tool) are reliable measures for IPV (Arkins et al., 2016).
7. Be prepared with written referral options in the community that you can give to the woman at the time of the visit, including a number she can call 24/7.
8. Make a follow-up appointment with her. If the woman is abused but does not disclose this information to you, your demonstration of concern for her may encourage her to disclose information at a future visit or seek assistance for IPV.
9. A visit in which a pelvic examination is planned offers an opportunity to ask about past or current IPV, since this type of examination may be traumatic/emotional for some women.

D. Remember
1. The woman herself knows how safe she is and whether she wants to leave the situation.
2. Leaving the abusive partner may not be the solution, or even an option, for many women.
3. The time immediately after a woman leaves her abuser is potentially the greatest period of risk for abused women.
4. Do not encourage the woman to leave her abuser unless she wants to. Instead, listen to the woman, provide her with referrals, tell her how courageous she is, provide her with a safety plan, and encourage her to come back and see you. These actions are interventions.
5. Pregnant women should be screened for past and current abuse during pregnancy. Abuse may begin or worsen during pregnancy and may result in placental abruption, fetal injury, pre-term delivery, or low birth weight (American College of Obstetricians and Gynecologists, 2012).
6. The presence of children in the home should be considered, and appropriate action taken to report child abuse/neglect.

HEALTH CONSEQUENCES OF INTIMATE PARTNER VIOLENCE

A. Many physical and psychological health problems have been associated with IPV.
1. In addition to physical injuries as a direct result of physical abuse, chronic health conditions and infections are related to IPV, including headaches, pelvic pain, dyspareunia, gastrointestinal reflux, sexually transmitted infections, and urinary tract infections.
2. Psychological conditions such as anxiety, depression, eating disorders, and sleep disturbances have also been associated with IPV.
3. Children who witness IPV in the household have poorer health throughout their lives.

CONCLUSION

A. IPV is the most common cause of injury among women of child-bearing age and their children (CDC, 2021).
B. Healthcare professionals should screen for IPV and learn the abuse indicators, supportive care, safety planning, and community resources available to support women victims of IPV.
C. Most states have laws to protect women from their abusers. The courts in most states try to prosecute perpetrators.

D. The cost of IPV in the United States is estimated at between $5.8 and $12.6 billion annually (National Coalition Against Domestic Violence, 2020).

E. IPV is clearly a problem that is deserving of the clinical time spent to screen and counsel women.

BIBLIOGRAPHY

Alvarez, C., Fedock, G., Grace, K. T., & Campbell, J. (2017). Provider screening and counseling for intimate partner violence: A systematic review of practices and influencing factors. *Trauma, Violence & Abuse, 18*(5), 479–495. https://doi.org/10.1177/1524838016637080

Arkins, B., Begley, C., & Higgins, A. (2016). Measures for screening for intimate partner violence: A systematic review. *Journal of Psychiatric and Mental Health Nursing, 23*(3–4), 217–235. https://doi-org.silk.library.umass.edu/10.1111/jpm.12289

Association of Women's Health, Obstetric and Neonatal Nurses. (2019). Intimate Partner Violence. *Journal of Obstetric, Gynecologic, and Neonatal Nursing: JOGNN, 48*(1), 112–116. https://doi-org.silk.library.umass.edu/10.1016/j.jogn.2018.11.003

Centers for Disease Control and Prevention. (2021). *Preventing intimate partner violence.* https://www.cdc.gov/violenceprevention/intimatepartnerviolence/fastfact.html

Chisholm, C. A., Bullock, L., & Ferguson, J. E. J. (2017). Intimate partner violence and pregnancy: Screening and intervention. *American Journal of Obstetrics and Gynecology, 217*(2), 145–149. doi:10.1016/j.ajog.2017.05.043

Clark, C. J., Renner, L. M., Wang, Q., Flowers, N. I., Morrow, G., & Logeais, M. (2021). Longitudinal trends in screening males and females for intimate partner violence as part of a systemic multi-specialty health system intervention. *BMC Research Notes, 14*(1), 344. https://doi-org.silk.library.umass.edu/10.1186/s13104-021-05754-x

National Coalition Against Domestic Violence. (2020). *Domestic violence.* https://assets.speakcdn.com/assets/2497/domestic_violence-2020080709350855.pdf?1596811079991.

Renner, L. M., Wang, Q., Logeais, M. E., & Clark, C. J. (2021). Health care providers' readiness to identify and respond to intimate partner violence. *Journal of Interpersonal Violence, 36*(19–20), 9507–9534. https://doi-org.silk.library.umass.edu/10.1177/0886260519867705

Smith, S. G., Zhang, X., Basile, K. C., Merrick, M. T., Wang, J., Kresnow, M., & Chen, J. (2018). *The National Intimate Partner and Sexual Violence Survey (NISVS): 2015 data brief updated release.* National Center for Injury Prevention and Control, Centers for Disease Control and Prevention.

U.S. Preventive Services Task Force. Curry, S. J., Krist, A. H., Owens, D. K., Barry, M. J., Caughey, A. B., Davidson, K. W., Doubeni, C. A., Epling, J. W., Jr, Grossman, D. C., Kemper, A. R., Kubik, M., Kurth, A., Landefeld, C. S., Mangione, C. M., Silverstein, M., Simon, M. A., Tseng, C. W., & Wong, J. B. (2018). Screening for intimate partner violence, elder abuse, and abuse of vulnerable adults: US preventive services task force final recommendation statement. *Journal of the American Medical Association, 320*(16),1678–1687. https://doi.org/10.1001/jama.2018.14741

36

ASSESSMENT AND RESPONSE TO HUMAN TRAFFICKING

HEATHER QUAILE AND SARAH L. PEDERSON

TRAFFICKING DEFINED

A. Human trafficking, also known as trafficking in persons or modern-day slavery, is a crime that involves compelling or coercing a person to provide labor or services or to engage in commercial sex acts. The coercion can be subtle or overt, physical or psychological. The exploitation of a minor for commercial sex is human trafficking, regardless of whether any form of force, fraud, or coercion was used. A person does not need to be physically transported from one location to another to fall within the definition of human trafficking.

B. Sex trafficking is the recruitment, harboring, transportation, provision, obtaining, patronizing, soliciting, or advertising of a person for a commercial sex act. A commercial sex act is induced by force, fraud, or coercion. Sex trafficking is divided into two distinct subcategories: adult sex trafficking and child sex trafficking. Under the law, an adult is sex trafficked when induced to perform sex through force, fraud, or coercion. However, when a person younger than 18 years of age is induced to perform a commercial sex act, it is a crime regardless of whether there is any force, fraud, or coercion.

1. Subset of child/minor sex trafficking
   a. **Domestic minor sex trafficking (DMST; also known as child sex trafficking):** The recruitment, harboring, transportation, provision, or obtaining of a person of a commercial sex act where the person is a U.S. citizen or lawful permanent resident under the age of 18 years
   b. **Commercial sexual exploitation of children (CSEC):** Sexual activity involving a child in exchange for something of value or promise thereof, to the child or another person where the child is being treated as a commercial sexual object

C. Labor trafficking is the recruitment, harboring, transportation, provision, or obtaining of a person for labor or services, through the use of force, fraud, or coercion for the purpose of subjection to involuntary servitude, peonage, debt bondage, or slavery.

ETIOLOGY AND INCIDENCE

A. Global
   1. 600,000 to 800,000 people are trafficked annually, worldwide.
   2. 80% of transnational victims are women and girls.
   3. For every 10 female victims identified globally, five were women and two were girls.
   4. About one third of overall detected victims were children (girls and boys).
   5. 77% of women detected for trafficking were sexually exploited.
   6. 14% of women were detected for labor trafficking.
   7. 9% of women were detected for other forms of exploitation.
   8. 19% of girls detected for trafficking were sexually exploited.
   9. $15.5 billion is generated in industrialized countries alone.
   10. Sex trafficking alone nets an estimated $7 billion to $19 billion annually.

B. United States
   1. 22,326 human trafficking victims were identified in 2019.
   2. 14,597 were victims of sex trafficking.
      a. **Types (identified):** Escort services (1,278); illicit massage, health, and beauty (1,247); pornography (733)
      b. **Risk factors:** Substance use concerns (510), runaway homeless youth (473), recent migration/relocation (416), unstable housing (366), mental health concerns (334)
      c. **Forms of force, fraud and coercion:** Induces/exploits substance abuse issues (1,898), physical abuse (1,780), sexual abuse (1,184), intimidations/displays/threatens weapons (1,102), emotional abuse/intimacy related (1,019)
      d. **Recruitment tactics:** Intimate partner/marriage proposition (1,067), familiar (981), job offer/advertisement (515), posing as a benefactor (438), false promises/fraud (353)
   3. 4,934 were labor trafficking.
      a. **Types (identified):** Domestic work (218), agriculture and animal husbandry (108), traveling sales crews (107)
      b. **Risk factors:** Recent migration/relocation (2,364), unstable housing (91), criminal record/criminal history (90), physical health concern (53), substance use concern (32)
      c. **Forms of force, fraud and coercion:** Withholds pay/earning (2,279), excessive working hours (2,043), threat to report to immigration (1,866), verbal abuse (1,640), withholds/denies needs (1,254)
      d. **Recruitment tactics:** Job offer/advertisement (2,557), false promises/fraud (805), smuggling-related (221), familial (168), passing as a benefactor (132)
   4. 1,048 were sex and labor trafficking.
      a. Illicit massage, health, and beauty (123)
      b. Illicit activities (81)
      c. Bars, strip clubs, and cantina (43)
   5. 15,222 were women.
   6. Women are exploited more in the United States than in any other country.
C. Children
   1. A family member inflicts 34% of child sexual abuse.
   2. 94% of sex trafficking survivors reported childhood sexual abuse.
   3. Of the 94%, 70% were sexually abused by a family member as a child.

RISK FACTORS (BOX 36.1)

A. **Age:** 12 to 16 years
B. Runaway or homeless
C. History of sexual or physical abuse or neglect
D. Dysfunctional families
E. Interactions with Child Protective Services or the Juvenile Justice System
F. Marginalized communities; e.g., LGBTQIA+
G. Substance abuse, behavioral, mental health issues
H. Economically vulnerable
I. Learning disabilities
J. Living in high crime areas, poverty, transient male populations
K. Living in countries with political or social unrest or corruption
L. Living in societies with gender bias and discrimination or glorification of pimp culture
M. Undocumented individuals
N. Individuals with mental illness

BOX 36.1 Red Flags

- Difficulties seeing patient alone or the accompanying individual is answering questions
- Refusal to use interpreters
- Unexpected material things/significant change in appearance
- History of foster care or repeatedly living in group homes
- Overly familiar with sex
- Tattoo that the patient is unwilling to discuss
- Body language indicating fear, anxiety, or distrust
- Physical injuries in various stages of healing
- A physical examination that does not match the patient's history
- Scripted or memorized history
- Vague or inconsistent answers
- Patient being unaware of their address or current location, the date, or time
- Lack of identification documents
- Multiple sexual partners, unintended pregnancies, sexually transmitted infections, or repeated visits for emergency contraception

GUIDELINES FOR PRIMARY CARE PROVIDERS RESPONDING TO SUSPICION OR DISCLOSURES OF HUMAN TRAFFICKING

A. Assessment for signs and symptoms of persons that are trafficked/abused
  1. Verbal indicators
     a. Expresses lack of knowledge of a given community/whereabouts
     b. Does not speak/refusal of interpretation services
     c. Discloses an inconsistent history
     d. The claim of "just visiting"
     e. Discloses suicidal or homicidal ideation
     f. Provides vague background information
  2. Behavioral indicators
     a. Demeanor (e.g., fearful, anxious, submissive, flat affect)
     b. Defers to or seeks permission from the person accompanying them to speak
     c. Uncomfortable leaving without their escort or being alone with the examiner
     d. Hypervigilant
     e. Body language indicating fear, anxiety, trust issues
     f. Drug-seeking behaviors
  3. Physical indicators
     a. Branding/tattoo that the patient is unwilling to discuss
     b. Drug overdose or abuse
     c. Signs of malnourishment, neglect, or dehydration
     d. Poorly controlled/untreated medical conditions
     e. Multiple or recurrent sexually transmitted infections (STIs)
     f. Unintended pregnancy, pregnancy complications
     g. Female genital mutilation (FGM)
     h. Injuries that are suspicious of abuse
        (1) Oral and dental
        (2) Strangulation
        (3) Central body
        (4) Sustained during pregnancy

      (5) Pelvic injuries

      (6) Defensive posturing

      (7) Bilateral or multiple types (e.g., bruising, lacerations, abrasions)

      (8) Different stages of healing of injuries

      (9) **Burns:** chemical, cigarette, heated liquid burns

     (10) Patterned injuries with identifiable markings that allow a provider to discern that they were caused by a specific or unknown object and or by a specific mechanism of injuries

    4. Other indicators

      a. Limited or no healthcare

      b. Not in control of personal identification

      c. Third party insists on being present or interpreting for the person being trafficked

      d. Multiple visits to the emergency department

      e. Few or no personal possessions

      f. Difficulty seeing patient alone

      g. Under 18 and in the sex industry

      h. Has an unstable living situation

      i. A history of domestic/interpersonal violence

TRAUMA-INFORMED CARE

A. What is trauma? A universal definition of trauma does not exist, but overall trauma refers to any experience that causes an intense psychological or physical stress reaction. It may occur due to violence, abuse, neglect, loss, disaster, war, and other emotionally harmful experiences. Trauma can result in a wide range of responses, including intense feelings of fear, loss of trust in others, decreased sense of personal safety, guilt, and shame. Trauma does not discriminate, and it bridges itself across age groups, gender, socioeconomic status, race, ethnicity, geography, and sexual orientation.

B. What is trauma-informed care (TIC)? TIC is a strength-based service delivery approach. This approach can improve patient engagement, treatment adherence, health outcomes, and provider and staff wellness. TIC integrates a comprehensive approach, which includes providing a safe environment for all patients and staff, identifying survivors of trauma, and implementing practices to avoid retraumatization.

C. Fundamental principles to trauma-informed response (see Box 36.2)

D. Provide trauma-informed training for staff and providers

E. Provide TIC to all patients using the six key principles of trauma

    1. Safety

    2. Trustworthiness and transparency

    3. Peer support

    4. Collaboration and mutuality

BOX 36.2 Critical Principles for a Trauma-Informed Care Response

- Reduce the impact of trauma on individuals, families, and communities.
- Develop/implement a trauma-informed approach across systems and workplaces, for users and providers of services.
- Make trauma-informed screening, early intervention, and treatment common practice.
- Promote recovery, well-being, and resilience.

BOX 36.3 Provider Screening Tools for Trauma-Informed Care Assessment

The Brief Trauma Questionnaire (BTQ): https://www.ptsd.va.gov/professional/assessment/documents/BTQ.pdf

Stressful Life Events Screening Questionnaire (SLESQ):
https://georgetown.app.box.com/s/nzprmm2bn5pwzdw1l62w

The Traumatic Life Events Questionnaire (TLECQ) (the scale is in the appendix of the article):
https://www.ncbi.nlm.nih.gov/pmc/articles/PMC3115408

The PTSD Checklist (PCL): https://www.ptsd.va.gov/professional/assessment/documents/PCL5_criterionA_form.PDF

PEARR Tool: Trauma-Informed Approach to Victim Assistance in Health Care Settings: https://www.dignityhealth.org/content/dam/dignity-health/pdfs/pearrtoolm15nofield2019.pdf

A Short Screening Tool to Identify Victims of Child Sex Trafficking in Health Care Setting:
https://healtrafficking.org/2018/05/a-short-screening-tool-to-identify-victims-of-child-sex-trafficking-in-the-health-care-setting

Family Justice Center Alliance Human Trafficking Questionnaire and Guide for Frontline:
https://www.familyjusticecenter.org/resources/human-trafficking-questionnaire-and-guide-for-frontline-staff

National Human Trafficking Resource Center - Framework for a Human Trafficking Protocol in Healthcare Settings: Framework for a Human Trafficking Protocol in Healthcare Settings | National Human Trafficking Hotline

Administration for Children and Families: Office on Trafficking in Persons. (2018). Adult human

Trafficking screening tool and guide: https://www.acf.hhs.gov/sites/default/files/documents/otip/adult_human_trafficking_screening_tool_and_guide.pdf

---

5. Empowerment, voice, and choice
6. Cultural, historical, and gender issues

F. Trauma-informed screening and assessment tools (see Box 36.3)

TREATMENT AND MANAGEMENT

A. Identify human trafficking indicators.

B. Treat the chief complaint/illness and the emergent issue (e.g., STI and HIV testing and treatment at the time of visit as often trafficked persons do not come back for care).

C. Offer and provide (if patient-desired) referrals and appropriate treatment for the unsafe environment (Box 36.4).

D. Offer forensic evidence collection or referral to a sexual assault or human trafficking center (respect if the patient declines a forensic exam, but do not withhold medical treatment).

E. Document assessment as well as indicators of potential findings on exam.

OTHER CONSIDERATIONS FOR RESPONSE

A. Implement internal protocols

B. Ongoing training for the response to human trafficking

C. Culturally sensitive care and training

D. Safety plan and protocol to protect patients, providers, staff

BOX 36.4 Screening Questions

- Can you leave your job or situation if you choose?
- Can you move about freely?
- Have you been threatened if you tried to leave?
- Have you been physically or sexually harmed?
- Has your family been threatened?
- Has your identification been taken away?
- Where do you sleep?
- Do you have enough food to eat or water to drink?
- Are you afraid to leave?
- Are you being forced to do anything that you do not want to do?

E. Knowledge about community resources and referrals

F. Process in place for persons of trafficking to self-identify/disclose

G. Pamphlets and resources in patient bathroom areas

DEFINITION AND TYPES OF FEMALE GENITAL MUTILATION

A. FGM comprises procedures involving partial or total removal of external female genitalia. FGM may also include injuries to the female genital organs for nonmedical concerns. FGM is most commonly performed on young females between infancy and adolescence. FGM violates several human rights issues and is a global concern.

B. FGM is classified into four major types.
1. Type 1 is the partial or total removal of the clitoral glans (the external and visible part of the clitoris, which is a sensitive part of the female genitals) and the prepuce/clitoral hood (the fold of skin surrounding the clitoral glans).
2. Type 2 involves the partial or total removal of the clitoral glans and the labia minora (the inner folds of the vulva), with or without removal of the labia majora (the outer folds of skin of the vulva).
3. Type 3 is also known as infibulation; this is the narrowing of the vaginal opening through the creation of a covering seal. The seal is formed by cutting and repositioning the labia minora, or labia majora, sometimes through stitching, with or without removal of the clitoral prepuce/clitoral hood and glans (Type I FGM).
4. Type 4 also includes all other harmful procedures to the female genitalia for nonmedical purposes (e.g., pricking, piercing, incising, scraping, and cauterizing the genital area).

BIBLIOGRAPHY

Allert, J. L. (2021). Justice professionals' lens on familial trafficking cases. The samaritan women institute for shelter care. *Criminal Justice Review.*

Faugno, D., Speck, P. M., Spencer, M. J., & Giardino, A. P. (2016). *Sexual assault quick reference* (2nd ed.). STM Learning.

Greenbaum, V. J., Dodd, M., & McCracken, C. (2018). A short screening tool to identify victims of child sex trafficking in the health care setting. *Pediatric Emergency Care, 34*(1), 33–37. https://doi.org/10.1097/PEC.0000000000000602. Retrieved from A Short Screening Tool to Identify Victims of Child Sex Trafficking in the Health Care Setting | HEAL Trafficking: Health, Education, Advocacy, Linkage

Hammer, R. M., Moynihan, B., & Pagliaro, E. M. (2013). *Forensic nursing: A handbook for practice* (2nd ed.). Jones & Bartlett Learning

Kelsey, B. M., & Nagtalon-Ramos, J. (2021). *Midwifery & women's health nurse practitioner certification review guide.* Springer Publishing Company.

Office of Juvenile Justice and Delinquency Prevention. (2018). Human trafficking resources. https://human trafficking resources | office of juvenile justice and delinquency prevention (ojp.gov)

Polaris. (2019). 2019 Data report: The US national human trafficking hotline. https://polarisproject.org/wp-content/uploads/2019/09/Polaris-2019-US-National-Human-Trafficking-Hotline-Data-Report.pdf

Quaile, H. C. (2020). Trauma-informed care for the primary care provider. *Women's Healthcare, 8*(4), 6–12. Retrieved from https://www.npwomenshealthcare.com/trauma-informed-care-for-the-primary-care-provider

Quaile, H. C., & Benyounes-Ulrich, J. (2021). Trauma-informed care. Part 1: The road to its operationalization. *Women's Healthcare, 9*(3), 32–36. https://www.npwomenshealthcare.com/trauma-informed-care-part-1-the-road-to-its-operationalization

Scannell, M. J. (2019). *Fast facts about forensic nursing.* Springer Publishing Company.

Substance Abuse and Mental Health Services Administration. (2014a). *TIP 57: Trauma-Informed Care in Behavioral Health Services.* SAMHSA.

Substance Abuse and Mental Health Services Administration. (2014b). *SAMHSA's Concept of Trauma and Guidance for a Trauma-Informed Approach.* SAMHSA's Trauma and Justice Strategic Initiative. SAMHSA.

United Nations Office on Drugs and Crime. (2020). *Global report on trafficking in persons: Global overview.* https://www.unodc.org/documents/data-and-analysis/tip/2021/GLOTiP_2020_Global_overview.pdf

U.S. Department of Health and Human Services. (2016). *Agency for Healthcare Research and Quality. Trauma-informed care.* https://www.ahrq.gov/professionals/prevention-chronic-care/healthier-pregnancy/preventive/trauma.html.

U.S. Department of Justice. (2020). *What is human trafficking?* https://www.justice.gov/humantrafficking

World Health Organization. (2020). *Female genital mutilation.* https://www.who.int/news-room/fact-sheets/detail/female-genital-mutilation

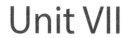

Unit VII

INFERTILITY AND SUBFERTILITY ASSESSMENT

37

INITIAL EVALUATION OF INFERTILITY

CAROL LESSER

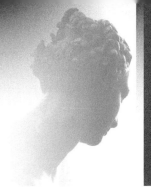

INFERTILITY EXPLAINED

A. Infertility affects the ability to conceive and carry a pregnancy to term.
1. Infertility affects approximately 7.4 million women and their partners or approximately 15% of the reproductive-age population in the United States.
2. Infertility affects both females and males. Both should be evaluated.
3. Most patients are not infertile, but instead, subfertile. Choice of words can affect patient self-perception.
4. Primary infertility refers to trying to conceive with no prior history of pregnancy.
   a. Trying to conceive for 12 months if younger than 35 years
   b. Trying to conceive for 6 months or longer if 35 years and older
   c. Also includes those with known problems that prevent pregnancy, such as blocked tubes, anovulation, or male factor problems
5. *Secondary infertility* refers to women who have trouble conceiving a child after prior success.
   a. The National Center for Health Statistics estimates more than 12% of women of reproductive age in the United States have secondary infertility.
   b. Age is most often a factor. Post-delivery complications can be relevant.
6. The number of infertility clinics in the United States is more than 480.
   a. Since the birth of the first in vitro fertilization (IVF) baby in 1978, IVF centers have offered comprehensive evaluation and treatments with significant advances in the field of reproductive medicine.
   b. Worldwide, more than 8 million babies have been born as a result of IVF.
7. *Assisted reproductive technology* (ART) is the term used for fertility-related treatments.
8. Physicians who offer these services work in the field of reproductive endocrinology and infertility and are called *REIs* (reproductive endocrinology and infertility).
   a. Advanced practice clinicians can play a key role in the assessment and treatment of the fertility patient.
   b. Advanced practice clinicians can facilitate prompt referral to ART services when appropriate.
9. Most individuals with a fertility-related problem never seek evaluation or treatment. IVF and its associated technologies remain an underutilized mode of treatment, often due to misconceptions that treatments are too painful and too costly. Clinicians can help redress.
10. The clinician's goal is to help diagnose, treat, and resolve infertility, and find the best resources to assist patients in moving forward. These include:
    a. Helping those who prefer adoption
    b. Third-party reproduction
    c. Child-free living
B. More women than ever before are seeking diagnosis and treatment of fertility-related problems. Several factors have contributed to this increase.

1. Delayed childbearing has become the norm for increasing numbers of women who start trying to conceive after 35 years when natural fertility rates have already declined.
2. Infertility centers are increasingly caring for women who are past their reproductive prime and as a result may require more intensive treatments.
3. Third-party reproduction, including donor egg and gestational carriers, is available in most centers.
4. The development of egg banks similar to sperm banks has made donor egg treatment more affordable and attractive to more individuals.
5. Singles and same-sex couples are increasingly requesting fertility-related services as our societal acceptance of alternative ways for family building increases.
6. Single women who are not ready to procreate as well as women diagnosed with cancer are requesting egg freezing in increasing numbers. No longer considered experimental, freezing one's own oocytes has become an insurance policy for women who are aging and concerned they will run out of competent oocytes once ready to start a family.
7. Availability of adoptable babies remains a challenge as costs, screening requirements, and numbers of healthy infants limit access for many. This has contributed to the popularity of ART treatments.
8. Infertility causes significant stress and affects every aspect of a woman's life and relationship. Increasingly, fertility centers offer a range of mental health and stress reduction programs and services to address these needs.

C. Causes of infertility
1. The cause may be due to female or male factors and often is a combination of both. Counsel patients to avoid blame. Infertility is a "couple's" issue unless a single person is seeking care.
2. Female factors include advanced age, ovulation disorders, tubal and uterine factors. Female age is a prime contributor, often causing subfertility or premature ovarian insufficiency (POI).
3. Male factor includes obstructive and nonobstructive causes of absent sperm (azoospermia).
   a. Males are evaluated for potential anatomic and/or endocrine issues, prior infection or trauma, genetics, lifestyle, and environmental/occupational exposure as causes of subfertility, infertility, or sterility.
   b. The initial female workup (for those who present with a partner) always includes a semen analysis (SA).
4. The single most important factor that influences the ability to conceive is maternal age. Remember, fertility starts to measurably decline in a woman's 20s.
5. Monthly fecundity in the general population has been estimated to be between 15% and 20%, decreasing exponentially with advanced age. Most individuals overestimate their monthly chances to conceive and equate ovulation with fertility. Women tend to equate overall good health and physical fitness with the ability to procreate without impediment.
6. Unexplained infertility accounts for a small percentage of cases. In general, unexplained infertility can be attributed to age.
7. Box 37.1 contains a summary of the causes of infertility.

HEALTH ASSESSMENT OF THE INFERTILE WOMAN/COUPLE

A. Initiate a workup for anyone trying to conceive if there is a known fertility problem such as anovulation or blocked tubes, recurrent miscarriage, or any reason to question the ability to conceive. There is no good reason to turn a patient away who wants reassurance regarding her fertility potential.
B. Increasingly, younger women present for fertility preservation if they are diagnosed with cancer requiring gonadotoxic treatments during their reproductive years.
1. Learn where to refer these patients. Fertility preservation programs are often regional.
2. The national organization Fertile Hope can assist with patient support and referrals.

BOX 37.1 Causes of Infertility and Subfertility

- Advanced maternal age
- Cervical factor
- Combined
- Male factor
- Ovulatory factor
- Tubal factor
- Unexplained
- Uterine factor

C. Take a thorough history of both parties.
  1. Be sensitive to issues of confidentiality.
  2. Women may not want partners to know about a previous therapeutic termination.
D. When treatment is started, informed consent involves both parties. If couples disagree on treatment, counseling is strongly recommended.
E. Identify risk factors
  1. Gynecologic factors—prior intrauterine device (IUD) use, loop electrosurgical excision procedure (LEEP) or conization of the cervix, pelvic inflammatory disease (PID), irregular cycles, menorrhagia, severe dysmenorrhea or dyspareunia—might suggest endometriosis.
  2. Reassure the patient that cervical polyps will not adversely affect fertility. If they are annoying and friable, they may be removed for those reasons. However, endometrial polyps may interfere with implantation and most often should be removed and sent for pathology.
  3. Smoking is the most deleterious habit to screen for but check for any substance abuse.
  4. Occupational exposures, such as nitrous oxide, are associated with reduced fertility and spontaneous abortions. Dry-cleaning chemicals and mercury have also been associated with decreased fecundity.
F. Be aware that the level of stress associated with infertility is similar to what is experienced in a terminal illness.
  1. Anger, depression, frustration, and anxiety are commonly reported. Try to remain nonreactive and offer timely support and appropriate referrals as needed.
  2. A well-informed patient who understands her treatment options and prognosis will be easier to care for. Support groups or individual counseling resources are available.
  3. Accommodating patient requests for appointments in a timely manner is important. Patients feel that time is running out. Tests are often cycle-day dependent and patients are very sensitive to "losing a month" while waiting to be seen.
G. A thorough history must be obtained initially.
H. See Appendix 37.1 for assessment forms for females and males.

PHYSICAL EXAMINATION OF THE INFERTILE WOMAN

A. A complete physical examination is recommended before treatment is initiated.
  1. Check height, weight, and body mass index (BMI) or another method of evaluating body-fat composition.
    a. Women of very short stature may need evaluation for Turner's (XO) syndrome. Check karyotype.

b. Extremes in weight (BMI) are associated with health risks as well as infertility or subfertility and lower rates of success with ART.

c. Extremely low BMI may be associated with anovulation secondary to hypothalamic hypogonadism, which baseline hormones can usually detect.

d. Elevated BMI is often associated with polycystic ovarian syndrome (PCOS), hyperinsulinemia, and, in severe cases, metabolic syndrome, requiring a multidisciplinary approach.

2. Check for hirsutism/androgen excess.

a. The Ferriman–Gallwey grading system can be helpful. Many women seek electrolysis or laser treatment, so ask whether they have had these procedures done (Box 37.2).

b. Hyperandrogenic states are often associated with PCOS and less often with congenital adrenal hyperplasia (CAH), which can affect ovulation.

c. Excessive hair growth on the upper torso and back can suggest more significant hyperandrogenism.

d. If acanthosis nigricans (leathery brown discoloration of skin at back of neck, axilla, or other skin folds) is found, this suggests severe hyperandrogenism associated with hyperinsulinemia and metabolic syndrome.

e. These sequelae are seen in more severe cases of PCOS. Similarly, facial acne or more extensive acne on the upper torso and back are associated with PCOS or other hyperandrogenic states. Check for clitoromegaly or male pattern baldness, which also suggests significant hyperandrogenism

3. Thyroid examination should be performed.

a. Thyroid nodules or enlargement may provide an explanation for difficulty in conceiving.

b. Thyroid function tests should always be performed, including test of thyroid antibodies, if the patient is hypothyroid or has a strong family history as the presence of thyroid antibodies may be more significant than the finding of subclinical hypothyroidism.

4. Perform a breast examination with attention to nipple discharge (galactorrhea), either spontaneous or expressive.

a. May be associated with hyperprolactinemia, which can block ovulation, thus preventing pregnancy.

b. If appropriate, a mammogram or other breast imaging should be ordered. Always check a prolactin level.

5. A pelvic examination should be performed.

a. If cervical motion tenderness or unusual discharge are noted, then sexually transmitted infection (STI) testing should be performed.

b. Chlamydia is the most common notifiable STI in the United States. If untreated, it can cause tubal factor infertility.

c. If a Pap test has not been done, then either perform one or arrange for this to be done.

BOX 37.2 Ferriman–Galwey Tool to Assess Hirsutism

- Hair growth is rated from 0 (no growth of terminal hair) to 4 (complete and heavy cover).
- Nine locations: upper lip, chin, chest, upper back, lower back, upper abdomen, lower abdomen, the upper arms, and the thighs
- Maximum score of 36
- In White women, a score of 8 or higher is regarded as indicative of androgen excess.
- With other ethnic groups, the amount of hair expected for that race should be considered.

6. Blood pressure, cardiac, and lung auscultation should be performed. Abdominal examination and skin evaluation are also required.
7. The time of the examination can be an optimal opportunity to check for smoking or drug use. Often the smell of cigarettes will be noted on the serious smoker.
   a. Fertility is adversely affected for both males and females, and this issue should be addressed at the outset.
   b. Women who smoke are at risk for earlier menopause and embryo quality is negatively affected by nicotine.
   c. Miscarriage rates are higher for smokers.
   d. Signs of drug abuse may prompt permission for toxicology tests and counseling.
8. Women of advanced age, usually described as older than 45 years, are often required to have a more thorough initial examination, including mammogram, EKG, and oral glucose tolerance testing, as well as a request for clearance from her OB/GYN for pregnancy-related treatments and ability to carry a pregnancy.
9. Ensure that vaccinations are up to date, including rubella and varicella, as well as seasonal flu vaccination. It is always best to address these concerns prior to attempting pregnancy. COVID-19 vaccines are now added to this list.

THE INITIAL WORKUP

A. The infertility evaluation begins with a visit, ideally with both parties if a couple is involved. Allotting a full hour is reasonable. This allows for history, physical examination, discussion, and ordering of appropriate tests.
1. Evaluative tests should be accomplished within 1 to 2 months.
2. Patients often present with unnecessary fears of tests and treatments. A thorough review of the basic tests, including blood, ultrasound, and x-ray for females and SA and blood tests for men, can help patients feel less anxious.
3. Make yourself available to answer patient questions and concerns promptly.
4. Educate patients about sexual intercourse.
   a. Inform patients that only sperm-safe lubricants are acceptable and that many over-the-counter (OTC) lubricants are not recommended. Sperm-safe pH-balanced lubricants mimic midcycle secretions. When in doubt, natural oils work well, without interfering with sperm.
   b. Do not tell patients how often to have intercourse. There are no data to suggest that too-frequent ejaculations will have a negative effect on conception.
   c. There is no need for women to remain on their backs or with raised hips or in bed after intercourse.
   d. Douching after intercourse is not permitted.
5. A menstrual cycle history will suggest whether a woman is ovulatory.
   a. Regular cycles are highly correlated with ovulation. For those with regular cycles, midcycle secretions suggest preovulation.
   b. Instructing the couple to have intercourse twice a week should be adequate to cover her ovulation.
   c. It is stressful to give overly restrictive advice that is not based in fact.
6. Taking a thorough history will reveal particular risk factors. Query for:
   a. Prior and current medical, surgical, gynecologic, infectious, and genetic problems for the patient, her partner, and immediate family
   b. Previous cervical conization or loop electrosurgical excision procedure (LEEP) may have affected cervical mucus secretory glands or caused stenosis. Typically, this interferes with catheter-based procedures, but microscopic sperm should not be affected.

c. Significant dysmenorrhea and/or dyspareunia might be associated with endometriosis.

d. Menstrual history, including age at menarche and interruptions to normal cyclicity and for how long. Obtain a karyotype if menarche was delayed.

e. Ask about normal pubertal milestones.

f. Check for history of irregular or dysfunctional bleeding, eating disorder, excessive athleticism, or obesity.

g. Prior methods of birth control:

    (1) IUD use and positive STI history may have caused tubal damage.

    (2) Hydrosalpinges reduce implantation most likely due to the adverse effect of backflow of the intratubal fluid on the endometrium. Prior history of peritonitis or ruptured appendix may affect tubal status.

h. Previous obstetrical history, including parity, miscarriages, ectopics, terminations, premature deliveries

i. Gynecologic procedures such as laparoscopy, laparotomy, or hysteroscopy with surgical findings

j. Fibroids, endometriosis, and adenomyosis

    (1) Submucosal fibroids can have the greatest impact on fertility.

    (2) Fibroids that impinge on the cavity and measure greater than 5 cm may need to be removed but surgical advice must be individualized.

k. Endometriosis should be staged. There is no clear evidence that medical or surgical treatment enhances fertility. IVF is generally recommended to best address this issue, although gonadotropin-releasing hormone (GnRH) suppressive treatments may be initiated prior to ART to increase the odds of success.

l. Screen for OTC, prescription, or recreational drug use or abuse that might impact fertility. For example, nonsteroidal anti-inflammatory drugs (NSAIDs) are not recommended when trying to conceive.

7. Preconception counseling includes explaining to patients the importance of carrier testing before conception.

a. The American College of Obstetricians and Gynecologists (ACOG) and other professional organizations recommend screening every patient for cystic fibrosis and spinal muscular atrophy (*SMN1*) gene before conception.

b. Check Tay–Sachs for those of Ashkenazi, French Canadian, and Cajun descent.

c. Check a hemoglobin electrophoresis to rule out thalassemias for those of Mediterranean descent and sickle cell trait for those of African descent.

d. Patients are increasingly unsure or mistaken of their ethnicity, so consider pan screening to be on the safe side.

e. For those with premature ovarian failure and insufficiency, check for fragile X, as premutation carrier status can affect ovarian reserve.

8. If BMI is greater than 30 to 35, refer to nutritionist or primary care for further evaluation and intervention. Elevated BMI is associated with hyperinsulinemia in PCOS patients and adversely affects ability to conceive and carry pregnancy to term. If accompanied by amenorrhea or irregular bleeding, a pelvic scan to check the endometrial lining should be performed. In some cases, a significantly thickened endometrial lining may be noted. This would prompt the need for an endometrial biopsy to rule out endometrial hyperplasia.

a. As a general rule, an endometrial biopsy is no longer considered part of the basic infertility evaluation. In part, this is because the concept of luteal phase deficiency is no longer considered relevant. However, endometrial biopsy is still performed routinely for abnormal uterine bleeding (AUB) when age 45 years or older to rule out endometritis and endometrial hyperplasia.

BOX 37.3 Summary of Basic Fertility Evaluation

- Ovarian reserve testing: "Day 3" FSH, estradiol, AMH level
- If anovulatory: Complete hormonal workup, including TSH, prolactin, LH, testosterone, DHEA-S
- Hysterosalpingogram
- SA
- Preconception blood work: omit CBC, STI panel, rubella, varicella, blood type, and antibody screen
- Genetic screening: CF, SMA, and fragile X, Ashkenazi panel, and Hgb electrophoresis as indicated by ethnicity or consider pan screening since reported ethnicity is often in error.

Note: Consider broader screening if patient is uncertain of ethnicity.

AMH, anti-Müllerian hormone; CBC, complete blood count; CF, cystic fibrosis; DHEA-S, dehydroepiandrosterone sulfate; FSH, follicle-stimulating hormone; Hgb, hemoglobin; LH, luteinizing hormone; SA, semen analysis; SMA, spinal muscular atrophy; STI, sexually transmitted infection; TSH, thyroidstimulating hormone.

---

9. Couple should leave their first visit aware of what tests they need and why. Speaking with a financial counselor will help them address any financial- or insurance-based concerns.
10. Give patients reading materials or online links, as the first visit is usually overwhelming due to information overload.
11. Box 37.3 summarizes the basic infertility evaluation.

MALE ASSESSMENT

A. SA
1. Check for volume, count, motility, and morphology.
2. Better results if specimen is produced at home under more relaxed circumstances than a medical office or bathroom. There are at-home SA kits that can be shipped to men who cannot find a close laboratory for analysis with a clinician order to Reprosource (www .reprosource.com).
3. General recommendations: Up to 2 days of abstinence is recommended but should not last more than 5 to 7 days as this can adversely affect quality due to less frequent ejaculations.
4. Use a nontoxic specimen container for the collection.
5. Transportation of semen
   a. Keep out of direct sunlight while transporting.
   b. Avoid extreme temperatures.
   c. Best to keep warm next to body.
   d. Do not refrigerate the specimen.
   e. Do not use lubricants when producing the specimen.
6. If the specimen was partially lost, report this, as it will affect the findings.
7. If abnormal, repeat, as sperm parameters can vary widely in the same individual. A single abnormal test is not conclusive.
8. If two abnormal semen analyses are reported, refer to a reproductive urologist.

B. History and screening

1. Take a thorough male history, including undescended testes (bilateral cryptorchidism); mumps orchitis; urologic infections; prior urologic surgeries, including hernia repair; sports injuries; endocrine disorders such as diabetes mellitus; diethylstilbestrol (DES) exposure of his mother; epilepsy; obesity.

2. Screen for use of recreational drugs, including nicotine and alcohol as well as testosterone supplements, which can stop sperm production, including anabolic steroids and performance-enhancing substances that may contain testosterone or its derivatives. A skilled RE or reproductive urologist can tell if a male is using anabolic steroids without disclosure from the semen analysis indices.

3. Ask whether he has close male relatives with infertility or males who have never fathered children.

4. Take a full sexual history, including ejaculatory problems and whether he has fathered a child or been involved in any prior pregnancies.

5. Certain prescription drugs are detrimental to sperm production such as calcium channel blockers, cimetidine, Dilantin, sulfasalazine, allopurinol, colchicine, nitrofurantoin, and certain chemotherapy agents.

6. Perform STI testing as there is still significant STI transmission due to lack of detection and awareness.

7. Screen for varicoceles, or varices of the testes, which are more common on the left side.
   a. Varioceles are controversial as they are common and also found in fertile men.
   b. In some cases, they are large and cause pain.
   c. They should be evaluated by a reproductive urologist to determine whether they are clinically significant.

8. If male is unable to produce a specimen for SA, he may require a collection condom, available from specialty pharmacies or online. These condoms are not toxic to sperm and allow intercourse to take place for collection.

9. Refer males for a complete examination with primary care physician or urologist to check for normal virilization, testes size and consistency (including presence of varicoceles), presence or absence of the vas deferens, and phimosis.

10. Box 37.4 lists the organizations that offer support for infertility and subfertility.

BOX 37.4 National Advocacy Groups

Resolve: The National Infertility Association
   703-556-7172
   www.rrsolve.org
American Fertility Association (AFA)
   888-917-3777
   www.theafa.org
The American Society for Reproductive Medicine (ASRM)
   205-978-5000
   www.asrm.org
National Council for Adoption
   703-299-6633
   www.adoptioncouncil.org
Fertile Hope
   855-220-7777
   www.fertilehope.org

BIBLIOGRAPHY

ACOG Committee Opinion No. 749. American College of Obstetricians and Gynecologists. (2018). Marriage and family building equality for lesbian, gay, bisexual, transgender, queer, intersex, asexual, and gender nonconforming individuals. *Obstetrics & Gynecology, 132*(2), e82–86. https://doi.org/10.1097/AOG.0000000000002765

ACOG Committee Opinion No. 762. American College of Obstetrcians and Gynecologists. (2019). Prepregnancy counseling. *Obstetrics & Gynecology, 133,* e78–89

ACOG Committee Opinion. (2019). Infertility workup for the women's health specialist. *Obstetrics & Gynecology, 133*(6), e377–384. https://doi.org/10.1097/AOG.0000000000003271

Bayer, S. R., Alper, M. M., & Penzias, A. S. (Eds.). (2017). *The Boston IVF handbook of infertility: A practical guide for practitioners who care for infertile couples* (3rd ed.). Taylor & Francis.

Brinsden, P. R. (Ed.). (2005). *Textbook of in vitro fertilization and assisted reproduction: The Bourn Hall guide to clinical and laboratory practice* (3rd ed.). Taylor & Francis.

Carcio, H. A., & Secor, M. C. (2018). *Advanced health assessment of women: Clinical skills and procedures* (2nd ed.). Springer Publishing.

Carr, S. C. (2011). Ultrasound for nurses in reproductive medicine. *Journal of Obstetric, Gynecologic, and Neonatal Nursing, 40*(5), 638–653. https://doi.org/10.1111/j.1552-6909.2011.01286.x

Committee on Gynecologic Practice of the American College of Obstetricians and Gynecologists and The Practice Committee of the American Society for Reproductive Medicine. (2008). Age-related fertility decline: A committee opinion. *Fertility and Sterility, 90*(3), 486–487. https://doi.org/10.1016/j.fertnstert.2008.08.006

Committee on Gynecologic Practice of the American College of Obstetricians and Gynecologists and The Practice Committee of the American Society for Reproductive Medicine. (2020a). Testing and interpreting measures of ovarian reserve: A committee opinion. *Fertility and Sterility, 114*(6), 1151–1156. https://doi.org/10.1016/j.fertnstert.2020.09.134

Committee on Gynecologic Practice of the American College of Obstetricians and Gynecologists and The Practice Committee of the American Society for Reproductive Medicine. (2020b). Diagnosis and treatment of infertility in men: AUA/ASRM guideline part I and II. *Fertility and Sterility, Article in Press.*

Committee on Gynecologic Practice of the American College of Obstetricians and Gynecologists and The Practice Committee of the American Society for Reproductive Medicine. (2021). Evidence-based outcomes after oocyte cryopreservation for donor oocyte in vitro fertilization and planned oocyte cryopreservation: A guideline. *Fertility and Sterility, 116*(1), 36–46. https://doi.org/10.1016/j.fertnstert.2021.02.024

Coutifaris, C., Myers, E. R., Guzick, D. S., Diamond, M. P., Carson, S. A., Legro, R. S., McGovern, P. G., Schlaff, W. D., Carr, B. R., Steinkampf, M. P., Silva, S., Vogel, D. L., & Leppert, P. C.; NICHD National Cooperative Reproductive Medicine Network. (2004). Histological dating of timed endometrial biopsy tissue is not related to fertility status. *Fertility and Sterility, 82*(5), 1264–1272. https://doi.org/10.1016/j.fertnstert.2004.03.069

Crawshaw, M., & Balen, R. (Eds.). (2010). *Adopting after infertility: Messages from practice, research and personal experience.* Jessica Kingsley Publishers.

Cronister, A., Teicher, J., Rohlfs, E. M., Donnenfeld, A., & Hallam, S. (2008). Prevalence and instability of fragile X alleles: Implications for offering fragile X prenatal diagnosis. *Obstetrics and Gynecology, 111*(3), 596–601. https://doi.org/10.1097/AOG.0b013e318163be0b

DeCherney, A., Nathan, L., Goodwin, T. M., Laufer, N., & Roman, A. (2013). *Current diagnosis and treatment obstetrics & gynecology* (11th ed.). McGraw-Hill.

Domar, A. D., & Kelly, A. L. (2004). *Conquering infertility: Dr. Alice Domar's mind/body guide to enhancing fertility and coping with infertility.* Penguin Books.

Feinberg, E. C. (2017). Tests used in the diagnostic evaluation of infertility: From ubiquitous to obsolete. *Fertility and Sterility, 107*(5), 1147. https://doi.org/10.1016/j.fertnstert.2017.02.117

Fritz, M. A., & Speroff, L. (2011). *Clinical gynecologic endocrinology and infertility* (8th ed.). Lippincott Williams & Wilkins.

Goldstein, M., & Schlegel, P. N. (Eds.). (2013). *Surgical and medical management of male infertility.* Cambridge University Press.

Gordon, J. D., Rydfors, J. T., & Druzin, M. L. (2001). *Obstetrics, gynecology and infertility: Handbook for clinicians–resident survival guide* (5th ed.). Scrub Hill Press.

Gunn, D. D., & Bates, G. W. (2016). Evidence-based approach to unexplained infertility: A systematic review. *Fertility and Sterility, 105*(6), 1566–1574.e1. https://doi.org/10.1016/j.fertnstert.2016.02.001

Lebovic, D., Gordon, J. D., & Taylor, R. (2013). *Reproductive endocrinology and infertility, handbook for clinicians* (2nd ed.). Scrub Hill Press.

Lipshultz, L. I., Howards, S. S., & Niederberger, C. S. (Eds.). (2009). *Infertility in the male* (4th ed.). Cambridge University Press.

Marrs, R., Bloch, L. F., & Silverman, K. K. (2011). *Dr. Richard Marrs' fertility book: America's leading infertility expert tells you everything you need to know about getting pregnant.* Dell.

Practice Committee of American Society for Reproductive Medicine. (2008). Vaccination guidelines for female infertility patients. *Fertility and Sterility, 90*(5), S169–S171. https://doi.org/10.1016/j.fertnstert.2008.08.056

Practice Committee of the American Society for Reproductive Medicine. (2012a). Diagnostic evaluation of the infertile female: A committee opinion. *Fertility and Sterility, 98*(2), 302–307. https://doi.org/10.1016/j.fertnstert.2012.05.032

Practice Committee of the American Society for Reproductive Medicine. (2012b). Diagnostic evaluation of the infertile male: A committee opinion. *Fertility and Sterility, 98*(2), 294–301. https://doi.org/10.1016/j.fertnstert.2012.05.033

Practice Committee of the American Society for Reproductive Medicine. (2018). Smoking and infertility: A committee opinion. *Fertility and Sterility, 110*(4), 611–18. https://doi.org/10.1016/j.fertnstert.2018.06.016

Practice Committee of the American Society for Reproductive Medicine. (2020). Testing and interpreting measures of ovarian reserve: A committee opinion. *Fertility and Sterility, 98*(6), 1407–1415. https://doi.org/10.1016/j.fertnstert.2012.09.036

Practice Committee of the American Society for Reproductive Medicine. (2021) Diagnosis and treatment of luteal phase deficiency: A committee opinion. *Fertility and Sterility, 115*(6), 1416–1422. https://doi.org/10.1016/j.fertnstert.2021.02.010

Schoolcraft, W. (2010). *If at first you don't conceive: A complete guide to infertility from one of the nation's leading clinics.* Rodale Press.

Sedaka, M., & Rosen, G. (2011). *What he can expect when she's not expecting: How to support your wife, save your marriage, and conquer infertility.* Skyhorse Publishing.

Speroff, L., Glass, R. H., Kase, N. G., & Seifer, D. B. (2001). *Clinical gynecologic endocrinology & infertility: Text, self-assessment and study guide* (6th ed.) [CD-ROM]. Lippincott Williams & Wilkins.

Stadtmauer, L., & Tur-Kaspa, I. (Eds.). (2013). *Ultrasound imaging in reproductive medicine: Advances in infertility workup, treatment, and ART.* Springer.

Wardell, H. (2003). *Childfree after infertility: Moving from childlessness to a joyous life.* iUniverse.

Wilcox, A. J, Dunson, D., & Baird, D. D. (2000). The timing of the "fertile window" in the menstrual cycle: Day specific estimates from a prospective study. *British Medical Journal, 321*(7271), 1259–1262. https://doi.org/10.1136/bmj.321.7271.1259

Wright, H. (2010). *The PCOS diet plan: A natural approach to health for women with polycystic ovary syndrome.* Celestial Arts.

APPENDIX 37.1 ASSESSMENT FORMS

Health History

Female Fertility Evaluation

Please complete the following:

Name: _____

Member #: _____

Date of birth: _____ Age: _____

Partner's name: _____ Member #: _____

Date of birth: _____ Age: _____

Primary care provider: _____

OB/GYN provider: _____

How long have you been trying to get pregnant? _____

Weight: _____ Height: _____ Current medications: _____

Allergies: _____ Reaction: _____

Menstrual History

Date of last menses:

Age at onset of your menstrual period:

Average length between cycles:

Any history of irregular menses, spotting, or missed menses? If yes, please explain (include dates):

Painful menses?

List any medications you take for cramps.

Ovulation

Do you experience:

Premenstrual cramps?	Yes ❏	No ❏
Clear discharge midcycle?	Yes ❏	No ❏
Monthly cycles?	Yes ❏	No ❏
Pain at midcycle?	Yes ❏	No ❏

Have you ever used the following?

Basal body temperature: _____ months Temperature shift: _____

Day of shift: _____

Ovulation predictor kit:

Name of kit: _____

Number of cycles: _____

Day of surge: _____

Luteinizing hormone (LH) surge seen? Yes ❏ No ❏

Birth Control

Have you ever used any of the following?
Birth control pills, intrauterine device (IUD), diaphragm, condoms, Norplant, Depo-Provera, foam, sponge, other (please describe)

METHOD	DATES	HOW LONG	WHY STOPPED	COMPLICATIONS

Obstetric History

PREGNANCY NUMBER	YEAR	TIME TO CONCEIVE	TYPE OF FERTILITY TREATMENT? (IF ANY) WEEKS CARRIED	OUTCOME	TYPE OF DELIVERY (VAGINAL/C-SECTION)	COMPLI-CATIONS	CURRENT PARTNER

Gynecologic History

Please include dates and treatment if you ever had:

> Pelvic infection
>
> Chlamydia/gonorrhea
>
> Herpes
>
> Vaginitis
>
> Endometriosis
>
> Ovarian cysts
>
> Genital warts
>
> Ectopic pregnancy
>
> Miscarriage
>
> Abortion
>
> List date and nature of any pelvic surgery: Have you had a tubal ligation? If so, when was it reversed? Were you ever treated for an abnormal Pap test? If yes, list date and nature of treatment.

Sexual History

Please describe any positive responses.

> Do you have painful intercourse?
>
> Do you use vaginal lubricants or douches?

Hormonal Assessment

Have you experienced any of the following?

> Weight gain/loss of 10+ pounds
>
> Discharge from nipples

Change in vision

Unusual sensitivity to hot or cold

Excessive change in hair growth/loss

Thyroid disease, diabetes, or other hormonal abnormalities

Medical History

Please list any medical or psychiatric conditions that you have or had in the past and any medications used in treatment. List dates.

Surgical/Hospitalization History

Please list any surgeries or hospitalizations you have had. List dates.

Family History

Please list any family history of infertility, genetic problems, thyroid disease, diabetes, cancer, or any other major medical problems.

Social History

Occupation: Travel for work?   Frequency?

Caffeine intake:

Do you smoke cigarettes?   _____ packs per day

Alcohol consumption: _____ drinks/week   Type:

Medications

  Prescription:

  Over the counter:

  Recreational (marijuana, hallucinogens, crack/cocaine, other addictive drugs; if yes, explain):

  List the form and frequency of any regular exercise. Have you ever been told you have or suspected you have an eating disorder?

  Have you recently traveled to Zika-infected areas?

Previous Infertility Treatment

Describe results. Include dates.

Name of physician/practice:

  Has your partner ever had an SA?

  Have you had any hormonal blood tests?

  Have you ever had an endometrial biopsy?

  Have you ever had an x-ray of your tubes and uterus (hysterosalpingogram [HSG])?

  Have you ever had a laparoscopy?

  Have you ever taken medications to stimulate ovulation?

  Have you ever had intrauterine insemination?

  Have you ever had advanced reproductive technology procedures performed via intrauterine device (IVF) or associated procedures?

  Why do you think you are not getting pregnant?

Female Partner Fertility Evaluation

Please complete the following:

Name:_____ Member #: _____

Date of birth: _____ Age: _____

Partner's name: _____ Member #: _____

Gynecologic History

Please include dates and treatment if you ever had

  Pelvic infection

  Chlamydia/gonorrhea

  Herpes

  Vaginitis

  Genital warts

Were you ever treated for an abnormal Pap test? If yes, list date and nature of treatment.

38

METHODS TO DETECT OVULATION

CAROL LESSER

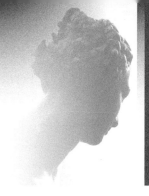

METHODS TO DETECT OVULATION

A. Key concepts
1. Take a menstrual history.
   a. Determine whether there is a history of amenorrhea or long cycles that are greater than 35 to 40 days or short cycles less than 25 days.
   b. A sign of perimenopause is the shortening of cycle length, so determine whether short cycles are chronic or a new occurrence.
2. Previously, women were instructed to check their basal body temperature (BBT) using a digital thermometer to record their early-morning temperature before taking food or drink, every day of the menstrual cycle.
   a. The BBT rises 0.4°F to 0.8°F after ovulation and a biphasic pattern emerges due to a thermal shift.
   b. After ovulation, the temperature remains elevated until the corpus luteum recedes and stops making progesterone. Menses ensues, accompanied by a BBT drop.
   c. If pregnancy occurs, the BBT remains elevated for the duration of pregnancy.
3. Checking for spinnbarkeit (clear, stretchy secretions) is difficult for many women to grasp and is highly subjective. However, this information can be useful if other testing is not available.
4. These older methods have been replaced by other more reliable methods of determining midcycle (Box 38.1) for fertility patients.

BOX 38.1 Basic Fertility Evaluation

- Ovarian reserve testing: "Day 3" FSH, estradiol, AMH level
- If anovulatory: complete hormonal workup including androgen panel
- Hysterosalpingogram or FemVue also known as HyCoSy
- Semen analysis
- Preconception blood work: TSH, prolactin, CBC, STI panel, rubella, varicella, blood type and antibody screen. Consider vitamin D.
- Genetic screening: CF, SMA, and fragile X, Ashkenazi panel, and thalassemia panel with Hgb electrophoresis. Consider broader screening since knowledge of one's ethnicity may be incorrect. And expanded panels are more affordable. Fragile X permutations are associated with POF so should be checked if there is a personal or family history of POF.

AMH, anti-Müllerian hormone; CBC, complete blood count; CF, cystic fibrosis; FSH, follicle-stimulating hormone; Hgb, hemoglobin; POF, premature ovarian failure; SMA, spinal muscular atrophy; STI, sexually transmitted infection; TSH, thyroid-stimulating hormone.

---

   a. While useful to understand this method, most clinicians no longer recommend BBT charting as it is time-consuming and confusing.
   b. BBT charting gives better information retrospectively than prospectively.
5. Mobile applications are available to help women track their cycles and symptoms. There are multiple free applications available.

B. Ovulation predictor kits (OPKs)
   1. OPK or ovulation predictor kits and monitors are widely used.
   2. No home-based method is completely reliable, so care must be taken to educate the patient in their proper use. Urine strips and fertility monitors are available. Some kits work better for individuals than others requiring a trial-and-error approach. Women frequently complain that their kits are hard to read and interpret.
   3. Cost varies and often affects decision on which to use.
   4. All kits detect the luteinizing hormone (LH).
   5. The LH surge precedes ovulation.
      a. A color change or positive indicator indicates that ovulation is approaching, usually in 12 to 36 hours.
      b. Must follow instructions for the kit or monitor being used. Some are daily and others focus on a more limited window of testing.
      c. Most urine-testing kits instruct that the first-morning void be discarded, as it may be too concentrated.
      d. Read instructions carefully and familiarize yourself with the kits you recommend.
   6. Testing too late in the cycle will miss the surge and chance to conceive. This is the most common error. Remaining sexually active is a safeguard against this for those who have a partner and can do so.
   7. If a woman has regular cycles and knows when she is ovulating, then kits are not necessary.
   8. Timing of intercourse does not have to be so precise.
      a. Pregnancy occurs if exposure to sperm takes place in a 5- to 6-day window leading up to and including ovulation.
      b. Wilcox et al. (2000) confirmed the greatest chance of pregnancy occurred with intercourse beginning 2 days before ovulation. No pregnancies occurred if intercourse took place after ovulation.
      c. Sperm can live for up to 5 days in the reproductive tract while the oocyte lives for less than 24 hours.
      d. This is why intercourse or exposure to sperm postovulation is ineffective but preovulation can be effective.

HORMONAL EVALUATION OF OVULATION

A. Estradiol rises as the follicle matures. At ovulation, the estradiol level is usually between 150 and 250 pg/mL per follicle. Estradiol is checked with a blood test. Newer saliva tests have been developed and hold promise for the future.
B. As the follicle reaches maturity, LH rises. At its peak, a surge occurs.
C. A rise in progesterone is diagnostic for postovulation.
   1. Laboratories use different assays and cutoffs, so it is important to know what the periovulatory and postovulatory levels are for your laboratory.
   2. Generally, progesterone greater than 1.5 ng/mL is diagnostic for post ovulation.
   3. Progesterone levels dip right before menses. A low progesterone level can mean menses is approaching or is suggestive of anovulation or preovulation.
   4. Progesterone is released in pulses every 2 to 3 hours. Levels can vary widely, making a single level less diagnostic.

BOX 38.2 Presumptive Signs That Ovulation Is Occurring (Molimina)

Molimina (Premenstrual Signs) That Signify Ovulation

Menstrual characteristics

- Predictable bleeding pattern every 21 to 35 days
- Bleeding that lasts 3 to 5 days
- Breast tenderness that resolves with menses
- Mild-to-moderate cramps

Periovulatory characteristics

- Spinnbarkeit, midcycle stretchy cervical secretions resembling clear egg white
- Mild cramping (Mittelschmerz)
- Occasional midcycle spotting (Hartman's sign)
- Increase in sexual desire

D. Moliminal premenstrual symptoms (Box 38.2) are highly diagnostic for ovulation. Regular menstrual cycles are also highly diagnostic for ovulation.
E. Luteal-phase defect is a concept now considered controversial and outdated.
  1. Infertility centers rarely check for this anymore.
  2. An exception is a patient who has failed multiple in vitro fertilization (IVF) cycles despite the creation of high-quality embryos. Specialized tests can be ordered that go far beyond the endometrial dating assessed during a routine endometrial biopsy.

THE ENDOMETRIAL BIOPSY

A. The issues
  1. In the past, endometrial biopsy was routinely performed to rule out a luteal-phase deficiency (LPD).
  2. It was theorized that some ovulatory women had inadequate progesterone production in the luteal phase, negatively impacting endometrium maturation and receptivity for implantation and ongoing pregnancy.
  3. The luteal phase can be between 13 and 16 days long but the tests were interpreted in light of a 14-day luteal phase, leading to overdiagnosis.
  4. For these reasons, endometrial biopsies are no longer routinely offered in fertility centers.
  5. See Chapter 49 regarding gynecologic indications for this test.
  6. May still be used and important to rule out endometritis and hyperplasia or atypia (see Chapter 39). More sophisticated endometrial dating biopsies may be offered by in vitro fertilization (IVF) centers while addressing issues of failed implantation or recurrent miscarriage.

UTERINE CAVITY AND FALLOPIAN TUBE ASSESSMENT

A. The basics
  1. Pregnancy without assistance of IVF depends on normal uterine and fallopian tube anatomy.
  2. Pregnancy can occur if only one fallopian tube is present or open.
  3. Advanced practice practitioners perform these tests.
  4. Check for Müllerian defects such as unicornuate, bicornuate, or didelphys uterus; fibroids, polyps, or Asherman's syndrome; as well as tubal disease, most notably hydrosalpinges.

5. In the case of fibroids, the cavity evaluations are looking for impingement on the cavity or large myomas that are close to the endometrial border that could interfere with implantation or pregnancy advancement.

B. Tests include

1. Pelvic ultrasound to rule out any obvious pathology, including fibroids, ovarian cysts or dermoids, or obvious structural defects. Evidence of polycystic ovarian syndrome (PCOS) like ovaries with their characteristic "string of pearls" appearance ringing the perimeter should be noted.

2. Hysterosalpingogram used to assess tubal patency and assess the internal uterine cavity for fibroid impingement, polyps, Müllerian defects, or Asherman's syndrome. Done in a radiology-equipped room or facility after menstrual flow but before ovulation if trying to conceive that cycle. Ovaries are not visualized with this test.

3. HyCoSy or FemVue is an ultrasound procedure that examines the internal uterine cavity as well checks for tubal patency. The practitioner places a balloon catheter or FemVue catheter that allows the administration of saline and bubbles to accomplish this. Since it is an ultrasound, patients tend to be less anxious. They can take ibuprofen prior to both hysterosalpingogram (HSG) and HyCoSy to minimize cramping. Timing is the same as HSG. Results are immediately available. Varies can be assessed at the same time.

4. Sonohysterogram is a procedure done in the office in which a small amount of saline is instilled into the uterus via a catheter placed through the internal os.
   a. Often used to rule out any uterine pathology such as polyps, fibroids, and adhesions. Also used to assess abnormal bleeding or recurrent miscarriage. Done after menstrual flow but before ovulation if trying to conceive that cycle (see Chapter 55).

5. Perform office hysteroscopy when defects need further evaluation and possible treatment such as polypectomy or lysis of adhesions from Asherman's syndrome.

6. Operative hysteroscopy may be indicated based on findings if more extensive surgery is needed.

7. Laparoscopy may be indicated if the patient has significant pelvic pain or a history of endometriosis or large fibroids that need intervention. Hydrosalpinges may be removed, drained, or ligated to increase the probability of implantation. Hydrosalpinges have been associated with lower rates of implantation.

OVARIAN RESERVE TESTING

A. Background

1. This is an integral part of the infertility evaluation. Commonly refers to oocyte quantity, quality, and reproductive potential.

2. Ovarian reserve (OR) testing offers valuable information to help determine appropriate diagnosis and treatment. Interpretation takes extra care and results must be interpreted in light of all patient factors.

3. Can be assessed by blood and ultrasound, often interpreted together in the context of patient history (e.g., age, how long trying to conceive, obstetrical history).

4. Chronologic age and genetics determine oocyte quality and quantity, and younger patients tend to have more and better quality eggs.
   a. The highest number of eggs is present in the ovaries at 20 weeks of gestational age with a steady decline until menopause and a precipitous drop in the later reproductive years.
   b. Fertility measurably declines in a woman's 20s but is usually not of concern.

5. OR tests measure the relative quantity of eggs remaining, but chronologic age is still an excellent predictor of success. Therefore, younger patients whose levels suggest decreased OR tend to fare better than older patients, even if their levels look superior. There are

TABLE 38.1 Interpretation of AMH Levels

AMH	LEVEL	OR
1–3	ng/mL	Normal
<1	ng/mL	Reduced
<0.83	ng/mL	Further reduced
<0.1	ng/mL	Poor prognosis

Note: AMH level reflects the remaining follicular pool.

AMH, anti-Müllerian hormone; OR, ovarian reserve.

multiple cases of young women with reduced anti-Mullerian hormone (AMH) levels who conceive spontaneously. However, menopause may be hastened so if they want additional children, they should be counseled to shorten the wait period between pregnancies.

B. The tests
  1. AMH
     a. The newest OR test that many find to be the most helpful predictor of OR. Expressed by the granulosa cells of the ovary.
     b. Can be done on any cycle day, including while on oral contraceptives, when anovulatory, breastfeeding, or postpartum, but best done off of oral contraceptives for at least 1 month.
     c. This test is often used when screening potential oocyte donors or women interested in elective egg freezing to see if they will be a good candidate for egg freezing.
     d. Generally, higher numbers are reassuring and are associated with PCOS. Lower numbers are associated with perimenopause and premature ovarian insufficiency and failure or when ovarian surgery has been performed (Table 38.1).
     e. The AMH test is the earliest known marker for detecting ovarian aging and decline.
     f. Some studies suggest that results from younger women can be predictive of age at onset of menopause.
  2. Follicle-stimulating hormone (FSH) and estradiol
     a. Basal FSH concentrations increase with advancing age until their peak at menopause.
     b. An elevated FSH is associated with decreased *or* premature ovarian insufficiency. Menopausal FSH levels in a younger woman indicate premature ovarian failure (POF; Table 38.2).
        (1) Younger patients with FSH elevations should be counseled to seek reproductive treatments as soon as possible if childbearing is desired.

TABLE 38.2 Interpretation of Cycle Day 3 Hormone Levels

FSH (MIU/ML)	ESTRADIOL (PG/ML)	OR
>10	<70	Reduced
>10	>70	Reduced
2–10	>70	Reduced
2–10	<70	Normal

Note: An ovulatory younger woman with an elevated FSH has a significantly higher chance of pregnancy than an older woman with the same level. Provide general guidelines: No level can predict pregnancy. OR tests are quantitative not qualitative assessment tools.

FSH, follicle-stimulating hormone; OR, ovarian reserve.

      (2) If ovulatory, check in the early follicular phase, typically on days 2, 3, or 4. This is when basal FSH levels should be at their lowest, before follicle recruitment.

      (3) If anovulatory, basal FSH levels can be drawn on any day since follicle recruitment is not taking place.

    c. Estradiol suppresses FSH. Best to interpret the FSH level with an estradiol level drawn at the same time.

    d. If the estradiol is significantly elevated, this can be associated with perimenopause.

      (1) Levels greater than 70 pg/mL are considered elevated and lower the FSH level.

      (2) FSH would need to be repeated on a future cycle when the estradiol was within the normal range.

    e. Elevations in estradiol are common in perimenopause and can happen intermittently or frequently.

    f. OR testing from a specialty laboratory can be arranged by the patient.

    g. Most important, there is no single test that can accurately predict pregnancy even when decreased OR is documented.

  3. Basal antral follicle (BAF) count

    a. This is technician dependent and must be done by trained personnel.

    b. A simple test that measures antral follicles, which are small follicles (2–8 mm in size) that are visible on the ovaries via ultrasound. They are also known as *resting follicles* and give a representation of the pool of primordial follicles that remain.

    c. The higher the number of antral follicles, the greater the OR potential. Lower counts are associated with decreased OR ovarian insufficiency. Very high levels are associated with PCOS.

BASELINE HORMONE TESTING

A. What to test and when

  1. Hormones are best checked in the early follicular phase if including OR tests. Otherwise, any cycle day will suffice.

  2. Check FSH, estradiol, and AMH as described previously.

  3. Check LH. Although it was previously taught that LH and the FSH:LH ratio are increased in PCOS, this is not always the case. A normal LH does not preclude the diagnosis of PCOS.

  4. Check prolactin if there is menstrual irregularity or anovulation or galactorrhea.

  5. Check TSH for all patients with infertility. If the TSH is elevated, check for thyroid antibodies as they are associated with infertility and miscarriage.

  6. If oligo or anovulatory, screen for hyperandrogenism. Check LH, free testosterone, testosterone, and consider adrenal hormones such as 17 hydroxyprogesterone (17-H-P) and dehydroepiandrosterone sulfate (DHEA-S).

  7. If congenital adrenal hyperplasia (CAH) is suspected, further testing will be indicated. Consider a 24-hour urinary cortisol or CAH (adrenocorticotropic hormone [ACTH]) challenge test.

  8. Most patients with oligo or anovulation have PCOS. They often have elevated basal estradiol levels produced by their active ovaries. This artificially suppresses FSH and interpretation must be done carefully. Fasting insulin and glucose levels can be useful since there has been an increase in insulin resistance, obesity, and PCOS. Practitioners may find it useful to recommend metformin if the PCOS patient is prediabetic along with nutrition counseling and recommendations for diet/exercise modifications.

POSTCOITAL TEST: NO LONGER PART OF THE CURRENT DAY INFERTILE EVALUATION

  1. Microscopically tests the survival of sperm postcoitus in cervical mucus at midcycle.

2. Cervical mucus was examined under microscope and graded for its degree of ferning, which peaks at midcycle as estradiol levels rise.
3. Test was not found to be reliable or predictive so has been dropped.

OVULATION INDUCTION

A. Define the cause.
   1. If oligo or anovulatory due to PCOS, offer ovulation induction medication.
      a. Most popular oral agent is no longer clomiphene citrate (CC), a selective estrogen receptor modulator (SERM). While CC is still prescribed, first line ovulation induction for PCOS patients is with letrozole, an aromatase inhibitor (AI) prescribed off-label.
         (1) Both CC and letrozole are prescribed for those with open tube(s) and normal semen parameters or using donor sperm.
         (2) **Letrozole dose:** 2.5–7.5 mg for 5 consecutive days.
         (3) **CC dose:** 50–150 mg for 5 consecutive days. This can start on day 2, 3, 4, or 5 of the menstrual cycle. Lowest effective dose is typically prescribed. For severe PCOS with impaired glucose tolerance (IGT), metformin is often also prescribed. Some patients benefit from the addition of over-the-counter inositol, a B-vitamin derivative that also induces insulin sensitivity and is better tolerated by patients.
      b. If anovulatory, assess the uterine lining to rule out hyperplasia. If normal, can prescribe with or without a withdrawal bleed. CC can thin the endometrium due to its hypoestrogenic effect. Some studies suggest better implantation without a prior induced bleed, which can further diminish the lining. Letrozole does not thin the lining or decrease mid cycle cervical mucus as CC can.
      c. Efficacy can be assessed by waiting for a menstrual cycle to occur within 35 days, highly correlated with ovulation. If the patient experiences molimina for the first time, this too is reassuring.
      d. A progesterone level can be obtained after day 21 to see whether it is within the postovulatory level, generally greater than 1.5 ng/mL, but check your laboratory cutoff.
      e. An OPK checks for an LH surge. If a woman's baseline LH is always elevated, then the kit may initially test positive and is not the best way to assess letrozole or clomiphene's efficacy or the woman's ovulatory status if she inadvertently tests too early.
      f. Fertility centers can offer serum monitoring of estradiol, LH, and progesterone as well as pelvic ultrasound to track mature follicle(s) if necessary.
      g. CC has approximately a 10% to 15% success rate per cycle and a 10% chance of causing twins.
         (1) Side effects, including hypoestrogenic complaints such as hot flashes, moodiness, and thinning of endometrium and cervical secretions, have been described.
         (2) The off-label aspect of letrozole is the chief factor limiting its broader use. Patients prefer letrozole to CC and it continues gaining in popularity.
         (3) Prescribed in the same way as CC for 5 days starting on days 2, 3, 4, or 5. Dose is 2.5 to 7.5 mg daily. Lowest effective dose is typically prescribed.
      h. Advantage of artificial insemination is lack of hypoestrogenic side effects and slightly lower risk of twins.
   2. Hypothalamic amenorrhea
      a. Hypogonadotropic hypogonadism, although not common, is most often self-inflicted and associated with eating disorders, low body mass index (BMI), and excessive athleticism now or in the past. Rarely, Kallmann syndrome will be the cause, characterized by anosmia and deficiency of gonadotropin-releasing hormone (GnRH).
      b. Psychological counseling is often indicated for eating disorders, but can be a very difficult disorder to treat.

    c. Hormonal assays reveal depressed FSH, LH, and estradiol. Panhypopituitarism is sometimes seen with lowered TSH and as well as prolactin.

    d. Treatment is usually injectable gonadotropin therapy, which patient can self-administer subcutaneously, delivering a combination of FSH and LH in a 1:1 ratio. A trigger shot of human chorionic gonadotropin (hCG) acting as an LH surrogate is also needed to complete final follicle maturation and ovulation.

        (1) Main risks are hyperstimulation syndrome and multiple births. Offering IVF with single embryo transfer ameliorates these concerns.

        (2) Requires careful monitoring and extremely low dose to decrease these risks. Patients with low BMI can become ovulatory with modest weight gain.

BIBLIOGRAPHY

Bayer, S. R., Alper, M. M., & Penzias, A. S. (Eds.). (2017). *The Boston IVF handbook of infertility: A practical guide for practitioners who care for infertile couples* (5th ed.). Taylor & Francis.

Brinsden, P. R. (Ed.). (2005). *Textbook of in vitro fertilization and assisted reproduction: The Bourn Hall guide to clinical and laboratory practice* (3rd ed.). Taylor & Francis.

Burns, L. H., & Covington, S. N. (Eds.). (2000). *Infertility counseling: A comprehensive handbook for clinicians.* Parthenon Publishing Group.

Carcio, H. A., & Secor, M. C. (2018). *Advanced health assessment of women: Clinical skills and procedures* (4th ed.). Springer Publishing.

Carr, S. C. (2011). Ultrasound for nurses in reproductive medicine. *Journal of Obstetric, Gynecologic, and Neonatal Nursing, 40*(5), 638–653. https://doi.org/10.1111/j.1552-6909.2011.01286.x

Cedars, M. I. (2005). *Infertility: Practical pathways in obstetrics & gynecology.* McGraw-Hill.

Committee on Gynecologic Practice of the American College of Obstetricians and Gynecologists and The Practice Committee of the American Society for Reproductive Medicine. (2008). Age-related fertility decline: A committee opinion. *Fertility and Sterility, 90*(3), 486–487. https://doi.org/10.1016/j.fertnstert.2008.08.006

Crawshaw, M., & Balen, R. (Eds.). (2010). *Adopting after infertility: Messages from practice, research and personal experience.* Jessica Kingsley Publishers.

Cronister, A., Teicher, J., Rohlfs, E. M., Donnenfeld, A., & Hallam, S. (2008). Prevalence and instability of fragile X alleles: Implications for offering fragile X prenatal diagnosis. *Obstetrics and Gynecology, 111*(3), 596–601. https://doi.org/10.1097/AOG.0b013e318163be0b

DeCherney, A., Nathan, L., Goodwin, T. M., Laufer, N., & Roman, A. (2013). *Current diagnosis & treatment obstetrics & gynecology* (11th ed.). McGraw-Hill.

Domar, A. D., & Kelly, A. L. (2004). *Conquering infertility: Dr. Alice Domar's mind/body guide to enhancing fertility and coping with infertility.* Penguin Books.

Dreyer, Kim, D., Out, R., Hompes, P. G. A., & Mijatovic, V. (2014). Hysterosalpingo-foam sonography, a less painful procedure for tubal patency testing during fertility workup compared with (serial) hysterosalpingography: A randomized controlled trial. *Fertility and Sterility, 102*(3), 821–825. https://doi.org/10.1016/j.fertnstert.2014.05.042

Ecochard, R., Duterque, O., Leiva, R., Bouchard, T., & Vigil, P. (2015). Self-identification of the clinical fertile window and the ovulation period. *Fertility and Sterility, 103*(5), 1319–25. e3. https://doi.org/10.1016/j.fertnstert.2015.01.031

Evans-Hoeker, E., Pritchard, D. A., Long, D. L., Herring, A. H., Stanford, J. B., & Steiner, A. Z. (2013). Cervical mucus monitoring prevalence and associated fecundability in women trying to conceive. *Fertility and Sterility, 100*(4), 1033–1038. e1. https://doi.org/10.1016/j.fertnstert.2013.06.002

Fritz, M. A., & Speroff, L. (2011). *Clinical gynecologic endocrinology and infertility* (8th ed.). Lippincott Williams & Wilkins.

Goldstein, M., & Schlegel, P. N. (Eds.). (2013). *Surgical and medical management of male infertility.* Cambridge University Press.

Gordon, J. D., Rydfors, J. T., & Druzin, M. L. (2001). *Obstetrics, gynecology and infertility: Handbook for clinicians— Resident survival guide* (5th ed.). Scrub Hill Press.

Lebovic, D., Gordon, J. D., & Taylor, R. (2013). *Reproductive endocrinology and infertility, handbook for clinicians* (2nd ed.). Scrub Hill Press.

Lipshultz, L. I., Howards, S. S., & Niederberger, C. S. (Eds.). (2009). *Infertility in the male* (4th ed.). Cambridge University Press.

Marrs, R., Bloch, L. F., & Silverman, K. K. (2011). *Dr. Richard Marrs' fertility book: America's leading infertility expert tells you everything you need to know about getting pregnant.* Dell Publishing.

Mejia, R. B., Summers, K. M., Kresowik, J. D., & Voorhis, B. J. V. (2019). A randomized controlled trial of combination letrozole and clomiphene citrate or letrozole alone for ovulation induction in women with polycystic ovary syndrome. *Fertility and Sterility, 111*(3), 571–578. e1. https://doi.org/10.1016/j.fertnstert.2018.11.030

Practice Committee of American Society for Reproductive Medicine. (2008). Vaccination guidelines for female infertility patients. *Fertility and Sterility, 90*(5), S169–S171. https://doi.org/10.1016/j.fertnstert.2008.08.056

Practice Committee of the American Society for Reproductive Medicine. (2012a). Diagnostic evaluation of the infertile female: A committee opinion. *Fertility and Sterility, 98*(2), 302–307. https://doi.org/10.1016/j.fertnstert.2012.05.032

Practice Committee of the American Society for Reproductive Medicine. (2012b). Diagnostic evaluation of the infertile male: A committee opinion. *Fertility and Sterility, 98*(2), 294–301. https://doi.org/10.1016/j.fertnstert.2012.05.033

Practice Committee of the American Society for Reproductive Medicine. (2012c). Smoking and infertility: A committee opinion. *Fertility and Sterility, 98*(6), 1400–1406. https://doi.org/10.1016/j.fertnstert.2012.07.1146

Practice Committee of the American Society for Reproductive Medicine. (2012d). Testing and interpreting measures of ovarian reserve: A committee opinion. *Fertility and Sterility, 98*(6), 1407–1415. https://doi.org/10.1016/j.fertnstert.2012.09.036

Practice Committee of the American Society for Reproductive Medicine. (2012e). The clinical relevance of luteal phase deficiency: A committee opinion. *Fertility and Sterility, 98*(5), 1112–1117. https://doi.org/10.1016/j.fertnstert.2012.06.050

Practice Committee of the American Society for Reproductive Medicine. (2016). Optimizing natural fertility: A committee opinion. *Fertility and Sterility, 107*(1), 52–58. https://doi.org/10.1016/j.fertnstert.2016.09.029

Racowsky, C., Schlegel, P. N., Fauser, B. C., & Carrell, D. T. (Eds.). (2011). *Biennial review of infertility* (Vol. 2). Springer.

Schoolcraft, W. (2010). *If at first you don't conceive: A complete guide to infertility from one of the nation's leading clinics.* Rodale Press.

Sedaka, M., & Rosen, G. (2011). *What he can expect when she's not expecting: How to support your wife, save your marriage, and conquer infertility.* Skyhorse Publishing.

Speroff, L., Glass, R. H., Kase, N. G., & Seifer, D. B. (2021). *Clinical gynecologic endocrinology & infertility: Text, self-assessment and study guide* (6th ed.) [CD-ROM]. Lippincott Williams & Wilkins.

Stadtmauer, L., & Tur-Kaspa, I. (Eds.). (2013). *Ultrasound imaging in reproductive medicine: Advances in infertility work-up, treatment, and ART.* Springer.

Tulandi, T., & DeCherney, A. H. (2007). Limiting access to letrozole—is it justified? *Fertility and Sterility, 88*(4), 779–780. https://doi.org/10.1016/j.fertnstert.2007.01.115

Wardell, H. (2003). *Childfree after infertility: Moving from childlessness to a joyous life.* iUniverse, Inc.

Wilcox, A. J, Dunson, D., & Baird, D. D. (2000). The timing of the "fertile window" in the menstrual cycle: Day specific estimates from a prospective study. *British Medical Journal, 321*(7271), 1259–1262. https://doi.org/10.1136/bmj.321.7271.1259

Wright, H. (2010). *The PCOS diet plan: A natural approach to health for women with polycystic ovary syndrome.* Celestial Arts.

Zimon, A., Lannon, B., Sakkas, D., Ulrich, M., & Alper, M. (2013). Venopuncture-free IVF: Measurement of estrogen in controlled ovarian stimulation IVF cycles using a "patient-friendly" saliva-based estradiol assay. *Fertility and Sterility, 100*(3), 1677.

39

INTRAUTERINE INSEMINATION

CAROL LESSER

INTRAUTERINE INSEMINATION

A. Indications for intrauterine insemination (IUI; Box 39.1)
1. Ejaculatory problems requiring masturbation and insemination of either a fresh or frozen specimen
2. If male partner is unavailable at midcycle, frozen sperm can be inseminated.
3. Certain fertility medications
   a. Clomiphene citrate (CC) may reduce midcycle secretions after several cycles. This is not an issue with other fertility medications.
4. Reduced sperm parameters
   a. If a couple is not ready for in vitro fertilization (IVF), IUI may improve outcome.
5. Avoid HIV or other sexually transmitted infection (STI) transmission; affected partner's sperm may be sequestered, processed, and stored separately for future IUI or assisted reproductive technologies such as IVF.
6. Male fertility preservation in the case of a cancer diagnosis or when gonadotoxic therapy or surgery may be planned
7. Unexplained infertility or those not ready for IVF
8. If using donor sperm
9. Retroversion or retroflexion of the uterus is not an indication for IUI.
10. Previous vasectomy with cryopreserved sperm
11. Female sexual dysfunction preventing intercourse. Referral to a pelvic floor physical therapist is important. Simultaneously offering IUI with as small a speculum as possible while maintaining visualization of cervical os can be helpful.
12. Do not offer IUI in the presence of a known hydrosalpinx as the possibility of causing an infection is increased.
    a. It is advised to bank sperm in case the need for it arises in the future if the partner frequently travels or has medical issues interfering with ejaculation or intercourse.
    b. In these cases, IUI or assisted reproductive technology (ART) may be recommended to optimize sperm performance after cryopreservation.

BOX 39.1 Factors That Impact Success of Intrauterine Insemination

- Age/ovarian reserve
- History of unilateral tube and/or ovary. Even if only one tube or ovary is present, conception can still occur on the contralateral side.
- Total motile sperm count
- Fertility medications versus natural cycle

B. Technique
   1. **Fresh IUI:** Obtain the specimen.
      a. The specimen is most often obtained via masturbation into a sterile container that has been tested to be nontoxic to sperm.
      b. Can be collected at home or office if there is a private collection room.
      c. Generally, it is recommended to collect at home for privacy and a more relaxed atmosphere, which may improve the specimen. Men reportedly prefer at-home collection.
         (1) Try to transport the specimen within 1.5 hours but 2 hours is generally acceptable.
         (2) When transporting, body warmth, if possible, provides the best temperature.
         (3) Avoid excessive heat, like the heater of the car, or excessive cold.
      d. Proper specimen identification is required. A driver's license is usually best.
      e. Once the specimen is identified and dropped off, it will require processing before the IUI can be performed.
         (1) Ask couple to return at the appointment time.
         (2) Processing usually takes at least 45 minutes.
         (3) If specimen is placed in an incubator, it will retain its motility for several hours in case there is a delay in the insemination. Patients become anxious if there is a delay in IUI so reassure them that a reasonable period of delay will not negatively impact quality or success.
      f. If the male has performance anxiety or will be out of town at midcycle
         (1) Specimen can be frozen for future use.
         (2) If the male has performance anxiety on the day of the IUI, be supportive and recommend going home and attempting intercourse later that day. If they can have intercourse at home, encourage this since timed intercourse can still bring success.
         (3) Provide sildenafil or other phosphodiesterase (PDE) inhibitors if needed.
         (4) Consider rescheduling to the next day if not postovulatory.
   2. If frozen specimen is used, woman must properly identify it.
C. Preparing the woman
   1. Have the woman empty her bladder for comfort. Occasionally a full bladder will be helpful in catheter insertion, so this must be individualized.
   2. Ensure that her last menses was normal and that her midcycle surge has been detected.
      a. IUI is performed up to and including day of ovulation.
      b. The day of ovulation predictor kit (OPK) color change as well as the next 2 days are good choices.
   3. A single insemination is adequate unless the specimen or timing proves to be suboptimal.
   4. If any symptom or concern for a pelvic infection, do not proceed. In the case of a monilial vaginal infection, it is okay to proceed if tolerated by the patient.
   5. Some offices encourage gentle music or anything that encourages a more relaxed and less impersonal environment.
D. Insemination technique
   1. Bring prepared or thawed specimen into the room with catheter in sterile wrapper. Name should be visible. Draw up specimen when patient has identified the sperm source as that of her partner or sperm donor.
   2. Partner may be present. If partner is uncomfortable watching procedure, have the partner stand at head of table to offer support.
   3. Review the procedure and what can be expected. Emphasize the process takes only a few minutes and is usually painless.
   4. Record specimen parameters, especially the total motile number of sperm if provided by the laboratory.
   5. Document whether fertility medications have been used and the menstrual cycle day.

TABLE 39.1 Timing of Intrauterine Insemination	
OPK or urinary LH kit	Day of, or up to 2 days after, color change
	Most centers suggest day after
Ultrasound	If mature follicle (18–24 mm diameter) is seen: 24–36 hours later

ILH, luteinizing hormone; OPK, ovulation predictor kit.

6. Document the method of ovulation detection used. Most women use an OPK that detects a luteinizing hormone (LH) surge or another monitoring method that includes blood and ultrasound (Table 39.1).
7. Review potential complications and symptoms to report.
   a. Bleeding or cramping rarely occur.
   b. Prostaglandin reaction or vasovagal response is also rare with newer methods of sperm preparation. If this does occur, it is typically self-limiting. In rare cases giving an NSAID can be helpful.
   c. Vasovagal reaction occurs rarely if the procedure is difficult to perform and a tenaculum was needed to straighten out the canal. Tenaculums can be applied gently. It is not necessary to ask the patient to cough. Instead, applying gently pressure at the apex of the cervix until the area blanches and then clicking the instrument into place slowly can suffice.
8. Obtain written consent.
   a. Many states require written consent from both partners.
   b. Usually completed before the first insemination is performed and may need to be updated annually or if any change in relationship status.
   c. Consents should be prepared and properly worded for single, heterosexual, bisexual, and same-sex couples.
9. Help woman into the lithotomy position.
   a. Use of stirrups is optional, as long as speculum placement is efficient and comfortable.
   b. Use nonlatex gloves if known latex allergy.
10. Assess the uterine size and position.
11. Insert speculum; use smallest speculum that allows proper visualization and entry of catheter.
12. Assess cervical appearance.
    a. Note cervical secretions.
    b. Swab cervical secretions if copious to enable better access to os for catheter placement.
    c. Not necessary to examine the cervical mucus under the microscope because the patient is periovulatory.
    d. Cervical secretions are a healthy sign of impending ovulation. Cervix is wiped with a large cotton scopette.
13. A variety of catheters exist for the purpose of IUI.
    a. Use the narrowest gauge for patient comfort.
    b. Catheters with "memory" can be bent to follow uterine flexion as needed.
14. Thread the preloaded syringe through the os.
    a. Do not force.
    b. Once fundus is felt, pull back to prevent bleeding and trauma.
    c. This brings sperm closer to the tubal ostia.
15. Avoid a tenaculum except if entry is difficult as in the case of severe ante- or retroversion of the uterus, as it can cause cramping. Although if needed, tenaculum-induced cramping/bleeding will not adversely affect success rates.

16. If the cervix is stenotic, use the narrowest gauge possible.
    a. Tom cat catheters work well and are cost-effective. Otherwise, narrow catheters with memory can work well.
    b. Occasionally, dilatation with a narrow dilator or os finder will help guide passage for the catheter to follow.
17. The patient should feel no more than mild cramping and no pain.
18. Slowly inject the sperm over 30 to 60 seconds to avoid cramping or retrograde flow.
19. Any excess specimen should be allowed to collect near the os.
20. Leaving the catheter in place or removing it if there is no backflow is acceptable.
21. Bleeding
    a. Friable cervices often bleed on contact.
    b. This should not affect the success of an IUI procedure.
    c. Bleeding from the tenaculum also is external bleeding and should not affect success.
    d. Avoid heavy bleeding with catheter placement.
22. Remove catheter in a way that avoids spillage.
23. Remove speculum sideways so any excess specimen will collect in the vagina.
24. Resting after IUI is controversial. It may be pleasant for the patient but is not medically necessary.
    a. Best not to rush the patient and give her the choice to rest.
25. A rare complication is a prostaglandin reaction.
    a. This was more common in the past when unwashed sperm was used for IUI.
    b. For vasovagal and prostaglandin reaction, do not leave the patient unattended.
    c. The patient will benefit from nonsteroidal anti-inflammatory drugs (NSAIDs); reassure her that this will pass. Acetaminophen is generally not helpful.
    d. In rare cases with vasovagal reactions, patients can lose consciousness or have a mild seizure. (This is true for all gynecologic procedures when the cervical os is traversed.)
    e. Occasionally, ammonium salts or even atropine will be administered.
    f. Monitor vital signs and discharge once stable and symptom free.
    g. When frozen sperm is used, the volume tends to be very low, and incidence of prostaglandin reaction is also low.
    h. However, when this occurs, it is similar to a vasovagal reaction and the patient can be in extreme pain with cramping.
26. Instruct patient to call if fever, chills, unusual discharge, or bleeding develop.
27. Single versus double IUI is frequently debated. Single IUI is cost-effective, and studies suggest comparable success rates. Couples can supplement with intercourse when able.
28. Instruct her to schedule or check for pregnancy in 2 weeks.

BIBLIOGRAPHY

Blumenthal, P. D., & Berek, J. C. (2013). *A practical guide to office gynecologic procedures.* Lippincott, William & Wilkins.

Craig, L. B., Arya, S., Burks, H. R., Warta, K., Jarshaw, C., Hansen, K. R., & Peck, J. D. (2021). Relationship between semen regurgitation and pregnancy rates with intrauterine insemination. *Fertility and Sterility, 116*(6), 1526–1531. https://doi.org/10.1016/j.fertnstert.2021.07.1183

Goldstein, M., & Schlegel, P. N. (Eds.). (2013). *Surgical and medical management of male infertility.* Cambridge University Press.

Gordon, J. D., Rydfors, J. T., & Druzin, M. L. (2001). *Obstetrics, gynecology and infertility: Handbook for clinicians-resident survival guide* (5th ed.). Scrub Hill Press.

Johal, J. K., Gardner, R. M., Vaughn, S. J., Jaswa, E. G., Hedlin, H., & Aghajanova, L. (2021) Pregnancy success rates for lesbian women undergoing intrauterine insemination. *Fertility and Sterility Reports, 2*(3), 275–281. https://doi.org/10.1016/j.xfre.2021.04.007

Lebovic, D., Gordon, J. D., & Taylor, R. (2013). *Reproductive endocrinology and infertility: Handbook for clinicians* (2nd ed.). Scrub Hill Press.

Lipshultz, L. I., Howards, S. S., & Niederberger, C. S. (Eds.). (2009). *Infertility in the male* (4th ed.). Cambridge University Press.

Zarek, S. M., Hill, M. J., Richter, K. S., Wu, M., DeCherney, A. H., Osheroff, J. E., & Levens, E. D. (2014). Single-donor and double-donor sperm intrauterine insemination cycles: Does double intrauterine insemination increase clinical pregnancy rates? *Fertility and Sterility, 102*(3), 739–743. https://doi.org/10.1016/j.fertnstert.2014.05.018

Unit VIII

CONTRACEPTION

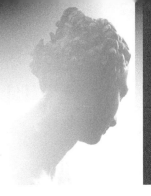

40

THE CONTRACEPTIVE CONSULT

KOMKWUAN P. PARUCHABUTR

REPRODUCTIVE JUSTICE

A. Introduced by Black feminist scholars and health activists to bring light to structural racism and reproductive health outcomes in the United States (Ross & Solinger, 2017).
B. It is a "human right to maintain personal bodily autonomy, have children, not have children, and parent the children we have in safe and sustainable communities" (SisterSong, 2022).
C. Addressing structures and systems that can pose as barriers for those who seek access to contraceptive services can help prevent poor reproductive health outcomes.

CONTRACEPTION

A. On average, U.S. women will spend approximately 3 years of her life pregnant, postpartum, or attempting pregnancy (Guttmacher Institute, 2019).
B. On average, U.S. women will spend approximately three decades or three quarters of her reproductive years avoiding pregnancy (Guttmacher Institute, 2019).
C. Approximately 45% of pregnancies in the United States are unintended (Curtis et al., 2016).
D. Unintended pregnancies are associated with (Curtis et al., 2016):
   1. Adverse and maternal health outcomes
   2. Increased healthcare costs
E. The Centers for Disease Control and Prevention (CDC) published the first U.S. Medical Eligibility Criteria (U.S. MEC) in 2010.
   1. U.S. MEC provides recommendations for safe use of contraceptive methods with various medical conditions and other characteristics (Curtis et al., 2016).
   2. U.S. MEC was adapted from the global recommendations of the World Health Organization Medical Eligibility Criteria (WHO-MEC).
   3. U.S. MEC is a companion document to the U.S. Selected Practice Recommendations for Contraceptive Use (U.S. SPR).
   4. U.S. SPR provides guidance on how to use contraceptive methods safely and effectively once found to be medically appropriate (Curtis et al., 2016).
   5. U.S. MEC has been updated to this current 2016 version with updates on the CDC website (Figure 40.1).

KEY CONSIDERATIONS TO CONTRACEPTION

A. Efficacy (Figure 40.2)
   1. Introduce women to contraceptive options in order of most efficacious (Curtis et al., 2016).
   2. Failure rates represent a way to assess efficacy of a contraceptive option.

Summary Chart of U.S. Medical Eligibility Criteria for Contraceptive Use

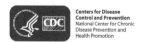

Centers for Disease Control and Prevention
National Center for Chronic Disease Prevention and Health Promotion

Condition	Sub-Condition	Cu-IUD		LNG-IUD		Implant		DMPA		POP		CHC	
		I	C	I	C	I	C	I	C	I	C	I	C
Age		Menarche to <20 yrs:**2**		Menarche to <20 yrs:**2**		Menarche to <18 yrs:**1**		Menarche to <18 yrs:**2**		Menarche to <18 yrs:**1**		Menarche to <40 yrs:**1**	
		≥20 yrs:**1**		≥20 yrs:**1**		18-45 yrs:**1**		18-45 yrs:**1**		18-45 yrs:**1**		≥40 yrs:**2**	
						>45 yrs:**1**		>45 yrs:**2**		>45 yrs:**1**			
Anatomical abnormalities	a) Distorted uterine cavity	4		4									
	b) Other abnormalities	2		2									
Anemias	a) Thalassemia	2		1		1		1		1		1	
	b) Sickle cell disease‡	2		1		1		1		1		2	
	c) Iron-deficiency anemia	2		1		1		1		1		1	
Benign ovarian tumors	(including cysts)	1		1		1		1		1		1	
Breast disease	a) Undiagnosed mass	1		2		2*		2*		2*		2*	
	b) Benign breast disease	1		1		1		1		1		1	
	c) Family history of cancer	1		1		1		1		1		1	
	d) Breast cancer‡												
	i) Current	1		4		4		4		4		4	
	ii) Past and no evidence of current disease for 5 years	1		3		3		3		3		3	
Breastfeeding	a) <21 days postpartum					2*		2*		2*		4*	
	b) 21 to <30 days postpartum												
	i) With other risk factors for VTE					2*		2*		2*		3*	
	ii) Without other risk factors for VTE					2*		2*		2*		3*	
	c) 30-42 days postpartum												
	i) With other risk factors for VTE					1*		1*		1*		3*	
	ii) Without other risk factors for VTE					1*		1*		1*		2*	
	d) >42 days postpartum					1*		1*		1*		2*	
Cervical cancer	Awaiting treatment	4	2	4	2	2		2		1		2	
Cervical ectropion		1		1		1		1		1		1	
Cervical intraepithelial neoplasia		1		2		2		2		1		2	
Cirrhosis	a) Mild (compensated)	1		1		1		1		1		1	
	b) Severe‡ (decompensated)	1		3		3		3		3		4	
Cystic fibrosis‡		1*		1*		1*		2*		1*		1*	
Deep venous thrombosis (DVT)/Pulmonary embolism (PE)	a) History of DVT/PE, not receiving anticoagulant therapy												
	i) Higher risk for recurrent DVT/PE	1		2		2		2		2		4	
	ii) Lower risk for recurrent DVT/PE	1		2		2		2		2		3	
	b) Acute DVT/PE	2		2		2		2		2		4	
	c) DVT/PE and established anticoagulant therapy for at least 3 months												
	i) Higher risk for recurrent DVT/PE	2		2		2		2		2		4*	
	ii) Lower risk for recurrent DVT/PE	2		2		2		2		2		3*	
	d) Family history (first-degree relatives)	1		1		1		1		1		2	
	e) Major surgery												
	i) With prolonged immobilization	1		2		2		2		2		4	
	ii) Without prolonged immobilization	1		1		1		1		1		2	
	f) Minor surgery without immobilization	1		1		1		1		1		1	
Depressive disorders		1*		1*		1*		1*		1*		1*	

Key:

1 No restriction (method can be used)	**3** Theoretical or proven risks usually outweigh the advantages
2 Advantages generally outweigh theoretical or proven risks	**4** Unacceptable health risk (method not to be used)

FIGURE 40.1 (continued)

Summary Chart of U.S. Medical Eligibility Criteria for Contraceptive Use

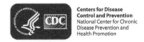

Centers for Disease Control and Prevention
National Center for Chronic Disease Prevention and Health Promotion

Condition	Sub-Condition	Cu-IUD		LNG-IUD		Implant		DMPA		POP		CHC	
		I	C	I	C	I	C	I	C	I	C	I	C
Diabetes	a) History of gestational disease	1		1		1		1		1		1	
	b) Nonvascular disease												
	i) Non-insulin dependent	1		2		2		2		2		2	
	ii) Insulin dependent	1		2		2		2		2		2	
	c) Nephropathy/retinopathy/neuropathy‡	1		2		2		3		2		3/4*	
	d) Other vascular disease or diabetes of >20 years' duration‡	1		2		2		3		2		3/4*	
Dysmenorrhea	Severe	2		1		1		1		1		1	
Endometrial cancer‡		4	2	4	2	1		1		1		1	
Endometrial hyperplasia		1		1		1		1		1		1	
Endometriosis		2		1		1		1		1		1	
Epilepsy‡	(see also Drug Interactions)	1		1		1*		1*		1*		1*	
Gallbladder disease	a) Symptomatic												
	i) Treated by cholecystectomy	1		2		2		2		2		2	
	ii) Medically treated	1		2		2		2		2		3	
	iii) Current	1		2		2		2		2		3	
	b) Asymptomatic	1		2		2		2		2		2	
Gestational trophoblastic disease‡	a) Suspected GTD (immediate postevacuation)												
	i) Uterine size first trimester	1*		1*		1*		1*		1*		1*	
	ii) Uterine size second trimester	2*		2*		1*		1*		1*		1*	
	b) Confirmed GTD												
	i) Undetectable/non-pregnant ß-hCG levels	1*	1*	1*	1*	1*		1*		1*		1*	
	ii) Decreasing ß-hCG levels	2*	1*	2*	1*	1*		1*		1*		1*	
	iii) Persistently elevated ß-hCG levels or malignant disease, with no evidence or suspicion of intrauterine disease	2*	1*	2*	1*	1*		1*		1*		1*	
	iv) Persistently elevated ß-hCG levels or malignant disease, with evidence or suspicion of intrauterine disease	4*	2*	4*	2*	1*		1*		1*		1*	
Headaches	a) Nonmigraine (mild or severe)	1		1		1		1		1		1*	
	b) Migraine												
	i) Without aura (includes menstrual migraine)	1		1		1		1		1		2*	
	ii) With aura	1		1		1		1		1		4*	
History of bariatric surgery‡	a) Restrictive procedures	1		1		1		1		1		1	
	b) Malabsorptive procedures	1		1		1		1		3		COCs: 3 / P/R: 1	
History of cholestasis	a) Pregnancy related	1		1		1		1		1		2	
	b) Past COC related	1		2		2		2		2		3	
History of high blood pressure during pregnancy		1		1		1		1		1		2	
History of Pelvic surgery		1		1		1		1		1		1	
HIV	a) High risk for HIV	1*	1*	1*	1*	1		1		1		1	
	b) HIV infection					1*		1*		1*		1*	
	i) Clinically well receiving ARV therapy	1	1	1	1	If on treatment, see Drug Interactions							
	ii) Not clinically well or not receiving ARV therapy‡	2	1	2	1	If on treatment, see Drug Interactions							

Key:	
1 No restriction (method can be used)	3 Theoretical or proven risks usually outweigh the advantages
2 Advantages generally outweigh theoretical or proven risks	4 Unacceptable health risk (method not to be used)

FIGURE 40.1 (*continued*)

Summary Chart of U.S. Medical Eligibility Criteria for Contraceptive Use

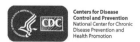

Centers for Disease Control and Prevention
National Center for Chronic Disease Prevention and Health Promotion

Condition	Sub-Condition	Cu-IUD I	Cu-IUD C	LNG-IUD I	LNG-IUD C	Implant I	Implant C	DMPA I	DMPA C	POP I	POP C	CHC I	CHC C
Hypertension	a) Adequately controlled hypertension	1*	1*	1*	1*	1*	1*	2*	2*	1*	1*	3*	3*
	b) Elevated blood pressure levels *(properly taken measurements)*												
	i) Systolic 140-159 or diastolic 90-99	1*	1*	1*	1*	1*	1*	2*	2*	1*	1*	3*	3*
	ii) Systolic ≥160 or diastolic ≥100‡	1*	1*	2*	2*	2*	2*	3*	3*	2*	2*	4*	4*
	c) Vascular disease	1*	1*	2*	2*	2*	2*	3*	3*	2*	2*	4*	4*
Inflammatory bowel disease	*(Ulcerative colitis, Crohn's disease)*	1	1	1	1	1	1	2	2	2	2	2/3*	2/3*
Ischemic heart disease‡	Current and history of	1	1	2	3	2	3	3	3	2	3	4	4
Known thrombogenic mutations‡		1*	1*	2*	2*	2*	2*	2*	2*	2*	2*	4*	4*
Liver tumors	a) Benign												
	i) Focal nodular hyperplasia	1	1	2	2	2	2	2	2	2	2	2	2
	ii) Hepatocellular adenoma‡	1	1	3	3	3	3	3	3	3	3	4	4
	b) Malignant‡ (hepatoma)	1	1	3	3	3	3	3	3	3	3	4	4
Malaria		1	1	1	1	1	1	1	1	1	1	1	1
Multiple risk factors for atherosclerotic cardiovascular disease	(e.g., older age, smoking, diabetes, hypertension, low HDL, high LDL, or high triglyceride levels)	1	1	2	2	2*	2*	3*	3*	2*	2*	3/4*	3/4*
Multiple sclerosis	a) With prolonged immobility	1	1	1	1	1	1	2	2	1	1	3	3
	b) Without prolonged immobility	1	1	1	1	1	1	2	2	1	1	1	1
Obesity	a) Body mass index (BMI) ≥30 kg/m²	1	1	1	1	1	1	1	1	1	1	2	2
	b) Menarche to <18 years and BMI ≥ 30 kg/m²	1	1	1	1	1	1	2	2	1	1	2	2
Ovarian cancer‡		1	1	1	1	1	1	1	1	1	1	1	1
Parity	a) Nulliparous	2	2	2	2	1	1	1	1	1	1	1	1
	b) Parous	1	1	1	1	1	1	1	1	1	1	1	1
Past ectopic pregnancy		1	1	1	1	1	1	1	1	2	2	1	1
Pelvic inflammatory disease	a) Past												
	i) With subsequent pregnancy	1	1	1	1	1	1	1	1	1	1	1	1
	ii) Without subsequent pregnancy	2	2	2	2	1	1	1	1	1	1	1	1
	b) Current	4	2*	4	2*	1	1	1	1	1	1	1	1
Peripartum cardiomyopathy‡	a) Normal or mildly impaired cardiac function												
	i) <6 months	2	2	2	2	1	1	1	1	1	1	4	4
	ii) ≥6 months	2	2	2	2	1	1	1	1	1	1	3	3
	b) Moderately or severely impaired cardiac function	2	2	2	2	2	2	2	2	2	2	4	4
Postabortion	a) First trimester	1*	1*	1*	1*	1*	1*	1*	1*	1*	1*	1*	1*
	b) Second trimester	2*	2*	2*	2*	1*	1*	1*	1*	1*	1*	1*	1*
	c) Immediate postseptic abortion	4	4	4	4	1*	1*	1*	1*	1*	1*	1*	1*
Postpartum *(nonbreastfeeding women)*	a) <21 days					1	1	1	1	1	1	4	4
	b) 21 days to 42 days												
	i) With other risk factors for VTE					1	1	1	1	1	1	3*	3*
	ii) Without other risk factors for VTE					1	1	1	1	1	1	2	2
	c) >42 days					1	1	1	1	1	1	1	1
Postpartum *(in breastfeeding or non-breastfeeding women, including cesarean delivery)*	a) <10 minutes after delivery of the placenta												
	i) Breastfeeding	1*	1*	2*	2*								
	ii) Nonbreastfeeding	1*	1*	1*	1*								
	b) 10 minutes after delivery of the placenta to <4 weeks	2*	2*	2*	2*								
	c) ≥4 weeks	1*	1*	1*	1*								
	d) Postpartum sepsis	4	4	4	4								

Key:

1 No restriction (method can be used)	**3** Theoretical or proven risks usually outweigh the advantages
2 Advantages generally outweigh theoretical or proven risks	**4** Unacceptable health risk (method not to be used)

FIGURE 40.1 *(continued)*

Summary Chart of U.S. Medical Eligibility Criteria for Contraceptive Use

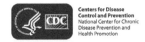

Centers for Disease Control and Prevention
National Center for Chronic Disease Prevention and Health Promotion

Condition	Sub-Condition	Cu-IUD I	Cu-IUD C	LNG-IUD I	LNG-IUD C	Implant I	Implant C	DMPA I	DMPA C	POP I	POP C	CHC I	CHC C
Pregnancy		4*	4*	4*	4*	NA*	NA*	NA*	NA*	NA*	NA*	NA*	NA*
Rheumatoid arthritis	a) On immunosuppressive therapy	2	1	2	1	1	1	2/3*	2/3*	1	1	2	2
	b) Not on immunosuppressive therapy	1	1	1	1	1	1	2	2	1	1	2	2
Schistosomiasis	a) Uncomplicated	1	1	1	1	1	1	1	1	1	1	1	1
	b) Fibrosis of the liver‡	1	1	1	1	1	1	1	1	1	1	1	1
Sexually transmitted diseases (STDs)	a) Current purulent cervicitis or chlamydial infection or gonococcal infection	4	2*	4	2*	1	1	1	1	1	1	1	1
	b) Vaginitis (including trichomonas vaginalis and bacterial vaginosis)	2	2	2	2	1	1	1	1	1	1	1	1
	c) Other factors relating to STDs	2*	2	2*	2	1	1	1	1	1	1	1	1
Smoking	a) Age <35	1	1	1	1	1	1	1	1	1	1	2	2
	b) Age ≥35, <15 cigarettes/day	1	1	1	1	1	1	1	1	1	1	3	3
	c) Age ≥35, ≥15 cigarettes/day	1	1	1	1	1	1	1	1	1	1	4	4
Solid organ transplantation‡	a) Complicated	3	2	3	2	2	2	2	2	2	2	4	4
	b) Uncomplicated	2	2	2	2	2	2	2	2	2	2	2*	2*
Stroke‡	History of cerebrovascular accident	1	1	2	2	2	3	3	3	2	3	4	4
Superficial venous disorders	a) Varicose veins	1	1	1	1	1	1	1	1	1	1	1	1
	b) Superficial venous thrombosis (acute or history)	1	1	1	1	1	1	1	1	1	1	3*	3*
Systemic lupus erythematosus‡	a) Positive (or unknown) antiphospholipid antibodies	1*	1*	3*	3*	3*	3*	3*	3*	3*	3*	4*	4*
	b) Severe thrombocytopenia	3*	2*	2*	2*	2*	2*	3*	2*	2*	2*	2*	2*
	c) Immunosuppressive therapy	2*	1*	2*	2*	2*	2*	2*	2*	2*	2*	2*	2*
	d) None of the above	1*	1*	2*	2*	2*	2*	2*	2*	2*	2*	2*	2*
Thyroid disorders	Simple goiter/ hyperthyroid/hypothyroid	1	1	1	1	1	1	1	1	1	1	1	1
Tuberculosis‡ (see also Drug Interactions)	a) Nonpelvic	1	1	1	1	1*	1*	1*	1*	1*	1*	1*	1*
	b) Pelvic	4	3	4	3	1*	1*	1*	1*	1*	1*	1*	1*
Unexplained vaginal bleeding	(suspicious for serious condition) before evaluation	4*	2*	4*	2*	3*	3*	3*	3*	2*	2*	2*	2*
Uterine fibroids		2	2	2	2	1	1	1	1	1	1	1	1
Valvular heart disease	a) Uncomplicated	1	1	1	1	1	1	1	1	1	1	2	2
	b) Complicated‡	1	1	1	1	1	1	1	1	1	1	4	4
Vaginal bleeding patterns	a) Irregular pattern without heavy bleeding	1	1	1	1	2	2	2	2	2	2	1	1
	b) Heavy or prolonged bleeding	2*	2*	1*	2*	2*	2*	2*	2*	2*	2*	1*	1*
Viral hepatitis	a) Acute or flare	1	1	1	1	1	1	1	1	1	1	3/4*	2
	b) Carrier/Chronic	1	1	1	1	1	1	1	1	1	1	1	1
Drug Interactions													
Antiretrovirals used for prevention (PrEP) or treatment of HIV	Fosamprenavir (FPV) — All other ARVs are 1 or 2 for all methods.	1/2*	1*	1/2*	1*	2*	2*	2*	2*	2*	2*	3*	3*
Anticonvulsant therapy	a) Certain anticonvulsants (phenytoin, carbamazepine, barbiturates, primidone, topiramate, oxcarbazepine)	1	1	1	1	2*	2*	1*	1*	3*	3*	3*	3*
	b) Lamotrigine	1	1	1	1	1	1	1	1	1	1	3*	3*
Antimicrobial therapy	a) Broad spectrum antibiotics	1	1	1	1	1	1	1	1	1	1	1	1
	b) Antifungals	1	1	1	1	1	1	1	1	1	1	1	1
	c) Antiparasitics	1	1	1	1	1	1	1	1	1	1	1	1
	d) Rifampin or rifabutin therapy	1	1	1	1	2*	2*	1*	1*	3*	3*	3*	3*
SSRIs		1	1	1	1	1	1	1	1	1	1	1	1
St. John's wort		1	1	1	1	2	2	1	1	2	2	2	2

CS314239-A

Key:

1 No restriction (method can be used)	3 Theoretical or proven risks usually outweigh the advantages
2 Advantages generally outweigh theoretical or proven risks	4 Unacceptable health risk (method not to be used)

Abbreviations: ARV = antiretroviral; C=continuation of contraceptive method; CHC=combined hormonal contraception (pill, patch, and, ring); COC=combined oral contraceptive; Cu-IUD=copper-containing intrauterine device; DMPA = depot medroxyprogesterone acetate; I=initiation of contraceptive method; LNG-IUD=levonorgestrel-releasing intrauterine device; NA=not applicable; POP=progestin-only pill; P/R=patch/ring; SSRI=selective serotonin reuptake inhibitor; ‡ Condition that exposes a woman to increased risk as a result of pregnancy. *Please see the complete guidance for a clarification to this classification: https://www.cdc.gov/reproductivehealth/contraception/contraception_guidance.htm.

Updated in 2020. This summary sheet only contains a subset of the recommendations from the U.S. MEC. For complete guidance, see: https://www.cdc.gov/reproductivehealth/contraception/contraception_guidance.htm. Most contraceptive methods do not protect against sexually transmitted diseases (STDs). Consistent and correct use of the male latex condom reduces the risk of STDs and HIV.

FIGURE 40.1 Summary chart of U.S. medical eligibility criteria for contraceptive use.

Source: CDC. https://www.cdc.gov/reproductivehealth/contraception/pdf/summary-chart-us-medical-eligibility-criteria_508tagged.pdf.

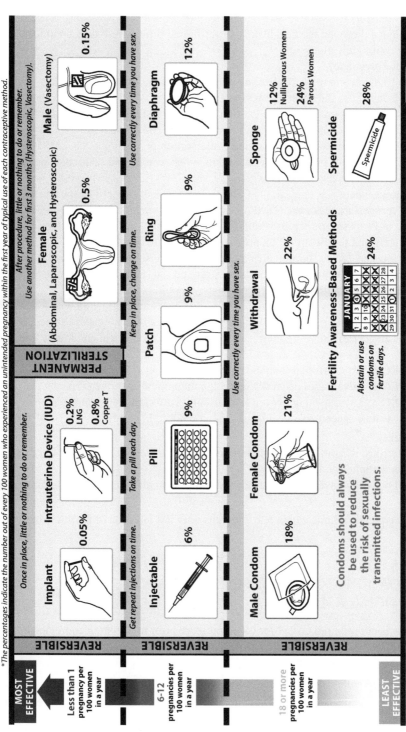

FIGURE 40.2 Effectiveness of family planning methods.

Source: CDC. https://www.cdc.gov/reproductivehealth/unintendedpregnancy/pdf/family-planning-methods-2014.pdf.

B. Safety
   1. U.S. MEC categorizes the safety of each method in accordance with specific health concerns or diagnoses.
   2. Past medical history
      a. Ensure that a thorough medical history is performed prior to initiating contraception to identify contraindications.
      b. Assess for pregnancy
         (1) The CDC recommends confirming at least one of the following criteria:
            - ≤7 days after the onset of a period
            - No sexual intercourse since the first day of the last menstrual period
            - Correct and consistent use of a reliable contraceptive method
            - ≤7 days after a miscarriage or induced abortion procedure
            - Exclusively or primarily breastfeeding, amenorrheic, and <6 months postpartum
            - Is within 4 weeks postpartum
      c. In situations where it is unclear, the CDC recommends the benefit of starting depot medroxyprogesterone acetate (DMPA), combined hormonal contraception (CHC), implant, or Progestin-only pills (POPs) likely exceed any risks and to initiate treatment immediately and follow up with a pregnancy test in 2 to 4 weeks.
      d. For intrauterine device (hormonal and nonhormonal) insertions, if patient has had unprotected intercourse since her last menstrual period (LMP) and within the last 5 days, risks/benefits of insertion with early pregnancy should be discussed.
         (1) If the patient still would like to proceed, then insert and follow up with a home pregnancy test or office test within 2 weeks (Reproductive Access Project, 2021)
   3. U.S. MEC categorizes safety for contraceptive options with medical conditions into four categories
      a. **U.S. MEC 1:** No restriction (method can be used)
      b. **U.S. MEC 2:** Advantages generally outweigh theoretical or proven risks.
      c. **U.S. MEC 3:** Theoretical or proven risks usually outweigh the advantages.
      d. **U.S. MEC 4:** Unacceptable health risk (method not to be used)
C. Return to fertility
   1. Return to fertility is rapid after discontinuation of a contraceptive method with both hormonal and nonhormonal methods
   2. DMPA will typically have a slower return to fertility than all other methods (Mansour et al., 2011).
      a. Fertility typically returns within 5 to 7 months after last injection of DMPA (Mansour et al., 2011).

KEY CENTERS FOR DISEASE CONTROL AND PREVENTION RECOMMENDATIONS TO LIMIT BARRIERS FOR ACCESS TO CONTRACEPTION (CASEY, 2020)

A. Physical exam is not required except for blood pressure prior to initiating combined hormonal contraception (CHC).
B. Laboratory tests are not required prior to initiating contraception.
C. Cervical cancer screening is not required prior to insertion of IUDs.
D. IUD removal is not indicated for women who develop pelvic inflammatory disease. Treatment with antibiotics and signs of clinical improvement are sufficient.

CONTRACEPTIVE METHODS

A. Lactational amenorrhea

1. Mechanism of action
   a. Elevated prolactin levels and an interruption of gonadotropin-releasing hormone by the hypothalamus lead to the suppression of ovulation (Hatcher, 2018).
   b. The duration of ovulation suppression has variable rates and is dependent on frequency and duration of breastfeeding.
2. Method requires all criteria listed in the following:
   a. Feeding every 4 hours during the day and every 6 hours at night
   b. No supplementing with formula or food
   c. Menses has not returned.
   d. Infant must be younger than 6 months old (Casey, 2020).
3. Efficacy
   a. Perfect use failure rate is 0.1% and 2% for typical use (Casey, 2020).
B. Coitus interruptus (withdrawal) method
   1. Mechanism of action
      a. Withdrawal of entire penis prior to ejaculation thereby preventing fertilization by lacking contact of spermatozoa and ovum.
   2. Efficacy
      a. Largely depends on the man being able to entirely withdraw prior to ejaculation and therefore varies widely.
      b. Perfect use failure rate is 4% within the first year and 22% with typical use within the first year (Casey, 2020).
C. Chemical barriers
   1. Spermicidal agents containing nonoxynol-9 (N-9) or octoxynol
      a. **Forms:** vaginal foams, creams, suppositories, films, jellies, foaming tablets
         (1) Must be inserted into vagina prior to each coital act
         (2) Over-the-counter (does not require prescription)
      b. Mechanism of action
         (1) It is a surfactant that disrupts sperm cell wall membrane, effecting the flagella and body of sperm decreasing motility and fructolytic activity (Baker & Chen, 2022; Casey, 2020).
         (2) N-9 is toxic to lactobacilli and disrupts normal vaginal flora and potentially increases risk of infections (i.e., sexually transmitted infections, *Escherichia coli*).
      c. Efficacy
         (1) Perfect use failure rate is 6% and typical use failure rate within the first year is 26% (Casey, 2020).
   2. Vaginal pH regulator
      a. Phexxi/lactic acid-citric acid-potassium bitartrate vaginal (FDA approved May 2020)
         (1) Single dose applicator 5 g gel administered vaginally up to 1 hour prior to each sexual episode (Baker & Chen, 2022)
         (2) Requires a prescription
            • Mechanism of action
               ▪ Vaginal pH regulator containing lactic acid, citric acid, and potassium bitartrate
               ▪ Maintains natural acidic vaginal environment to reduce sperm motility and potentially enhance the antimicrobial environment of the vagina (Baker & Chen, 2022).
               ▪ Currently being evaluated as a microbicide (Baker & Chen, 2022)
         (3) Efficacy
            • Perfect use failure rate is 7% and typical use failure rate is 14% (Baker & Chen, 2022; Planned Parenthood, 2022).

(4) Adverse effects (Baker & Chen, 2022)
- Vulvovaginal burning (20%)
- Pain (3.8%)
- Genitourinary tract infections (5.7%)
- Vulvovaginal complaints to include pruritis (11.2%)

D. Barrier method
1. Male/female condoms (Casey, 2020)
   a. **Mechanism of action:** prevents pregnancy by preventing semen into the vagina by acting as a barrier
   b. Not recommended for male/female barrier concomitant use due to adherence to both products and dislodgement of barriers
   c. **Efficacy:** Failure rate of perfect use is 3% and typical use within a year is 14%.
   d. Benefits
      (1) Nonhormonal
      (2) Cost-effective
      (3) Effective against STIs
   e. Disadvantages
      (1) May decrease sexual pleasure during intercourse
      (2) Some users may have an allergy to latex
      (3) Breakage and slippage can decrease effectiveness
      (4) Oil-based lubricants can damage the condom
2. Diaphragm
   a. Mechanism of action: Prevents pregnancy by preventing semen from going into the vagina by acting as a barrier
   b. Inserted up to 6 hours prior to intercourse with penile penetration covering the posterior fornix and sitting beyond the pubic bone (Casey, 2020)
   c. Spermicidal agent is placed on the interior dome which covers the cervix (Casey, 2020).
   d. Efficacy
      (1) Failure rate of approximately 20%
   e. Benefits
      (1) Nonhormonal
      (2) Controlled by the woman
   f. Disadvantages
      (1) Prolonged use during multiple acts of intercourse may increase the risk of genitourinary infections
      (2) Not recommended for >24 hours due to risk of toxic shock syndrome (TSS)
      (3) Requires a fitting
      (4) Poor fitting may lead to vaginal erosions.
      (5) Must be cleansed after use.
3. Cervical cap (Casey, 2020)
   a. Mechanism of action: Prevents pregnancy by preventing semen to pass through the cervix
      (1) Cap must be filled one-third full of spermicide
      (2) May be placed up to 8 hours prior to coitus and may stay in as long as 48 hours
   b. Efficacy: Failure rate with typical use is 20% nulliparous to 40% of parous women
   c. Benefits
      (1) Continuous contraceptive protection regardless of number of intercourse acts
      (2) Nonhormonal
   d. Disadvantages
      (1) Cervical erosion may lead to vaginal spotting.
      (2) Theoretical risk of TSS if left longer than 48 hours

(3) Requires professional fitting and training.

(4) Morbid obesity may make placement difficult.

(5) Must have normal pap smears.

E. Combined hormonal contraceptives

1. Mechanism of action

a. CHCs have both estrogenic and progestin effects

b. Estrogen inhibits ovulation by suppressing the follicle-stimulating hormone (FSH), preventing the dominant follicle to mature (Hatcher, 2018).

c. Progestin prevents the luteinizing hormone (LH) surge inhibiting ovulation. It also thickens cervical mucus to decrease penetration of sperm and creates an atrophic endometrium to impair implantation (Hatcher, 2018).

2. Contraindications

a. Cerebral vascular disease or coronary artery disease

b. Hypertension

(1) Blood pressures ≥160/100 absolute contraindication

(2) Blood pressures 140/90 to 159/99, theoretical or proven risks usually outweigh advantages

c. Diabetes with vascular complications

d. Active liver disease

e. Estrogen dependent neoplasia

f. Breast cancer

g. Undiagnosed abnormal vaginal bleeding

h. Known/suspected pregnancy

i. Age ≥35 and cigarette smoking

j. Known thrombogenic mutation

k. Drospirenone has antimineralcorticoid properties

(1) Contraindicated in patients with kidney, adrenal gland insufficiency, or liver problems

(2) Must evaluate potassium levels during first month of use, especially if taken in concordance with drugs that increase potassium levels (i.e., nonsteroidal anti-inflammatory drugs [NSAIDs], ACE inhibitors; CDC, 2016;Casey, 2020)

3. CHC pills

a. Use

(1) Take one tablet daily every day (preferably same time each day).

(2) Better adherence with "quick start" method; start on day of visit without increased incidence of irregular bleeding (Britton et al., 2020).

(3) **Extended and continuous use:** Utilizing the CHC continuously without taking placebo pills (Nappi et al., 2016)

- Improved unscheduled bleeding rates
- Fewer hormone withdrawal symptoms (Nappi et al., 2016)
- Safety profile similar to 28-day regimens. Myocardial infarctions, stroke, thrombosis rates did not increase with extended use (Nappi et al., 2016).
- Prescribe up to 1 year, an initial visit or routine visits (thirteen 28-day pill packs). This has been shown to have better adherence to regimen.

(4) Missed pill

- If the patient missed one pill, take missed pill as soon as it is remembered followed by the regularly scheduled pill.
- If missed two or more consecutive pills, take one pill and continue one pill a day until pack is finished and skip placebo pills.

- Use a backup method of contraception and could require an emergency contraceptive method dependent upon cycle timing (especially during the first week of active pills)

b. **Efficacy:** Correlated with individual compliance
   (1) Ranges from 0.1% perfect use failure rate to 5% failure rate with typical use (Casey, 2020)

c. Adverse events
   (1) Nausea
   (2) Breast tenderness
   (3) Breakthrough bleeding
   (4) Headaches
   (5) Amenorrhea

d. Benefits
   (1) Ability to manipulate cycles with reduction of heavy menses
   (2) Acne improvement
   (3) Prevention of epithelium endometrial and ovarian carcinoma (Casey, 2020)
   (4) Prevention of benign breast disease and pelvic inflammatory disease (PID), ectopic pregnancy

4. CHC transdermal patch

   a. Xulane/norelgestromin-ethinyl estradiol transdermal patch, 150 mcg/day norelgestromin and 35 mcg/day ethinyl estradiol
      (1) Ortho Evra discontinued in United States due to availability of generic version of Xulane.

   b. Twirla/levonorgestrel-ethinyl estradiol transdermal patch, 120 mcg/day levonorgestrel and 30 mcg/day ethinyl estradiol; FDA approved February 2020
      (1) Developed to address the gap in a lower dose transdermal system with same benefits.
      (2) May be less efficacious in those who are overweight compared to those with normal weight (Baker & Chen, 2022)

   c. Use
      (1) Weekly application for 3 weeks, fourth week no patch is worn, and withdrawal bleed occurs.
      (2) Alternating sites recommended
         - Stomach, upper arm, buttock, or back

   d. Efficacy
      (1) FDA noted 1% failure rate for transdermal system in 2002 (Casey, 2020)
      (2) Twirla noted failure rate of 5.8%; however, this differed by BMI. Therefore, counseling for decreased efficacy for those overweight may be indicated; however, it is not a contraindication (Baker & Chen, 2022).

   e. Benefits
      (1) More stable hormone levels compared to pill users
      (2) Decreased loss of drug bioavailability by bypassing hepatic first-pass metabolism
      (3) Potential improvement with compliance due to weekly dosing (Baker & Chen, 2022)

   f. Adverse events
      (1) Nausea
      (2) Headache
      (3) Skin irritation

5. CHC vaginal ring

   a. NuvaRing/etonogestrel-ethinyl estradiol vaginal, 15 mcg/day ethinyl estradiol and 120 mcg/day etonogestrel
      (1) Use
         - Placed vaginally for 21 days and removed for 7 days

        (2) Efficacy
- With typical use, although no studies have been published, it is presumed to be less than 1 out of 100 pregnancies (Casey, 2020).

   b. Annovera/segesterone acetate-ethinyl estradiol vaginal, 13 mcg/day ethinyl estradiol and 150 mcg/day segesterone acetate. FDA approved in 2018
      (1) 1-Year ethinyl estradiol and segesterone acetate contraceptive vaginal system
      (2) Use
- Ring is placed vaginally for 21 days and removed for 7 days each cycle over 1 year.
- Re-used for 13 consecutive cycles and no refrigeration is required

      (3) Efficacy
- Failure rate of 2 to 4 pregnancies out of 100 per year (Casey, 2020)

   c. Benefits
      (1) Steady release of hormones
      (2) Effective and reversible

   d. Disadvantages
      (1) NuvaRing may only be removed for up to 3 hours and placed in cool or lukewarm water prior to reinsertion (Britton et al., 2020)
      (2) Annovera may only be removed up to 2 hours during the active phase (Baker & Chen, 2022)

   e. Adverse events (Britton et al., 2020)
      (1) Headache
      (2) Nausea
      (3) Vaginal discharge/irritation

F. Progestin only methods
  1. Progestin-only pills
   a. Available formulations
      (1) Norethindrone 350 mcg
- Mechanism of action
  - Ovulation suppression in about 50% of users
  - Increases cervical mucous viscosity
- Efficacy
  - Failure rate of 7% with typical use
- Disadvantage
  - Three-hour missed window period
  - Must have strict adherence to maintain efficacy
  - Unscheduled bleeding
- Benefits
  - Safe for those with contraindications to estrogen

      (1) Drospirenone (Slynd) 4 mg, FDA approved 2019 (Baker & Chen, 2022)
- Mechanism of action
  - Ovulation suppression
  - Analog of spironolactone with antimineralcorticoid activity
  - Half-life 25 to 30 hours
- Formulation comes in a 28-day pack with 24 hormonal pills and 4 days of inert pills
  - Hormone-free interval (HFI) is intended to provide a scheduled withdrawal bleed
- Efficacy
  - Failure rate of 4%
- Benefits
  - 24-hour missed window
  - Safe for those with contraindications to estrogen
  - Few contraindications and almost no drug interactions (Britton et al., 2020)

- Disadvantages
  - Unscheduled bleeding in 50% of users (Baker & Chen, 2022)
  - 0.5% cases of hyperkalemia

2. DMPA, Depo-provera injection
   a. Mechanism of action
      (1) Inhibits ovulation by suppressing FSH and LH and eliminating LH surge
   b. Formulation
      (1) DMP-IM (intramuscular), 150 mg/mL IM every 12 to 13 weeks
         - Single pre-filled dose or vial
         - Provider administration
      (2) DMPA-SQ (subcutaneous), 104 mg/mL SQ every 12 to 13 weeks
         - The CDC adopts WHO's recommendation of self-administration in 2021 for DMPA-SQ (Curtis et al., 2021)
         - Single pre-filled dose
         - Higher rates of continuation were observed with self-administration (Curtis et al., 2021)
   c. Efficacy
      (1) Failure rate with first year of perfect use 0.3%
   d. Benefits
      (1) Safe for breastfeeding mothers
      (2) Safe for those with contraindications to estrogen
      (3) Risks for endometrial and ovarian carcinoma decreased
   e. Disadvantages
      (1) Delay of return to fertility
      (2) Unscheduled bleeding
   f. Adverse effects
      (1) Increased hunger sensation may result in weight gain
      (2) Impaired glucose metabolism
      (3) Headache
      (4) Mood changes (depression)
      (5) The FDA issued a black box warning in 2004 for potentially nonreversible bone loss; however, since then studies have not really seen nonreversible bone loss. Teenagers regained bone loss at a faster rate than older women (Casey, 2020; Curtis et al, 2021)

3. Implant (Implanon/etonogestrel subdermal and Nexplanon/etonogestrel subdermal)
   a. Implanon FDA approved in 2001 and Nexplanon FDA approved in 2011. Implanon is no longer available.
   b. Nexplanon, etonogestrel, 68 mg
      (1) Single rod implant measuring 40-mm long and 2-mm in diameter
      (2) Inserted in the upper arm above tricep muscle subcutaneously
      (3) Remains in place for up to 3 years
   c. Mechanism of action
      (1) Ovulation suppression, inhibits LH surge
      (2) Increases cervical mucus viscosity
   d. Efficacy
      (1) Failure rates are better than surgical sterilization of 0.5% (Casey, 2020)
   e. Benefits
      (1) Fertility returns once removed.
      (2) No adverse effects on breast milk production
      (3) Longevity of its effectiveness while still inserted
   f. Disadvantages
      (1) Requires minor surgical procedure

TABLE 40.1 Progestin Intrauterine Devices

TYPE	FDA-APPROVED DURATION	TOTAL PROGESTIN	INITIAL RELEASE OF PROGESTIN/DAY	INSERTION DEVICE DIAMETER	AMENORRHEA RATE BY 1 YEAR
Skyla	3 years	13.5 mg	14 mcg	3.8 mm	6%–12%
Kyleena	5 years	19.5 mg	17.5 mcg	3.8 mm	12%–20%
Mirena	7 years	52 mg	20 mcg	4.4 mm	20%–40%
Liletta	6 years	52 mg	20 mcg	4.4 mm	19%–30%

g. Adverse effects (Britton et al., 2020; Casey, 2020)
  (1) Unscheduled bleeding (corrected with NSAIDs or short course of low-dose COC or estrogen, if not contraindicated)
  (2) Headaches
  (3) Breast tenderness
  (4) Emotional labilities
4. Intrauterine devices (see Table 40.1)
  a. Hormonal and nonhormonal
    (1) Nonhormonal
      • Copper T380 (ParaGard), introduced in 1988
        ▪ Mechanism of action: Foreign-body reaction creating a toxic intrauterine environment, preventing fertilization
        ▪ Copper ions are spermicidal (Britton et al., 2020)
        ▪ Contraceptive effectiveness continues for 10 years.
        ▪ Efficacy
          ◦ Failure rates of 0.6% with typical and perfect use
        ▪ Benefits
          ◦ Effectiveness for 10 years
          ◦ Highly efficacious
        ▪ Disadvantages
          ◦ Heavier bleeding and dysmenorrhea during the first few months after insertion
          ◦ Must be inserted by a skilled provider
          ◦ Does not prevent STIs
        ▪ Contraindicated for those with copper allergies, uterine cancer, uterine infections (Britton et al., 2020)
    (1) Hormonal IUDs
      • Mechanism of action (Casey, 2020):
        ▪ Increases cervical mucous viscosity
        ▪ Creates endometrial suppression
      • Efficacy
        ▪ Failure rate is 0.1% with typical and perfect use
      • Benefits
        ▪ No systemic side effects
        ▪ Menstrual bleeding is decreased overall
        ▪ Dysmenorrhea is decreased overall
        ▪ Lowers risk for endometrial and ovarian cancer
      • Disadvantages
        ▪ Increased risk (1%) uterine perforation

- Requires a skilled provider for insertion
- Does not prevent STIs
  - Adverse events
    - Cramping/pain
    - Headaches
    - Irregular bleeding which may improve after 6 months
    - Acne
    - Emotional lability
  - Contraindications
    - Current purulent cervicitis
    - Current PID, chlamydia or gonorrhea at time of insertion
    - If PID occurs after insertion, may give antibiotic therapy and assess for clinical improvement. If improvement is noted removal is not indicated (Britton et al., 2020)
    - May be discouraged for those with liver disease

G. Emergency contraception (Casey, 2020; CDC, 2018)
  1. Cu-IUD
     a. Inserted within the first 5 days of unprotected intercourse
     b. Additionally, when the day of ovulation can be estimated, may insert >5 days after unprotected intercourse, as long as it is not >5 days after ovulation
  2. Emergency contraceptive pills (ECP)
     a. Ella/ulipristal, 30 mg single dose
        (1) Progesterone agonist/antagonist
        (2) Taken as soon as possible within 120 hours (5 days) of unprotected sexual intercourse or contraceptive failure
        (3) Efficacy
           - If taken within 72 hours, it is considered as effective as levonorgestrel with pregnancy rates 0.9% to 1.8%
        (4) Adverse effects, similar profile to other ECPs
           - Headache
           - Abdominal pain
           - Nausea
        (5) Contraindications
           - No absolute contraindications
           - Pregnancy
           - Allergy or severe asthma treated by oral glucocorticoids
           - Severe liver disease
     b. Plan B/Levonorgestrel, single dose 1.5 mg or 0.75 mg first dose and 0.75 mg second dose 12 hours later
        (1) Taken within the first 72 hours of unprotected intercourse
        (2) Off-label use to 96 hours
        (3) Mechanism of action blunts the LH surge and delaying or inhibiting ovulation. It also thickens cervical mucus.
        (4) Efficacy
           - With failure rate up to 5% to 13% if taken within 24 to 72 hours.
        (5) Adverse effects
           - Headaches
           - Nausea
           - Acne
           - Menstrual abnormalities

(6) Contraindications
- No absolute contraindications
- Allergy/hypersensitivity
- Severe liver disease
- Drug/drug interactions with liver enzyme-inducing drugs
- Pregnancy

c. Combined estrogen and progestin in two doses (Yuzpe regimen; CDC, 2018)
(1) One dose of 100 mcg of ethinyl estradiol plus 0.50 mg of levonorgestrel followed by a second dose of 100 mcg of ethinyl estradiol plus 0.50 mg of levonorgestrel 12 hours later
(2) Ideally taken immediately after unprotected intercourse or failed method
(3) Taken within 120 hours (5 days)
(4) Efficacy
- Failure rate approximately 2% (Bosworth et al., 2014)
(5) Adverse effects
- Nausea/vomiting
- Irregular vaginal bleeding
- Fatigue
(6) Contraindications
- No absolute contraindications

H. Permanent contraception (Casey, 2020)

1. Female permanent contraception
   a. Surgical procedure on fallopian tubes thereby interrupting fertilization by disrupting the fallopian tubes or performing a hysterectomy
   b. Efficacy
      (1) Failure rate of 0.5%
   c. Benefits
      (1) Same-day procedure
      (2) Nonhormonal and does not affect hormones
   d. Disadvantage
      (1) Regret rate for those under 30 years of age is approximately 26%
      (2) Less than 20% seek reversal
      (3) 10% actually undergo procedure
      (4) Does not prevent STIs

2. Male permanent contraception
   a. Vasectomy
      (1) Outpatient procedure involving transection of the vas deferens and occluded both severed ends; must meet criteria with sperm-free ejaculate (15–20 ejaculations) with semen analysis
      (2) Efficacy
         - Failure rate of 0.1%
      (3) Benefits
         - No hormone
         - Permanent
         - Outpatient procedure with minimal risks
      (4) Disadvantages
         - Patients may regret
         - Short term discomfort
         - Does not prevent STIs

TABLE 40.2 Resources for Contraceptive Consultation

RESOURCE	PROVIDER	LOCATION
Bedsider Birth Control Reminder App	Bedsider	Apple Store: https://apps.apple.com/us/app/bedsider-birth-control-reminders/id1059779792 Google Play Store: https://play.google.com/store/apps/details?id=bedsider.reminders
Birth Control	Planned Parenthood	https://www.plannedparenthood.org/learn/birth-control
CDC Contraception App (U.S. MEC and SPR)	CDC	Apple Store: https://apps.apple.com/app/contraception/id595752188?OCID=MY01SV&form=MY01SV Google Play Store: https://play.google.com/store/apps/details?id=gov.cdc.ondieh/nccdph.contraception2&form=MY01SV&OCID=MY01SV
Decide + Be Ready	Defense Health Agency	Apple Store: https://apps.apple.com/us/app/decide-be-ready/id1451879300 Google Play Store: https://play.google.com/store/apps/details?id=mil.dha.decidebeready&hl=en_US&gl=US
Quick Start Algorithm for Hormonal Contraception	Reproductive Access Project	https://www.reproductiveaccess.org/wp-content/uploads/2014/12/QuickstartAlgorithm.pdf
Summary Chart of U.S. Medical Eligibility Criteria for Contraceptive Use	CDC	https://www.cdc.gov/reproductivehealth/contraception/pdf/summary-chart-us-medical-eligibility-criteria_508tagged.pdf

SELECTING A CONTRACEPTIVE METHOD

A. Shared decision-making with the patient is important with all factors considered.

B. Providing resources for patients to make informed choices is imperative (Table 40.2).

BIBLIOGRAPHY

Baker, C. C., & Chen, M. J. (2022). New contraception update—annovera, phexxi, slynd, and twirla. *Current Obstetrics and Gynecology Reports, 11*(1), 21–27. https://doi.org/10.1007/s13669-021-00321-4

Bosworth, M. C., Olusola, P. L., & Low, S. B., (2014). An update on emergency contraception. *American Family Physician, 89*(7), 545–550.

Britton, L. E., Alspaugh, A., Greene, M. Z., & McLemore, M. R. (2020). An evidence-based update on contraception: A detailed review of hormonal and nonhormonal methods. *The American Journal of Nursing, 120*(2), 22.

Casey, F. E. (2020). *Contraception.* https://emedicine.medscape.com/article/258507-print

Centers for Disease Control and Prevention. (2016). *Summary Chart of U.S. Medical Eligibility Criteria for Contraceptive Use.* https://www.cdc.gov/reproductivehealth/contraception/pdf/summary-chart-us-medical-eligibility-criteria_508tagged.pdf

Curtis, K. M., Nguyen, A., Reeves, J. A., Clark, E. A., Folger, S. G., & Whiteman, M. K. (2021). Update to US selected practice recommendations for contraceptive use: Self-administration of subcutaneous depot medroxyprogesterone acetate. *Morbidity and Mortality Weekly Report, 70*(20), 739–743. https://doi.org/10.15585/mmwr.mm7020a2

Curtis, K. M., Tepper, N. K., Jatlaoui, T. C., Berry-Bibee, E., Horton, L. G., Zapata, L. B., Simmons, K. B., Pagano, H. P., Jamieson, D. J., & Whiteman, M. K. (2016). U.S. medical eligibility criteria for contraceptive use, 2016. *Morbidity and Mortality Weekly Report Recommendations and Reports, 65*(3), 1–104. https://doi.org/10.15585/mmwr.rr6503a1external icon.

Guttmacher Institute. (2019). *Fact sheet: Unintended pregnancy in the United States.* https://www.guttmacher.org/sites/default/files/factsheet/fb-unintended-pregnancy-us.pdf

Hatcher, R. A. (2018). *Contraceptive technology* (21st ed.). Ayer Company Publishers, Inc.

Holland, A. C., Strachan, A. T., Pair, L., Stallworth, K., & Hodges, A. (2018). Highlights from the US selected practice recommendations for contraceptive use. *Nursing for Women's Health, 22*(2), 181–190. https://doi.org/10.1016/j.nwh.2018.02.006

Klein, D. A., Arnold, J. J., & Reese, E. S. (2015). Provision of contraception: Key recommendations from the CDC. *American Family Physician, 91*(9), 625–637.

Knight, K. R., Duncan, L. G., Szilvasi, M., Premkumar, A., Matache, M., & Jackson, A. (2019). Reproductive (In)justice — Two patients with avoidable poor reproductive outcomes. *The New England Journal of Medicine, 381*(7), 593–596. https://doi.org/10.1056/NEJMp1907437

Lee, A. L. (2020). Segesterone acetate and ethinyl estradiol vaginal ring (Annovera) for contraception. *American Family Physician, 101*(10), 618–620.

Mansour, D., Gemzell-Danielsson, K., Inki, P., & Jensen, J. T. (2011). Fertility after discontinuation of contraception: A comprehensive review of the literature. *Contraception (Stoneham); Contraception, 84*(5), 465–477. https://doi.org/10.1016/j.contraception.2011.04.002

Nappi, R. E., Kaunitz, A. M., & Bitzer, J. (2016). Extended regimen combined oral contraception: A review of evolving concepts and acceptance by women and clinicians. *The European Journal of Contraception & Reproductive Health Care, 21*(2), 106–115. https://doi.org/10.3109/13625187.2015.1107894

Nelson, A. L., Kaunitz, A. M., Kroll, R., Simon, J. A., Poindexter, A. N., Castaño, P. M., Ackerman, R. T., Flood, L., Chiodo III, J. A., & Garner, E. I. (2021). Efficacy, safety, and tolerability of a levonorgestrel/ethinyl estradiol transdermal delivery system: Phase 3 clinical trial results. *Contraception, 103*(3), 137–143. https://doi.org/10.1016/j.contraception.2020.11.011

Ross, L., & Solinger, R. (2017). *Reproductive justice: An introduction.* University of California Press.

Schreiber, C. A., Teal, S. B., Blumenthal, P. D., Keder, L. M., Olariu, A. I., & Creinin, M. D. (2018). Bleeding patterns for the Liletta® levonorgestrel 52 mg intrauterine system. *The European Journal of Contraception & Reproductive Health Care, 23*(2), 116–120. https://doi.org/10.1080/13625187.2018.1449825

Scott, K. A., Britton, L., & McLemore, M. R. (2019). The ethics of perinatal care for black women: Dismantling the structural racism in "mother blame" narratives. *The Journal of Perinatal & Neonatal Nursing, 33*(2), 108–115. https://doi.org/10.1097/JPN.0000000000000394

Serfaty, D. (2019). Update on the contraceptive contraindications. *Journal of Gynecology Obstetrics and Human Reproduction, 48*(5), 297-307. https://doi.org/10.1016/j.jogoh.2019.02.006

Sergison, J. E., Maldonado, L. Y., Gao, X., & Hubacher, D. (2019). Levonorgestrel intrauterine system associated amenorrhea: A systematic review and metaanalysis. *American Journal of Obstetrics and Gynecology, 220*(5), 440–448.e8. https://doi.org/10.1016/j.ajog.2018.12.008

SisterSong. (2022). *SisterSong; Women of color reproductive justice collective.* https://www.sistersong.net

Steinberg, J., & Lynch, S. E. (2021). Lactic acid, citric acid, and potassium bitartrate (Phexxi) vaginal gel for contraception. *American Family Physician, 103*(10), 628–629.

Tepper, N. K., Curtis, K. M., Cox, S., Whiteman, M. K. (2020). Update to U.S. medical eligibility criteria for contraceptive use, 2016: Updated recommendations for the use of contraception among women at high risk for HIV infection. *Morbidity and Mortality Weekly Report, 69*, 405–410. https://doi.org/10.15585/mmwr.mm6914a3external icon.

Torres, L. N., Turok, D. K., Clark, E. A. S., Sanders, J. N., & Godfrey, E. M. (2018). Increasing IUD and implant use among those at risk of a subsequent preterm birth: A randomized controlled trial of postpartum contraceptive counseling. *Women's Health Issues, 28*(5), 393–400. https://doi.org/10.1016/j.whi.2018.05.003

What Is New in Contraception? (2021). *Contraceptive Technology Update, 43*(11).

41

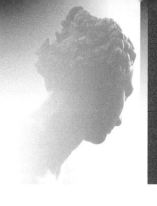

MEDICAL ELIGIBILITY CRITERIA FOR CONTRACEPTIVE USE

R. MIMI SECOR AND IRIS STENDIG-RASKIN

THE CENTERS FOR DISEASE CONTROL AND PREVENTION MEDICAL ELIGIBILITY CRITERIA EXPLAINED

A. In 2010, the Centers for Disease Control and Prevention (CDC) issued the first ever U.S. medical eligibility criteria (MEC) for contraceptive use.
   1. These guidelines were issued in response to the 2009 World Health Organization (WHO) contraceptive guidelines.
   2. The CDC MEC guidelines provide evidence-based guidance on whether women and men with particular medical conditions or physical characteristics can safely use certain methods of contraception.
   3. Two-page summary charts are available and can be printed double-sided, laminated, and used by healthcare providers as a reference and when counseling women.
   4. The categories of risk are based on a scale of 1 to 4; these categories are summarized in Table 41.1.

B. In 2020, the CDC updated the 2016 MEC guidelines and Selected Practice Recommendations (SPR)
   1. For the Use of Contraception Among Women at High Risk for HIV infection. Updated recommendations include the following:
      a. Progestin-only injectable contraception (including depot medroxyprogesterone acetate [DMPA]) and intrauterine devices (including levonorgestrel-releasing and copper-bearing) are safe for use without restriction to the amount with women at high risk for HIV infection.
      b. New U.S. SPR on self-administration of DMPA-SC

TABLE 41.1 Categories for Medical Eligibility Criteria for Contraceptive Use

RATING	DEFINITION
1	A condition for which there is no restriction for the use of the contraceptive method
2	A condition for which the advantages of using the method generally outweigh the theoretical or proven risks
3	A condition for which the theoretical or proven risks usually outweigh the advantages of using the method
4	A condition that represents an unacceptable health risk if the contraceptive method is used

Source: Centers for Disease Control and Prevention. (2016) U.S. medical eligibility criteria for contraceptive use, 2016. *Morbidity and Mortality Weekly Report, 65(3),* 1–108. Retrieved from https://www.cdc.gov/reproductivehealth/contraception/mmwr/mec/summary.html

C. In 2016, the CDC updated the 2010 MEC guidelines for combined hormonal contraceptive. Notable updates and revisions include the following:
1. Added contraceptive usage for women diagnosed with cystic fibrosis
2. Added contraceptive usage for women with multiple sclerosis
3. Added category regarding concomitant usage of certain psychotrophic drugs and St. John's wort
4. Revision of emergency contraceptive pill (ECP) use, including addition of ullipristol acetate (ella)
5. Other revisions/updates include:
   a. Postpartum women who are lactating
   b. Women with dyslipidemia
   c. Women diagnosed with migraine headaches
   d. Women with superficial venous disease
   e. Women with a history of gestational trophoblastic disease
   f. Women diagnosed with HIV receiving or not receiving antiretroviral therapy therapy
6. Utilizing the new CDC MEC app (see the following), multiple conditions may be selected.
D. Issued in 2013, U.S. SPR for contraceptive use is a companion document to the CDC MEC and addresses how to use contraceptive methods.
1. Although the CDC MEC provides guidance on who can use various methods of contraception, the U.S. SPR provides guidance on how contraceptive methods can be used and how to remove unnecessary barriers for patients in accessing and successfully using contraceptive methods.
2. The section entitled Special Practice Recommendations (SPR) includes the following topics: initiation, examinations and tests, routine follow-up, late or missed doses (for combined hormonal contraception [CHC]), and bleeding irregularities (for many methods).
E. New app, "CDC MEC 2021," was released in May 2021.
1. The new U.S. MEC and U.S. SPR App is an easy-to-use reference for the CDC's contraception guidance for healthcare providers.
2. Includes the full guidelines, is free, is kept updated and includes the following sections: MEC by method, MEC by condition, SPR, About this App, Full Guidelines, Provider Tools, and Resources.
3. Includes new features that allow for the selection of multiple conditions and methods.

BIBLIOGRAPHY

Altshuler, A. L., Gaffield, M. E., & Kiarie, J. N. (2015). The WHO's medical eligibility criteria for contraceptive use: 20 years of global guidance. *Current Opinion in Obstetrics & Gynecology, 27*(6), 451–459. https://doi.org/10.1097/GCO.0000000000000212

American Congress of Obstetricians and Gynecologists. (2011). Understanding and using the U.S. Medical eligibility criteria for contraceptive use 2010. *Obstetrics and Gynecology, 118*(3), 754–760. https://doi.org/10.1097/AOG.0b013e3182310cd3

Curtis, K. M., Jatlaoui, T. C., Tepper, N. K., Zapata, L. B., Horton, L. G., Jamieson, D. J., & Whiteman, M. K. (2016). U.S. selected practice recommendations for contraceptive use, 2016. *MMWR. Recommendations and Reports: Morbidity and Mortality Weekly Report. Recommendations and Reports, 65*(4), 1–66. https://doi.org/10.15585/mmwr.rr6504a1

Curtis, K. M., Tepper, N. K., Jatlaoui, T. C., Berry-Bibee, E., Horton, L. G., Zapata, L. B., Simmons, K. B., Pagano, H. P., Jamieson, D. J., & Whiteman, M. K. (2016). U.S. medical eligibility criteria for contraceptive use, 2016. *Morbidity and Mortality Weekly Report, 65*(3), 1–108. https://www.cdc .gov/mmwr/volumes/65/rr/rr6503a1.htm?s_cid=rr6503a1_w

Division of Reproductive Health, National Center for Chronic Disease Prevention and Health Promotion. (2013). U.S. selected practice recommendations for contraceptive use, 2013: Adapted from the World Health Organization *Selected Practice Recommendations for Contraceptive Use,* 2nd Edition. *Morbidity and Mortality Weekly Report: Recommendations and Reports, 62*(RR05), 1–46. https://www.cdc.gov/mmwr/preview/mmwrhtml/rr6205a1.htm

Tepper, N. K., Phillips, S. J., Kapp, N., Gaffield, M. E., & Curtis, K. M. (2016). Combined hormonal contraceptive use among breastfeeding women: An updated systematic review. *Contraception, 94*(3), 262–274. https://doi.org/10.1016/j .contraception.2015.05.006

U.S. Department of Health and Human Services. (2015), *Healthy people 2020: Maternal, infant, and child health objectives.* US Department of Health and Human Services. http://www.healthypeople.gov/2020/topics-objectives/topic/maternal -infant-and-child-health/objectivesexternal icon

World Health Organization. (2009). *Medical eligibility criteria for contraceptive use* (4th ed.). http://whqlibdoc.who .int/publications/2010/9789241563888_eng.pdf

42

CERVICAL CAP AND THE ONE-SIZE DIAPHRAGM

ASHTON TUREAUD STRACHAN AND REBECCA KOENIGER-DONOHUE

THE CERVICAL CAP AND ONE-SIZE DIAPHRAGM EXPLAINED

The brand names for these products are FemCap and Caya. These barrier contraceptive methods are ideal for women of childbearing age who cannot or do not want to use hormonal contraceptives or an intrauterine device (IUD) and may be interested in using a female barrier contraceptive, especially one that requires no involvement by the male partner.

A. FemCap (Figure 42.1) and Caya (Figure 42.2) are both nonhormonal, latex-free, female-controlled barrier contraceptives.

B. Both are available by prescription with no side effects (unlike hormonal methods).

C. The FemCap comes in three sizes. Proper size selection is based on a woman's obstetric history because pregnancy and delivery are the two major factors that have the greatest impact on the elasticity of the vagina and the size of the cervix. Caya is available in one size and fits most females. No formal fitting is necessary.

D. FemCap was approved by the U.S. Food and Drug Administration (FDA) in March 2003. Caya was FDA cleared in September 2014.

E. FemCap offers a unique design: Brim designed to flare outward like an inverted funnel—flaring of the brim is met by the physiological inward concentric contraction of the vagina. FemCap is held in place by the vaginal contraction, which allows the vagina to hold and support the FemCap without causing any pressure over the cervix. Caya is made from a silicone membrane, which covers the cervix to prevent sperm from reaching the uterus. Grip dimples help to facilitate vaginal insertion. A flexible rim helps to ensure correct position. The removal dome aids in removal from the vagina

F. FemCap is reusable for 1 year. Caya is reusable for 2 years.

G. Neither FemCap or Caya interfere with the menstrual cycle, libido, or sexual pleasure for either partner.

H. Both devices are easy to insert and remove, but practicing placement before use should be performed.

I. FemCap and Caya are both designed to cover the cervix completely and deliver spermicide on the cervical and—most important—on the vaginal side, to mechanically block sperm.

J. Both are effective in preventing pregnancy when used as directed and are safe to use, with no systemic side effects.

K. **Cost:** The retail price for a single FemCap kit is $100.99. The cost for Caya is $120.39. The devices could possibly be cheaper with coupons and/or insurance coverage.

L. It is recommended that the FemCap be replaced every year (or sooner if it shows signs of deterioration). The Caya diaphragm can be used for 2 years.

M. For information and orders, please visit www.femcap.com and www.caya.us.com

N. The advantages and disadvantages of both methods are summarized in Box 42.1.

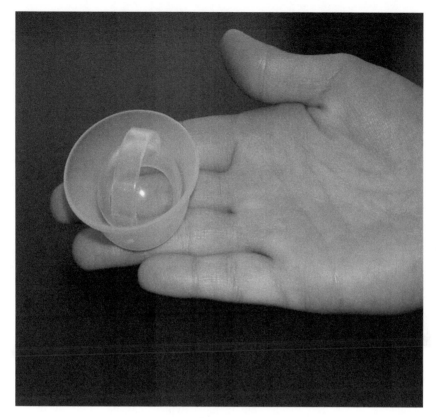

FIGURE 42.1 FemCap.
Source: http://www.femcap.com, Copyright 2022 FemCap Inc.

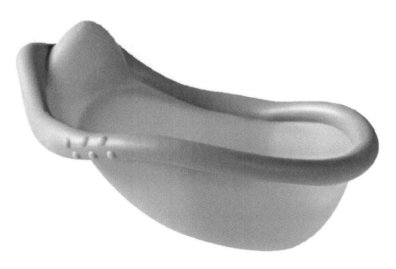

FIGURE 42.2 Caya.
Source: http://www.caya.us.com © 2022 HPSRx Enterprises.

BOX 42.1 Advantages and Disadvantages of the FemCap and Caya

Advantages
- Easy to use
- No systemic side effects or local effects
- Silicone rubber has a longer shelf life than latex rubber
- Safe for latex-allergic women or partners with a latex allergy
- Can be left in place for up to 48 hours (FemCap) and 24 hours (Caya)
- FemCap does not breakdown with petroleum-based products. Caya diaphragm should only be used with water-soluble lubricants.
- Does not absorb odors; easy to clean
- Immediately reversible if and when pregnancy is desired
- When compared with diaphragms—, FemCap isassociated with fewer UTIs, needs less spermicide, is more comfortable.
- Caya is 88% effective. FemCap is 86% effective in women who have not given birth and 71% effective in women who have given birth.
- Compared with IUDs—both methods are less invasive.
- Compared with hormonal contraceptives—does not have systemic or serious side effects, does not change the menstrual cycle, does not decrease libido.
- Compared with male condom—does not interrupt spontaneity or reduce sexual pleasure for either partner; is under the user's control.

Disadvantages
- Both FemCap and Caya require a prescription.
- Necessitates that the user touch their genitalia, which may be culturally or personally unacceptable.
- Theoretical risk of toxic shock syndrome if left in place longer than recommended.

IUD, intrauterine device; UTI, urinary tract infection.

DESCRIPTION OF THE CERVICAL CAP AND ONE-SIZE DIAPHRAGM

A. FemCap is made of soft, durable, hypoallergenic silicone rubber. Caya is a soft silicone device with a nylon rim.

B. FemCap resembles a sailor's hat with an upturned brim that lies against the vaginal walls around the cervix. Caya comes in a dome shape with a built-in notch.

C. FemCap conforms to the anatomy of the cervix and the physiologic changes of the vagina that occur during sexual arousal. The dome of the FemCap fits over the cervix "like a glove," covering it completely. Caya completely covers the cervix and the notch slides just behind the pubic symphysis.

D. Complete cervical coverage prevents sperm from entering the cervix and the uterus of both devices.

E. Components
  1. FemCap
     a. The rim of the cervical cap provides a snug fit into the vaginal fornices and covers the vaginal vault; the brim covers the vaginal walls surrounding the cervix.
     b. The brim is longer posteriorly to conform to the unique anatomy of the vaginal walls.

    c. The out flaring of the brim facing the vaginal opening has a unique groove that acts as a trap for sperm and a reservoir for any spermicide, or any microbicidal/spermicide that will soon be developed in the future, to reinforce the mechanical barrier of the FemCap.

    d. The FemCap is held in place by the muscular walls of the vagina and does not have to be snug around the cervix or hinge behind the pubic bone.

    e. The FemCap has a strap over the dome to facilitate the removal of the device and provide added protection to the vaginal walls and cervix from possible fingernail abrasions during removal.

    f. When the FemCap is placed correctly, users should rarely, if ever, be aware of its presence. During the several clinical trials, fewer than 2% of women and 22% of men reported a sense of awareness of the FemCap and it did not interfere with their sexual pleasure.

2. Caya

    a. Cervical cup is made of a thin silicone material that covers the cervix and accommodates a range of cervical sizes.

    b. Rim is flexible, provides stability, and helps guide Caya deep into the vagina as you push on the anterior edge. The rim holds the diaphragm in place and ensures that it is positioned correctly.

    c. Grip dimples orient your finger and provide a tactile cue for where to hold and squeeze the rim.

    d. Removal dome allows for easy removal; a finger can fit under or over the dome to remove the device.

    e. A palpable center point for a better positioning of the diaphragm.

SIZE SELECTION

A. Selecting the correct size is based on obstetric history (FemCap) and pelvic examination (not required for Caya, but may be useful).

B. The pelvic examination is essential to estimate the size of the cervix and to exclude women who have contraindications such as cancer, laceration, infection, or a flat cervix (FemCap). Box 42.2 summarizes contraindications to the FemCap.

C. FemCap is available in three sizes.

    1. Small (22-mm internal diameter) for nulligravida women

    2. Medium (26 mm) for women who have been pregnant but have had a miscarriage, therapeutic abortion, or delivered by cesarean section.

    3. Large (30 mm), for women who have had at least one full-term vaginal delivery.

    4. If the woman denies ever having been pregnant, but the cervix looks bigger on pelvic examination than a nulligravida cervix, then provide her with the 26-mm FemCap. If in doubt about the fit, it is safest to use the 26-mm size.

PROTECTION AGAINST STIs AND HIV/AIDS

A. Using the FemCap with spermicide, or Caya with spermicide, has *not* been shown to protect against STIs.

B. Studies have not yet demonstrated a protective effect against HIV or other STIs.

C. Nonoxynol-9 spermicide alone does not provide protection against HIV, chlamydia, and gonorrhea.

D. Frequent use of large doses of spermicide alone can cause disruption of the single-layer endocervical columnar epithelium. This disruption creates micro abrasions or ulcerations that, at least in theory, could *increase* susceptibility to HIV transmission.

BOX 42.2 Contraindications

FemCap
- Adhesions between the cervix and the vaginal walls
- Third-degree uterine prolapse
- Flat cervix
- Acute cervicitis
- Cancer of the cervix
- Active pelvic inflammatory disease
- History of toxic shock syndrome
- Cut or tear in the vagina or cervix visualized on pelvic examination
- Allergy to spermicide
- Women who are adverse to touching their genitals (cultural norms or personal preference)

Caya
- Within 6 weeks of childbirth
- Previously measuring <60 mm for a traditional diaphragm or >85 mm (Caya)
- Allergy to spermicide
- Acute or chronic/recurrent urinary tract infections
- Active pelvic infections
- Third-degree uterine prolapse
- Cystocele with obliteration of the retropubic niche in the vagina
- Weakly formed or absent retropubic niche
- Women who are adverse to touching their genitals (cultural norms or personal preference)

FEMCAP PROTOCOL

One can request information on the FemCap, as well as request a kit, by logging on to www.femcap.com.

A. The clinician should
1. Schedule a 30- to 45-minute visit for cap fitting and instructions.
2. Perform a pelvic examination to exclude any anatomical or pathological contraindications.
3. Allow privacy and time to practice inserting and removing the FemCap, making sure the client can identify and cover their cervix with the FemCap.
4. Encourage the client to practice insertion and removal several times.
5. Have the client leave the FemCap in place so clinician can recheck for proper fit by digital examination.
6. Use speculum examination (if needed for further confirmation).
7. Use only a plastic disposable speculum as it has blunt tips and allows good lighting.
8. Insert the speculum halfway into the vagina and open it enough at this point to be able to see the FemCap covering the cervix without dislodging it.
9. Some comments
   a. Unlike the diaphragm, the bulk of the spermicide is stored in the grooved area between the dome and brim of the FemCap, facing the vaginal opening, to expose sperm to the spermicide when deposited into the vagina.
   b. The FemCap does not require measurement for custom fitting.
   c. The client can most easily insert and remove the FemCap in a squatting position.

CAYA PROTOCOL

A. A traditional fitting is not required for the Caya diaphragm.

B. If a client has any concerns of whether they are too big or too small for Caya, a "test fit" sample can be ordered.

C. The provider can have the client practice placing the diaphragm in the vagina and then confirm the correct location of the device.

D. The test fit is a single-use device.

DIRECTIONS FOR USE

A. Insertion
  1. FemCap
     a. Place ½ teaspoon of spermicide in the groove between the dome and the brim of the FemCap and ¼ teaspoon of the spermicide over the rim and in the bowl of the device.
     b. Spread a thin layer all over the brim of the FemCap except for the spots where the finger and the thumb are holding the device.
     c. Squeeze and flatten the device, insert it into the vagina with the bowl facing upward and the long brim entering first.
     d. The FemCap is inserted downward toward the rectum and then downward and back as far as possible in the vagina to be sure the cervix is covered.
     e. It is important to ensure that the FemCap is not partway between the vaginal opening and the cervix.
     f. With repeated acts of intercourse, check the position of the FemCap and insert ½ teaspoon of spermicide (without removing the device).
     g. If the FemCap is placed correctly, the woman should not be aware of its presence during intercourse or daily activities. It should fit comfortably over the cervix, with the rim fitting snugly to the vaginal fornices and the brim adhering to the vaginal walls.
     h. It *must* be placed in the vagina *before* any sexual stimulation and may be worn for up to 48 hours maximum. The device should remain in place for at least 6 hours after sexual intercourse, but no longer than 48 hours total.
  2. Caya
     a. Before insertion, Caya is folded using grip nubs on each side. About 4 mL (one teaspoon) of contraceptive gel is poured into each fold of the Caya.
     b. A small amount of contraceptive gel is spread on the rim. This will help facilitate insertion into the vagina.
     c. The Caya diaphragm and contraceptive gel can be applied up to 2 hours before coitus.
     d. The diaphragm is held in one hand. During insertion, the arrow on it points toward the body.
     e. Caya is pushed past the vaginal portion of the cervix into the posterior fornix. The recessed grip fills the retropubic space completely.
     f. Caya is correctly placed when the cervix is completely covered by the diaphragm and placed between the retropubic arch and the niche on the pubic bone.
     g. The placement should be controlled with the finger after insertion. It is correct when the cervix can be felt through the membrane of the diaphragm (feels like the tip of a nose). Otherwise, the diaphragm must be removed and inserted again.
     h. In case of repeated sexual intercourse, the diaphragm remains in the vagina. To ensure continued safety, before the second coitus, additional gel must be introduced into the vagina using a gel applicator.

i. The diaphragm must remain in the vagina at least 6 hours before it is removed. (Otherwise, motile sperm might ascend into the then unprotected cervical canal.) Important: The Caya diaphragm should never remain in the vagina for more than 24 hours.

A. Removal
   1. FemCap
      a. The client should squat and bear down, which will bring the removal strap closer to the fingers, facilitating removal of the device.
      b. The device can then be rotated and removed comfortably by pushing the tip of the finger against the dome of the FemCap to dimple it. This will break the suction and allow room for the finger to be inserted between the dome and the removal strap and then it can be pulled out gently by hooking a finger into the removal strap.
      c. The client should develop a routine for insertion and removal, such as after daily shower.
      d. The FemCap should be washed with antibacterial soap and rinsed thoroughly with tepid tap water and air dried or patted dry with a clean, soft towel. It should be stored in the plastic container supplied with it and kept in a cool, dry place. Powder should be avoided. It should never be placed in a microwave or cleaned by synthetic detergents, organic solvents, or sharp objects.
   2. Caya
      a. The client should remove the Caya diaphragm from the vagina using the recessed grip.
      b. After removal from the vagina, the Caya diaphragm is rinsed with water and soap and dried in the open case.
      c. For protection against external influences, the Caya should always be stored in the case provided.

BIBLIOGRAPHY

Abdool Karim, Q., Abdool Karim, S. S., Frohlich, J. A., Grobler, A. C., Baxter, C., Mansoor, L. E., Kharsany, A. B., Sibeko, S., Mlisana, K. P., Omar, Z., & Gengiah, T. N. (2010). Effectiveness and safety of tenofovir gel, an antiretroviral microbicide for the prevention of HIV infection in women. *Science, 329*(5996), 1168–1174. doi:10.1126/science.1193748

Caya US. (2021). *Caya.* https://www.caya.us.com

Contraceptive Technology Update. (2015). Single-size Caya diaphragm is available by prescription in U.S. https://www.reliasmedia.com/articles/136004-single-size-caya-diaphragm-is-available-by-prescription-in-us

Koeniger-Donohue, R. (2006). The FemCap: A non-hormonal contraceptive. *Women's Health Care, 5*(4), 79–91.

Planned Parenthood. (n.d.). *Birth control.* https://www.plannedparenthood.org/learn/birth-control

Shihata, A. (n.d.). *FemCap.* http:// www.femcap.com

Shihata, A., & Brody, S. (2011). HIV/STIs and pregnancy prevention: Using a cervical barrier and microbicide. *World Journal of AIDS, 1*, 131–135. https://doi.org/10.4236/wja.2011.14018

43

INTRAUTERINE CONTRACEPTION

KELLEY STALLWORTH BORELLA, AIMEE CHISM HOLLAND,
MARCIA DENINE, AND R. MIMI SECOR

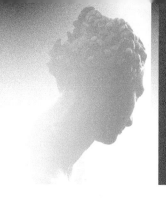

THE INTRAUTERINE CONTRACEPTIVE EXPLAINED

A. The intrauterine contraceptive (IUC) is a plastic contraceptive device that is inserted into the uterine cavity through the cervical canal.
 1. There are five IUCs available in the United States. All types have a two-strand, polyethylene monofilament string that protrudes from the cervical os.
  a. Copper IUC (ParaGard; www.paragard.com) with white strings
  b. Levonorgestrel (LNG)-containing IUC (Mirena; www.mirena .com) with brown strings
  c. LNG-containing IUC (Skyla; www.skyla-us.com) with blue strings
  d. LNG-containing IUC (Liletta; www.liletta.com) with blue strings
  e. LNG-containing IUC (Kyleena; www.kyleena-us.com) with blue strings
 2. The IUC is for contraceptive use only. No IUC is intended to offer any protection against sexually transmitted infection (STI) transmission. If there is STI risk, encourage consistent use of condoms.
 3. IUC efficacy is equivalent to sterilization yet reversible.
 4. It is cost-effective.
B. The ParaGard T380A is a copper-releasing IUC (Cu-IUC).
 1. Manufactured by Cooper Surgical
 2. One size; fine copper wire is wound around the vertical limb of T-shaped device
 3. Releasing free copper and copper salts, affecting the endometrium
 4. Advantages
  a. Is the longest acting contraceptive method available
  b. Metabolically neutral
  c. Can remain in place for 10 years; off-label for 12 years
  d. Has the lowest expulsion rates
  e. Can be inserted into nulliparous women
  f. Safety and efficacy have been established in women older than 16 years
  g. Mechanisms of action (MOA): ParaGard works by preventing sperm from reaching the egg, preventing sperm from fertilizing the egg, and possibly preventing the egg from attaching (implanting) in the uterus. ParaGard does not stop your ovaries from releasing an egg (ovulating) each month. ParaGard is not an abortifacient.
 5. Contraindicated in women with known allergy to copper or a diagnosis of Wilson's disease
 6. **Disadvantage:** May alter bleeding pattern and increase menstrual flow, as well as increase cramping associated with menses
C. The Mirena IUC is an levonorgestrel-containing IUC (LNG-IUC).
 1. Manufactured by Bayer HealthCare
 2. Progestin-only hormone-releasing device

3. The progestin is contained in a vertical limb that releases low-dose progestin locally into the endometrial cavity.
4. Offers continuous contraceptive protection for 7 years
5. Thins endometrial lining
6. Thickens cervical secretions
7. Decreases menstrual flow
8. Reduces dysmenorrheal and menstrual blood loss; after 8 months, 50% of women have no menstrual bleeding, only monthly spotting; 20% of women have amenorrhea within the first year.
9. Food and Drug Administration (FDA)-approved indications include contraception and treatment of heavy menstrual bleeding for women who choose to use intrauterine contraception as their method of contraception.
10. Mirena is appropriate for parous women or nulliparous women with dysmenorrhea or menorrhagia.

D. Skyla IUC is a progestin-releasing LNG-IUC.
1. Skyla is manufactured by Bayer HealthCare.
2. It releases LNG at a rate of 14 mcg/day after 24 days and declines to 5 mcg/day after 3 years.
3. It provides continuous contraceptive protection for 3 years.
4. MOA are the same as the Mirena LNG-IUC (as described previously).
5. LNG-IUC is not FDA approved for postcoital contraception.
6. It is appropriate for parous or nulliparous women
7. Skyla is a smaller device (28-mm horizontally) than the Mirena and is the preferred LNG-IUC for a nulliparous woman because it is smaller and therefore usually easier to insert into a smaller uterus.

E. Liletta is an LNG-containing IUC device.
1. Liletta is manufactured by Odyssea Pharmaceuticals, an AbbVie company.
2. It contains 52 mg of LNG and provides an initial release rate of 18.6 mcg/day of LNG, diminishing over a 3-year period to an average of 15.6 mcg/day.
3. Liletta provides continuous contraceptive protection for 3 years.
4. MOAs are similar to Mirena and Skyla,
5. Per the FDA, should not be used for postcoital contraception.
6. It should not be inserted during the first 7 days of the menstrual cycle.
7. Is appropriate for parous or nulliparous women.

F. Kyleena is an LNG-IUC system.
1. Kyleena is manufactured by Bayer Corporation.
2. It contains 19.5 mg of LNG and releases approximately 17.5 mcg/day of LNG after 24 days.
3. It provides continuous contraceptive protection for 5 years.
4. MOAs are similar to Mirena and Skyla.
5. A silver ring visible on ultrasound distinguishes Kyleena from other IUCs.
6. Insertion following postpartum or after second-trimester terminations should be withheld for a period of 6 weeks or until full involution of the uterus.

G. Contraindications for IUC use
1. Cu-IUCs and all LNG-IUCs
   a. Pregnancy or suspicion of pregnancy
   b. Congenital or acquired uterine anomaly if it distorts the uterine cavity
   c. Acute pelvic inflammatory disease (PID); initiation only is category 4; past history of PID is not a contraindication if no known current risk factors for STIs; increased risk of STIs is category 3 for both IUCs for initiation only.
   d. Defer until post-septic abortion or peurperal sepsis is resolved.
   e. Known or suspected uterine or cervical neoplasia (while awaiting treatment)

   f. Unexplained vaginal bleeding (initiation only is category 4)
   g. Current untreated acute cervicitis or chlamydia or gonorrhea infection (initiation only is category 4); vaginitis, including *Trichomonas vaginalis* and bacterial vaginosis are not a contraindication (category 2).
   h. Severe cirrhosis, benign hepatocellular adenoma, malignant hepatoma (LNG-IUC only is category 3); Cu-IUC is category 1 for these conditions.
   i. A previously inserted IUC that has not been removed (per package insert)
   j. Breast cancer (LNG-IUC only), current disease is category 4, past history, and no evidence of current disease for 5 years is category 3.
   k. Systemic lupus erythematosus (SLE) with positive or unknown antiphospholipid antibodies (category 3 for LNG-IUC only)
   l. Solid organ transplantation; complicated graft failure (initiation only for both is category 3)
   m. Pelvic tuberculosis (initiation only is category 4 for both IUCs)
   n. HIV is *not* a contraindication for either IUC; these guidelines were updated in 2012.
   o. Past history of syncope especially with medical procedures
   p. History of cardiac problems that might impact tolerating procedure
2. Mirena should be used with caution in patients who have
   a. Coagulopathy or are receiving anticoagulants
   b. Migraine, focal migraine with asymmetrical visual loss, or other symptoms indicating:
      (1) Transient cerebral ischemia
      (2) Severe headaches
      (3) Significantly elevated blood pressure
      (4) Significant arterial disease, such as stroke or myocardial infarction
      (5) Topomax (topiramate) doses greater than 200 mg/day
H. Historical perspective on IUCs listed chronologically
1. The first intrauterine device was a ring-shaped device described in 1909 by a German gynecologist, Ernest Grafenberg.
2. During the 1960s and 1970s, 10% of women in the United States who used contraception chose the IUC.
3. The Dalkon Shield was introduced in 1970.
   a. Within 3 years, a high incidence of PID was recognized.
   b. It was documented that the braided multifilament tail of the Dalkon Shield provided a pathway for bacteria to pass through the protective cervical mucus and ascend into the uterus.
   c. A large number of women sued the manufacturer.
   d. The number of IUCs used decreased in proportion to the increase in IUC litigation.
4. The controversy and litigation surrounding the Dalkon Shield tainted the image of all IUCs.
5. In addition, two studies in the mid-1980s reported that the use of IUCs was associated with infertility, which further frightened women.
6. Many IUCs were removed from the market in 1986 because of the concern regarding medical liability, giving the message that IUCs are unsafe.
7. Women became distrustful because they remember the Dalkon Shield.
8. The number of women using IUCs in the United States declined by two thirds from 1981 to 1989.
9. Today, manufacturers have made great strides to protect the product.
   a. Package materials include an informed consent.
   b. Strict patient-selection criteria are listed.
   c. Appropriate clinician/patient dialogue is strongly encouraged.
   d. Product label comes with extensive warnings.

10. Despite the previously mentioned measures, IUCs now account for less than 10% of the contraception used in the United States among childbearing women.
11. Worldwide, IUC is the most popular method of reversible contraception.

I. Some comments and considerations regarding selection of contraception
   1. Prescribing contraceptives should be individually tailored.
   2. Patient selection and proper insertion technique are vital.
      a. Group A streptococcal infection has been reported following IUC insertion. Strict aseptic technique is essential during insertion (per package insert).
   3. Factors that influence a woman's choice of contraceptive:
      a. Sexual lifestyle
      b. Number of partners and frequency of coitus
      c. Status of marriage or relationship
      d. Cultural or religious beliefs
      e. Motivation of the woman and her partner
      f. Degree of comfort with one's body
      g. Lactation status
      h. Confidence in the method
      i. Effectiveness
      j. Safety
      k. Access to healthcare
      l. Convenience
      m. Temporary or permanent nature of the method
      n. Previous experience or experience of others
      o. Educational and cognitive status
      p. Cost
      q. Health concerns
      r. Allergies

J. The advantages of the IUC in general include
   1. It is safe, highly effective, and economical.
   2. It offers long-term contraceptive protection with few compliance issues.

THE INSERTION

A. Timing of insertion is controversial.
   1. Can occur at any time as long as contraindications have been considered and potential pregnancy have been ruled out
   2. Insertion during menses
      a. Insertion may be easier because the cervical canal is lubricated with menstrual blood.
      b. Must be relatively sure that the patient is not pregnant.
      c. Os is slightly dilated.
      d. The disadvantage is that menstrual blood may provide a medium for bacterial growth. The infection rate and expulsion rate are higher when the IUC is inserted during menses.
      e. Menstrual insertion is not recommended for Liletta.
   3. Insertion at midcycle
      a. Cervical os is dilated.
      b. Must have used protection the previous week
   4. Insert immediately on the removal of another IUC.
   5. Following delivery or abortion, may be inserted following these procedures. Expulsion rate is lower if the clinician waits until 4 to 8 weeks postpartum visit.
      a. Waiting until full involution of the uterus is recommended for Kyleena.

B. The "U.S. Selected Practice Recommendations for Contraceptive Use" encourage same-day insertion if possible.
   1. Complete history
      a. Rule out contraindications.
      b. Note date of last menses, length, flow, and any associated pain.
      c. Ask whether any odor or change in vaginal discharge is present.
      d. Rule out pregnancy.
      e. Determine past and present sexual partners.
      f. Assess behavioral risk of STIs.
   2. Pelvic examination, including bimanual examination
      a. Inspect vulva, vagina, and cervix, noting any signs of infection or cervical stenosis.
      b. Note size, shape, contour, and position of uterus or any tenderness or masses on palpation.
      c. Rule out infection, pregnancy, or neoplasia.
   3. Use the Centers for Disease Control and Prevention (CDC) STI treatment guidelines to assess for STIs and consider a wet mount to assess for vaginitis, if indicated.
      a. If white blood cells (WBCs) are present, culture for gonorrhea and chlamydia. Delay insertion of the IUC until after treatment if culture is positive. Explain the risks.
      b. If bacterial vaginosis (BV) is present, the IUC may still be inserted and BV treated, preferably with oral metronidazole or oral clindamycin per the CDC STI treatment guidelines.
   4. Counsel regarding disadvantages and advantages
   5. Encourage questions
   6. Explain procedure
   7. The patient may read and sign informed consent, or may bring to next visit
   8. Explain the necessity of proper protection against pregnancy until insertion visit
   9. Laboratory tests
      a. Hemoglobin and hematocrit measurement recommended, particularly if the patient has a history of heavy menses.
      b. Pap test per the American Cancer Society (ACS) Pap HPV screening guidelines, the American Society for Colposcopy and Cervical Pathology (ASCCP), and the American Society for Clinical Pathology (ASCP) consensus guidelines.
      c. Test sedimentation rate, STI testing per the CDC STI guidelines, and vaginal microscopy if PID suspected.
      d. Perform routine urinalysis and urine pregnancy test as needed.
      e. Request chlamydia and gonorrhea screening per CDC STI guidelines according to age, risk, and symptoms present, especially if the patient is 25 years of age or younger or their sexual partner is 25 years of age or younger.
   10. Discuss analgesia and consider a prostaglandin inhibitor, such as ibuprofen, for discomfort
      a. Take a nonsteroidal anti-inflammatory drug (NSAID) one-half hour before appointment.
   11. Discuss use of antibiotics
      a. There is no consensus regarding the effectiveness of antibiotics in reducing postinsertion infection.
      b. If subacute endocarditis is present, most clinicians do not recommend use of IUC.
C. Insertion visit
   1. Healthcare provider should be reasonably certain that a woman is not pregnant; if irregular or absent menses are noted, perform sensitive (within 10 days postovulation) pregnancy test.
   2. Review previous laboratory results on electronic medical record; confirm negative STI screening per CDC STI guidelines.
   3. Obtain informed consent prior to insertion.
   4. Allow time for questions.

D. Helpful comments and considerations
 1. Move slowly and gently during all phases of IUC insertion to minimize the chance of perforation and vasovagal reaction.
 2. Use strictest sterile technique.
 3. Always read the manufacturer's instructions included in the IUC package because they vary slightly and are updated
 4. The withdrawal technique may minimize the risk of uterine perforation.
 5. Explain the procedure carefully to help the patient relax.
 6. Show the IUC and review the insertion technique.
 7. Vasovagal reactions may occur in women who
    a. Have not been pregnant for many years
    b. Are nulliparous
    c. Are very nervous and fearful
    d. Have an empty stomach
    e. Have a history of previous episodes of fainting
    f. Reactions are usually transient and spontaneously subside
    g. Are wearing a mask covering the nose and mouth
 8. Slow manipulation with the instruments decreases the risk of syncope
 9. Patient discomfort
    a. The woman may feel menstrual-type cramps during the sounding of the uterus and the actual insertion of the IUC.
    b. The tenaculum may cause a pinching sensation.
E. Equipment
 1. Sterile gloves
 2. Bivalve speculum
 3. Ring forceps
 4. Six to eight large swabs
 5. Tenaculum
 6. Uterine sound
 7. Antiseptic solution
 8. Sterile IUC in unopened package
 9. Scissors to trim string after insertion
 10. **Optional:** Paracervical block tray if approved by state to perform
F. Technique of the examination
 1. Perform a bimanual examination to reassess the position of the uterus (although this was done previously). Consistently observe patient for stability and comfort throughout the entire procedure. Warning: Perforations occur most often in an anteflexed or retroflexed uterus that was not diagnosed before the IUC was inserted.
 2. Visualize the cervix. If no signs of STI, proceed by cleaning with an antiseptic solution. If iodine is present in the antiseptic solution, rule out an allergy to iodine. If observe potential signs of STI, then halt procedure, screen for STI, and have patient return at a later date after confirming negative STI screening before proceeding.
 3. Next, a topical local anesthetic such as (Novocaine or Hurricane) may be applied to area where tenaculum is placed.
 4. Grasp the anterior lip of the cervix with a tenaculum about 1.5 to 2.0 cm from the os. Close the single-toothed tenaculum slowly, one notch at a time. (Use of a tenaculum is not always necessary, although it is generally recommended based on package insert.) Apply gentle traction to stabilize the uterus and straighten the canal.
    a. Warn that the woman may feel a pinching sensation.
    b. The tenaculum should avoid areas of blood vessels on the cervix.

      (1) If the cervix is anteverted, apply tenaculum at the 10-o'clock and 2-o'clock positions.

      (2) If the cervix is retroverted, apply the tenaculum to the cervix at the 4-o'clock and 8-o'clock positions.

5. Sound uterus slowly and gently until the resistance of the fundus is felt, to determine depth, direction, and configuration.

6. Measure the depth of the fundus by sounding the uterus.

   a. Place a cotton swab at the cervix when the sound is all the way in.

   b. Remove sound and swab while holding swab against sound.

   c. Measure distance between end of swab and end of sound.

   d. If the distance is less than 6 cm, expulsion, bleeding, pain, and perforation are more likely.

   e. If the distance is greater than 10 cm, decreased contraceptive effectiveness (increased cavity surface) may occur.

   f. No resistance may indicate perforation.

   g. Leave sound in place for a few seconds to dilate the cervix.

7. Load the contraceptive device into the inserter barrel under sterile conditions following package insert directions.

8. IUC loading instructions differ in how the T-shaped plastic frame is loaded into the inserter. ParaGard IUC folds the ends of the wings down into the inserter, whereas the Mirena, Skyla, Lyletta, and Kyleena IUCs fold the wings up into the inserter as they are pulled through with a gentle tug on the threads. Check the loading instructions on the product packaging before loading the device.

9. Apply steady, gentle traction on the tenaculum with nondominant hand.

   a. If it is anteverted, pull downward and outward.

   b. If it is retroverted, pull upward and outward.

10. Slowly advance insertion tube toward the top of the fundus following package insert instructions.

11. Release the device from the inserter into uterus following the directions in the package insert for each device type.

12. Remove insertion tube from vagina.

13. Remove tenaculum.

14. Use sterile, long scissors to trim the device strings perpendicular across, leaving 3 cm outside of cervical os.

15. Remove the speculum from vagina.

16. Assist patient to upright sitting position.

17. Assess patient for a few minutes prior to standing.

18. Assist patient to upright standing position. Observe for syncopal episode.

19. Some possible causes of string disappearance include:

   a. Retraction of strings into the cervical canal or uterus

   b. Cut too short during insertion

   c. Rotation of the device within the uterus

   d. If the string has disappeared, try to grasp strings with uterine forceps (no further than 1 in.) and pull them down into the vagina. A cytobrush may also be gently inserted in an attempt to retrieve the string.

   e. Perforation; recommend transvaginal ultrasound (3D is best) and possibly pelvic/abdominal x-ray

G. Postinsertion instructions

1. Teach the patient to feel for the string of the IUC before leaving the examining room.

   a. She should be instructed to feel for the IUC string similarly after each menses.

   b. May use a mirror to show the patient the placement in the os.

   c. Instruct the woman how to feel for the string.

      (1) Wash hands.

      (2) Assume a comfortable position, either lie down with knees on chest; standing with one leg on a chair, toilet, or stool; or sit on toilet.

      (3) Insert finger into vagina toward the cervix and feel for the strings.

      (4) Call the healthcare provider if no string is felt. It may simply be curled up in the cervix.

      (5) Avoid tugging on the string.

2. Call the clinician if moderate to severe uterine cramping occurs.

    a. Mild cramping over 1 to 3 days is normal. Treat with over-the-counter pain medication as needed.

    b. Cramping may occur intermittently 1 to 3 months after insertion.

3. Avoid use of tampons for the first 48 hours.

4. May want to avoid strenuous activity within 24 hours of insertion.

5. Call the clinician if you miss a period. This may occur with the LNG-IUC (Mirena, Skyla, Liletta, and Kyleena).

6. Condom use is always encouraged with sexual activity.

7. Chances of accidental pregnancy, although low, are highest during the first month. The patient may use additional contraception but this is usually not necessary.

8. A follow-up visit is encouraged anytime the strings are not felt or woman has concerns.

9. Keep a careful menstruation calendar.

10. Warn the woman that for the first few menstrual periods bleeding may be unchanged or heavier than normal. Over time, this will likely then be followed by reduced menstrual bleeding and possibly no menstrual bleeding.

11. Reinforce that the woman is at greatest risk of infection during the first month.

    a. Patient should observe for early signs of pelvic inflammatory disease (PID) and return immediately if present.

    b. Report increased and abnormal vaginal discharge, fever, or lower abdominal pain.

12. Review need for consistent use of condoms if at risk for STIs.

H. Postinsertion documentation. Clearly document the following:

1. Teaching and counseling provided

2. Uterine size, shape, and tenderness

3. Depth of uterine sounding

4. Type of IUC device used

5. Ease of insertion

6. How patient tolerated the procedure

7. Length of string

8. Any pregnancy screening results

9. Document device lot number

MANAGEMENT OF SIDE EFFECTS

A. Increased cramping. If this should occur:

1. Avoid strenuous exercise, and rest when possible.

2. Using a hot water bottle or heating pad placed on lower abdomen may be helpful.

3. Use over-the-counter analgesics as needed.

4. Call provider if concerned.

B. If partner feels string, return for evaluation.

1. **String too long:** Trim shorter.

2. **String too short:** If the device placement in the uterus is confirmed by ultrasound or x-ray, then removal is not required.

C. **Missed menses:** Return for a pregnancy test. May occur with Mirena, Skyla, Lyletta, and Kyleena *and is considered normal.*

D. **Increased vaginal discharge:** Evaluate for vaginitis, cervicitis, PID, and STIs.

E. **Heavy menses, anemia:** Monitor and workup as indicated.
   1. Treat anemia as indicated.

FOLLOW-UP VISIT AS NEEDED

A. If woman desires a follow-up visit
   1. Assess satisfaction with IUC.
   2. Review menstruation calendar.
   3. Check for the strings and trim if needed.
      a. If no strings are visualized, they can be extracted from the cervical canal by rotating two cotton-tipped applicators or inserting a Pap test cytobrush in the endocervical canal.
      b. If further maneuvers are required, the clinician should refer the patient to a gynecologist.
   4. Return in 1 year for annual well-woman exam (with or without a Pap per current guidelines).

B. Elicit information regarding the presence of:
   1. Foul-smelling vaginal discharge
   2. Lower backache
   3. Menorrhagia
   4. Dysmenorrhea
   5. New sexual partner(s)
   6. Fever

C. Evaluate for possible STIs and/or a vaginal infection by performing vaginal pH, amine/potassium hydroxide (KOH) testing, and wet mount/vaginal microscopy if infection is suspected.

D. Patient instructions as follows:
   1. Reinforce previous teaching.
   2. Return for annual well-woman visit.

REMOVAL

A. Reasons for removal
   1. Patient choice
      a. Desire to switch to alternative method of contraception
      b. Desires pregnancy
      c. Contraception no longer required
      d. Uncomfortable with side effects
      e. Patient preference for whatever reason
   2. Possible medical indications
      a. Accidental pregnancy
      b. Severe anemia resulting from persistent bleeding
      c. PID—controversial
      d. Excessive cramping and bleeding
      e. Development of a malignancy
      f. Pain with intercourse
      g. Partial expulsion of the device
      h. Cervical or fundal perforation
      i. Approximately 7% of women with IUCs will have actinomyces identified on their Pap tests and this may represent colonization, not infection. Symptomatic women with IUCs

should have the IUC removed and should receive antibiotics. However, the management of the asymptomatic carrier is controversial because actinomyces can be found normally in the genital tract cultures in healthy women without IUDs. False-positive findings of actinomycosis on Pap tests can be a problem. When possible, consider a confirmatory diagnostic test such as a culture, wet mount, or other appropriate screening test, per the CDC.

B. Technique
1. Insert speculum and visualize os.
2. Grasp tail with ring forceps.
3. If the IUD is embedded, the patient may require hysteroscopy.
4. Apply gentle, steady traction, being careful not to break the strings, and remove. Having the patient cough during this procedure may reduce her perception of any pain and distract her if there is pain with removal.
5. If gentle traction does not lead to IUC removal, refer to gynecologist.
6. Remove the speculum.
7. Examine the device for missing parts and for unusual discharge. *If unusual discharge is present, consider sending for culture.*
8. Instruct woman to remain sitting on the table for a few minutes. Observe for any dizziness.

MANAGEMENT OF SIDE EFFECTS AND COMPLICATIONS

A. PID
1. Positive cultures and IUC in place with no symptoms—treat without removal.
2. If PID, treat per CDC STI treatment guidelines, but if *not* improved within 72 hours, the device may be removed. Prudent clinical judgment must be used. Consider consulting a gynecologist if you are not sure about your plan of action.

B. **Bacterial vaginosis (BV):** Consider treating the patient with oral antibiotics (metronidazole) to prevent BV-associated endometritis; the IUC may remain in place.

C. **Endometritis:** Treat per CDC STI treatment guidelines for PID.

D. Pregnancy
1. Risk of pregnancy is very low.
2. Irregular menses commonly occur. With IUCs, lack of menses is no longer an indicator of pregnancy.
3. Routine pregnancy testing is not necessary.
4. Testing is indicated in a patient who has an abrupt change in bleeding patterns or who develops symptoms of pregnancy.
5. Although rare, women who conceive need to have ultrasonographic localization of the gestational sac to rule out ectopic pregnancy. This is because pregnancy in the context of an IUC is more likely to be ectopic.
6. In pregnancy, the IUC should be removed because the risk of miscarriage, sepsis, premature labor, and delivery increase. In this context, referral to a gynecologist for IUC removal must be considered.

E. Actinomyces
1. Actinomyces may be reported on the Pap test in up to 7% of IUC users. This may be normal colonization (not infection).
2. If the patient is asymptomatic and the clinical examination indicates no infection, then no treatment is needed and the clinician may leave the device in place.
3. If the patient is symptomatic, the device should be removed and oral antibiotics given. Penicillin 500 mg orally four times a day for 1 month is recommended.

4. May replace device after repeat culture performed 3 months later shows absence of actinomyces.
5. LNG-IUCs are less likely than copper intrauterine devices to harbor actinomyces-like bacteria as identified on Pap test.

EXPULSION

A. Removal of partially expelled IUC
   1. Grasp the string or tip with ring forceps.
   2. Evaluate the patient for infection or pregnancy.
   3. Reinsert another IUC if the woman desires.

BIBLIOGRAPHY

American Cancer Society. (2021). The American Cancer Society guidelines for the prevention and early detection of cervical cancer. https://www.cancer.org/cancer/cervical-cancer/detection-diagnosis-staging/cervical-cancer-screening-guidelines.html

Bayer Healthcare. (2021a). *Kyleena* [package insert]. https://labeling.bayerhealthcare.com/html/products/pi/Kyleena_PI.pdf

Bayer Healthcare. (2021b). *Mirena* [package insert]. https://labeling.bayerhealthcare.com/html/products/pi/Mirena_PI.pdf

Bayer Healthcare. (2021c). *Skyla* [package insert]. https://labeling.bayerhealthcare.com/html/products/pi/Skyla_PI.pdf

Centers for Disease Control and Prevention. (2021). Sexually transmitted infections treatment guidelines, 2021. https://www.cdc.gov/std/treatment-guidelines/default.htm

Curtis, K. M., Jatlaoui, T. C., Tepper, N. K., Zapata, L. B., Horton, L. G., Jamieson, D. J., & Whiteman, M. K. (2016). U.S. selected practice recommendations for contraceptive use, 2016. *MMWR Recommendations and Reports, 65*(4), 1–66. https://doi.org/10.15585/mmwr.rr6504a1

Holland, A. C., Shah, B., Metcalf, N., & Pridgen, K. (2020). Preparing for intrauterine device consults and procedures. *Women's Healthcare, 8*(6), 37–43.

Odyssea Pharma, Belgium. (2021). *Liletta* [product insert]. Allergan Pharmaceuticals. https://media.allergan.com/actavis/actavis/media/allergan-pdf-documents/product-prescribing/liletta_pi.pdf

Pocius, K. D., & Bartz, D. A. (2018). Intrauterine contraception: Management of side effects and complications. In C. A. Schreiber (Ed.), *UpToDate*. https://www.uptodate.com/contents/intrauterine-contraception-management-of-side-effects-and-complications

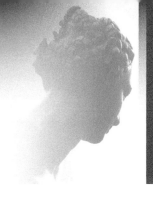

44

CONTRACEPTIVE IMPLANTS

AIMEE CHISM HOLLAND, KATHLEEN PRIDGEN,
NICOLE METCALF, MEGHAN M. WHITFIELD, R. MIMI SECOR,
AND KAHLIL A. DEMONBREUN

ETONOGESTREL IMPLANT (NEXPLANON) EXPLAINED

A. Nexplanon is a progestin-only, single-rod, subdermal contraceptive implant that utilizes the third-generation progestin 3-keto-desogestrel (etonogestrel) and has a reported efficacy of up to 3 years.
  1. Over 11 million implants have been inserted worldwide in more than 60 countries since 1998.
  2. The etonogestrel implant was initially approved by the Food and Drug Administration (FDA) in the United States in 2006 and marketed under the product name Implanon. Nexplanon (approved in 2011) differs from Implanon in the following ways: It is impregnated with barium sulfate, rendering it radiopaque, and utilizes an improved specialized insertion system that reduces the risk of inserting the device too deeply.
  3. Consists of a 4-cm long by 2-mm wide (1.57 × 0.078 in.) rod with a rate-controlling membrane of 37% ethylene vinyl acetate (EVA) copolymer, 3% barium sulfate (15 mg), and 60% etonogestrel (68 mcg).
  4. The progestin is released at a rate of 60 mcg to 70 mcg initially and then decreases to 25 mcg to 30 mcg by the third year.
  5. Is a long-acting, low-dose, quickly reversible, progestin-only method of contraception.
  6. Average retail cost ranges from $600 to $1300 for the device, and insertion charges range from $125 to $300.
  7. Many private insurers cover all or some of the cost of the device as well as insertion and removal. Merck offers a program that will investigate patients' insurance policies to determine coverage and copays.
  8. Many state Medicaid programs cover the device as well as insertion and removal in full.
  9. A careful and correct subdermal placement technique is crucial to successful insertion and facilitates removal.
  10. Per FDA requirements, all providers must complete a free educational program on Nexplanon provided by the manufacturer before inserting or removing these implants. Clinician training can be requested here: https://www.nexplanontraining.com/request-clinical-training/in-person-training
B. Effectiveness
  1. Six pregnancies were reported in 20,648 cycles. Each conception was likely to have occurred before removal or within 2 weeks after removal.
  2. The cumulative Pearl Index is 0.38 pregnancies per 100 woman-years of use.
  3. The efficacy of Nexplanon in women who weighed more than 130% of their ideal body weight has not been defined because such women were not studied in clinical trials.
C. Mechanism of action
  1. Primarily inhibits ovulation
  2. Secondarily increases viscosity of cervical mucus

3. Thins the lining of the endometrium
4. It is *not* an abortifacient

D. Indications
1. Nexplanon can be used by any woman who:
   a. Seeks a safe, highly effective, long-term, reversible form of contraception
   b. Cannot take estrogen because of contraindications or intolerance of side effects
   c. Has a history of poor compliance with other methods of contraception
   d. Does not desire future pregnancies but is unsure of permanent sterilization
   e. Because of health problems or medication use should not become pregnant

E. Advantages
1. Does not contain estrogen, hence can be used for effective hormonal contraception in women who cannot use estrogen.
2. Can be used postpartum in breastfeeding women. Less than 0.2% estimated absolute maternal dose is excreted in breast milk. Does not affect production or quality of breast milk.
3. Effective immediately when inserted at the proper time (see manufacturer's insert)
4. Causes stable hemoglobin levels with use because menstrual blood loss is less than in women who are not using this method.
5. A highly effective, safe, and rapidly reversible method that requires little adherence from user.
6. Free 2- to 3-hour training program offered to teach product insertion and removal.
7. Method is paid for up front. If patient's financial or insurance status changes in those 3 years, contraception is already paid for.
8. Nexplanon is discreet and does not affect sexual spontaneity.

F. Disadvantages
1. May cause unpredictable bleeding patterns throughout the duration of the 3 years of use.
2. Weight changes may occur in women who use Nexplanon. Some women gain weight, and some women lose weight. The number of women who gain is about equal to the number of those who lose weight. Total weight gain is minimal, that is, less than 2 to 3 pounds per year.
3. Cost can be a disadvantage for some women as all the costs for this method are paid up front.
4. Some women do not like that they cannot start or stop this method without the assistance of a clinician and so feel less in control.
5. Some women do not like the idea of a foreign object being inserted into their bodies.
6. The implant may be slightly noticeable.
7. The implant offers no protection from acquiring sexually transmitted infections.

G. Irregular bleeding
1. Bleeding is the most common reason for removal. The patient needs to be educated that this is to be expected and that it is a normal side effect. If the patient is intolerant of irregular bleeding, she may not want to choose implants.
2. Counsel patient that bleeding may be light or heavy, last for a few days or many days in a row, or be absent for several months.
3. Bleeding patterns are not necessarily similar to other progestin-only methods of contraception. Patients' experiences with other methods of progestin-only contraception do not predict what the experience with Nexplanon will be.
4. Typically, the mean bleeding days per 90-day reference time show that using Nexplanon is associated with fewer total bleeding and/or spotting days than not using any hormones.
5. Prostaglandin inhibitors (nonsteroidal anti-inflammatory drugs [NSAIDs]), combined oral contraceptives (COCs; if medically eligible), or a trial of supplemental estrogen (if applicable) have been shown to be effective in the management of abnormal bleeding.

BOX 44.1 Contraindications of Nexplanon Use

- Known or suspected pregnancy
- Hypersensitivity to any components of etonogestrel implant
- Known, suspected, or past personal history of breast cancer
- Current or past history of thrombolytic disease
- Hepatic tumor or active liver disease
- Undiagnosed genital bleeding
- Allergic reaction to Nexplanon components

---

    a. The preferred option is NSAIDs (e.g., naproxen) 440 mg stat, then repeat every 6–8 hours bid tid x 5 to 7 days (taken with food).

    b. Another option is one pack of COCs x 1 month

    c. Another option is to administer oral estradiol 20 to 25 mcg daily x 1 month (off label).

H. Contraindications/warnings/precautions are summarized in Boxes 44.1 and 44.2.

I. Drug interactions

    1. Women who take drugs that are potent inducers of hepatic enzymes should not use etonogestrel, as these drugs potentially can decrease the efficacy of etonogestrel and therefore may result in an unintended pregnancy.

    2. Examples of these drugs include griseofulvin, barbiturates, rifampin, phenytoin, carbamazepine, felbamate, oxcarbazepine, topiramate, and modafinil.

J. Special considerations

    1. To assist clinicians in the decision-making process for providing the etonogestrel implant to women, the Centers for Disease Control and Prevention (CDC) U.S. medical eligibility criteria for contraception use (U.S. MEC) defined the following conditions affecting eligibility for the use of progestin-only contraceptive implants.

        a. 1 = A condition for which there is no restriction for the use of the contraceptive method

        b. 2 = A condition for which the advantages of using the method generally outweigh the theoretical or proven risks

        c. 3 = A condition for which the theoretical or proven risks usually outweigh the advantages of using the method

        d. 4 = A condition that represents an unacceptable health risk if the contraceptive method is used

        e. The full summary chart can be obtained from www.cdc.gov/reproductivehealth/contraception/pdf/summary-chart-us-medical-eligibility-criteria_508tagged.pdf

---

BOX 44.2 Warning and Precautions for Nexplanon Use

- Arterial cardiovascular disease
- History of cerebrovascular accident
- Systemic lupus erythematosus (antibody positive or unknown)
- Smoking
- Diabetes mellitus
- Severe cirrhosis
- Current and history of ischemic heart disease

2. Recommendations for use in postpartum women (nonbreastfeeding/breastfeeding)
   a. Less than 21 days   U.S. MEC category 1/U.S. MEC category 2
   b. 21 days to less than 30 days   U.S. MEC category 1/U.S. MEC category 2
   c. 30 to 42 days   U.S. MEC category 1/U.S. MEC category 2
   d. Greater than 42 days   U.S. MEC category 1/U.S. MEC category 1
3. Recommendations for use postabortion
   a. First trimester   U.S. MEC category 1
   b. Second trimester   U.S. MEC category 1
   c. Immediate postseptic abortion   U.S. MEC category 1

NEXPLANON INSERTION

A. Counseling
   1. Appropriate counseling is essential for proper selection of implants for contraception.
   2. It is best to do this during a visit separate from product insertion.
   3. Explain what it is, how it works, its advantages and disadvantages, bleeding patterns, what to expect at insertion and removal, contraindications, and costs.
   4. Informed consent may be obtained at this visit or at the time of insertion.
B. When to insert. Pregnancy must be excluded before insertion.
   1. Before clinicians can insert or remove Nexplanon, they must complete a training program provided at no cost by the manufacturer per FDA regulations.
   2. If the patient is not using any hormonal contraception, it can be inserted on days 1 to 7 of her menstrual cycle.
   3. If the patient is switching from combined oral contraceptive, Nexplanon can be inserted any time within 7 days from the last dose of active hormone pill.
   4. If the patient is switching from a progesterone-only pill and has not skipped any pills that month, Nexplanon can be inserted at any time while still taking the progestin-only pills. They can be stopped after the device is inserted.
   5. If the patient has a Nexplanon insert that is due for removal and wishes to continue with Nexplanon, a new one can be inserted right after removal through the same incision.
   6. If the patient is switching from medroxyprogesterone acetate injections, Nexplanon can be inserted during the 2-week window when the next injection would have been due.
   7. Nexplanon can be inserted within the first 7 days after a spontaneous or induced abortion (U.S. MEC 1).
   8. It can be inserted any time postpartum and breastfeeding exclusively (U.S. MEC category 2 if less than 1-month postpartum and U.S. MEC category 1 if greater than 1-month postpartum).
   9. If Nexplanon is inserted according to the preceding guidelines, it is effective immediately.
   10. If the patient has an intrauterine contraceptive (IUC), Nexplanon can be inserted the same day as the device's removal.
   11. If switching from an IUC and the women has had sexual intercourse since the start of her current menstrual cycle and it has been more than 5 days, the following options should be considered:
       a. Advise her to retain the IUC for at least 7 days after insertion of the implant.
       b. Advise her to abstain from sexual intercourse or use a barrier contraception for 7 days before removing the IUC.
       c. Advise her to use emergency contraception at the time of IUC removal.
   12. If Nexplanon is being inserted outside these guidelines, the patient should be advised to use a nonhormonal form of backup contraception for 7 days.
C. Equipment required

1. Comes in a sterile, disposable, preloaded applicator
2. A comfortable table with support for the patient's arm (a pillow works well) is needed.
3. Sterile gloves, antiseptic solution, local anesthetic, sterile gauze, skin closures, paper tape, and elastic gauze dressing are needed.

D. Insertion procedure
1. Nondominant arm is used.
2. Insertion site is overlying the triceps muscle about 8 to 10 cm (3–4 in.) from the medial condyle of the humerus and 3 to 5 cm (1.25–2 inches) posterior to the sulcus between the biceps and triceps muscles. This location is recommended to avoid the large blood vessels and nerves surrounding the sulcus. If unable to insert in this location, then insert the implant as far posterior as possible from the sulcus.
3. Insertion is always subdermal.
4. Approved clinicians should follow the insertion procedure directions found in the package insert.
5. Experienced clinicians can insert Nexplanon in 1 to 2 minutes.
6. Correct placement must be confirmed right after insertion by palpation.
7. Careful and correct subdermal insertion is necessary for successful placement and will facilitate removal.
    a. Three years after insertion, if the patient wants to continue with an etonogestrel implant, a new rod can be inserted at the time the initial rod is removed, at the same site.

E. Postinsertion instructions
    a. Request the patient to palpate the implant.
    b. Apply a pressure bandage to minimize bruising.
    c. Complete the user card and give to the patient to keep.
    d. Document insertion note in the patient's medical record.

F. Postinsertion complications
1. Pain at insertion site occurred in fewer than 3% of women.
2. Redness, swelling, and hematoma were reported in less than 1% of women.

IMPLANT REMOVAL PROCEDURE

A. **When to remove:** The etonogestrel implant should be removed at the patient's request or when the time period has expired (Box 44.3).

B. Patient education points
1. Most removals take about 5 to 10 minutes.
2. Minor to no discomfort is experienced at the time of removal.
3. Postremoval, the patient may have some bruising and tenderness at the site.

C. Changing to another method of contraception
1. Another method of contraception can be initiated immediately postremoval without loss of contraceptive efficacy; that is, oral contraceptives, contraceptive ring, patches, or IUC.

BOX 44.3 Circumstances for the Removal of the Implant

Nexplanon should be removed:
1. If the patient wants to conceive
2. If patient wants to change to another form of contraception
3. If there are side effects, such as inability to tolerate unscheduled vaginal bleeding, allergic reaction, or other unexpected adverse reactions

PATIENT AND PROVIDER RESOURCES

A. The manufacturer has a comprehensive program for provider and patient education and support that can be accessed by visiting www.Nexplanon-USA.com or calling 1-877-467-5266.

B. For full prescribing information, see the package insert available on the manufacturer's website.

BIBLIOGRAPHY

American College of Obstetricians and Gynecologists. (2021). ACOG Practice Bulletin No. 186: *Long-acting reversible contraception: Implants and intrauterine devices.* https://www.acog.org/clinical/clinical-guidance/practice-bulletin/articles/2017/11/long-acting-reversible-contraception-implants-and-intrauterine-devices

Bahamondes, L., Fernandex, A., Monterior, I., & Bahamondes, M. V. (2020). Long-acting reversible contraceptive methods. *Best Practice & Research Clinical Obstetrics & Gynecology, 66*, 28–40. https://doi.org/10.1016/j.bpobgyn.2019.12.002.

Curtis, K. M., Jatlaoui, T. C., Tepper, N. K., Zapata, L. B., Horton, L. G. Jamieson, D. J., & Whiteman, M. K. (2016). U.S. selected practice recommendations for contraception use. *Morbidity and Mortality Weekly Report, 65*(4), 1–66. Retrieved from https://www.cdc.gov/mmwr/volumes/65/rr/rr6504a1.htm

Curtis, K. M., Tepper, N. K., Jatlaoui, T. C., Berry-Bibee, E. Horton, L. G., Zapata, L. B., Simmons, K. B., Pagano, H. P., Jamieson, D. J., & Whiteman, M. K. (2016). U.S. medical eligibility criteria for contraception use, 2016. *Morbidity and Mortality Weekly Report, 65*, 1–108. https://doi.org/10.15585/mmwr.rr6503a1 https://www.cdc.gov/mmwr/volumes/65/rr/pdfs/rr6503.pdf

Darney, P. D. (2022). *Etonogestrel contraceptive implant.* UpToDate. https://www-uptodate-com.ezproxy3.lhl.uab.edu/contents/etonogestrel-contraceptive-implant?search=nexplanon&source=search_result&selectedTitle=2~49&usage_type=default&display_rank=1

Organon Global Inc. (2021). *Nexplanon prescribing information.* https://www.organon.com/product/usa/pi_circulars/n/nexplanon/nexplanon_pi.pdf

Tepper, N. K., Curtis, K. M., Jamieson, D. J., & Marchbanks, P. A. (2011). Update to *CDC's U.S medical eligibility criteria for contraceptive use, 2010:* Revised recommendations for the use of contraceptive methods during the postpartum period. *Morbidity and Mortality Weekly Report, 60*(26), 878–883. http://www.cdc.gov/mmwr/pdf/wk/mm6026.pdf

Unit IX

INVESTIGATIVE PROCEDURES

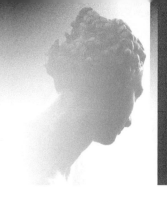

45

CERVICAL CANCER SCREENING AND COLPOSCOPY

NANCY R. BERMAN, KIM CHOMA, AND REBECCA KOENIGER-DONOHUE

SCREENING FOR CERVICAL CANCER

A. According to the American Cancer Society (ACS), cervical cancer is fourth to breast cancer as a leading type of cancer in women globally (ACS, 2021a). In the United States, cervical cancer is the second leading cause of death in women aged 20 to 39 years (Luvero et al., 2020). Since the introduction of the Pap test in the 1950s, cervical cancer rates in the United States have been reduced by 75%. While the Pap test alone has reduced cervical cancer in well-screened populations, the incidence of cervical cancer in the United States in 2021 was still reported to be 14,480 cases with 4,290 deaths, with a higher incidence in unscreened and underscreened women, and with geographic disparities. Screening women who have never been screened or have not been screened adequately will make the biggest impact on reducing cervical cancer rates. In addition, primary prevention of human papillomavirus (HPV) infection by vaccination and the addition of HPV testing in screening allows for increased prevention of cervical cancer and detection of precancerous lesions.

B. The approach to cervical cancer screening is based on the knowledge that the majority of women will be exposed to one or more types of oncogenic HPV (high-risk types), and most infections will be cleared by 24 months. Some women will not clear their infections and long-term persistent infection is a necessary cause of cervical cancer. Cervical cytology will identify women with abnormal cells caused by HPV. HPV testing will identify women who may have persistent infection and may have disease that was missed by the Pap or are at future risk for the development of neoplasia and progression to cancer as long as the virus persists.

1. The Pap
   a. The Pap test cytologic sampling technique, or Pap test, named for Dr. George Papanicolaou, was invented in 1941. It is a screening tool only and it is not diagnostic for disease. Tissue obtained from the cervix through directed biopsy or excision by scalpel, laser, or electrical loop is necessary for making a diagnosis of cervical cell pathology.
      (1) During the Pap test, the clinician collects desquamated cells of the female cervix.
      (2) The sample is sent to a pathologist where the cells are evaluated for size, shape, and regularity. Should an abnormality be reported, the clinician will determine whether a diagnostic procedure is needed.
   b. The most common diagnostic procedure used to confirm the results of the Pap test is a colposcopy.
      (1) The provider looks through the colposcope at the cervical or vaginal tissue after acetic acid (vinegar) has been applied.
      (2) Directed biopsies can be taken during the colposcopy and the tissue is analyzed.
      (3) Treatment decisions are based on the histological results of the tissue biopsy and correlation with the cytology and colposcopic impression.

   c. The Pap test results are reported using the 2001 Bethesda system of cytologic classification (Nayar & Wilbur, 2014; Solomon et al., 2002.). The gold standard used to interpret the Pap test findings are the algorithms developed by American Society for Colposcopy and Cervical Pathology (ASCCP; Perkins et al., 2020).

   d. There are two acceptable ways to prepare the collected cells for examination. The first is the conventional dry slide method in which collected cells are fixed onto a slide immediately and the second is to use a liquid-based medium. In using liquid-based cytology (LBC), the cells are mixed into a vial of liquid and a slide is prepared in the laboratory from the cells in the vial. The residual solution may be used for HPV testing, and in some laboratories gonorrhea, chlamydia, and trichomonas testing may be performed from the sample as well.

   e. The Pap test is intended to detect the changes in cervical cells caused by infection with HPV and are graded according to the degree of abnormality and the cell type that is involved. This may range from an equivocal change to either a low- or high-grade change (precancerous) to cancer.

   f. The Pap test is a valuable screening test because it is relatively inexpensive and can detect precancerous conditions long before they become cancerous.

   g. The limitations of the Pap test are:
      (1) Errors in Pap tests can be broadly categorized as errors in sampling and preparation, screening, or interpretation.
      (2) Sampling and preparation represent the greatest limitation because the sample must contain a representative cellular smear.

2. High-risk HPV testing
   a. In 2003, the U.S. Food and Drug Administration (FDA) approved high-risk HPV testing along with Pap testing to screen women 30 years and older.

   b. Testing women for high-risk HPV starting at age 30 years along with the Pap test is called *co-testing*. The FDA-approved age for co-testing women starting at 30 years was based on data in 2003.

   c. The peak age for HPV prevalence is in the mid-20s and the majority of infections are cleared by 24 months.

   d. HPV infections have two potential outcomes; the virus is no longer detected or persistence. Infections that persist increase the risk of the development of neoplasia and progression to pre-cancer or invasive cancer over time. If a woman 30 years and older is positive for high-risk HPV, this is most likely due to a persistent infection.

   e. Long-term persistent infection is necessary for the development of significant neoplasia and progression to cancer.

   f. Co-testing will identify women with persistent infection who may have neoplastic change that was missed by the Pap.

   g. Co-testing will identify women at future risk, who may develop neoplasia as long as they remain high-risk HPV positive and should be followed diligently as long as they remain positive.

3. Primary HPV screening for cervical cancer
   a. On April 25, 2014, the FDA approved the Roche cobas HPV test (Roche Diagnostics, Indianapolis, Indiana) for the primary screening of women 25 years and older. This means testing with a stand-alone high-risk HPV test first instead of a Pap test.
      (1) Data from the ATHENA Trial, which led to FDA approval, identified a significant number of women 25 to 29 years of age with high-grade disease and the age of approval was based on that data. The ATHENA trial enrolled more than 47,000 women and demonstrated that one in four women who are HPV 16 positive will have cervical disease within 3 years and that nearly one in seven women with normal cytology, who were HPV positive, actually had highgrade cervical disease that was missed by cytology.

b. The Roche cobas test provides a positive or negative result for a panel of 12 high-risk HPV types and a separate result for HPV 16 and 18 that are associated with most cervical cancers. It also has an internal control for specimen adequacy.

c. In 2018, the FDA approved a second HPV test for HPV primary screening: the BD Onclarity test (BD Onclarity test, Franklin Lakes, New Jersey). The Onclarity test has been FDA approved for expanded genotyping that includes 16, 18, 31, 45, 51, 52 and a grouped result of eight other types, though expanded genotyping is not yet included in management algorithms.

d. The Roche test was approved for primary screening after data from the Addressing the Need for Advanced HPV Diagnostics (ATHENA) trial was presented to a panel at the FDA.

e. Primary screening by HPV testing identifies not only women at risk for disease, but also identifies women who have future risk.

f. Clinical guidance for the management of the results of this testing was affirmed in 2021 by The American College of Obstetricians and Gynecologists (ACOG). This Practice Advisory supports the role of primary HPV screening and the strategies for reflexing to a Pap test on all HPV positive screens and referral to colposcopy.

4. Statistics
   a. Since 1941, cervical cancer incidence rates have decreased approximately 75% and mortality rates 70%.
   b. The Pap test has reduced the disease burden from cervical cancer by 75% since its introduction. However, cervical cancer continues to be a significant health issue (Box 45.1).
   c. More Black and Hispanic women are diagnosed with cervical cancer and are diagnosed at later stages of the disease than women of other races (incidence rates 9.0 cases/100,000 women and 9.5 cases/100,000 women, respectively), possibly due to decreased access to Pap testing or follow-up treatment (ACS, 2021b).
   d. Cancers missed by laboratories represent only a tiny fraction of cervical cancers. Many women diagnosed with cervical cancer have not been screened recently prior to their diagnosis (ACS, 2021).

5. HPV epidemiology
   a. HPV is widespread. In the United States, approximately 1,700 new HPV infections occur daily, with 6.2 million new infections every year (incidence), and there are 20 million active infections every year (prevalence).
   b. Approximately 75% to 80% of both males and females will be infected in their lifetime.
   c. The Centers for Disease Control and Prevention (CDC) estimates $8 billion per year is spent in direct medical costs for preventing and treating HPV-associated disease.
   d. Up to 40% of women are infected with HPV within 24 months of first sexual intercourse.
   e. HPV is the most common STI in the world, having a negative impact on an individual's social life (CDC, 2021a). Condoms can reduce the incidence by 70%.
   f. Infection rates peak in the mid-20s, with highest prevalence in 20- to 24-year-olds, then decrease as the woman ages. In women ages 14 to 19 years, the prevalence of HPV infection is 35%. Conversely, the prevalence in women 50 to 65 years is just 6%.
   g. Long-term persistence of HPV infection may lead to the development of high-grade neoplasia and progression to cancer.

BOX 45.1 Women Who Died of Cancer of the Cervix Uteri

In 2021, an estimated 14,480 American women were diagnosed with cervical cancer, and 4,290 women died of cancer of the cervix uteri (ACS, 2021a).

h. Most lesions caused by HPV are transient and will regress spontaneously. Research indicates that 91% of HPV infections in women older than 18 years resolve within 2 years (Massad et al., 2013); 61% of low-grade squamous intraepithelial lesions (LSILs) in young women regress at 12 months and 91% regress at 36 months; 3% of LSILs progress to high-grade SILs (HSILs).

6. Development of cervical abnormalities: Understanding the transformation zone (TZ)

   a. There are two types of cervical cells.

      (1) **Columnar epithelial cells:** The interior of the cervical canal is lined with columnar tissue that contains mucus-secreting glands.

      (2) **Squamous epithelial cells:** The ectocervix is covered with a different type of flat tissue, called *squamous epithelial tissue*. This tissue is pink and shiny.

   b. These two types of tissue meet at the squamocolumnar junction, or the transformation zone (TZ). Where these cell types abut, due to the acidity of the vagina, there is a change process during which the villous tips of columnar cells are burned (by the acidic vaginal pH) and begin a transformation process to become mature squamous cells after becoming metaplastic cells. The endocervical cells (ECs) are located in the TZ (Figure 45.1).

   c. Significance of the TZ

      (1) The majority of malignant and premalignant diseases arise in the TZ. This is an area of rapidly changing metaplastic cells that vary with hormonal status (Table 45.1).

      (2) The presence of these cells on the Pap suggests that the area where most lesions occur has been represented in the sample.

   d. These cells are absent in 10% of Pap tests in premenopausal women and in 50% of postmenopausal women.

   e. The TZ shifts in response to age and hormone levels.

   f. Infection of the cervix with high-risk HPV is a requirement for the development of virtually all cervical carcinomas (squamous cell and adenocarcinoma).

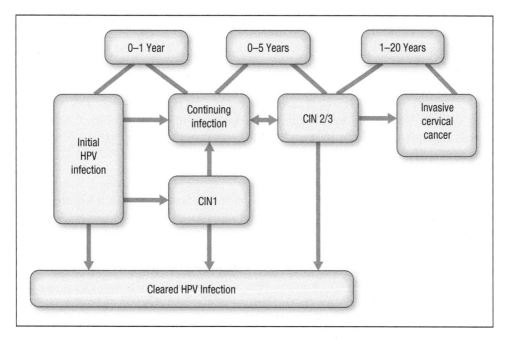

FIGURE 45.1 Progression of invasive carcinoma.

CIN, cervical intraepithelial neoplasia; HPV, human papillomavirus.

TABLE 45.1 Transformation Zone (Squamocolumnar Junction) Shifts in Response to Age and Hormonal Alterations

DEVELOPMENTAL PERIOD	PATHOPHYSIOLOGIC PROCESS	LOCATION OF TRANSFORMATION ZONE
Puberty	Squamous tissue slowly replaces the glandular tissue on the ectocervix under the influence of estrogen	Junction on the surface of the cervix
Early to middle years	Remains relatively stable	Junction at the cervical os
Menopause	Continued maturation of the transformation zone may lead to migration of mature squamous epithelium proximally up the cervical canal	Junction recedes inside the os

g. HPV has a unique mechanism of infection in that it can only bind to the outermost layer of the cervical epithelium. It then requires capsid proteins to infect deeper layers of the epithelium and complete its life cycle.

  (1) LSILs are characterized by abnormalities in the cells of the lower third of the epithelium. Most of these lesions are transient and will regress over time.

  (2) HSILs occur when abnormal cells proliferate into the basal layer of the cervical epithelium. A percentage of these lesions will progress to invasive cancer over time.

h. The addition of co-factors may trigger malignant transformation (Box 45.2)

i. Of the more than 100 known HPV types that may infect humans, approximately 40 infect the female genital tract. Fourteen of these are considered oncogenic or high-risk carcinogenic types for cervical carcinoma.

j. Two high-risk types, HPV-16 and HPV-18, account for nearly 70% of cervical carcinomas. Two low-risk types, HPV-6 and HPV-11, cause 90% of anogenital warts.

k. HPV testing should target only high-risk carcinogenic cancer-associated types.

l. Types of cancer detected

  (1) Squamous cell carcinomas, 70%

  (2) Adenocarcinomas, 18%

  (3) Adenosquamous carcinomas, 4%

  (4) Other carcinomas or malignancies, 6.5%

m. HSIL may progress to cervical cancer and become invasive (see Figure 45.1).

n. The peak incidence of HSIL occurs between the ages of 35 and 45 years.

o. **It generally takes 10 to 15 years from precancer to the development of invasive cancer. Rapid development of invasive carcinoma is rare** (see Figure 45.1).

7. Symptoms

a. **Most cervical cancer is asymptomatic.**

b. Abnormal uterine/cervical bleeding is the most significant finding. It is usually associated with friability of the diseased cervix, occurring as postcoital or midcycle spotting.

BOX 45.2 Possible Cofactors That Trigger Malignant Transformation

- Coinfection with or exposure to other sexually transmitted infections
- HIV
- Smoking
- Nutritional deficiencies

BOX 45.3 Risk Factors for Cervical Cancer

- Unprotected sex, particularly if with multiple partners
- Early coitarche (age of first intercourse <16 years)
- A sexual partner with more than one sexual partner or a history of multiple sexual partners
- Exposure to or infection with other sexually transmitted diseases
- HPV, particularly if concomitant smoking
- DES exposure
- Previous abnormal cervical cancer screening test
- HIV
- Malnutrition
- Infrequent screening
- Lack of access to regular screenings

DES, diethylstilbestrol; HPV, human papillomavirus.

---

8. Risk factors and prevention
   a. The clinician should assess each patient for cervical cancer risk factors (Box 45.3).
   b. Women should be taught measures to reduce the risk for cervical cancer (Box 45.4).
   c. Clinicians should use strategies for increasing the use of the Pap test and age-appropriate HPV testing.
      (1) Speak regularly to all female patients about the risk of cervical cancer and the need for regular screening.
      (2) Reduce the costs associated with the procedure.
      (3) Provide easy access to screening.
9. Screening
   a. Screening recommendations are age dependent (see guidelines from the U.S. Preventive Services Task Force [USPSTF], ACOG, ACS, and ASCCP).
   b. Screening options: All specimens are collected into a liquid-based vial:
      (1) **Pap test only:** Ordered on the requisition with option to request reflex to an HPV test for any ASC-US Pap (reflex HPV test)
      (2) **Co-testing:** Both Pap and HPV test are ordered at time of screening
      (3) **Primary HPV screening:** Only an HPV test is ordered. In current guidelines, a Pap is performed in the laboratory from the residual liquid in the vial on any positive HPV test (reflex Pap).
   c. Initiation of screening
      (1) Women younger than 21 years should *not* be screened.

BOX 45.4 Measures to Reduce the Risk of Cervical Cancer

- Get an HPV vaccine
- Avoid early coitarche (age of first intercourse)
- Limit the number of sexual partners
- Use condoms consistently and correctly with every episode of oral, vaginal, or anal intercourse
- Cervical cancer screening test screening per ASCCP guidelines
- Avoid smoking cigarettes

ASCCP, American Society for Colposcopy and Cervical Pathology; HPV, human papillomavirus.

(2) Start screening at age 21 years, regardless of coitarche
- An exception is the new 2020 ACS recommendation to delay the start of screening to age 25.
- The ACOG, ASCCP, and The Society of Gynecologic Oncologists (SGO) still recommend initiating the first screening at age 21.

d. Age 21 to 25 years
   (1) Screening is recommended with cytology alone every 3 years.

e. Age 25 to 65 years
   (1) ACS guideline preferred screening: HPV test every 5 years

OR

f. Age 30 to 65 years
   (1) Preferred screening—Primary HPV testing every 5 years.
   - Co-testing every 5 years is acceptable.
   - Pap alone may be used if HPV testing is not available.

g. There are two options in managing co-testing results
   (1) Women who are Pap/negative and HPV/positive
   - Perform Pap and HPV in 12 months.
   - If the HPV test is still positive, and the Pap is negative, refer for colposcopy.
   (2) Genotyping may be performed for HPV-16 and HPV18
   - If positive for HPV-16 or HPV-18, immediate referral for colposcopy is needed.
   (3) Sexual history does not alter the frequency of co-testing. Guidelines indicate that exposure to a new partner does not require that screening be obtained earlier than the next routine screen.

h. Age to start co-testing or primary HPV screening
   (1) Co-testing with Pap and HPV begins at age 30 years and the age to start was determined by data at the time of FDA approval in 2003.
   (2) Stand-alone primary HPV screening begins at age 25 years and the age to start was due to data at the time of its FDA approval in 2014.
   (3) HPV testing should be performed with an FDA-approved test. There are currently five tests on the market.
   - Hybrid Capture 2 (QIAGEN)
     - Tests for a panel of 13 high-risk types
     - Reported as positive or negative for the panel
   - Cobas (Roche; FDA-approved test for primary HPV)
     - Tests for a panel of 12 high-risk types and uses a separate test for HPV-16/HPV-18
     - Reported as positive or negative for the panel and individually for HPV-16 and HPV-18
   - Cervista (Hologic)
     - Tests for a panel of 14 high-risk types
     - Reported as positive or negative for the panel
     - If the panel is positive, a test for 16/18 may be ordered.
   - Aptima HPV mRNA (Hologic)
     - Tests for a panel of 14 high-risk types
     - If the panel is positive, a test for HPV-16 and HPV-18 may be ordered
   - BD Onclarity (FDA-approved test for primary HPV)
     - Tests for HPV-16, HPV-18, HPV-31, HPV-45, HPV-51, HPV-52, and a grouped result of eight other types
   (4) Acceptable screening—Cytology alone every 3 years.

i. Age greater than 65 years
   (1) It is *not* recommended to screen this age group when there has been adequate negative screening in the previous 10 years.

- Adequate negative screening occurs when there have been three negative Pap tests or two negative co-tests (Pap and HPV) in the past 10 years with no history of an abnormal result during this time.
  - If at 65 years, the Pap is reported as atypical squamous cells of undetermined significance (ASC-US) and the HPV is negative, an accelerated repeat co-testing at 12 months is recommended. If negative on both, the patient may be exited out of screening.
  - (2) Once testing has stopped, it should not be started again, regardless of sexual history.
  - (3) **Women with a history of treatment for precancer should continue to be tested for at least 25 years after that diagnosis, even if testing continues past age 65 years (per ASCCP guidelines).**
- j. Women exposed to diethylstilbestrol (DES)
  - (1) There are differing guidelines regarding the frequency of Pap tests in this group of women. At a minimum, these women should have an annual pelvic, bimanual, and rectal examination. The most frequently these women should have a Pap test is every year, but they may also need a colposcopy as well to visualize the lower genital tract (National Cancer Institute [NCI], 2021b). Ob/gyn consult may be appropriate.
- k. DES offspring
  - (1) Use of DES was discontinued by the FDA in 1971; therefore, treatment of DES offspring includes those women who are born before that year and older.
  - (2) Women whose mothers took DES while pregnant may have an extension of glandular and metaplastic epithelium on the ectocervix and into the upper vagina. This epithelium called *adenosis* is at risk for neoplastic change and should be sampled. The cervix may have structural abnormalities such as a collar, cervical hood, and hypoplastic cervix.
  - (3) **Recommended testing:** Yearly cervical and four-quadrant vaginal Pap tests. During a four-quadrant smear, the provider is instructed to sample from four different quadrants of the vagina, maximizing the surface area tested. Ob/gyn Consult may be appropriate.
- l. HIV-infected women
  - (1) These women should begin screening within 1 year of first insertional sexual activity and continue throughout the patient's lifetime: annually for 3 years, then every 3 years with cytology alone. Once 30 years old, cytology alone or cotesting can continue every 3 years (Perkins et al., 2020).
- m. Women who have undergone hysterectomy
  - (1) Elicit reason(s) why the hysterectomy was performed.
    - **Benign:** ACS, USPSTF, and ASCCP guidelines recommend stopping routine Pap screening for women who have undergone total hysterectomy for benign disease (such as fibroids, uterine prolapse, or endometriosis).
    - **Malignancy:** Women with hysterectomy resulting from cervical intraepithelial neoplasia (CIN 2) or higher, involves HPV-based testing at 3-year intervals for 25 years, regardless of whether the patient has had a hysterectomy either for treatment or at any point during the surveillance period (Perkins et al., 2020).
    - In women whose cervix remains intact after a hysterectomy, regularly scheduled Pap tests should be performed as indicated, per ASCCP.
    - Women may not know whether they had a supracervical hysterectomy and the absence or presence of a cervix should be determined by examination.
- n. A woman who has been vaccinated against HPV should still follow the screening recommendations for her age group.
10. Obtaining the Pap test
  - a. **Patient instructions:** When the patient schedules her appointment for a Pap test, she should be instructed in the following:

(1) Do not schedule a Pap test during menses, because the presence of blood may obscure the results.

(2) Avoid intercourse for 48 hours before the test.

(3) Abstain from vaginal douches, creams, or medications for 48 hours before the test. Douching and medications may remove or contaminate the cells necessary for collection. Pap tests can be obtained under these conditions if absolutely necessary, but the woman must understand that the results may be altered.

(4) **Postpartum:** Schedule the Pap test for 6 to 8 weeks after delivery, by which time the cervix will have undergone reparative changes.

b. **Equipment:** The following equipment should be assembled in advance.

(1) Nonsterile gloves

(2) Speculum (metal or plastic)

(3) A good light source (a speculum with a light is ideal)

(4) Liquid-based container or one frosted glass slide

(5) A pencil for labeling the frosted portion with the woman's name or a label for the liquid-based container

(6) A single or double cardboard slide cover

(7) Ideally a "notched" plastic spatula (Figure 45.2) paired with a cytobrush or a broom (cotton swabs are no longer recommended). A broom may be used alone as it combines endo- and ectocervical sampling.

(8) Aerosol fixative for the conventional smear

c. Liquid-based Pap

(1) The FDA approved a test in May 1996 as a replacement for the conventional Pap test (ThinPrep Pap Test, Hologic Corporation; Surepath, Becton Dickinson Company).

(2) It was the first such advance in 50 years.

(3) Liquid-based testing reduces the chance that the Pap test will need to be repeated, but it does not seem to find more precancers than a conventional Pap test.

(4) The liquid helps remove some of the mucus, bacteria, yeast, and pus cells in a sample. It also allows the cervical cells to be spread more evenly on the slide (monolayer) and keeps them from drying and distorting.

(5) A key point is that the residual solution may be tested for HPV in the laboratory either at the time of the Pap or as a reflex test done because of the results of the Pap.

(6) Additional testing for chlamydia, gonorrhea, and trichomonas may be performed from the residual solution.

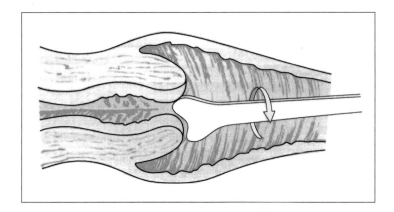

FIGURE 45.2 Collecting an ectocervical sample with a plastic spatula.

d. **The technique:** Careful sampling techniques are vital to ensure an adequate sample for accurate interpretation by the pathologist. This is true for both liquid-based and conventional Pap tests.

(1) Endocervical brush and spatula protocol
- Insert a speculum (water-soluble gel lubricant can be applied sparingly on the posterior blade of the speculum if needed).
- Gently open the speculum to visualize the entire cervix and cervical os.
- Insert the plastic spatula and, using the contoured end, make contact with the outer surface of the cervix. Keeping firm pressure on the cervix, rotate the spatula 360° around the entire ectocervix while maintaining light contact with the cervix.
- Place the spatula and endocervical brush sample into the liquid-based medium.
- Remove the spatula and immediately place it in the vial of solution. Agitate the spatula to remove sample by swirling it vigorously in the liquid 10 times. Discard the spatula.
- Insert the endocervical brush into the vagina. Gently insert the tip of the brush into the cervical os until only the bottom-most fibers are exposed. Slowly rotate one-quarter or one-half turn in one direction. Take care to sample the squamocolumnar junction (Figure 45.3; TZ). This may appear as the area where smooth contiguous epithelium meets irregular, red tissue.
- Remove the brush and place it immediately into the same vial of solution. Remove the sample from the brush by rotating the brush in the solution 10 times while pushing against the vial wall. Swirl the brush vigorously several more times to further release material. Discard the brush.
- **Another option:** The spatula and brush may be placed into the liquid-based vial and rubbed together 10 times as an alternative mixing option. All mucus may *not* be removed from the brush and this is acceptable.
- Tighten the cap so that the torque line (marker) on the cap passes the torque line on the vial.
- Record the patient's name and ID number on the vial. Record the patient information and medical history on the cytology request form. Place the vial and requisition form in a specimen bag for transport to the laboratory.

(2) Endocervical broom-like device protocol
- Insert a speculum (water-soluble gel lubricant can be applied sparingly on the posterior blade of the speculum if needed) into the vaginal canal.
- Gently open the speculum and visualize the entire cervix and cervical os.

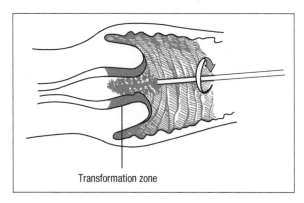

Transformation zone

FIGURE 45.3 Ectocervical sampling using a brush to obtain cells from the transformation zone/endocervix.

- Insert the central bristles of the broom into vagina and make contact with the cervix. Push the tip of the broom into the endocervical canal deep enough to allow the shorter bristles to fully contact the ectocervix. Push gently and rotate the broom five times.
- Remove the broom from the vagina and place it immediately in the vial of solution. Agitate the sample off the broom by pushing it into the bottom of the vial 10 times, forcing the bristles apart. As a final step, swirl the broom vigorously in the liquid to remove additional cellular material. Discard the broom. Some laboratories request the broom tip be included in the vial, so check with your laboratory.
- Tighten the cap so the torque line marker on the cap passes the torque line on the vial.
- Record the patient's name and ID number on the vial, and the patient information and medical history on the cytology requisition form. Place the vial and requisition in a specimen bag for transport to the laboratory.
- Place the sample on a conventional slide using spatula and endocervical brush.
- The cells on the slide must be clearly visible to be accurately interpreted. Characteristics of an adequate conventional smear include:
  - An adequate number of squamous epithelial cells
  - Lack of excessive amounts of blood, inflammatory exudate, or ovulatory discharge
  - Good fixation of smear, with minimal air-drying artifact
- Insert a speculum (water-soluble gel lubricant can be applied sparingly on the posterior blade of the speculum if needed) into the vaginal canal.
- Gently open the speculum; visualize the entire cervix and cervical os.
- Insert the plastic spatula and, using the contoured end, make contact with the outer surface of the cervix. Keeping firm pressure on the cervix, rotate the spatula 360° around the entire exocervix while maintaining light contact with the exocervical surface.
- Hold the horizontal surface of the spatula with the sample on it in the upright position and carefully withdraw from the vagina.
- Place the flat side of the spatula against the labeled glass slide and smear uniformly across two thirds of the side, using one firm motion. A counterclockwise, circular, or zigzag pattern may be used. Avoid excessive pressure because it may alter or destroy the cell structure.
- Insert the endocervical brush into the vagina. Gently insert the tip of the brush into the cervical os until only the bottom-most fibers are exposed. Slowly rotate onehalf turn in one direction. Take care to sample the squamocolumnar junction (TZ; see Figure 45.3).
- Unroll the specimen on the slide in the opposite direction of that taken when collecting the specimen. Add to the remaining third of the slide, being careful not to overlap with the ectocervical sample.
- Apply fixative to the entire slide. Hold the aerosol bottle approximately 6 to 12 inches away from the slide and spray enough times to saturate the sample.

(3) Conventional slide using the broom
- Insert a speculum (a water-soluble gel lubricant can be applied sparingly on the posterior blade of the speculum if needed).
- Gently open the speculum; visualize the entire cervix and cervical os.
- With a large swab, carefully clear any excessive cervical mucus from the cervix.
- Insert the central bristles of the broom into vagina and make contact with the cervix. Insert the tip of the broom into the endocervical canal deep enough to allow the shorter bristles to fully contact the ectocervix. Push gently and rotate the broom in a clockwise direction five times.

- Transfer the sample to the slide with two single paint strokes, applying first one side of the bristles, then the other side, painting the slide again in exactly the same area.
  - Apply fixative to the entire slide. Hold the aerosol bottle approximately 6 to 12 inches away from the slide and spray enough times to saturate the sample.
- e. **Follow-up:** The system of communicating Pap test results to women varies by clinic and facility.
  - (1) The patient is informed that the results may take up to a couple of weeks, and in some cases even longer. The patient should be advised to contact the practitioner if she does not receive the results.
  - (2) A good practice is to send a negative test result via a letter, secure messaging, or using the patient portal. This should be documented in the patient's medical record.
  - (3) Abnormal results need to be verbally and clearly communicated by the clinician to the patient as the woman may misinterpret written information or have immediate questions. This should be documented in the patient's medical record.
- f. Special considerations
  - (1) Because the os tends to bleed with use of the cytobrush, it is best to obtain the ectocervical sample first with the spatula before it becomes obscured with blood.
  - (2) If the patient is symptomatic or the vaginal discharge is abnormal, the clinician may consider obtaining a pH test of the secretions and/or performing a potassium chloride (KOH)/amine test and/or a wet mount in addition to the Pap test. Sexually transmitted infection (STI) testing may also be indicated.
  - (3) The 2021 CDC guidelines on STIs recommend that women with abnormal vaginal discharge should have a diagnostic test for trichomonas.
  - (4) If a trichomonas infection is present on the Pap, the condition should be retested with sensitive diagnostic tests and the infection treated if confirmed.
  - (5) If the examiner is obtaining additional samples from the cervix, obtain the Pap test first. STI testing may utilize cervical, vaginal, or urine samples.
  - (6) Box 45.5 compares the different collection devices.
11. LBC versus conventional Pap tests
    - a. Pros and cons
      - (1) Liquid-based pros
        - Less risk of air-drying artifact
        - More sensitive
        - May have lower risk of "partially obscuring inflammation"
        - HPV testing can be performed from the same specimen.
      - (2) Liquid-based cons
        - May be more false positives
        - Uses more cytopathology resources so more expensive
    - b. LBC is *not* more sensitive than conventional Pap tests for the detection of HSIL[+] and CIN 2[+] regardless of age. However, LBC decreases the rate of inadequate smears, has increased rates of low-grade cytology detection for women younger than 40 years, and has a decreased total rate of abnormal smears in women older than 40 years (Sigurdsson, 2013).
12. Management of abnormal Pap results using the Bethesda Classification System (please refer to the end of the chapter for the management of Pap test results using the 2019 "ASCCP Risk-Based Management Guidelines"; Perkins et al., 2020)
    - a. The Bethesda Classification System (Solomon et al., 2002) is the most widely used protocol for classifying Pap tests. This is an abbreviated summary.
      - (1) **Adequacy of specimen:** Satisfactory for evaluation (ECs and TZ present or not) or unsatisfactory for evaluation (reason).

BOX 45.5 Comparison of Brush and Broom for Cervical Sampling

Brush: Advantages and Disadvantages

Advantages

- Highly efficacious for collection of endocervical cells
- Can insert into a narrow os more easily than broom
- Cochrane review found brush is safe in pregnancy.

Disadvantages

- May cause more bleeding and discomfort
- Controversy regarding safety in pregnancy
- Manufacturer warns *not* to use brush after 10 weeks of pregnancy.

Broom: Advantages and Disadvantages

Advantages

- Causes less bleeding
- Usually effective for endocervical cell collection
- Simultaneously collects both the endocervical and ectocervical sample
- May be used in pregnancy

Disadvantages

- More expensive if must purchase
- May not be as effective in obtaining endocervical cells if narrow cervical os and/or if the transformation zone is high in the canal (common in older women)
- Sampling errors may occur if the clinician does not complete five rotations.

---

(2) **Interpretation/result:** Negative for intraepithelial lesion or malignancy (NILM). Can include the following findings: *Trichomonas*; bacterial, viral, and fungal infection; nonneoplastic findings, including reactive cellular changes associated with inflammation, radiation, and intrauterine devices (IUDs); glandular cells (post-hysterectomy); and atrophy.

(3) **Squamous cell abnormalities:** Atypical squamous cells (ASCs)
   - **ASC-US:** ASCs of undetermined significance
   - **ASC-H:** Cannot exclude HSIL
   - **LSIL:** Refers to cervical cancer precursors, including HPV, CIN 1, lesion involves the initial one third of the epithelial layer.
   - **HSIL:** Refers to cervical cancer precursors, including CIN 2 (lesion involves one third to two thirds of the epithelial layer), CIN 3 (lesion involves two thirds to full thickness)
   - **Squamous cell carcinoma:** Malignant cells penetrate basement membrane of cervical epithelium and infiltrate stromal tissues. If advanced can invade other parts of the body proximal and distant.

(4) Glandular cells
   - **Atypical glandular cell (AGC):** Specify as endocervical, endometrial, or not otherwise specified (NOS).
   - **AGC favor neoplastic:** Specify as endocervical or NOS.

(5) Endocervical adenocarcinoma in situ (AIS)

(6) Adenocarcinoma

(7) Other

- **Endometrial cells:** These are cells shed from the lining of the uterus.
  - If the Pap test was taken during the time of menstruation, this finding is normal.
  - This finding is abnormal in postmenopausal women. Endometrial biopsy and possibly transvaginal ultrasound are necessary to rule out endometrial cancer.

13. Management of cytologic abnormalities including surveillance, colposcopy or expedited treatment; see ASCCP Risk-Based Management Guidelines (Perkins et al., 2020).

a. Management of Pap test results and HPV status if known, is based on the current risk of CIN 3+ (pre-cancer) calculated from current and past results if known in an app or on-line and clinical action thresholds provided by the ASCCP (Apple or Android; Perkins, et al., 2021) or on-line (ASCCP quick start guide; available at: asccp.org/quickstart).

14. Adequate colposcopy

a. Visualizes the entire TZ and the entirety of all lesions

15. HPV vaccines

a. HPV vaccines contain virus-like particles (VLPs) that are not infectious, but stimulate the development of anti-HPV antibodies

(1) The younger population of 11- and 12-year-olds has the most robust immune response when vaccinated and develop the highest antibody levels.

(2) The HPV vaccines are noninfectious and nononcogenic.

(3) The vaccines produce higher levels of neutralizing antibody than natural infection.

b. There is one available HPV vaccine in the United States.

(1) Gardasil 9, a 9-valent vaccine, targets HPV-6, HPV-11, HPV-6,HPV-18, HPV-31, HPV-33, HPV-45, HPV-52, and HPV-58.

c. HPV vaccine dosing schedule

(1) In the United States, recommended dosing schedule depends on age

(2) Gardasil 9

- 9 to 14 years of age: Can be given on a two- or three-dose schedule.
  - Dose schedule: The second dose should be given 6 to 12 months after the first dose.
  - If the second dose is less than 5 months after the first dose, the third dose should be given at least 4 months after the second dose.
- For those 15 to 45 years of age: Vaccination is usually given on a three-dose schedule.

(3) Can be administered at same visit as other age-appropriate vaccines (e.g., tetanus, diphtheria, and pertussis [Tdap]; adult diphtheria and tetanus [TD]; meningococcal conjugate [MCV4]; and hepatitis B)

(4) Not recommended for use in pregnancy though no known risks with inadvertent administration during pregnancy

(5) Can be given to lactating women

(6) Do not restart the series if the schedule is interrupted.

(7) Education regarding the 9-valent vaccine

- Educate women who received the HPV vaccine regarding the importance of cervical cancer screening.
- Sexually active women may have been infected before vaccination. Nonvaccine HPV types could subsequently infect vaccinated women.

d. Contraindications to vaccination

(1) Moderate for severe acute illnesses: Defer until after illness improves.

(2) It is acceptable to administer during minor acute illnesses (e.g., diarrhea or mild upper respiratory infection with or without fever).

(3) History of immediate hypersensitivity or severe allergic reaction to yeast or to any vaccine component

e. Vaccine safety

(1) The most common adverse events are mild, including injection-site reactions.

(2) The CDC maintains an ongoing system for reporting adverse events called the *Vaccine Adverse Event Reporting System* (VAERS), which is available online and anyone can report an adverse event.

(3) Analyses from VAERS and Vaccine Safety Datalink have not demonstrated unexpected safety problems related to Gardisil 9.

16. Cervical cancer screening guidelines

a. Cervical cancer can be prevented through periodic screening and the prompt management of abnormal results.

b. Clinicians should follow updated evidence-based cervical cancer screening recommendations for individuals of average risk as endorsed by ACOG (2021), ACS (2020), and the USPFTF (2018; Perkins et al., 2021).

c. Routine average-risk patients do not include patients with exposure to DES, those under surveillance for abnormal screening tests, or treatment for precancer or cancer.

d. Individuals at high risk of cervical cancer should follow ASCCP recommendations for special populations (Perkins et al., 2020).

17. 2019 ASCCP Risk-Based Management Consensus Guidelines

a. Developed with experts representing 19 professional societies, national and international health organizations, federal agencies and for the first time, patient advocacy groups.

b. The 2019 guidelines have evolved from the 2012 guidelines to further align management recommendations with current understandings of how prior results affect risk (Perkins et al., 2020).

c. Recommendations are based on risk, not results.

d. Colposcopy can be deferred for certain patients.

e. Guidance for expedited treatment is expanded.

f. Excisional treatment is preferred to ablative treatment for CIN 2 or 3.

g. Observation is preferred for histological CIN 1.

h. LAST terminology (Lower Anogenital Squamous Terminology) is used for histopathology results.

i. All primary HPV screening tests that are positive should have additional reflex triage testing performed from the same laboratory.

j. Surveillance with cytology alone is acceptable when HPV primary and co-testing are not available.

k. New data demonstrate that prior history is a very important factor when considering management of low-grade results: HPV positive ASC-US or LSIL.

18. The risk-based algorithms may be downloaded from ASCCP at: www.asccp.org. There is also a web-based application you can access on the website at https://app.asccp.org.

a. iPhone and Android are available in the app store or the Goggle play store.

b. Patient education handouts are free to download from the CDC

(1) https://www.cdc.gov/cancer/gynecologic/resources/print.htm

BIBLIOGRAPHY

American Cancer Society. (2021a). *Cancer facts and figures 2021*. https://www.cancer.org/content/dam/cancer-org/research/cancer-facts-and-statistics/annual-cancer-facts-and-figures/2021/cancer-facts-and-figures-2021.pdf

American Cancer Society. (2021b). *Key statistics for cervical cancer*. http://www.cancer.org/cancer/cervicalcancer/detailed-guide/cervical-cancer-key-statistics

American College of Obstetricians and Gynecologists. (2021) *Updated cervical cancer screening guidelines*. https://www.acog.org/clinical/clinical-guidance/practice-advisory/articles/2021/04/updated-cervical-cancer-screening-guidelines

Arbyn, M., Weiderpass, E., Bruni, L., de Sanjose, S., Saraiya, M., Ferley, J., & Bray, F. (2021). Estimates of incidence and mortality of cervical cancer in 2018: A worldwide analysis. *The Lancet Global Health, 8*(2), e191–e203. https://doi.org/10.1016/s2214-109x(19)30482-6.

Buskwofie, A., David-West, G., & Clare, C. A. (2020). A review of cervical cancer: incidence and disparities. *Journal of the National Medical Association, 112*(2), 229–232. https://doi.org/10.1016/j.jnma.2020.03.002

Centers for Disease Control and Prevention. (2021a). *Epidemiology and prevention of vaccine—preventable diseases. The Pink Book: Course textbook* – (14th ed.). https://www.cdc.gov/vaccines/pubs/pinkbook/index.html

Centers for Disease Control and Prevention. (2021b). *United States Cancer Statistics (USCS)*. https://www.cdc.gov/uscs

Centers for Disease Control and Prevention. (2021c). *2021 STI Treatment Guidelines*. https://www.cdc.gov/std/treatment-guidelines/default.htm

Curry, S. J., Krist, A. H., Owens, D. K., Barry, M. J., Caughey, A. B., Davidson, K. W., Doubeni, C. A., Epling, J. W. Jr., Kemper, A. R., Kubik, M., Landefeld, C. S., Mangione, C. M., Phipps, M. G., Silverstein, M., Simon, M. A., Tseng, C. W., & Wong, J. B. (2018). Screening for cervical cancer: US preventive services task force recommendation statement. *Journal of the American Medical Association, 320*(7), 674–686. https://doi.org/10.1001/jama.2018.10897

Demarco, M., Hyuan, N., Carter-Porkas, O., Raine-Bennette, T., Cheung, L., Chen, X., Hammer, A...Schiffman, M. (2020). A study of type-specific HPV natural history and implications for contemporary cervical cancer screening programs. *EClinicalMedicine, 22,* 100293. https://doi.org/10.1016/j.eclinm.2020.100293. https://reader.elsevier.com/reader/sd/pii/S2589537020300377?token=D0344C3009B0DBD7A4B6035528F4DCC586F01AF8EBB0E03B1402074F73200905EFF7BE6E03242688C2756CAB57B994BA&originRegion=us-east-1&originCreation=20210930214358

De Sanjose, S., Brotons, M., & Pavon, M. A. (2018). The natural history of human papillomavirus infection. *Best Practice & Research Clinical Obstetrics & Gynaecology, 47,* 2–13. https;//doi.org/10.1016//j.bpongyn. 2017.08.

Fontham, E. T. H., Wolf, A. M. D., Church, T. R., Etzioni, R., Flowers, C. R., Herzig, A., Guerra, C. E., Oeffinger, K. C., Shih, Y. T., Walter, L. C., Kim, J. J., Andrews, K. S., DeSantis, C. E., Stacey A Fedewa, S. A., Manassaram-Baptiste, D., Saslow, D., Wender, R. C., & Smith, R. A. Cervical cancer screening for individuals at average risk: 2020 guideline update from the American Cancer Society. *CA: A Cancer Journal for Clinicians, 70*(5), 321–346. https://doi.org/10.3322/caac.21628

Freedman, M. S., Ault, K., & Bernstein, H. (2021). Advisory committee on immunization practices recommended immunization schedule for adults aged 19 years or older--United States. *Morbidity and Mortality Weekly Report, 70*(6), 193–196. https://pubmed.ncbi.nlm.nih.gov/33571173. https://doi.org/10.15585/mmwr.mm7006a2.

Ho, G. Y., Bierman, R., Beardsley, L., Chang, C. J., & Burk, R. D. (1998). Natural history of cervicovaginal papillomavirus infection in young women. *The New England journal of medicine, 338*(7), 423–428. https://doi.org/10.1056/NEJM199802123380703

Lewis, R., Laprise, J. F., Gargano, J., Unger, E., Querec, T., Chesson, H., Brisson, M., & Markowitz, L. (2021). Estimated prevalence and incidence of disease-associated human papillomavirus types among 15–59-year-oldsin the United States. *Sexually Transmitted Diseases 48*(4), 273–277. https://doi.org/10.1097/OLQ.0000000000001356

Luvero, D., Lopez, S., Bogani, G., Raspagliesi, F., & Angioli, R. (2020). From the infection to the immunotherapy in cervical cancer: Can we stop the natural course of the disease? *Vaccine, 8*(4), 597. https://www.mdpi.com/2076-393X/8/4/597/htm

Marcus, J. Z., Cason, P., Downs, L. S, Jr., Einstein, M. H., & Flowers, L. (2021). The ASCCP cervical cancer screening task force endorsement and opinion on the american cancer society updated cervical cancer screening guidelines. *Journal of Lower Genital Tract Disease, 25*(3), 187–191. https://doi.org/10.1097/LGT.0000000000000614

Meites, E., Szilagyi, P., Chesson, H., Unger, E., Romero, J. R., Markowitz, L. S. (2019). Human papillomavirus vaccination for adults: Updated recommendations of the advisory committee on immunization practices. *Morbidity and Mortality Weekly Report Recommendations and Reports, 68*(32), 698–702. https://www.cdc.gov/mmwr/volumes/68/wr/mm6832a3.htm

Massad, L. S., Einstein, M. H., Huh, W. K., Katki, H. A., Kinney, W. K., Schiffman, M., Solomon, D., Wentzensen, N., & Lawson, H. W. (2013). 2012 updated consensus guidelines for the management of abnormal cervical cancer screening tests and cancer precursors. *Journal of Lower Genital Tract Disease, 17*(5 Suppl. 1), S1–S27. https://doi.org/10.1097/LGT.0b013e318287d329

Nayar, R., & Wilbur, D. (2015). *The Pap test and Bethesda 2014*. https://www.karger.com/Article/Pdf/381842

National Cancer Institute. (June 7, 2022, May 25, 2022, & May 4, 2022). *New ACS Cervical Cancer Screening Guideline*. Retrieved July 20, 2022, from https://www.cancer.gov/news-events/cancer-currents-blog/2020/cervical-cancer-screening-hpv-test-guideline

National Cancer Institute. (2021a). *HPV & cancer*. https://www.cancer.gov/about-cancer/causes-prevention/risk/infectious-agents/hpv-and-cancer#what-is-hpv

National Cancer Institute. (2021b). *DES & cancer*. National Cancer Institute. HPV & Cancer. https://www.cancer.gov/about-cancer/causes-prevention/risk/infectious-agents/hpv-and-cancer#what-is-hpv

Perkins, R. B., Guido, R. S., Castle, P. E., Chelmow, D., Einstein, M. H., Garcia, F., Huh, W. K., Kim, J. J., Moscicki, A. B., Nayar, R., Saraiya, M., Sawaya, G. F., Wentzensen, N., & Schiffman, M. (2020). 2019 ASCCP risk-based management consensus guidelines for abnormal cervical cancer screening tests and cancer precursors. *Journal of Lower Genital Tract Disease, 24*(2), 102–131. https://doi.org/10.1097/LGT.0000000000000628

Perkins, R., Guido R., Saraiya, M., Sawaya, G., Wentzensen, N., Schiffman, M., & Feldman, S. (2021). Summary of current guidelines for cervical cancer screening and management of abnormal test results: 2016–2020. *Journal of Womens Health, 30(1), 5–13.* https://doi.org/10.1089/jw.2020.8918

Plummer, M., Peto, J., & Franceschi, S. (2012). Time since first sexual intercourse and the risk of cervical cancer. *International Journal of Cancer, 130*(11), 2638–2644. https://doi.org/10.1002/ijc.26250

Saslow, D., Solomon, D., Lawson, H. W., Killackey, M., Kulasingam, S. L., Cain, J. M., . . . Waldman, J. (2012a). American cancer society, American society for colposcopy and cervical pathology, and American society for clinical pathology screening guidelines for the prevention and early detection of cervical cancer. *Journal of Lower Genital Tract Disease, 16*(3), 175–204. https://doi.org/10.1097/LGT.0b013e31824ca9d5

Saslow, D., Solomon, D., Lawson, H. W., Killackey, M., Kulasingam, S. L., Cain, J., . . . Myers, E. R. (2012b). American Cancer Society, American society for colposcopy and cervical pathology, and American Society for Clinical Pathology screening guidelines for the prevention and early detection of cervical cancer. *American Journal of Clinical Pathology, 137*(4), 516–542. https://doi.org/10.1309/AJCPTGD94EVRSJCG

Schiffman, M., Wentzensen, N., Perkins, R. B., & Guido, R. S. (2020). An introduction to the 2019 ASCCP risk-based management consensus guidelines. *Journal of Lower Genital Tract Disease, 24*(2), 87–89. https://doi.org/10.1097/LGT.0000000000000531

Shimabukuro, T., Su, J., Marquez, P., Mba-Jonas, A., Arana, J., & Cano, M. (2019). Saftery of the 9-valent Human Papilllomavirus Vaccine. *Pediatrics, 144(*6). https://pediatrics.aappublications.org/content/144/6/e20191791

Siegel, R. L., Miller, K. D., Fuchs, H. E., & Jemal, A. (2021). Cancer statistics, 2021. *CA: A Cancer Journal for Clinicians, 71*(1), 7–33. https://doi.org/10.3322/caac.21654

Sigurdsson, K. (2013). Is a liquid-based cytology more sensitive than a conventional Pap smear? *Cytopathology, 24*(4), 254–263. https://doi.org/10.1111/cyt.12037

Solomon, D., Davey, D., Kurman, R., Moriarty, A., O'Connor, D., Prey, M., Raab, S., Sherman, M., Wilbur, D., Wright, T. Jr., & Young, N. (2002). The 2001 Bethesda system: Terminology for reporting results of cervical cytology. *Journal of the American Medical Association, 287*(16), 2114–2119. https://doi.org/10.1001/jama.287.16.2114

Wodi, A. P., Ault. K., Hunter, P., McNally, V., Szilagi, P., & Bernstein, H. (2021). Advisory committee on immunization practices recommended immunization schedule for children and adolescents aged 18 years or younger—United States, 2021. *Morbidity and Mortality Weekly Report, 70*(6), 189–192. https://doi.org/10.15585/mmwr.mm7006a1

Wright, T. C., Stoler, M. H., Behrens, C. M., Apple, R., Derion, T., & Wright, T. L. (2012). The ATHENA human papillomavirus study: Design, methods, and baseline results. *American Journal of Obstetrics and Gynecology, 206*(1), 46.e1–46.e11. https://doi.org/10.1016/j.ajog.2011.07.024

46

GENETIC TESTING FOR HEREDITARY BREAST AND OVARIAN CANCER

CHRISTY MARTIN, CONSTANCE A. ROCHE, NANCIE PETRUCELLI, AND AIMEE CHISM HOLLAND

INTRODUCTION AND OVERVIEW: CANCERS OF THE BREAST AND OVARY IMPOSE A SIGNIFICANT BURDEN ON WOMEN'S HEALTH

A. Most cancers are sporadic (noninherited, occurring by chance, and due to acquired cellular changes) and there is limited ability to predict who will be affected.

B. Family history of cancer is common, but specific features in the family pedigree can suggest a hereditary pattern and increased cancer risk for family members.

C. Approximately 5% to 10% of breast cancers and 15% of ovarian cancers are hereditary, due to a single gene germline mutation.

   1. *BRCA1* and *BRCA2* gene mutations are responsible for hereditary breast and ovarian cancer syndrome, accounting for a large percentage of heritable cancers of the breast and ovary. A mutation in one of these genes has a profound impact on cancer risk.

   2. Mutations in other highly penetrant genes are also associated with less common cancer syndromes that predispose carriers to breast and/or ovarian cancers. These include *PTEN* (Cowden syndrome); *TP53* (Li-Fraumeni syndrome); *STK11* (Peutz–Jeghers syndrome); *PALB2, CDH1* (hereditary diffuse gastric syndrome); and *MLH1, MSH2, MSH6, PMS2,* or *EPCAM* (Lynch syndrome).

   3. Lower-penetrant genes also contribute to cancer risk.

      a. Testing of additional genes is now possible and may be warranted based on personal and family history.

D. Identification and screening of high-risk women are essential skills for healthcare practitioners.

   1. Cancer morbidity and mortality in high-risk women can be reduced with implementation of tailored screening, prevention, and treatment.

FACTS ABOUT BREAST AND OVARIAN CANCER

A. Breast cancer is the most frequently diagnosed cancer in women in the United States.

   1. According to the American Cancer Society, in 2022 among U.S. women, there were about 290,560 new cases of invasive breast cancer and about 43,780 breast cancer deaths.

   2. The average woman has a 12.5% risk of developing breast cancer in her lifetime (one in eight).

B. Breast cancer is the second most common cause of cancer death in women.

   1. Approximately 43,780 died from breast cancer in 2022.

C. Ovarian cancer is the ninth most common cancer in American women.

   1. About 19,880 cases were diagnosed in 2022.

   2. The average woman has a 1.5% (one in 78) lifetime risk of developing the disease.

D. Ovarian cancer ranks fifth in cancer deaths among women.

1. About 12,810 women died of the disease in 2022.

FACTS ABOUT *BRCA1* AND *BRCA2*

A. *BRCA1* cloned in 1994; *BRCA2* cloned in 1995

B. Two copies of these genes are in every human cell (one copy inherited from each parent).

C. Autosomal dominant pattern of inheritance

1. Child of mutation carrier has 50% chance of inheriting the mutation.

D. Classified as tumor-suppressor genes

1. Gene products involved in DNA repair

E. Thousands of mutations have been found in each of these genes

F. Prevalence of 1/300 to 1/800 in the general population

1. Some populations are at higher risk due to founder effects: Ashkenazi Jewish (1/40), Dutch, Icelandic, and others.

G. Commercial testing became available in 1996.

H. Lifetime cancer risk estimates are high for *BRCA* mutation cancers (Box 46.1).

1. One 2007 meta-analysis found risk to age 70 years.
   a. *BRCA1*
      (1) **Breast:** 57%
      (2) **Ovary:** 40%
   b. *BRCA2*
      (1) **Breast:** 49%
      (2) **Ovary:** 18%

I. Features associated with *BRCA* mutations

1. Several family members affected with breast and/or ovarian cancer
2. Young age (less than or equal to 50 years) at diagnosis (particularly breast cancer)
3. Bilateral breast cancer
4. Multiple primary cancers in single individual
5. Male breast cancer
6. Multiple generations affected
7. Related cancers such as pancreatic cancer and prostate cancer

J. *BRCA1* and *BRCA2* often grouped and tested together, but some differences in phenotype exist

1. *BRCA1* mutation carriers
   a. Younger onset breast cancers
   b. Triple negative (negative for estrogen and progesterone receptors and not overexpressing HER2/neu) breast cancer more common
2. *BRCA2* mutation carriers
   a. Breast cancer age at onset similar to that of sporadic cancers
   b. Histology similar to sporadic; more likely estrogen and progesterone receptor positive
   c. Ovarian cancer onset is on average 8 to 10 years later than in *BRCA1*
   d. Higher rate of male breast cancer, melanoma, and pancreatic cancer

---

BOX 46.1 Lifetime Cancer Risk for *BRCA* Mutation Carriers

Breast cancer risk: 41%–90%
Ovarian cancer risk: 8%–62%

IDENTIFICATION OF WOMEN WHO MAY BE CANDIDATES FOR TESTING

A. Obtain personal and family history (minimum three-generation pedigree, including affected and unaffected relatives is recommended; see Figure 46.1 for an example of pedigree with history of ovarian and breast cancer) to include:
  1. Cancers in the family
     a. Both maternal and paternal lineage
  2. Note whether bilateral disease
  3. Age at diagnosis
  4. Relevant surgical history (e.g., oophorectomy and reason for surgery)
B. Ontario Family History Assessment Tool (see Table 46.1)
  1. A screening tool recommended by the U.S. Preventive Services Task Force (USPSTF) to assess familial risk factors for specific cancers associated with a *BRCA* 1/2 gene mutation
C. Candidates for testing
  1. Individual whose relative has a known *BRCA* mutation
  2. Always preferable to first test the family member affected with cancer
     a. Counsel or refer women with
        (1) Breast cancer diagnosed at age 50 years or younger
        (2) Bilateral breast cancer
        (3) Breast cancer in Ashkenazi Jewish woman
        (4) Triple-negative breast cancer diagnosed before age 60 years
        (5) Breast cancer and relatives with breast or ovarian cancer
        (6) Any woman with ovarian cancer
        (7) Male with breast cancer
        (8) See National Comprehensive Cancer Network (NCCN) guidelines, updated regularly
  3. When no affected relative able to have testing
     a. Counsel or refer unaffected woman
        (1) With close relatives meeting aforementioned criteria

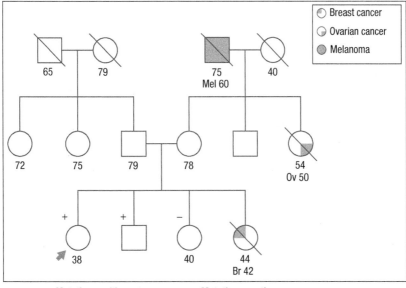

FIGURE 46.1 An example of a pedigree for patients with a familial risk for hereditary breast and ovarian cancer.

TABLE 46.1 Ontario Family Assessment Tool

RISK FACTOR	POINTS
Breast and ovarian cancer	
Mother	10
Sibling	7
Second-/third-degree relative	5
Breast cancer relatives	
Parent	4
Sibling	3
Second-/third-degree relative	2
Male relative (add to above)	2
Breast cancer characteristics	
Onset age, year	
20–29	6
30–39	4
40–49	2
Premenopausal/perimenopausal	2
Bilateral/multifocal	3
Ovarian cancer relatives	
Mother	7
Sibling	4
Second-/third-degree relative	3
Ovarian cancer onset age, year	
<40	6
40–60	4
>60	2
Prostate cancer onset	
Age <50 year	1
Colon cancer onset	
Age <50 year	1
Family total	
Referral*	≥10

*Referral with score of 10 or greater corresponds to doubling of lifetime risk for breast cancer (22%).

Source: https://www.uspreventiveservicestaskforce.org/uspstf/document/RecommendationStatementFinal/brca-related-cancer-risk
-assessment-genetic-counseling-and-genetic-testing

(2) With elevated risk as calculated by risk models such as BRCAPRO, Breast and Ovarian Analysis of Disease incidence and Carrier Estimation algorithm (BOADICEA), and Tyrer-Cuzick IBIS

(3) The National Cancer Institute Breast Cancer Risk Assessment tool (based on the Gail model) is not useful for assessing hereditary risk.

4. Consider factors impacting the pedigree
   a. Limited family structure
      (1) Young age at death due to noncancerous causes
      (2) Few females in the family
      (3) Paternal lineage with few females
   b. Unknown or inaccurate history
5. Testing is not recommended for individuals younger than 18 years.
6. Provide or refer for counseling any woman whose quality of life is affected by her anxiety about cancer risk, regardless of objective assessment.

PRETEST EDUCATION AND COUNSELING

A. Should be provided by healthcare professional with expertise and experience in cancer genetics
   1. Educate and counsel about hereditary cancer and the rationale, logistics, risks, and benefits of testing.
   2. Identify most informative family member to have testing.
      a. Once a familial mutation is identified, other family members can be tested for that family-specific mutation and obtain a definitive result.
   3. Discuss insurance implications.
      a. Genetic Information Nondiscrimination Act (GINA) and state laws prohibit health insurance and/or employment discrimination.
      b. Life, long-term, and disability insurers may use genetic information to change or deny coverage.
   4. Determine which genetic test(s) are appropriate to consider.
   5. Counsel about medical management.
      a. Discuss screening and prevention measures.
   6. Assist in formulating plans for management if positive.
   7. Discuss importance of sharing with family members and assist as needed.
   8. Obtain informed consent.
   9. Disclose and interpret results.
   10. Provide emotional support and guidance.

INTERPRETATION OF *BRCA* TEST RESULTS

A. Deleterious mutation
   1. **Breast cancer risk:** 41% to 90%
   2. **Ovarian cancer risk:** 8% to 62%
   3. No prediction if or when cancer might occur
      a. Penetrance may be mutation specific and/or affected by additional genetic or environmental factors.
   4. Increased risk for male breast cancer, melanoma, prostate cancer, and pancreatic cancer
   5. Family members at risk; first-degree relatives have 50% risk of carrying the mutation.
B. No mutation
   1. **True negative:** If known mutation in family
   2. **Uninformative negative:** If no known mutation in family

C. Variant of uncertain significance (VUS)
   1. Occurs in 3% to 5% overall
   2. Majority will be reclassified, most as benign polymorphisms/not disease causing

MANAGEMENT OPTIONS FOR THE UNAFFECTED WOMAN WHO TESTS *BRCA* POSITIVE

A. Management of cancer risk (Box 46.2)
   1. Breast
      a. Breast awareness/breast self-examination beginning at age 18 years
      b. Clinical breast examination, every 6 to 12 months, beginning at age 25 years
      c. Annual MRI screening with contrast or mammogram with consideration of tomosynthesis if MRI is not available, from ages 25 to 29 years, or individualized based on earliest age of breast cancer diagnosis in the family; annual mammogram with consideration of tomosynthesis and annual breast MRI with contrast from ages 30 to 75 years; management after the age of 75 years should be considered on an individual basis.
      d. Discuss option of risk-reducing mastectomy
         (1) Reduces risk by 90%
         (2) Counsel regarding effectiveness, limitations, reconstruction options, and psychological impact.
      e. Consider chemoprevention with tamoxifen or raloxifene.
         (1) Both demonstrated to reduce risk in high-risk women
         (2) Limited data on effect in *BRCA* mutation carriers
   2. Ovary
      a. Recommend risk-reducing salpingo-oophorectomy (RRSO) between age 35 and 40 years and after childbearing is complete. May individualize based on earliest age of ovarian cancer onset in family. In women with *BRCA2* mutations, it may be reasonable to delay RRSO until age 40 to 45 years.
         (1) It is believed that many ovarian cancers develop in the fallopian tube.
         (2) There is no reliable screening for early detection.
         (3) Reduces risk of *BRCA*-associated gynecologic cancer by 80% to 85%; there is residual risk of primary peritoneal cancer.
         (4) Reduces risk for breast cancer by 50% when premenopausal at the time of surgery.
         (5) Counsel regarding health risks of surgically induced early menopause: vasomotor and vaginal symptoms, osteoporosis, and increased risk for cardiovascular disease.
         (6) Short-term use of hormone replacement therapy (HRT) does not appear to mitigate the reduction in breast cancer risk.
         (7) Due to high rate of occult ovary or fallopian tube cancer, attention to sampling and pathologic review are important
      b. If RRSO not elected, or pending surgery, consider transvaginal ultrasound and CA-125 every 6 months starting at age 30 to 35 years, or 5 to 10 years younger than earliest age at ovarian cancer diagnosis in the family.
         (1) Counsel that this has not been demonstrated to be an effective screening strategy nor a substitute for surgery.

BOX 46.2 Recommended Lifestyle Factors to Reduce Breast Cancer Risk

- Achieve and maintain normal weight.
- 150 minutes of moderate-intensity exercise per week
- Limit alcohol to no more than one drink per day.

    c. Oral contraceptives
      (1) Reduce ovarian cancer risk by 50% in *BRCA* mutation carriers as well as in general population
      (2) May increase breast cancer risk after 5 years of use
      (3) Consider pending surgery, weigh pros and cons
  3. If childbearing age, consider referral to discuss prenatal diagnosis and/or preimplantation genetic testing
  4. Provide or refer for psychological counseling as needed for assistance with coping strategies
  5. Provide or refer for community resources such as FORCE (www.facingourrisk.org)

MANAGEMENT OPTIONS FOR THE WOMAN WITH BREAST OR OVARIAN CANCER WHO TESTS *BRCA* POSITIVE

A. Tested at time of breast cancer diagnosis
  1. Higher risk of ipsilateral breast tumor recurrence and contralateral breast cancer
    a. Consider bilateral mastectomy or recommend MRI screening
  2. Tailored treatment options or clinical protocol may be available
  3. Counsel regarding RRSO posttreatment
    a. Postsurgery HRT not recommended
    b. Oral contraceptives not recommended
  4. Address implications for family members

B. Tested at time of ovarian cancer diagnosis
  1. Tailored treatment options or clinical protocol may be available.
  2. Counsel regarding option of risk-reducing mastectomy or screening with MRI.
  3. Address implications for family members.

C. Tested following treatment for breast and/or ovarian cancer
  1. Consider surveillance and screening options in context of cancer history, prognosis, age, and life expectancy.
  2. Address implications for family members.

D. Provide or refer for counseling as needed.

IMPLICATIONS OF A NEGATIVE TEST OR VARIANTS OF UNCERTAIN SIGNIFICANCE

A. **True negative:** Negative result when known mutation in family
  1. Negative test indicates that the woman is at population risk for associated cancers unless she has personal risk factors (e.g., atypical ductal hyperplasia) elevating her risk.
  2. Counsel regarding the continued risk of sporadic cancer.
  3. Psychological adjustment to the change in risk status is needed.
  4. Possible to feel "survivor guilt"
  5. Refer for counseling as needed.

B. **Uninformative negative:** Negative results when no family member is known to have a mutation
  1. Risk assessment and management based on personal and family history

C. Variants of uncertain significance (VUS)
  1. Risk assessment and management based on personal and family history
  2. May warrant additional evaluation by an individual trained in cancer genetics
  3. Reclassification of VUS as either positive or negative by the laboratory may occur as evidence becomes available.

CONSIDER SYNDROMES OTHER THAN *BRCA*, HEREDITARY BREAST AND OVARIAN CANCER

A. Family history should also be assessed for less common syndromes associated with breast and ovarian cancer.
  1. Cowden syndrome
     a. Result of mutation in the *PTEN* gene
     b. Features include follicular thyroid cancer, breast cancer, endometrial cancer, macrocephaly
  2. Li-Fraumeni syndrome
     a. Result of mutation in the *TP53* gene
     b. Young-onset cancers, including soft tissue sarcoma, brain tumor, acute leukemia, breast cancer
  3. Peutz–Jeghers syndrome
     a. Result of mutation in the *STK11* gene
     b. Increased risk for breast, ovary, colon, small bowel, testicular, and other cancers
  4. Hereditary diffuse gastric cancer syndrome
     a. Result of mutation in the *CDH1* gene
     b. Stomach cancer (diffuse), breast cancer (lobular)
  5. Lynch syndrome
     a. Result of mutation in the *MLH1, MSH2, MSH6, PMS2,* or *EPCAM* genes
     b. Features include colon cancer, endometrial cancer, ovarian cancer, possibly breast cancer

EXPANDED TESTING OPTIONS WITH NEXT-GENERATION GENE SEQUENCING

A. Multigene panels
  1. Evolving technology changing landscape of genetic testing
  2. Panels identify genetic variation in multiple genes (20–40) at the same time
  3. Many moderately penetrant genes included to test for a range of genetic-related cancers
  4. May be considered as second-tier test when *BRCA* negative, or when family history suggests the possibility of more than one cancer syndrome
  5. No specific guidelines for eligibility, insurance reimbursement
  6. Limited data about risks associated with mutations with many of these genes
  7. Lack of clear guidelines for medical management for carriers of mutations in many of the low or moderately penetrant genes
  8. Should be interpreted by individuals trained in cancer genetics
  9. Research and increased use will elucidate risks and implications
B. Family pedigree with *BRCA* mutation
  1. No living affected family member, so proband had *BRCA* testing and deleterious *BRCA2* mutation found. Mother is unaffected and likely demonstrates incomplete penetrance but testing mother would be indicated to confirm her status. Inheritance potentially from maternal grandmother's lineage (she died young), or maternal grandfather (melanoma). Brother tested to provide information for future children, but also is at increased risk for breast cancer as well as pancreatic cancer, melanoma, and prostate cancer.

ACKNOWLEDGMENT

Special thanks to Dr. Quinetta Edwards for her special expertise in reviewing and editing this chapter.

BIBLIOGRAPHY

American Cancer Society. (2021). *Breast cancer*. https://www.cancer.org/cancer/breast-cancer

Aiello-Laws, L. (2011). Genetic cancer risk assessment. *Seminars in Oncology Nursing, 27*(1), 13–20. https://doi.org/10.1016/j.soncn.2010.11.003

Beitsch, P. D., Whitworth, P. W., Hughes, K., Patel, R., Rosen, B., Compagnoni, G., Baron, P., Simmons, R., Smith, L. A., Grady, I., Kinney, M., Coomer, C., Barbosa, K., Holmes, D. R., Brown, E., Gold, L., Clark, P., Riley, L., Lyons, S., ... Nussbaum, R. L. (2019). Underdiagnosis of hereditary breast cancer: Are genetic testing guidelines a tool or an obstacle? *Journal of Clinical Oncology, 37*(6), 453–460. https://doi.org/10.1200/JCO.18.01631

Berliner, J. L., Fay, A. M., Cummings, S. A., Burnett, B., & Tillmanns, T. (2013). NSGC practice guideline: Risk assessment and genetic counseling for hereditary breast and ovarian cancer. *Journal of Genetic Counseling, 22*(2), 155–163. https://doi.org/10.1007/s10897-012-9547-1

Centers, N., Ivanov, O., Buffington, C., & Caceres, A. (2017). Hormone Replacement Therapy (HRT) among BRCA mutation carriers. *Journal of Clinical Oncology, 35*(15_suppl), 1561–1561. https://doi.org/10.1200/JCO.2017.35.15_suppl.1561

Chen, S., & Parmigiani, G. (2007). Meta-analysis of *BRCA1* and *BRCA2* penetrance. *Journal of Clinical Oncology, 25*(11), 1329–1333. https://doi.org/10.1200/JCO.2006.09.1066

Domchek, S., & Robson, M. (2019) Broadening criteria for *BRCA1/2* Evaluation: Placing the USPSTF recommendation in context. *Journal of the American Medical Association, 322*(7), 619–621. https://doi.org/10.1001/jama.2019.9688

Domchek, S. M., Friebel, T. M., Singer, C. F., Evans, D. G., Lynch, H. T., Isaacs, C., ... Rebbeck, T. R. (2010). Association of risk-reducing surgery in BRCA1 or BRCA2 mutation carriers with cancer risk and mortality. *Journal of the American Medical Association, 304*(9), 967–975. https://doi.org/10.1001/jama.2010.1237

Domchek, S. M., Friebel, T., Neuhausen, S. L., Lynch, H. T., Singer, C. F., Eeles, R. A., ... , Rebbeck T. R.; PROSE Consortium. (2011). Is hormone replacement therapy (HRT) following risk-reducing salpingo-oophorectomy (RRSO) in *BRCA1* (B1)- and *BRCA2* (B2)-mutation carriers associated with an increased risk of breast cancer? *Journal of Clinical Oncology, 29*(15 Suppl), 1501–1501. https://doi.org/10.1200/jco.2011.29.15_suppl.1501

Dullens, B., de Putter, R., Lambertini, M., Toss, A., Han, S., Van Nieuwenhuysen, E., Van Gorp, T., Vanderstichele, A., Van Ongeval, C., Keupers, M., Prevos, R., Celis, V., Dekervel, J., Everaerts, W., Wildiers, H., Nevelsteen, I., Neven, P., Timmerman, D., Smeets, A., ... Punie, K. (2020). Cancer surveillance in healthy carriers of germline pathogenic variants in BRCA1/2: A review of secondary prevention guidelines. *Journal of Oncology, 2020*, 1–13. https://doi.org/10.1155/2020/9873954

Euhus, D. M. (2001). Understanding mathematical models for breast cancer risk assessment and counseling. *Breast Journal, 7*(4), 224–232. https://doi.org/10.1046/j.1524-4741.2001.20012.x

Gilpin, C. A., Carson, N., & Hunter, A. G. (2000). A preliminary validation of a family history assessment form to select women at risk for breast or ovarian cancer for referral to a genetics center. *Clinical Genetics, 58*(4), 299–308. https://doi.org/10.1034/j.1399-0004.2000.580408

Grann, V. R., Patel, P. R., Jacobson, J. S., Warner, E., Heitjan, D. F., Ashby-Thompson, M., Hershman, D. L., & Neugut, A. I. (2011). Comparative effectiveness of screening and prevention strategies among BRCA1/2-affected mutation carriers. *Breast Cancer Research and Treatment, 125*(3), 837–847. https://doi.org/10.1007/s10549-010-1043-4

Hilbers, F. S., Vreeswijk, M. P., van Asperen, C. J., & Devilee, P. (2013). The impact of next generation sequencing on the analysis of breast cancer susceptibility: A role for extremely rare genetic variation? *Clinical Genetics, 84*(5), 407–414. https://doi.org/10.1111/cge.12256

Jacobson, M., Coakley, N., Bernardini, M., Branco, K. A., Elit, L., Ferguson, S., & Kim, R. (2021). Risk reduction strategies for BRCA1/2 hereditary ovarian cancer syndromes: A clinical practice guideline. *Hereditary Cancer in Clinical Practice, 19*(1), 39–39. https://doi.org/10.1186/s13053-021-00196-9

Lynch, H. T., Snyder, C., & Casey, J. (2013). Hereditary ovarian and breast cancer: What have we learned? *Annals of Oncology, 24*(Suppl. 8), 83–95. https://doi.org/10.1093/annonc/mdt313

Manahan, E. R., Kuerer, H. M., Sebastian, M., Hughes, K. S., Boughey, J. C., Euhus, D. M., Boolbol, S. K., & Taylor, W. A. (2019). Consensus guidelines on genetic' testing for hereditary breast cancer from the American society of breast surgeons. *Annals of Surgical Oncology, 26*(10), 3025–3031. https://doi.org/10.1245/s10434-019-07549-8

Marchetti, C., De Felice, F., Boccia, S., Sassu, C., Di Donato, V., Perniola, G., Palaia, I., Monti, M., Muzii, L., Tombolini, V., & Benedetti Panici, P. (2018). Hormone replacement therapy after prophylactic risk-reducing salpingo-oophorectomy and breast cancer risk in BRCA1 and BRCA2 mutation carriers: A meta-analysis. *Critical Reviews in Oncology/hematology, 132*, 111–115. https://doi.org/10.1016/j.critrevonc.2018.09.018

Mavaddat, N., Peock, S., Frost, D., Ellis, S., Platte, R., Fineberg, E., ... Easton, D. F.; EMBRACE. (2013). Cancer risks for *BRCA1* and *BRCA2* mutation carriers: Results from prospective analysis of EMBRACE. *Journal of the National Cancer Institute, 105*(11), 812–822. https://doi.org/10.1093/jnci/djt095

McGuire, K. P., & Mamounas, E. P. (2020). Management of hereditary breast cancer: ASCO, ASTRO, and SSO guideline. *Annals of Surgical Oncology, 27*(6), 1721–1723. https://doi.org/10.1245/s10434-020-08396-8

National Comprehensive Cancer Network. NCCN Clinical Practice Guidelines in Oncology. (2017). *Genetic/familial high-risk assessment: Breast and ovarian (V1.2018)*. http://www.nccn.org/professionals/physician_gls/pdf/genetics_screening.pdf

Oncology Nursing Society. (2012). *Oncology nursing: The application of cancer genetics and genomics throughout the oncology care continuum.* https://www.ons.org/about-ons/ons-position-statements/education-certification-and-role-delineation/oncology-nursing

Pederson, H. J., & Noss, R. (2020). Updates in hereditary breast cancer genetic testing and practical high risk breast management in gene carriers. *Seminars in Oncology, 47*(4), 182–186. https://doi.org/10.1053/j.seminoncol.2020.05.008

Petrucelli, N., Daly, M. B., & Pal, T. (1998). *BRCA1-* and *BRCA2-*associated hereditary breast and ovarian cancer. [Updated 2016 Dec 15]. In M. P. Adam, H. H. Ardinger, R. A. Pagon, S. E. Wallace, L. J. H. Bean, K. Stephens, & A. Amemiya (Eds.), *GeneReviews® [Internet].* University of Washington. https://www.ncbi.nlm.nih.gov/books/NBK1247

Pouliot, M, Kothari, C., Joly-Beauparlant, C., Labrie, Y., Ouellette, G., Simard, J., Droit, A., & Durocher, F. (2017). Transcriptional signature lymphoblastoid cell lines of BRCA1, BRCA2, and nonBRCA ½ high risk breast cancer families. *Oncotarget, 8*(45), 78691 – 78712. https://doi.org/10.18632/oncotarget.20219

Rebbeck, T. R., Friebel, T., Wagner, T., Lynch, H. T., Garber, J. E., Daly, M. B., . . . Weber, B. L.; PROSE Study Group. (2005). Effect of short-term hormone replacement therapy on breast cancer risk reduction after bilateral prophylactic oophorectomy in *BRCA1* and *BRCA2* mutation carriers: The PROSE Study Group. *Journal of Clinical Oncology, 23*(31), 7804–7810. https://doi.org/10.1200/JCO.2004.00.8151

Robson, M. E., Bradbury, A. R., Arun, B., Domchek, S. M., Ford, J. M., Hampel, H. L., . . .Lindor, N. M. (2015). American society of clinical oncology policy statement update: Genetic and genomic testing for cancer susceptibility. *Journal of Clinical Oncology, 33*(31), 3660–3667. https://doi.org/10.1200/JCO.2015.63.0996

Tejada-Berges, T. (2016). Breast cancer: Genetics and risk assessment. *Clinical Obstetrics and Gynecology, 59*(4), 673–687. https://doi.org/10.1097/GRF.0000000000000236.

Tung, N. M., Boughey, J. C., Pierce, L. J., Robson, M. E., Bedrosian, I., Dietz, J. R., Dragun, A., Gelpi, J. B., Hofstatter, E. W., Isaacs, C. J., Jatoi, I., Kennedy, E., Litton, J. K., Mayr, N. A., Qamar, R. D., Trombetta, M. G., Harvey, B. E., Somerfield, M. R., & Zakalik, D. (2020). Management of hereditary breast cancer: American society of clinical oncology, American society for radiation oncology, and society of surgical oncology guideline. *Journal of Clinical Oncology, 38*(18), 2080–2106. https://doi.org/10.1200/JCO.20.00299

U.S. Preventive Services Task Force. (2019) Risk assessment, genetic counseling, and genetic testing for *BRCA*-related cancer: U.S. Preventive Services Task Force recommendation statement. *Journal of the American Medical Association, 322*(7), 652–665. https://doi.org/10.1001/jama.2019.10987

47

URINALYSIS AND URINARY TRACT INFECTIONS

LISA S. PAIR AND HELEN A. CARCIO

URINARY TRACT INFECTION

A. Urinary tract infections (UTIs) are common, mainly affecting healthy young women. UTIs are four times more frequent in women than in men.

B. Forty percent to 60% of women develop a UTI at least once in their lives; nearly 50% of these women develop a second infection.

C. UTIs generally have typical symptoms and are easy to diagnose. They can often be diagnosed by history alone. When the diagnosis is not clear a urinalysis is indicated. Usually, a urine culture is not necessary unless deciding on the type of antimicrobial treatment.

D. *Escherichia coli* causes 75% to 90% of all acute, uncomplicated infections. Refer to Box 47.1 for a list of the most organisms identified in urinary tract infection.

E. Definitions
  1. **Urethritis:** Inflammation of the urethra
  2. **Cystitis:** Inflammation of the bladder.
  3. **Pyelonephritis:** Inflammation of the kidney

F. Risk factors may predispose a woman to a UTI (Table 47.1). Women have shorter urethras than men and organisms can ascend the urethra into the bladder and result in UTIs.

G. Symptoms of cystitis include abrupt onset of
  1. **Dysuria:** Pain or stinging while urinating
  2. **Urinary frequency:** Voiding small amounts; producing only small amounts
  3. Urinary urgency
  4. Suprapubic pain, ache, pressure
  5. Gross hematuria
  6. Pyuria, odor, milky discharge
  7. Rare systemic symptoms but may occasionally present with low-grade fever (less than 101°F)
  8. Confusion and fatigue in women

URINARY EVALUATION

A. Assessment of urine in women in a primary care setting is often performed to identify or rule out UTI in the evaluation of dysuria, frequency, and suprapubic pain. Other conditions that relate specifically to the vulvovaginal area, such as those caused by *Candida, Chlamydia, Neisseria gonorrhoeae,* or *Trichomonas,* may also present with similar symptoms and must be explored.

B. A urine culture does not need to be ordered in young women with a history of previous uncomplicated UTIs who present with the usual symptoms. A dipstick test is sufficient.

C. Urinary assessment may include a comprehensive health history, physical examination, a urine dipstick test, microscopy, or culture.

BOX 47.1 Most Common Organisms Identified in Urinary Tract Infection

Gram-negative organisms (found in large intestine)
Escherichia coli (70%)
Proteus mirabilis
*Klebsiella*s
Pseudomonas aeruginosa

Gram-positive organisms (less commonly identified)
Streptococcus faecalis
Staphylococcus epidermidis

Organisms commonly found in the absence of disease
Lactobacillus
Corynebacterium
Micrococci
Neisseria

Organisms that are not found in routine cultures but can cause UTI
Chlamydia trachomatis
Neisseria gonorrhoeae
Herpes simplex virus
Mycoplasma hominis—less common
Urea plasma—less common

Symptomatic bacteriuria—8 to 10 WBC/HPF is diagnostic

Culture and sensitivity—indicates the specific pathologic bacteria in the urine
Determines which antibiotics will be effective against it

HPF, high-powered field; UTI, urinary tract infection; WBC, white blood cell.

D. A thorough evaluation should be performed
   1. For an initial episode
   2. If diagnosis is uncertain
   3. As an initial prenatal screen

TABLE 47.1 Factors That Contribute to Infection of the Urinary Tract

FACTOR	RESULT
Sexual activity	Introduction of bacteria into the urethra
Poor hygiene habits	Bacteria multiply in area of the urethra
Wiping from back to front	Introduces bacteria from the rectum into the urethra
Excessive stress	Reduces immune response
Contraception: Diaphragm use	Use of a diaphragm may press on bladder, causing stasis of urine Spermicides inhibit growth of lactobacilli
Voiding habits	Stasis of urine
Waiting long periods of time between urinating	Decreases flushing of bacteria from bladder

4. In elderly women

5. In immune-compromised women

E. A physical examination should include the following

1. Vital signs, especially temperature

2. Abdominal examination to palpate the suprapubic area for tenderness

3. Percussion of costal vertebral angle (CVA) tenderness (present in pyelonephritis)

4. Pelvic examination: Essential to rule out pelvic inflammatory disease, vaginitis, or sexually transmitted infections (STIs)

5. Wet mount if history or physical examination indicates risk factors for STI

F. The female anatomy predisposes a woman to bladder colonization with pathogens. This is related to

1. Short urethra (2.5 cm)

2. Proximity to the anal area

3. **Pregnancy:** Bladder enlarged with decreased tone; unable to empty completely

4. **Older age:** Lack of estrogen may cause urethral atrophy

PRINCIPLES RELATED TO THE PROCUREMENT OF URINE

A. A freshly voided concentrated specimen provides more useful information than a diluted specimen.

1. Use the first morning urine. However, a random specimen is more convenient (Box 47.2).

2. Bacteria must have been in the bladder at least 4 hours for accuracy.

B. Test within a few minutes of collection. (If this is not possible, cover tightly and refrigerate at 5°C [41°F].)

C. Do not allow specimen to stand at room temperature. Urine that is allowed to stand at room temperature begins to grow bacteria within 30 minutes; if more than 2 hours elapses, it will be highly contaminated by bacteria.

D. As urine sits, it becomes alkaline, decomposing important sediment.

E. Red blood cells (RBCs) and casts lyse quickly in diluted or alkaline urine.

THE CLEAN CATCH

A. Equipment

1. Sterile urine container

2. Three wipes saturated with soap

B. The following steps should be explained

1. Wash hands thoroughly.

2. Remove the cover of a sterile specimen container and put down with the lid side up. (Emphasize not to touch the inside of the lid or specimen container.)

3. Spread the labia with the nondominant hand and hold until after the specimen is collected.

4. Using the dominant hand, wipe one side of the vaginal area with a cleansing towelette.

5. Always use a single stroke, wiping the cleansing towelette from front to back.

BOX 47.2 Solutes in Random Urine

- Various solutes normally appear at different times of the day
- Glucosuria: More often after meals
- Proteinuria: After activity or assumption of orthostatic position from a recumbent position
- Hemoglobinuria: After severe physical exertion, such as working out at a gym

6. Cleanse the opposite side of the labia with the second towelette.
7. Cleanse the center area directly over the urethra downward.
8. Release a small amount of urine into the toilet to flush any bacteria from the distal portion of the urethra.
9. Place the specimen container under the urethra (be careful not to touch the vulva) and urinate into the sterile cup while the labia remain separated.
10. If there is heavy vaginal discharge, a tampon should be worn to absorb the vaginal secretions to avoid contamination of the urine sample.
11. Perform the urinalysis immediately or refrigerate the urine sample. Analysis in urine is performed via physical, chemical, and microscopic methods. The complete analysis of urine is a simple, noninvasive, and inexpensive means of detecting abnormalities and kidney and systemic disorders.

PHYSICAL EXAMINATION OF THE URINE

A. Assess the color, clarity, and odor of the urine.
  1. Description
     a. The amount of color depends on the density of urochromes (pigments formed by metabolism of bile). The intensity of the color is due to the concentration of the urine. Many substances may change the color of urine.
  2. Color
     a. Urine is often described as "straw colored" or yellow. Normal color ranges from almost colorless to deep yellow, depending on the concentration of urochrome pigment.
  3. Significance
     a. May be a sign of disease or may indicate the presence of a pigmented drug, dye, or food (Table 47.2).
        (1) Clarity
           • Clear
           • Urine that is cloudy or turbid may be normal or may indicate contamination, infection, semen, vaginal secretions, and so on.

TABLE 47.2 Appearance of Urine in Relation to Products

URINE APPEARANCE	ASSOCIATION
Colorless	Dilute urine associated with water diuresis or diabetes mellitus or insipidus
Red	RBCs or large amounts of free hemoglobin or myoglobin, bile pigments, food dyes, anthocyanin (pigment in beets and blackberries)
Red-brown	Porphyria, urobilinogen, bilirubin
Orange	Fever and dehydration
Yellow	Normal due to the presence of a yellow pigment, urochrome
Yellow-red	Pyridium, vegetables, or phenolphthalein
Blue or green	Beets, methylene blue in IV
Brown or black	Porphyrins, melanin, acidification of hemoglobin content, rhubarb
Turbid	Frequently secondary to urates or phosphates (benign), RBCs, WBCs
Foamy	Protein, bile acids
Milky white	Heavy WBC content or precipitation of amorphous phosphate salts in alkaline urine

IV, intravenous; RBCs, red blood cells; WBCs, white blood cells.

(2) Odor
- Fresh urine is aromatic; malodorous urine may be related to dietary substances or infection.

THE CHEMICAL ANALYSIS

A. **The dipstick:** Analysis of the urine is performed with the dipstick, a chemically impregnated plastic strip. When the dipstick is placed in urine, the color changes in the various reagent strips provide an approximate quantification of the amount of substance present.
   1. Principles
      a. Detects the presence of protein, occult blood, glucose, ketones, nitrites, leukocyte esterase, urobilinogen, and bilirubin in the urine.
      b. Determines the urinary pH.
      c. Color changes may be compared against a chart provided by the manufacturer.
      d. Store in a cool dry place and use before the expiration date.
   2. **Technique:** There are many rapid agent tests for routine and special urinalyses; most require dipping the stick into fresh, unspun urine and comparing each reagent area with the corresponding-colored area on the strip at varying suggested intervals (seconds to minutes). Important to read the strip color at the required time for accurate interpretation.
B. Dipstick urinalysis results
   1. **Specific gravity (SG):** Measures urine directly relative to the density of water
      a. **Description:** SG is used as in indirect measure of the kidneys' ability to concentrate the urine. The normal range is 1.010 to 1.025, with urine isotonic to plasma.
      b. **Diluted:** Less than 1.010
      c. **Concentrated:** More than 1.025
      d. **Significance:** If a first-morning specimen is SG 1.025 or greater, it is generally taken as evidence of adequate concentrating ability and, therefore, adequate renal function.
   2. pH
      a. Description: The dipstick is impregnated with various dyes that respond with different color changes to a pH in the range of 5 to 11. Measurement of pH on random urine samples has little clinical value.
      b. The normal range of urine pH is 4.5 to 8.5. The urine pH in a freshly voided urine sample from a woman on a healthy diet is about 6.0. Stale urine becomes alkaline.
         (1) Diffusion of carbon dioxide into the air
         (2) Bacteria converts urea to ammonia
      c. Significance: If fresh urine is alkaline, a UTI urea-splitting organism (e.g., *Proteus, Klebsiella, E. coli)* or bicarbonate excretion (e.g., renal tubular acidosis) must be considered.
   3. Protein
      a. Description: The dipstick is sensitive to as little as 5 to 20 mg/dL of albumin (the prominent protein in renal disease). Normal: Less than 50 mg/dL. Scored from trace to 4+, or by concentration. 5 to 20 mg/dL = trace, 30 mg/dL = 1+, 100 mg/dL = 2+, 300 mg/dL = 43+, greater than 2000 mg/dL = 4+.
   4. Significance
      a. Persistent proteinuria usually indicates renal disease or other systemic conditions.
      b. Transient proteinuria may be associated with stress, cold, exercise, and contamination of the specimen with menstrual blood as possible causes.
   5. Nitrites
      a. Description: Tests for bacteriuria and gram-negative bacteria convert urinary nitrate to nitrite, which will activate the chromogen of the dipstick. However, other organisms such as *Enterococcus, Streptococcus, E. faecalis,* or gonococci will not produce nitrite. In addition, urine must remain in the bladder for approximately 4 hours for production of nitrite from nitrate.

      b. **Significance:** Any degree of pink should be considered positive for the nitrite test, suggesting the presence of 10^5/mL.

      c. Be careful using a random sample making sure sufficient time (approximately 4 hours) has passed for conversion of nitrate to nitrite.

      d. More predictive of UTI than leukocyte esterase

  6. Leukocyte esterase

      a. **Description:** Leukocyte esterase is expressed in white blood cells (granulocytes) and will turn positive in the presence of >5 to 15 WBC/high-power field (HPF). However, it can be present with contamination.

  7. **Ketones:** Ketosis is seen in starvation (fad diets), nausea and vomiting, and with alcoholism, as well as in individuals with poorly controlled diabetes mellitus.

  8. **Blood:** Normal—RBCs may normally be seen in extremely small numbers in normal urine, particularly after strenuous exercise.

      a. The normal level is two or fewer RBCs per HPF.

      b. **Significance:** Hematuria is virtually always significant. Microhematuria should always be diagnosed on urine microscopy and not via urine dipstick. If positive, patients should be referred to urology for evaluation.

  9. Glucose

      a. **Description:** Can detect 100 mg/dL of glucose because the reaction relies on the enzyme glucose oxidase. However, results are qualitative.

      b. **Normal:** The absence of detectable glucose (negative dipstick) is considered a normal result.

      c. **Significance:** The dipstick method is extremely sensitive and specific for glucose. A positive finding of glucosuria indicated elevated blood glucose levels in the blood. Further evaluation is necessary to assess for diabetes mellitus.

 10. Bilirubin

      a. **Description:** Conjugated bilirubin should not be present in the urine. Bilirubin is a byproduct of RBC break down. Removed from the body via the liver. Presence may indicate liver disease.

 11. Urobilinogen

      a. **Description:** Urobilinogen is normally present in the urine in small amounts. Normal range is 0.2 to 1.0 mg/dL. Increased levels may indicate excess of bilirubin.

MICROSCOPIC EXAMINATION

A. **Description:** Evaluation of sediment for cellular elements, casts, crystals, and microorganisms.

  1. Performed in a laboratory setting when there is an abnormal finding on the urine dipstick results.

  2. APRNs can order microscopic urine evaluation to better quantify WBCs, RBCs, and so on.

  3. Common sediment in women (Table 47.3)

B. Casts

  1. **Description:** Casts usually occur in the distal convoluted tubule of the nephron and are so called because they are casts of the nephron. They are distinguished from other debris by smooth, parallel sides (which may show the trapezoidal narrowing of the nephron collecting system).

  2. Rarely normal. **Significance:** They are often difficult to interpret. They may indicate renal disease.

      a. RBC casts indicate proliferative glomerular disease or vasculitis.

      b. Hyaline casts that indicate proteinuria can be normal in concentrated urine.

      c. WBC casts indicate interstitial nephritis or pyelonephritis.

      d. Broad casts indicate tubular atrophy, with waxy casts indicating nephron death. Both are the successive changes in degeneration of cellular casts seen in renal failure.

TABLE 47.3 Common Urinary Sediments		
SEDIMENT	**DESCRIPTION**	**CLINICAL SIGNIFICANCE**
RBCs	Normal: Presence of 0–3/HPF; pale, biconcave discs; no nuclei; can be crenated; menses can contaminate and give false-positive results	Hematuria Cystitis most common cause of hematuria; can occur secondary to exertion, trauma, stress • 3 RBC/HPF is pathologic and needs referral to urology
WBCs	Normal: Presence of 0–5/HPF Polymorphonuclear leukocyte most common Segmented nuclei 1½ times as large as RBCs Cytoplasmic granules	Indicated infection or inflammation
Renal tubular epithelial cells	Round, single nucleus, slightly larger than WBCs	Renal tubular damage
Bladder epithelial cells	Varied shape: Flat to cuboidal; larger than renal cells	Normal
Squamous epithelial cells	Rectangular to round, flat cells; single small nuclei	Normal; usually due to vaginal contamination
Bacteria	Normal urine does not contain bacteria	Significant bacteria may indicate a urinary tract infection or contamination; send for culture and sensitivity if suspicious
Yeast cells	May be seen in urine (diabetics) Ovoid, budding Variable size Similar in size to RBCs	*Candida* or contamination from vulvovaginal candidiasis
Trichomonas	Most frequently seen parasite in urine Unicellular, ovoid with flagellate Undulates	Can be found in urine or urine contaminated from vaginal *Trichomonas*
Spermatozoa	Ovoid to round, with long tails; forward trajectory, spinning, immobile	May be seen after contamination by vaginal intercourse
Artifact	Starch granules (powder); cotton fibers	

HPF, high-powered field; RBCs, red blood cells; UTI, urinary tract infection; WBCs, white blood cells.

C. Crystals
1. **Description:** Crystals occur because of precipitated chemicals and cellular debris. Their interpretation depends on the clinical presentation involved and is beyond the scope of this chapter. Crystals are formed in normal (alkaline) urine as the specimen cools. Many different types of crystals are found in urine; however, a full discussion is beyond the scope of this chapter.

MANAGEMENT OF URINARY TRACT INFECTION

A. May prescribe phenazopyridine (Pyridium) 100 mg three times a day to relieve dysuria by preventing bladder spasm.
B. Uncomplicated cystitis (Table 47.4)

TABLE 47.4 Treatment of Uncomplicated Cystitis

NONPREGNANT WOMEN	PREGNANT WOMEN
First-line antibiotic treatment	First-line antibiotic treatment
Nitrofurantoin 100 mg BID for 5 days	Nitrofurantoin 100 mg BID for 5 days **NOTE: Avoid in first trimester due to possible teratogenic risk**
Trimethoprim-sulfamethoxazole 160/800 mg BID for 3–5 days	Amoxicillin 500 mg every 8 hours for 5–7 days or 875 mg BID for 3–7 days

BIBLIOGRAPHY

Abou Heidar, N. F., Degheili, J. A., Yacoubian, A. A., & Khauli, R. B. (2019). Management of urinary tract infection in women: A practical approach for everyday practice. *Urology Annals, 11*(4), 339–346. https://doi-org.ezproxy3.lhl.uab.edu/10.4103/UA.UA_104_19

Bono, M. J., & Reygaert, W. C. (2021). Urinary tract infection. In *StatPearls*. StatPearls Publishing.

Chu, C. M., & Lowder, J. L. (2018). Diagnosis and treatment of urinary tract infections across age groups. *American Journal of Obstetrics and Gynecology, 219*(1), 40–51. https://doi-org.ezproxy3.lhl.uab.edu/10.1016/j.ajog.2017.12.231113.

Flores-Mireles, A. L., Walker, J. N., Caparon, M., & Hultgren, S. J. (2015). Urinary tract infections: Epidemiology, mechanisms of infection and treatment options. *Nature Reviews. Microbiology, 13*(5), 269–284. https://doi.org/10.1038/nrmicro3432

Greenberg. (2014). Urinalysis and Urine Microscopy. In *National Kidney Foundation Primer on Kidney Diseases* (6th ed., pp. 33–41). https://doi.org/10.1016/B978-1-4557-4617-0.00004-2

Gupta, K., Grigoryan, L., & Trautner, B. (2017). Urinary Tract Infection. *Annals of Internal Medicine, 167*(7), ITC49–ITC64. https://doi-org.ezproxy3.lhl.uab.edu/10.7326/AITC201710030

Grigoryan, L., Zoorob, R., Wang, H., & Trautner, B. W. (2015). Low concordance with guidelines for treatment of acute cystitis in primary care. *Open Forum Infectious Diseases, 2*(4), ofv159. https://doi.org/10.1093/ofid/ofv159

Kavuru, V., Vu, T., Karageorge, L., Choudhury, D., Senger, R., & Robertson, J. (2020). Dipstick analysis of urine chemistry: Benefits and limitations of dry chemistry-based assays. *Postgraduate Medicine, 132*(3), 225–233. https://doi-org.ezproxy3.lhl.uab.edu/10.1080/00325481.2019.1679540

Lei, R., Huo, R., & Mohan, C. (2020). Current and emerging trends in point-of-care urinalysis tests. *Expert Review of Molecular Diagnostics, 20*(1), 69–84. https://doi-org.ezproxy3.lhl.uab.edu/10.1080/14737159.2020.1699063

Newman, D. K., Wyman, J. F. & Welch, V. W. (Eds.). (2017). *Society of Urologic Nurses and Associates core curriculum for urologic nursing* (1st ed). Anthony J. Jannetti, Inc.

Peck, J., & Shepherd, J. P. (2021). Recurrent urinary tract infections: Diagnosis, treatment, and prevention. *Obstetrics and Gynecology Clinics of North America, 48*(3), 501–513. https://doi-org.ezproxy3.lhl.uab.edu/10.1016/j.ogc.2021.05.005

Sigler, M., Leal, J. E., Bliven, K., Cogdill, B., & Thompson, A. (2015). Assessment of appropriate antibiotic prescribing for urinary tract infections in an internal medicine clinic. *Southern Medical Journal, 108*(5), 300–304. https://doi.org/10.14423/SMJ.0000000000000278.

Unit X

ADVANCED SKILLS

48

VULVAR BIOPSY

KELLEY STALLWORTH BORELLA, AIMEE CHISM HOLLAND, AND
HELEN A. CARCIO

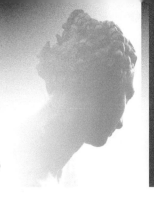

VULVAR CANCER EXPLAINED

A. Statistics
1. Accounts for 6% of all gynecologic cancers diagnosed in the United States
2. Causes 1,500 deaths annually in the United States
3. Women have a one in 333 chance of receiving the diagnosis during their life span.

B. Occurrence
1. Occurs most frequently in women older than 65 years
2. Incidence is rising in younger women
3. Usually diagnosed in the localized stage (about 60%)

C. Surgery is the usual treatment.

D. Most tumors are squamous cell in origin.

E. Long-standing pruritus is the most common complaint.

F. The most frequent site is the labia minora, in the middle or anterior portion.

G. Risk factors
1. History of HIV (human immunodeficiency virus) or HPV (human papillomavirus)
2. Multiple sexual partners
3. Smoking, especially if history of HPV
4. History of cervical cancer
5. History of lichen sclerosus (LSA); 4% of women who have LSA will later develop vulvar cancer

H. Early detection is key to reducing mortality rates.

I. Indications:
1. All white lesions of the vulva must undergo biopsy study if short-term medical treatment is unsuccessful; two thirds of the lesions appear acetowhite (white when vinegar is applied).
2. Any suspicious lesions of any color and persistent ulcerations should be excised.
3. Visible lesion for which definitive diagnosis cannot be made on clinical grounds
4. Suspicion of possible malignancy
5. Visible lesion with presumed clinical diagnosis that is not responding to topical therapy

NONNEOPLASTIC EPITHELIAL DISORDERS OF THE VULVAR SKIN AND MUCOSA

A. Squamous hyperplasia
1. This is a proliferative response to an irritant or allergen that has become chronic.
2. The presenting symptom is pruritus, with or without vulvodynia.
3. Suspect all substances that come in contact with the vulvar skin (see Box 48.1 for a list of vulvar irritants).

BOX 48.1 Substances That May Cause Vulvar Irritation

- Laundry detergents/fabric softeners
- Chlorine bleach
- Fiberglass particles (from residue in washing machine after washing fiberglass materials such as curtains)
- Propylene glycol in spermicides, lubricants, and vaginal medications
- Formalin found in the wool of permanent-press fabrics
- Nylon (can give off formaldehyde vapors)
- Deodorant substances on sanitary pads and liners
- Vaginal sprays and douches
- Creams in topical antifungal agents
- Synthetic-fiber underwear
- Fabric dyes, especially in colored underwear
- Saliva
- Semen
- Bromine and chlorine compounds in hot tubs and swimming pools
- Prescribed medications such as antifungals, antibacterials, crotamiton

Note: The distribution of lesions may provide a clue to which agent may be responsible for the allergic reaction.

4. Assessment includes
    a. Thick, white patches caused by localized thickening of the epidermis (lichenification)
    b. Raised lesions, often bilaterally symmetric
    c. Vulva may appear dusky red in color.
    d. Vulvar skin thickened with prominent skin markings (Perdu's sign)
5. Diagnosis
    a. Punch biopsy
    b. Histologic findings of acanthosis (irregular thickening of the Malpighian layer), hyperkeratosis, and inflammatory infiltrate

B. LSA
  1. Related to hormonal, genetic, and immunologic interactions
  2. Usually seen after a long period of self-diagnosis and treatment
  3. Symptoms include intractable itching, with or without vulvodynia
  4. Assessment includes
      a. Bluish-white papules, which progress to form thin white patches.
      b. Tissue is friable and may develop petechiae.
      c. Skin is thin and wrinkles like parchment paper.
  5. Diagnosis
      a. Punch biopsy
      b. Histologic findings include loss of rete layers, homogenization, and inflammatory infiltrate

C. Vulvar dermatologic manifestations that may be associated with systemic disease may not need to be excised if the systemic condition is well documented.
  1. Bechet's disease
      a. Small vesicles that ulcerate
      b. Systemic areas include oral ulcerations with uveitis and arthritis.

2. Pellagra
    a. A history of anorexia or poor dietary intake
    b. Hyperpigmentation and peeling of the vulva
    c. Systemic areas include dry scaly body skin with erythema of the mucous membrane.
3. Diabetes
    a. Chronic pruritus of vulva and erythema with a grey sheen
    b. Systemic areas include dry body skin and changes related to the kidney, retina, and heart.
4. Crohn's disease
    a. Knife-like slits in vulvar folds
    b. Associated with gastrointestinal problems of varying degrees.

DIFFERENTIAL DIAGNOSIS OF OTHER VULVAR DERMATOSES

A. Table 48.1 compares and contrasts other dermatoses.
B. A biopsy may be indicated because symptoms vary and may be cancerous.

TABLE 48.1 Differential Diagnosis of Other Vulvar Dermatoses

CONDITION	CLINICAL CHARACTERISTICS	OTHER SKIN AREAS AFFECTED
PAPULOSQUAMOUS LESIONS		
Contact dermatitis	Pruritus, history of exposure to irritant or allergen, erythema and edema in contact areas	Other areas in contact with irritant/allergen, although vulvar skin more sensitive
Lichen simplex chronicus	Pruritus, history of chronic irritation, thickened, leathery skin with accentuated skin markings	Not common
Lichen planus	Pruritus, purplish plaques defined by cross-hatched skin lines	Flat-topped papules on wrist, lumbar back, thighs, lacey pattern on buccal mucosa
Seborrheic dermatitis	Usually pruritus, yellow or red lesions covered by greasy scales in areas of sebaceous glands	Face, scalp, particularly eyebrows and hairline
Psoriasis	Mild pruritus, red plaques or silvery scales with bleeding points beneath	Silvery plaques on scalp, knees, elbows, sacrum
Tinea cruris	Variable, but usually dry, erythematous, annular lesions	May spread to buttocks and inner thighs
VESICULOBULLOUS LESIONS		
Erythema multiforme	History of recent genital herpes or drug allergy, "iris-shaped" lesions	Target lesions, especially on palms and soles
Pemphigus	Blisters and erosion	Any other skin areas on body
INFECTIONS		
Folliculitis	Tiny, red papules with white pustular center punctured by hair shaft	Any other skin in hairy areas
Impetigo	Superficial ulcer with yellow crust	Usually spread from infection of other body parts

VULVAR BIOPSY

A. Vulvar biopsy is a simple office procedure that is virtually free of complications and usually only causes minimal discomfort for the patient.

B. It is appropriate to use on lesions smaller than 0.5 cm. Refer larger lesions to a gynecologist.

C. The procedure takes approximately 15 minutes.

D. Excising all lesions, particularly fissures, ulcerations, or thick plaques, is mandatory because of the risk of cancer, no matter how small (only 1%–2% risk).

E. Biopsy sample must be full thickness.

F. Histologic findings are diagnostic.

ASSESSMENT

A. Ask about other dermatologic conditions on other parts of the body because a condition, such as psoriasis, can occur on the vulva.

B. Carefully evaluate the vagina and cervix, remembering that discharge from these areas bathes the vulvar tissues.

C. Perform a vaginal wet mount (see Chapter 6, "Vaginal Microscopy and Vaginal Infections") on any discharge.

INDICATIONS

A. To differentiate between benign and malignant conditions: Women who smoke or who are infected with HPV-16 are at higher risk for vulvar cancer.

   1. If the patient is seropositive, she is at even higher risk.

      a. Women with HPV seropositivity are 3-1/2 times more likely to develop in situ disease and more than 2-1/2 times more likely to develop invasive disease.

   2. The more a woman smokes and the longer she smokes, the greater the risk.

      a. Current smokers are at almost 6-1/2 times the risk for in situ disease and at 3 times the risk for invasive disease.

B. Confirm histologic characteristics.

PATIENT PREPARATION

A. Explain that discomfort during the procedure is usually minimal.

B. The reasons for the biopsy study should be explained and the technique should be outlined.

THE PROCEDURE

A. Some comments

   1. It is important to have good lighting.

   2. Use of 5% acetic acid can greatly enhance the identification of atypical areas, such as intraepithelial neoplasia or HPV infection, which will often turn aceto-white a few minutes after application on the vulva.

   3. Toluidine blue dye is no longer used owing to the high rate of false-positive and false-negative results.

   4. A large magnifying lens is essential to highlight abnormal areas for biopsy study.

   5. Colposcopy may be used and is particularly helpful in diagnosing HPV infection.

B. Equipment
   1. Hand magnifying lens (or colposcope)
   2. Betadine swabs
   3. Anesthetic agent
   4. A 25-gauge needle
   5. Syringe—0.3 mL
   6. No. 2-, 3-, or 4-mm Keyes's punch biopsy (disposable)
   7. Iris forceps
   8. Fine sterile scissors or no. 11 blade scalpel (disposable)
   9. Monsel's solution
   10. Sterile gauze sponges
   11. Labeled pathology container of formalin
   12. Paperwork for laboratory requisition
   13. Acetic acid (vinegar)
C. Identify area to be biopsied; multiple biopsy sites (two to three) may be indicated
D. Anesthesia
   1. Infiltrate skin locally with 1% xylocaine without epinephrine.
   2. Inject anesthetic solution subdermally with fine-gauge needle (0.5–1 mL per site).
   3. A wheal (4–5 mm) is created, which facilitates the biopsy by raising the lesion above the dermas and promotes local vasoconstriction, minimizing blood loss.
E. Biopsy procedure
   1. Cleanse area using antiseptic solution or iodine-soaked swabs.
   2. The dermal punch is like a corkborer.
   3. Place the punch biopsy over the site and rotate back and forth three or four times while holding the skin taut with the opposite hand (an assistant may be recruited to hold the skin).
   4. Bore out in a circular manner. Identify the location of the tissue sample once the punch is removed.
   5. Grasp the tissue sample with the forceps. Snip dermal skin areas transversely to sever the base with scissors or a scalpel.
   6. If the plug is lifted off and remains in the punch, dislodge the plug from the punch using a toothpick.
F. Control bleeding
   1. Bleeding is usually minimal because the dermis contains few blood vessels.
   2. Applying pressure with sterile gauze may be all that is required to stop any bleeding.
   3. If necessary, apply a small amount of Monsel's solution over the site for hemostasis.
   4. If bleeding persists, add a single suture using 4–0 Vicryl or Chromic.
   5. A sanitary pad may be used for additional pressure.
G. Laboratory preparation
   1. Gently place the sample in formalin and properly label the container.
   2. Complete required forms.
   3. Document the biopsy site(s) and the procedure itself, including the patient's response.
   4. If biopsy samples from different sites are obtained, place in separate containers and label with the site.

FOLLOW-UP

A. Care of the biopsy site
   1. The patient is instructed to keep the incision clean and dry.
   2. Showers should be taken daily until any soreness is gone.
   3. Blot dry. Be careful not to remove any healing scab.

4. Reassure the patient that the biopsy site will become practically invisible in 1 to 2 weeks.

5. Avoid intercourse for 2 or 3 days.

B. The patient is instructed to call if any redness or increasing discomfort occurs or the signs of infection develop such as malodorous or bloody drainage, uncontrolled pain, or a fever of 100.5° F or higher.

C. Return for follow-up to discuss the results and recommendations for treatment.

TEACH VULVAR SELF-EXAMINATION

A. Most vulvar malignancies are visible.

1. Vulvar examination should be performed monthly by women who are sexually active or who are older than 18 years.

2. The patient must recognize the importance of early detection of vulvar disease.

3. Understand the basic vulvar anatomy and function.

4. Learn the proper use of a handheld mirror to optimize viewing the vulva.

5. Perform the examination monthly between menses.

6. Report any new growths or changes.

BIBLIOGRAPHY

American Cancer Society. (2017). *What are the key statistics about vulvar cancer?* https://www.cancer.org/cancer/vulvar-cancer/about/key-statistics.html

American Cancer Society. (2021). *Vulvar cancer*. https://www.cancer.org/cancer/vulvar-cancer.html?utm_source=google&utm_medium=cpc&utm_campaign=Unassigned&utm_term=vulvar%20cancer&utm_id=go_cmp-10033843576_adg-97799932541_ad-434766943148_kwd-294909222373_dev-c_ext-_prd-_mca-_sig-CjwKCAiAvriMBhAuEiwA8Cs5lbZuzQKGmlHXWJvdRpNxXQxC7xEr8eYJZgSPhE4s3yMHkTtMTN_0IxoCpF0QAvD_BwE&gclid=CjwKCAiAvriMBhAuEiwA8Cs5lbZuzQKGmlHXWJvdRpNxXQxC7xEr8eYJZgSPhE4s3yMHkTtMTN_0IxoCpF0QAvD_BwE

Berek, J. & Karam, A. (2021). Vulvar cancer: Epidemiology, diagnosis, histopathology, and treatment. A. Chakrabarti (Ed.), *UpToDate*. https://www-uptodate-com.ezproxy3.lhl.uab.edu/contents/vulvar-cancer-epidemiology-diagnosis-histopathology-and-treatment?search=vulvar%20cancer&source=search_result&selectedTitle=1~97&usage_type=default&display_rank=1#H956750412

Holland, A. (2016). Using simulation to practice vulvar procedure skills. *Women's Healthcare, 4*(4), 24–28.

49

ENDOMETRIAL BIOPSY

KELLEY STALLWORTH BORELLA, AIMEE CHISM HOLLAND, AND
HELEN A. CARCIO

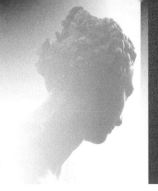

ENDOMETRIAL BIOPSY EXPLAINED

A. Endometrial biopsy examination is used mainly to diagnose two distinctly different conditions; endometrial caner and the presence of of luteal-phase defect. It is a method of removing a sample of representative tissue from the endometrium.
   1. It provides a histologic specimen of glandular epithelium from the uterine endometrial wall.
   2. It may be referred to as *endometrial sampling* because of the negative connotations that arise with the use of the word "biopsy."
   3. It is inexpensive and usually well tolerated by the woman.
   4. It is relatively easy to perform and can be performed appropriately by a trained healthcare provider.
   5. Advances in pipelles have made the procedure relatively simple to perform in the office, without the need for general anesthesia.
   6. Although the technique is relatively easy to perform by the clinician, it is often viewed as invasive by the patient.
   7. Its accuracy rate in identifying endometrial hyperplasia is greater than 90%. It is the only way to unequivocally diagnose endometrial cancer.

SOME COMMENTS CONCERNING ENDOMETRIAL CANCER

A. Survival rate
   1. **Local:** When endometrial cancer is diagnosed, if it is still confined to the area where it started, it is called *local*, and the 5-year survival rate is approximately 95%.
   2. **Regional:** If the cancer has spread regionally, the 5-year survival rate is approximately 69%.
   3. **Systemic spread:** If it is diagnosed after the cancer has spread into other areas of the body, the survival rate is 17%.
B. Incidence
   1. Endometrial cancer is the fourth most common cancer diagnosis in women in the United States and the sixth most frequent cause of death.
   2. In 2021, the American Cancer Society estimated 66,570 new diagnoses and 12,940 deaths from endometrial cancer.
   3. The median age at diagnosis is 60 years.
   4. Most uterine cancers are adenocarcinoma of the endometrium.
C. Risk factors
   1. **Age:** The incidence of endometrial cancer increases with age, particularly in those older than 65 years.
   2. It is rare in women younger than 45 years.

3. Obesity causes an increase in the presence of exogenous estrogens from peripheral conversions of estrogen in the fat cells.
   a. No progesterone is present to counterbalance the excess estrogen (unless on hormone replacement therapy [HRT]).
   b. Uterine cancer develops in women who are more than 50 pounds overweight 10 times more frequently than in women who are average weight.
4. Hyperestrogenic state is possibly related to the following
   a. Polycystic ovarian syndrome
   b. Early menarche
   c. Late menopause
5. Use of unopposed estrogen
   a. During the 1950s and 1960s, estrogen was given as replacement therapy without progesterone.
   b. This practice caused a dramatic increase in the occurrence of endometrial cancer.
   c. Clinicians are now aware of the need to use progesterone supplementation with estrogen replacement therapy (ERT) or to monitor the endometrium in a woman unwilling or unable to take progesterone.
6. Use of tamoxifen therapy as treatment for women with breast cancer
   a. It is antiestrogenic to breast tissue.
   b. It has an estrogenic effect on the lining of the uterus.
   c. It may contribute to endometrial stimulation, resulting in eventual hyperplasia and possible cancer.
   d. Its benefits in treating breast cancer probably outweigh the risk for development of endometrial cancer.
7. Endometrial hyperplasia and endometrial polyps put one at risk for endometrial cancer.
8. Previous breast or ovarian cancer are also risk factors.
9. A personal history of hypertension or diabetes put one at risk.
10. Consuming a diet high in fats puts one at risk.
D. Protective factors
   1. Progesterone use greatly diminishes hyperplasia of the endometrium; use of oral contraceptives, particularly if used during the later reproductive years, is protective.
   2. Breastfeeding
   3. Eating a diet low in fats and calories
E. Clinical features
   1. Abnormal uterine bleeding, particularly in postmenopausal women, including:
      a. Heavy menses
      b. Intermenstrual bleeding
      c. Frequent menstruation
   2. The older the woman, the higher the level of suspicion should be.
   3. Endometrial cells found on a Pap test

SOME COMMENTS CONCERNING LUTEAL-PHASE DEFECT

A. The condition exists when the corpus luteum secretes an inadequate amount of progesterone.
B. Approximately 3% to 4% of infertile women have LPD.
C. LPD is suspected when the luteal phase (the interval between ovulation and menstruation) is less than 11 days.
D. Causes
   1. Inadequate progesterone production by the granulosa cells of the ovary
   2. Hyperprolactinemia, which can cause an abnormal luteal phase

3. Psychogenic stress, nutritional factors, and exercise can cause a deficiency in the luteinizing hormone (LH) pulse
4. Kidney, liver, and immunologic diseases affect the corpus luteum cells

ENDOMETRIAL BIOPSY EXAMINATION EXPLAINED

A. Historical perspective
   1. Endometrial biopsy was first performed as early as the Ancient Greek era and was originally used as a treatment for abnormal uterine bleeding.
   2. In the 1950s, the normal characteristics of the endometrium were established, which led to the ability to apply endometrial dating to help diagnose LPDs.
B. Relationship to dilatation and curettage (D&C)
   1. Use of endometrial biopsy as a screen has replaced the need for D&C, which was previously the gold standard in many cases.
   2. Recent studies found that the results obtained by endometrial biopsy were histologically similar to specimens collected by D&C.
   3. Endometrial biopsy is more cost-effective and less invasive.

INDICATIONS FOR BIOPSY STUDY

A. Complaints of uterine bleeding in any postmenopausal woman: The level of concern should increase with the patient's advancing age, particularly if the woman:
   1. Is obese
   2. Is taking unopposed ERT
   3. Has had no spotting or bleeding for 12 months or longer
   4. The bleeding is excessive, prolonged, or irregular
   5. Is taking cyclic ERT with an increase in bleeding pattern
B. Postmenopausal women in whom bleeding begins or increases (if previously present) with the initiation of HRT that does not resolve after 3 to 6 months of therapy
   1. Some providers perform endometrial biopsy before the initiation of ERT, but most do not consider it necessary.
C. Monitoring endometrial response to hormonal influences of unopposed ERT in those women undergoing ERT who are unable or unwilling to take progesterone
   1. Progesterone protects the endometrium from the effects of unopposed estrogen.
      a. Women who are not taking progesterone are at increased risk for hyperplasia, which may lead to adenocarcinoma.
      b. Must monitor the patient yearly and document that the woman is aware of the increased risk for development of endometrial cancer.
      c. Biopsy study is sufficient, but the woman may choose to undergo ultrasonography to measure the width of the endometrial stripe.
         (1) The uterine lining is seen as a thin line or stripe.
         (2) The width of the stripe determines whether the lining of the uterus has thickened due to hyperplasia.
            - **Less than 5 mm:** No hyperplasia
            - **Between 5 and 10 mm:** Grey zone
            - **Greater than 10:** Hyperplasia
D. Endometrial cells found on a routine Pap test, especially
   1. If taken more than 10 days from the first day of the menstrual period
   2. In any patient older than 40 years
   3. In the presence of irregular bleeding

E. Infertile women with suspected LPD
   1. Documents endometrial response to progesterone
   2. Evaluates the luteal phase for endometrial dating in an infertile woman suspected of having an LPD
      a. A discrepancy of more than 2 days between the woman's endometrial histologic stage and menstrual dating is diagnostically significant.
   3. Also obtains valuable information about the patency of the cervical os
F. It is rarely performed before age 40 years because 95% of cancers occur in woman older than 40 years; Box 49.1 lists the exceptions.
G. Women who are undergoing tamoxifen treatment for breast cancer
H. Follow-up of abnormal ultrasound if endometrial thickness (stripe) is greater than 5 mm
I. Women in whom pelvic inflammatory disease (PID) is suspected (controversial)
   1. Endometritis is a fairly frequent cause of irregular bleeding in young women.
   2. Endometritis often precedes and then accompanies salpingitis.
   3. Endometrial biopsy offers an objective test in the diagnosis of PID to improve diagnostic accuracy.
      a. Positive if histologic findings of plasma cell endometritis are found

CONTRAINDICATIONS TO BIOPSY STUDY

A. Pregnancy or poorly involuted postpartum uterus (a sensitive pregnancy test can be performed before)
B. Infection
   1. Any infection can be passed into the uterine cavity and tubes as the pipelle passes through the cervical os.
   2. **Active or chronic cervicitis:** Defer until treated.
   3. **Active or chronic vaginitis:** Defer until treated.
C. Uterine abnormalities, such as a large myoma displacing the uterus, making obtaining of a sample impossible
D. Blood dyscrasias or suspected bleeding disorder
E. Woman is febrile. Note: If there is a history of valvular heart disease or rheumatic fever, bacterial endocarditis is a risk and antibiotic prophylaxis is appropriate.

Examination of the Woman

A. Subjective information must include
   1. Date of last menstrual period (LMP)
   2. Use of contraception; discuss compliance issues
   3. Risk-evaluation for sexually transmitted infections (STIs) and HIV
   4. History of any bleeding problems
   5. Presence of symptoms of vaginal or cervical infections

BOX 49.1 Indications for Biopsy Study Before Age 40 Years

Biopsy study before age 40 years is only indicated if the following factors are present:

- Obesity (may have higher levels of estrogen)
- Long-standing anovulation or irregular menstrual cycles
- History of other adenocarcinomas such as of the breast or colon
- Functional metrorrhagia with dysfunctional uterine bleeding

6. History of heart disease, especially rheumatic heart disease or mitral valve prolapse
7. Allergies, especially to lidocaine (Xylocaine) or povidone-iodine (Betadine)
8. Level of pain associated with previous Pap tests
9. History of vasovagal episode or hypoglycemia
10. Inquire about food eaten that day; offer sweetened juice to prevent a vasovagal reaction

B. Objective findings
1. Obtain vital signs, including temperature.
2. Perform pelvic examination to assess for any signs of infection.
3. Perform laboratory tests, if indicated.
   a. Sensitive pregnancy test
   b. Hematocrit
   c. Wet mount examination (see Chapter 6, "Vaginal Microscopy and Vaginal Infections")

SUPPLIES

A. Supplies
1. Nonsterile gloves
2. Vaginal speculum
3. Tenaculum
4. Aseptic solution (Betadine)
5. Cotton rectal swab
6. Sterile pipelle (two)
7. Biopsy sample container (10% formalin or other fixative)
8. Two percent to 10% viscous lidocaine gels and Hurricaine gel
9. Sterile lubricant

B. Characteristics of the pipelle
1. Advances in the pipelle have made the procedure relatively simple to perform in the office without the need for general anesthesia
2. Single-use, disposable, clear instrument with colored, graduated markings graded from 4 cm to 10 cm
3. Flexible polypropylene
4. **Size:** Small caliber, 3.1 cm (outside diameter) and 2.6 cm (inner diameter); 23.5 cm in length
5. **Use:** Histologic biopsy of uterine mucosal lining or sample extraction of uterine menstrual content
6. **Negative pressure:** Rapid movement of the piston creates a negative pressure within the lumen of the sheath, allowing for aspiration of the mucosal tissue through the curette opening and into the lumen of the tube as the curette scrapes against the endometrial walls while being moved within the uterine cavity; the piston cannot be fully pulled out.

PREPARATION

A. Timing in the evaluation of LPD
1. Performed 1 to 3 days before the expected onset of menses (take average of previous cycles)
2. Menses may begin on the day of the scheduled biopsy procedure because the timing is close; if this occurs, the biopsy procedure must be rescheduled for the next cycle, but a day or 2 earlier.

B. Can schedule evaluation of abnormal uterine bleeding or endometrial monitoring at any time.

C. Analgesia
1. Many clinicians suggest the use of nonsteroidal anti-inflammatory medication in the event that mild cramping occurs.
2. Administer ibuprofen, 400 mg, 30 to 60 minutes before the scheduled visit.

D. In patients who are very sensitive to pain, topical anesthesia, such as 20% benzocaine (Hurricaine), can be applied to the cervix a few minutes before the procedure.

INFORMED CONSENT AND EDUCATION

A. The clinician must clearly explain
   1. How much pain to expect
   2. Reasons for the procedure
   3. Risks involved, including perforation of the uterus, failure to obtain tissue, and infection
   4. Overall safety
   5. Realistic expectation of what will occur during the procedure
   6. What the results may indicate
B. Verbal or written consent should be obtained and documented.

THE PROCEDURE

A. **Position:** The woman is asked to assume a comfortable dorsal lithotomy position.
B. Bimanual examination
   1. A bimanual pelvic examination is first performed to determine the position and size of the uterus and to assess for any pelvic tenderness.
   2. A rectal examination may be necessary if the uterus is retroverted.
   3. The examination helps determine the direction of insertion of the catheter.
   4. It is important to assess the size of the uterus so that its proper depth can be determined.
C. **Use of lubricant:** A lubricant should not be used because it may prevent proper interpretation of cervical cytology tests.

TECHNIQUE

A. Put on gloves (sterile gloves are not necessary). Care should be taken not to touch the parts of the instruments that will come in contact with the cervix or the endometrial cavity.
B. The speculum is inserted into the vagina, and the cervical os is visualized.
   1. The cervix should be well positioned, facing directly outward, between the blades of the speculum. (This helps with the insertion technique.)
C. Inspection
   1. The vagina and cervix are inspected for the presence of any unusual discharge.
   2. If an infection is suspected, a wet mount examination should be performed.
      a. If white blood cells are present, the condition should be diagnosed and treated.
      b. Reschedule biopsy surgery for the next cycle.
D. Cleanse the area.
   1. Using a rectal swab, the cervix and upper vagina are next swabbed free of discharge and cleansed with an antiseptic such as Betadine.
   2. Any excess Betadine should be removed to prevent contamination of the specimen.
E. Use of a tenaculum for anteflexion or retroflexion
   1. A tenaculum is usually not necessary.
   2. It is only used 15% of the time.
   3. If it is used, a lidocaine gel should be placed at the site the tenaculum will grasp for 5 minutes, or 1% lidocaine (0.5–1.0 mL) should be injected at the tenaculum site via a spinal needle. Either method will significantly reduce the pain of tenaculum application.
   4. The tenaculum may be necessary to stabilize the cervix and straighten the uterus to facilitate passage of the pipelle if there is a marked degree of anteflexion or retroflexion.

  a. Anteflexion
   (1) Grasp the anterior upper lip of the cervix between the 2 o'clock and 10 o'clock positions. (Warn the patient that they will feel a pinch.)
   (2) This technique should compress approximately 1 cm of cervical tissue. (The tissue immediately turns white.)
   (3) Gently pull the cervix forward to straighten the cervical canal.
   (4) Guide the curved tip along the anterior surface of the endocervical canal.
  b. Retroflexion
   (1) Grasp the posterior lip of the cervix.
   (2) Guide the curved tip along the posterior surface of the endocervical canal.
  c. Remember that the uterine artery runs laterally at the 3 o'clock and 9 o'clock positions.
 5. The clinician may manually curve the tip of the pipelle while it is in the sterile package to accommodate the curvature of the uterus.
 6. If the tip is not curved, the straight tip may become embedded into the posterior or anterior wall of the canal.

F. Pipelle insertion
 1. If a topical anesthetic is being used, instill it into the cervical os using a swab.
 2. Once the position of the uterus has been assessed and the cervical os positioned, a thin pipelle or catheter is passed through the cervix, into the uterus to the fundus.
 3. The tip of the catheter can be bent manually for easier insertion to accommodate the natural curve of the endocervical canal.
 4. However, the clinician must be aware that the rigidness of the catheter may slightly increase chances of accidental perforation.
 5. It is usually not necessary to sound the uterus.
 6. Hold the pipelle lightly with a grip similar to that used to hold a pencil.
 7. As the pipelle is inserted through the cervix, the resistance of the internal os is felt as the pipelle is passed through.
 8. Slowly and gently advance the catheter the full depth of the endometrial cavity, until the resistance of the fundus is felt.
 9. Never use force against digitally felt resistance.
 10. Assess the length of the uterus by noting the centimeters marked on the pipelle.
  a. In premenopausal women, 6 cm or more
  b. Less than 6 cm in postmenopausal women
  c. The cavity has probably not been entered if only the 3 to 4 cm mark has been reached.
  d. The woman may feel mild uterine cramps at this point.
  e. Once the pipelle is fully inserted and the tip is positioned properly, release traction of the tenaculum, if it is used.

G. Aspiration
 1. The pipelle should be stabilized with the nondominant hand, using the dominant hand to pull the plunger fully back.
 2. Rapidly pull the piston firmly, using one full motion, as far toward the proximal end of the sheath as it will go. The piston cannot be pulled out completely.
 3. Slow, irregular pressure, or incomplete withdrawal of the plunger will not supply the suction required for an appropriate sample.
 4. Correct technique creates negative pressure inside the pipelle, which allows for aspiration of the endometrial tissue into the open tip of the pipelle.
 5. Next, the pipelle should be rotated continuously 360° by rolling or twisting it between thumb and index finger as it is rapidly, but gently, advanced and withdrawn between the fundus and internal os (Figure 49.1).
 6. Withdraw and advance the pipelle three or four times (for 30 seconds).

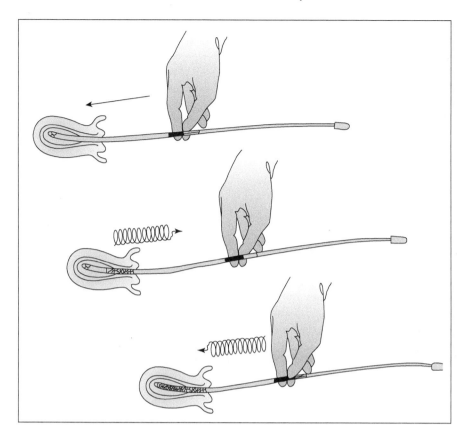

FIGURE 49.1 Simultaneously roll (twirl) sheath between fingers while moving sheath laterally and back and forth (in and out) between the fundus and internal os three or four times to obtain the sample.

7. As the tube is rotated, a column of tissue is seen as it is drawn into the tube, often filling it completely.
8. This suction from negative pressure generally yields an adequate sample.
9. If the pipelle is withdrawn from the os, the suction is lost.
10. If this occurs, the pipelle should be reinserted.
11. Once enough of a sample has been aspirated, the pipelle is slowly removed and the contents placed directly in preservative and sent to the pathology department for analysis.
12. If the instrument does not touch the container, it can be reinserted, if necessary.
13. Record the depth, ease of insertion, and patient response.
14. Any bleeding from the tenaculum site usually abates rapidly.
15. The patient should remain supine for a few minutes until any pain or dizziness passes.
16. Supply the woman with a perineal pad.

H. Sampling
1. Recent studies suggest that the most representative samples are obtained from high in the corpus from both the anterior and posterior walls.
2. The samples should be superficial rather than deep because the deeper tissues often show less intense reactivity to progesterone.
3. If a sufficient sample is not obtained, the procedure should be repeated at a later date.
4. The extent of the sample should correlate to the level of suspicion for malignancy.
5. For endometrial dating, only a single sample is necessary.

COMMON PROBLEMS

A. Difficulty entering the os due to cervical stenosis
   1. The cervix of a menopausal women is often tight. If this is the case, a smaller caliber (2–3 mm) pipelle should be used rather than the standard 4 mm.
   2. If the flexible cannula bends in the middle with any pressure during attempts to pass through a tight cervical canal, grasp the cannula about 4 cm from its end with a ring or uterine dressing forceps. (This method minimizes the bending in the middle of the cannula as pressure is applied and eases its passage through the cervix.)
   3. In addition, the pipelle, with the tip curved, can be placed in a freezer to increase rigidity. Remember, this stiffness may slightly increase the risk of perforation.
   4. A sterile lubricant can be placed on the pipelle to ease insertion in the elderly woman with a dry cervix.
   5. Some clinicians recommend a 2-week course of vaginal estrogen before the biopsy sample is taken, to open the cervical os.
   6. If the os it still too tight or if the woman has severe atrophy, in which the external os may no longer be patent, the clinician should refer the patient to a gynecologist to open the os after the administration of paracervical anesthesia.

B. Minimal tissue obtained
   1. Commonly seen in postmenopausal women evaluated for light spotting or bleeding
   2. Consider the presence of a scant amount of tissue diagnostically sufficient if the following apply:
      a. The pipelle has passed at least 6 cm into the uterus.
      b. There is a clear sensation of having reached the fundus.
      c. The patient is not at high risk for endometrial cancer (due to factors other than age).

AFTER THE BIOPSY PROCEDURE

A. Preparing the specimen for analysis
   1. After the specimen has been obtained, clip off the tip of the cannula with scissors.
   2. Advance the piston so that the endometrial sample is expressed into a vial containing fixative.
   3. Fill out the paperwork and label the specimen, including information about the patient's clinical status.
   4. Indicate any hormone therapy the woman is receiving.

B. Following the procedure, observe the woman for:
   1. Vasovagal response
      a. The woman should be closely observed for a vasovagal response.
      b. She should remain supine for a few minutes and then slowly be assisted to a sitting position.
      c. She should remain sitting until equilibrium is restored and any discomfort passes.
   2. Cramping
      a. Painful cramps usually subside rapidly and are well tolerated.
      b. If the cramps persist, an anti-inflammatory agent can be used.

C. Referral
   1. Patient with contraindications
   2. Patient with a severely stenotic os
   3. Confer with supervising physician to discuss a patient at risk for bacterial endocarditis

COMPLICATIONS (TABLE 49.1)

A. The client should be advised to monitor any bleeding and to return should any of the following develop:
 1. Severe cramping or worsening discomfort or pain
 2. Heavy bleeding and clots or any bleeding lasting longer than 2 days
 3. Any foul-smelling discharge, with or without fever and chills
 4. Uterine perforation
   a. Is very rare
   b. Usually without serious sequelae
   c. New catheters are very small and flexible, and carry little risk of perforation of the uterus
   d. If perforation is suspected, the patient needs to be closely monitored for heavy bleeding.
 5. Interruption of a pregnancy when evaluating LPD
   a. There is a slight chance of disturbing an early pregnancy.
   b. Interruption of a pregnancy is rare, occurring in 1/1,500 biopsy procedures total, and in 1/500 biopsy studies for evaluating LPD. (The resulting miscarriage rate is 20%.)
   c. The woman may choose to use contraception during the cycle preceding surgery, or she may elect to continue trying to conceive because the risk is slight.
   d. Nothing is worse than disrupting an established pregnancy during an endometrial biopsy study in an infertile couple.
   e. A sensitive pregnancy test is recommended.

FOLLOW-UP

A. LPD evaluation
 1. Ask the woman to call with the date that her next period begins.
 2. This information is essential for the accurate interpretation of results because they are based on the comparison of the histologic date to the day of menses.
 3. Normal results will confirm that ovulation has occurred and that there is adequate progesterone to support an early pregnancy.
B. Results are usually available in 7 to 10 days.
C. Have the client return in 2 weeks to discuss biopsy study results and any follow-up.

TABLE 49.1 Complications Associated With Endometrial Biopsy	
COMPLICATION	**RATE**
Cervical stenosis	12/28
Excessive bleeding	5/28
Fever	4/28
Excessive pain	2/28
Vasovagal reaction	2/28
Uterine perforation	2/28
Interrupted pregnancy	1/28

DIAGNOSIS

A. LPD
  1. LPD should be suspected if the endometrial tissue is "out of phase," demonstrating a lag of more than 2 days from the expected date of menses.
  2. The day of ovulation is counted forward to the date of the biopsy surgery.
  3. In addition, the onset of the next menses is counted as day 28, counting back to the day of the biopsy surgery, and comparing it with the histologic date provided.
  4. A normal basal body temperature (BBT) or LH surge and an "in-phase" biopsy support the adequacy of the hypothalamic–pituitary–ovarian axis.
  5. If the biopsy is out of phase, further hormonal assessment is warranted.
B. The case against the use of endometrial biopsy study in diagnosing LPD
  1. Endometrial biopsy examination is being used less and less because of the invasive nature of the test and the additional cost in both time and money.
  2. Some sources believe that there is a weak correlation between out-of-phase biopsy surgeries and infertility.
  3. Results are believed to be somewhat subjective, with different interpretations using the same sample.
  4. Other methods, such as the BBT, over-the-counter ovulation predictor kit, and serum progesterone test, are accurate in documenting luteal function.
  5. Although a normal in-phase endometrial biopsy sample is strongly suggestive of an adequate luteal phase, an abnormal result does not always indicate LPD because 25% to 30% of abnormal biopsy samples are found in normally fertile women.
C. Adenocarcinoma
  1. May note abundant friable fragments, which may appear as bits of rolled-up tissue in the endometrial sample.

BIBLIOGRAPHY

American Cancer Society. (2017). *Cancer facts and figures 2013*. American Cancer Society.
Del Priore, G. (2021). Endometrial sampling procedures. B. Goff (Ed.), *UpToDate*. https://www-uptodate-com.ezproxy3
  .lhl.uab.edu/contents/endometrial-sampling-procedures?search=endometrial%20biopsy&source=search_result
  &selectedTitle=1~149&usage_type=default&display_rank=1

50
ACROCHORDONECTOMY (SKIN TAG REMOVAL)

KELLEY STALLWORTH BORELLA, AIMEE CHISM HOLLAND, AND
HELEN A. CARCIO

ACROCHORDONECTOMY (REMOVAL OF SKIN TAGS) EXPLAINED

A. Acrochordonectomy is a simple technique for the advanced practice clinician to master.
1. Many women who are seen for their annual visit may complain of having a skin tag.
2. Although not painful, women often find them unsightly and bothersome as they may snag on clothes or jewelry, particularly if they are seen around the face and neck.
3. Because skin tags are harmless, often individuals may elect not to have them removed unless they cause chafing and irritation from the skin surfaces rubbing together, particularly in overweight individuals.

ACROCHORDON EXPLAINED

A. An acrochordon is a flesh-toned, papillomatous, cutaneous lesion.
1. If they are pedunculated, they are called *cutaneous papillomas* and *soft fibromas*.
2. **Histologically:** The lesion is hyperplastic epidermis enclosing a dermal connective tissue stalk.
3. Acrochordons usually range in size from 2 to 5 mm, although they can grow quite large.
4. Skin tags are generally harmless and do not enlarge over time.
5. Occurrence of skin tags
   a. Skin tags can occur almost anywhere on the body covered by skin. However, the two most common areas for skin tags are the neck and armpits; they also commonly occur in creases and skin folds.
   b. Other common body areas for the development of skin tags include the eyelids, upper chest (particularly under the female breasts), buttock folds, and groin folds.
   c. Tags are typically thought to occur where skin rubs against itself or clothing.
6. Generally speaking, skin tags are not precancerous or painful and are not associated with any other skin conditions. Patients often have cosmetic concerns and desire their removal.
7. There is no evidence that "seeding" occurs causing them to spread to other parts once they are removed.
B. Causes
1. A family history of acrochordons sometimes exists
2. Hormones during pregnancy
3. Obesity
4. High cholesterol
5. May serve as an important finding for people who have impaired carbohydrate metabolism and may alert them that they are at risk for type 2 diabetes.
C. There are many home remedies and products for acrochordon removal that can be found on the Internet; some women even try to snip them off themselves; caution should be advised because the stalk contains blood vessels and may bleed or become infected.

REMOVAL

A. The removal technique is easy, straightforward, and can be done during a routine physical examination.

B. Technique one
1. Identify the lesion to be removed.
   a. Cleanse the lesion and the surrounding area with an iodine swab.
   b. Rinse with sterile saline.
2. Anesthesia
   a. Use as needed. Use of 1% lidocaine (with or without epinephrine) is usually adequate.
   b. Use a 27-gauge needle.
   c. If the woman is opposed to the use of needles, a simple application of an ice cube over the lesion will provide enough numbness and seem less invasive to the patient.
3. Apply a surgical clamp, such as a Kelly clamp, at the base of the acrochordon. The stalk is usually easily identified.
   a. Keep clamp in place for approximately 5 to 10 minutes to decrease the blood flow.
   b. Remove the clamp.
4. Grasp the lesion with a small clamp and lift away from the skin.
5. Excise the lesion using fine-bladed scissors (iris scissors).
6. Cut in the middle of the approximately 2-mm compressed area left by the surgical clamp.
7. A small circular adhesive bandage may be applied, or the area may be left open.
8. The skin usually heals smooth.

C. Technique two
1. Identify the lesion to be removed.
2. Apply petroleum jelly around the lesion, being careful not to cover the lesion itself with the petroleum jelly.
3. Apply trichloroacetic acid (TCA) or bichloroacetic acid (BCA) or liquid nitrogen to the lesion until it turns white, being careful not to get any chemical on the surrounding skin. (The immediate area around it will turn red and a slight burning may occur, which usually subsides in a few minutes.)
4. Inform the patient that the lesion will turn black and eventually fall off.
5. There is a slight chance of scarring when and if some liquids make contact with healthy skin.
6. If the lesion is larger than 2 mm, the client may have to return for a second chemical application.
7. A lesion of more than 5 mm should be referred to a dermatologist.
8. Electrolysis destroys the lesion and the underlying skin.

D. If the woman has many tags, only three or four should be removed at one time.

FOLLOW-UP

A. The patient is advised to call should burning increase or signs of infection occur.

B. Return for removal of other lesions as needed.

C. Excision is quick and easy with immediate results that require little follow-up.

BIBLIOGRAPHY

Goldstein, A. (2021). Overview of benign lesions of the skin. R. Dellavalle (Ed.), *UpToDate*. https://www-uptodate-com.ezproxy3.lhl.uab.edu/contents/overview-of-benign-lesions-of-the-skin?search=acrochordon%20removal&source=search_result&selectedTitle=1~150&usage_type=default&display_rank=1

Hui, E. S., Yip, B. H., Tsang, K. W., Lai, F. T., Kung, K., & Wong, S. Y. (2016). Association between multiple skin tags and metabolic syndrome: A multicentre cross-sectional study in primary care. *Diabetes & Metabolism, 42*(2), 126–129. https://doi.org/10.1016/j.diabet.2015.11.004

Singh, P., John, A. M., Lee, B., Handler, M. Z., Schwartz, R. A., & Lambert, W. C. (2016). Deadly skin tags! *Skinmed, 14*(6), 441–443.

Srivastava, A., Khare, A. K., Gupta, L. K., Mittal, A., Mehta, S., Balai, M., & Bharti, G. (2017). A clinicoepidemiological study of skin tags and their association with metabolic syndrome. *Przeglad Dermatologiczy, 104*, 1–8. https://doi.org/10.5114/dr.2017.66216

51

CERVICAL POLYPECTOMY

KELLEY STALLWORTH BORELLA, AIMEE CHISM HOLLAND, AND
HELEN A. CARCIO

POLYPS EXPLAINED

A. Description
1. Polyps are the most common benign tumors of the cervix.
2. They are found most often during the menstruating years (parous women in their fifth decade).
3. Polyps are rare in young, nonmenstruating women.
4. They are soft, pear-shaped (finger-like), red to purple lesions, and are usually pedunculated growths from the surface of the cervical canal (Figure 51.1).
5. They are very friable and contain a large number of blood vessels, particularly near the surface.
6. Diameter varies from several millimeters to less than 3 cm.
7. They occur with overgrowth of one of the cervical folds.
8. They are usually asymptomatic but may be friable and bleed with intercourse.
9. Usually only one polyp is present, but in rare cases, there may be two.
10. Typically, polyps are not cancerous (benign) and are easy to remove. They are often removed during a routine pelvic examination.
11. Polyps do not usually grow back. However, women who have polyps once are at risk of growing more polyps.
12. During a pelvic examination, the healthcare provider will see smooth, red, or purple finger-like growths on the cervix. A cervical biopsy will most often show cells that are consistent with a benign polyp. Rarely, there may be abnormal, precancerous, or cancer cells in a polyp.
13. Although most cervical polyps are not cancerous (benign), the removed tissue should be sent to a laboratory and checked further.

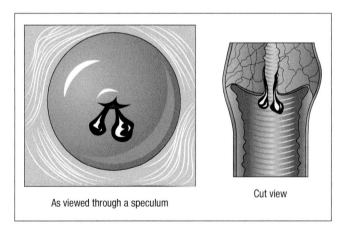

As viewed through a speculum

Cut view

FIGURE 51.1 Cervical polyps. Note how they are attached to a stalk.

B. Microscopic analysis
  1. Loose vascular connective tissue covered by endocervical epithelium is seen.
  2. Stroma may be inflamed and edematous.

C. Location
  1. Usually found in the lower endocervix; may protrude through the cervical os.
  2. May be found at the squamocolumnar junction or portio vaginal.

D. Cause
  1. Not completely understood
  2. May occur with
    a. An abnormal response to increased levels of estrogen
    b. Chronic inflammation
    c. Clogged blood vessels in the cervix

E. Symptoms
  1. Abnormally heavy periods (menorrhagia)
  2. Abnormal vaginal bleeding
    a. After douching
    b. After intercourse
    c. After menopause
    d. Between periods
    e. Polyps may not cause symptoms and do not need to be removed unless they are bothersome or cause heavy bleeding.

POLYPS ARE EASY TO REMOVE IN THE OFFICE AT THE TIME OF THE VISIT

A. Technique one
  1. Determine the site of origin.
  2. Grasp polyp with clamp.
  3. Twist until the polyp separates from the stalk.
  4. Apply silver nitrate or Monsel's solution for hemostasis.

B. Technique two (if polyp is large—greater than 5 mm)
  1. Determine the site of origin.
  2. Clamp approximately 0.5 cm above the origin of the pedicle.
  3. A surgical ligature is next tied between the clamp and the cervix.
  4. Remove the clamp.
  5. Using a pair of scissors with a fine blade, cut along the suture line to remove the polyp.
    a. Send specimen to the pathology department.
    b. All polyps should be sent to the pathology department because malignancy can occur in benign-appearing structures (0.2%–0.4% incidence).
  6. It may be left attached to undergo infarction and slough.

C. Referral
  1. Electrical current (loop electrosurgical excision procedure [LEEP]) or laser therapy is used for any polyp greater than 5 mm.
  2. If an endometrial polyp is suspected, dilation and curettage or a hysteroscope may be used to cut or scrap off the polyp.

D. Possible complications
  1. Bleeding and slight cramping may occur for a few days after the removal of a polyp.
  2. Rarely, cervical cancers may first appear as a polyp.
  3. Certain uterine polyps may be associated with uterine cancer.
  4. There is no need for special follow-up as polyps seldom recur after removal.

BIBLIOGRAPHY

Holland, A. (2016). Using simulation to practice and perfect gynecological procedure skills. *Women's Healthcare: A Clinical Journal for NPs*, *4*(1), 16–20.

Laufer, M. (2021). Benign cervical lesions and congenital anomalies of the cervix. R. Barbieri (Ed.), *UpToDate*. https://www-uptodate-com.ezproxy3.lhl.uab.edu/contents/benign-cervical-lesions-and-congenital-anomalies-of-the-cervix?-search=cervical%20polypectomy&source=search_result&selectedTitle=1~2&usage_type=default&display_rank=1

52

DRAINAGE OF BARTHOLIN'S ABSCESS

KELLEY STALLWORTH BORELLA, AIMEE CHISM HOLLAND, AND
HELEN A. CARCIO

BARTHOLIN'S GLANDS EXPLAINED

A. Bartholin's glands
 1. Pair of pea-sized mucus-secreting glands located on each side of the opening of the vagina, on the lips of the labia at 4 o'clock and 8 o'clock positions.
 2. Secrete a vaginal lubricating fluid during sexual stimulation to protect vaginal tissue from irritation.
 3. Lubricating fluid normally travels from the gland down tiny ducts about 0.8 inch.
 4. They are 2 cm long and drain into the lower part of the entrance to the vagina (Figure 52.1).
B. A Bartholin's gland cyst is a fluid-filled swelling on one of the glands.
 1. Commonly occur in younger women who are sexually active
 2. Usually not an infection but cellulitis may occur in the area
 3. Not sexually transmitted, but may be associated with gonorrhea
 4. Approximately 2% of women will develop a Bartholin's gland cyst in their lifetime.
 5. Usually develop in only one of the two glands
 6. Ducts become blocked and fluid accumulates, causing a cyst
 7. *Escherichia coli* is the most common pathogen
 8. Have a high rate of recurrence

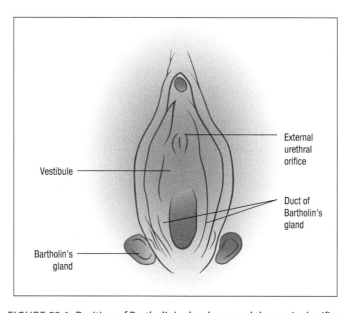

FIGURE 52.1 Position of Bartholin's glands around the vaginal orifice.

C. Symptoms
1. A woman may not even know she has it, and it may be picked up during a routine pelvic examination.
2. May note a large tender mass or lump in the vagina.
3. Pain is felt in the vaginal area especially during intercourse and movement such as sitting, walking, or sports activities.
4. Vulvar skin may be tender and red with swelling of the labia.
5. Causes enlarged, painful lymph nodes.

D. Treatment may not be needed if a Bartholin's gland cyst is small and does not cause any symptoms; if the cyst becomes swollen and painful, treatment may be necessary.

E. Home care
1. Sit in a warm bath a few times a day or apply a moist, warm compress. Helps the fluid to drain from the cyst
2. In many cases, home care may be enough to treat the cyst.

TREATMENT OF BARTHOLIN'S GLAND ABSCESS INVOLVES INCISION AND DRAINAGE OF CYST AND INSERTION OF WORD CATHETER

A. Equipment
1. 18- to 22-gauge needle
2. 5- to 10-mL syringe (catheter inflation) with normal saline
3. 25-gauge needle with 5-mL syringe (for application of anesthesia)
4. 1% Xylocaine
5. Antiseptic solution (betadine swabs)
6. Scalpel with #11 blade
7. Small hemostats (2)
8. 4 × 4 gauze pads
9. Silver nitrate sticks
10. Antiseptic solution
11. Bartholin's gland drainage catheter (Word)

PREPARATION

A. Position woman in a comfortable lithotomy position.
1. Cleanse area with antiseptic.
2. Palpate area to visualize the location and size of the abscess.
3. With needle bellow pointed upward, create a wheal by infiltrating the Xylocaine (5–10 mL) into the area of the duct.

THE PROCEDURE

A. The incision
1. Incise the vaginal side wall and create a 3-mm incision through the mucosa into the cysts.
2. Should be approximately 1 cm to 1.5 cm long to fit the Word catheter.
3. Stab wound should be deep enough to express fluid and allow for the flow of pus or mucus from the gland.
4. The catheter is put in place to drain the abscess and allow for re-epithelialization.

B. **Insertion of Word catheter:** A Word catheter is a small rubber catheter with an inflatable balloon tip that is inserted into the stab wound that has been drained.
1. Grasp the walls of the cyst with the hemostat to hold open.

     a. This stabilizes the walls.

     b. It prevents the creation of false tracts outside the cyst.

2. Using a second hemostat, insert into stab wound and move around to break up any loculations.

3. Allow for cyst contents to drain and then irrigate cyst with 5 mL of saline.

4. Test the balloon by filling with 3-mL sterile water and then deflate. (Do not use air.)

5. With syringe and needle still attached, insert the balloon tip into the Bartholin's gland through the incision.

6. Inflate the bulb with 2 to 3 mL of fluid through the sealed stopper.

7. Inflate to the point to ensure that it will not fall out.

8. The catheter should stay in place and comfortably fill the cavity.

9. Tuck the catheter stem into the vagina.

     a. The catheter rests perpendicular to the perineum to avoid tension on the tissue due to bending of the catheter stem.

     b. The catheter stem will not protrude out of the vagina, making it much more comfortable for the woman.

FOLLOW-UP

A. Call if discomfort or signs of infection occur.

    1. Woman should return in 3 weeks to remove the catheter once epithelialization occurs.

    2. The catheter balloon is deflated and easily removed.

    3. Antibiotic is not normally required except if cellulitis is present around the vulvar opening of the duct.

    4. The patient should call if the area has increased pain or swelling.

B. Refer to surgeon for marsupialization if the cyst recurs or the Word catheter does not resolve the abscess.

C. Complications

    1. Continuous pain

      a. Bulb may have been overinflated in the cavity and can cause pain once the anesthesia wears off.

    2. Infection at wound site

    3. Catheter may fall out

      a. If stab wound opening is too large

      b. If bulb not sufficiently inflated

    4. Catheter may deflate

      a. The stem of the catheter may be mistakenly punctured during insertion; catheter may gradually deflate and eventually fall out.

BIBLIOGRAPHY

Chen, K. (2021a). Bartholin gland masses: Diagnosis and management. R. Barbieri (Ed.), UpToDate. https://www-upto-date-com.ezproxy3.lhl.uab.edu/contents/bartholin-gland-masses-diagnosis-and-management?search=Incision%20 and%20drainage%20of%20bartholins%20abscess&source=search_result&selectedTitle=2~142&usage_type=de-fault&display_rank=2

Chen, K. (2021b). Bartholin gland cyst and abscess: Word catheter placement. R. Barbieri (Ed.), *UpToDate*. https:// www-uptodate-com.ezproxy3.lhl.uab.edu/contents/bartholin-gland-cyst-and-abscess-word-catheter-placement? search=Incision%20and%20drainage%20of%20bartholins%20abscess&source=search_result&selectedTi-tle=1~142&usage_type=default&display_rank=1

Holland, A. C., & Bibb, B. (2017). Treatment of a bartholin gland abscess: A step-by-step approach using simulation. *Women's Healthcare: A Clinical Journal for NPs, 5*(3), 22–27.

Mayo Clinic. (n.d. a). *Bartholin's cyst: Causes.* http://www.mayoclinic.com/health/bartholin-cyst/DS00667/DSECTION=causes

Mayo Clinic. (n.d. b). *Bartholin's cyst: Prevention.* http://www.mayoclinic.com/health/bartholin-cyst/DS00667/DSECTION =prevention

University of Maryland Medical Center. (n.d.). *Bartholin's cyst or abscess.* http://umm.edu/Health/Medical/Ency/Articles/ Bartholins-cyst-or-abscess

University of Michigan Health System. (n.d.). *Bartholin's gland cyst.* http://www.uofmhealth.org/health-library/tw2685 #tw2688

53

PESSARY INSERTION

LISA S. PAIR AND HELEN A. CARCIO

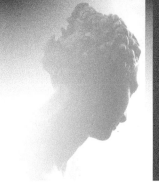

PESSARY

A. Overview
   1. The number of women 65 years and older will double in the next 20 years.
   2. Demand for pessary use is expected to grow by 45% in the next 30 years.
   3. A vaginal pessary should be considered as first-line treatment for all women presenting with a symptomatic pelvic organ prolapse and/or stress incontinence.
   4. Complications are rare with a properly fitted pessary, the most common being an increase in vaginal discharge.
      a. Complications can be minimized with simple vaginal hygiene and regular follow-up visits.
   5. Satisfaction rate is very high in the geriatric population.

B. Purpose
   1. To support the pelvic organs in close alignment to their proper anatomic position in the treatment of second- through fourth-degree prolapse
   2. To restore continence by stabilizing the bladder base
      a. Anchored behind the pubic symphysis and the posterior vaginal fornix
      b. Ring or knob of the pessary compresses the urethra and increases the closing pressure
      c. Provides a support to the redundant tissue of the prolapse
   3. To provide an alternative treatment for women who are at a high risk for surgical repair of the prolapse

C. Goals
   1. Can be used as a temporary measure for relief of symptoms while a patient delays surgery until a more opportune time, or until she decides whether to have surgery.
   2. Used as a permanent alternative to prolapse surgery, particularly in geriatric women who are at surgical risk.
   3. Used as a diagnostic aid to determine whether there is relief of symptoms with prolapse replacement. It serves as a useful predictor of a successful outcome from surgical management.
      a. Can uncover urinary incontinence, which is masked by obstruction of the urinary outflow tract.
      b. Can uncover incomplete bladder emptying from bladder outlet obstruction with normal voiding when prolapse is reduced. The patient may present with elevated post-void residual urine and with her prolapse reduced with a pessary, is able to completely empty.

D. Pessary practice pearls for the advanced practice provider
   1. When choosing pessary sizes, measuring the vagina is most helpful.
      a. The three or four sizes in the middle are most used.
      b. Most pessary wearers do well with the most common sizes.
   2. Modern use is a function of the provider's experience and training, along with the availability of the device.

3. With knowledge and practice, an advanced practice provider can become adept at fitting and caring for patients using the vaginal pessary.

4. Most pessaries come with printed material from the manufacturer that gives instructions regarding the insertion and care of the specific device.

5. Pessaries are available in various sizes, shapes, and materials.

6. If a pessary is made of latex rubber, the clinician needs to determine whether the woman has a sensitivity to latex before fitting. Very few pessaries are made of latex anymore.

7. Not all women can use a pessary (Box 53.1).

E. Coitus

1. It is important to identify if the patient is sexually active prior to pessary fitting as some pessaries are not conducive to sexual activity and must be removed prior to coitus.

2. The woman must have the dexterity to remove and reinsert the pessary.

3. Never assume that a geriatric patient is not sexually active.

4. Sexual intercourse is not possible with the following types of pessaries:

   a. Gellhorn
   b. Doughnut
   c. Shaatz
   d. Cube

GENERAL PRINCIPLES FOR FITTING A PESSARY

A. Choosing the right pessary

1. Pessaries are generally fit by trial and error. A pessary fitting kit is available but is usually not necessary because kits only give an approximation.

B. Clinicians soon develop favorite types that they become familiar with using.

1. The most commons pessaries used in clinical practice today are the ring with and without support, the cube, the Gellhorn, and the continence pessaries with and without support.

C. Perform a pelvic examination to assess for type of prolapse(s). Determine the size, shape, and position of the uterus and associated structures and assess for genitourinary syndrome of menopause.

1. Estrogen therapy

   a. Recommend estrogen therapy, preferably via the vaginal route, 2 to 6 weeks before the necessary fitting to:

      (1) Nourish the vaginal tissues.
      (2) Mature squamous epithelial tissues.
      (3) Increase pliability of submucosal connective tissue.
      (4) Improve perineal muscle tone.

   b. Routinely recommended as an adjunct to pessary use.

BOX 53.1   Reasons for Discontinuing Pessary Use

- Inconvenient to use
- Inadequate relief of symptoms
- Uncomfortable
- Elected for surgery
- Unable to remain in place
- Difficulty urinating (rare pessary-related issue)
- Incontinence increased

(1) May not be necessary in the postmenopausal woman receiving estrogen replacement therapy

(2) May be in the form of estrogen cream, suppositories, or estradiol vaginal ring (Estring)

(3) If Estring is used, insert before the pessary, and change every 3 months.

2. To measure for a pessary, insert the first two fingers deep into the vaginal canal to the posterior fornix behind the cervix or the apex of the vaginal vault and fold thumb against the forefinger where it touches the introitus or use forefinger from other hand to measure. Withdraw hand and measure against the pessary or the fitting kit (Figure 53.1).

a. The pessary should fit comfortably behind the pubic bone.

b. Once the proper size is found, the patient should be completely comfortable. She may feel the pessary, but it should never cause discomfort.

c. If the pessary fits properly, the examiner should be able to sweep the tip of the finger around the pessary and the vaginal wall. This prevents the breakdown of tissue.

3. Factors related to an unsuccessful fitting:

a. Client's lack of understanding regarding the pessary or commitment

b. A short vaginal length (less than 6 cm)

c. Wide vaginal introitus (greater than 4 finger breadths)

d. Previous pelvic surgery

e. Obesity (abdominal pressure may force pessary out)

GENERAL PESSARY INSERTION TECHNIQUE

A. Ask the client to empty her bladder and rectum, and to position herself as mentioned earlier.

1. With continence pessaries, some providers do not recommend voiding before fitting, to ensure that the woman has urine to void following the fitting. Another purpose is to assess for continence with coughing with the pessary in place.

B. Approximate the size of the pessary needed by using fingers to determine the length and depth of the vaginal vault (generally can predict within one size either way).

1. May use lubricant for a narrow or small introitus.

2. Lubricant may cause the pessary to be slippery and difficult to bend or hold.

3. It is best to lubricate only the entering edge.

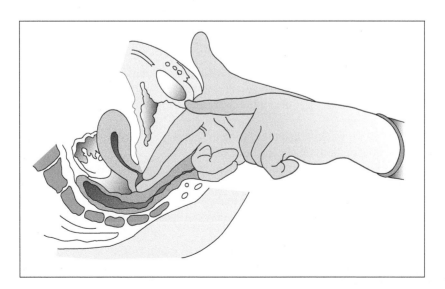

FIGURE 53.1 Measuring the vaginal canal for a pessary.

C. Spread the labia and pull downward with the nondominant hand.

D. Ask client to bear down.

E. Grade prolapse if present.

F. Reduce identified prolapse back inside the vagina using your fingers. Sometimes if the prolapse is large, you must reduce the prolapse with one hand and insert the pessary with the other hand.

G. Fit for various pessaries as described under each section that follows.

H. After pessary is placed:
   1. Separate the labia, observing the introitus.
   2. Ask the patient to bear down while being examined.
   3. The pessary may descend and become visible at the introitus but ascend with relaxation.
   4. Ask the patient to walk around the room, to sit, or to even use the toilet.
   5. Reassess fit.
   6. If the pessary has shifted, try a larger size.

I. A larger size may be necessary after using the pessary for a few weeks, due to an enlargement of the vault with the pessary in position.

RECOMMENDATIONS FOR POST-FITTING FOLLOW-UP

A. A return visit is important to:
   1. Recheck the fit.
   2. Question the patient regarding urination and defecation to assess status.
   3. Observe for a tissue reaction such as discharge, irritation, or ulceration.
   4. Reassure and support the woman.
   5. Determine the presence of any discomfort

B. Identify whether the client will be able to self-manage her pessary care or will clinically follow-up. Many pessaries are difficult for the client to remove and insert correctly, and those unable to self-manage will need to receive routine follow-up care directed by her provider.

C. Clients who can self-manage their pessary can return for follow up at 6 weeks and then as recommended by the provider.

D. Clients who are unable to self-manage their pessary will have scheduled return appointments at 4 to 6 weeks and increasing to up to 12 weeks depending on individual considerations.
   1. It is possible to forget or neglect a pessary. A list of pessary users within a given office must be kept and followed closely.
   2. Suggest a geriatric woman wear a medic-alert bracelet or have a card stating that she is wearing a pessary.
   3. Patient or clinician must routinely observe for any ulcerations or irritation from undue pressure (this can be minimized by vaginal estrogen use and properly fitted pessary or change to another pessary). If ulceration is present, the pessary needs to be removed for 3 to 4 weeks for healing.
   4. Return every 4 to 6 weeks when first fitting the pessary and then can extend to up to 12 weeks depending on individual considerations.
      a. May alter follow-up plan: If odor develops at 12 weeks, the patient needs to return earlier for next visit.
      b. Remember that a pessary is a foreign body and that there are limited nerve endings in the vagina and cervix. Therefore, a woman may not sense that any ulcerations are occurring.

E. All clients must return to clinic promptly if
   1. Urination or defecation is difficult.
   2. The pessary is uncomfortable in any way.
   3. The pessary falls out.

a. Reassure the client that this is a common event and to just clean the pessary, put in a plastic bag, and return with it.

b. Will most likely occur during the straining of a bowel movement.

F. A pessary should not be used in a noncompliant client or a woman unable to care for herself unless her caregivers understand the pessary is in place and that the client will receive routine follow-up care.

G. Because many pessary users are geriatric, it is important to keep in mind that a woman's status may change over the years (e.g., due to a stroke).

1. Caregivers (such as nursing home personnel) may not be aware that a pessary is in place.

H. There are very few contraindications for pessary use (Box 53.2).

I. Keep a list of all pessary users to make sure they are seen every 2 to 3 months. A forgotten pessary can cause serious complications.

J. The pessary may require sizing alterations or a complete change in style at subsequent visits.

K. Discuss with the client any possible problems.

1. Coital discomfort (if intercourse is allowable)
2. Disturbance in bowel or urinary function
3. Whether or not it remained in place
4. Overall comfort
5. Presence of any odor
6. Change in discharge

a. A yellow or white, or mild to moderate discharge is usually present.

b. If the discharge increases during subsequent visits, question the client's compliance with the vaginal care routine.

c. The discharge should never be foul smelling.

(1) Perform a wet mount and treat any infection.

(2) Replace the pessary after the infection is resolved.

L. At this point, one may discuss the possibility of the woman cleaning her own pessary.

1. Particularly if she is used to touching her own genitals

a. Geriatric women are not as familiar.

b. If the woman has previously used a diaphragm, it may be easy for her to learn how to use a pessary.

c. Observe her dexterity.

d. Evaluate compliance issues and ability to perform self-care.

2. Most pessaries are difficult to insert and remove, so a woman must not feel that she has failed if she is unable to do it herself.

3. Do not even raise the possibility if it is obvious that the woman is unable to manage the pessary.

M. Provide instructions regarding

1. Use of lubricant to ease insertion.

a. Nonpetroleum-based lubricants are not caustic and can be used.

BOX 53.2 Contraindications to Pessary Use

- Active vaginitis
- Abnormal Pap test
- Acute pelvic inflammatory disease
- Endometriosis (research varies)
- Noncompliant patient
- Woman with dementia without possibility of reasonable follow-up

2. Douching
   a. No consensus has been presented regarding its effectiveness.
   b. The woman should always consult with her clinician first.
   c. Mild vinegar may help to acidify the vagina.
3. Use of estrogen
   a. Vaginal estrogen, unless contraindicated, is recommended over systemic estrogen.
      (1) Vaginal cream or pill is inserted twice weekly.
      (2) Estring should be replaced every 3 months (should be inserted before pessary).
   b. May be used in conjunction with systemic preparations.
   c. The client may have difficulty using the applicator and inserting the cream.
   d. Estrogen will mature vaginal epithelium and improve perineal muscle tone.
4. Use of Trimo-San
   a. This is a cleansing, deodorant gel with a pH of 4 used to maintain antibacterial acid environment.
   b. The client should use one-half applicator two times per week.
   c. The active ingredient is oxyquinoline sulfate.

N. Pessary care and cleaning
   1. If the client is unable to remove the pessary, it should be removed, and the vagina should be observed for any excoriation, ulceration, or foul discharge.
   2. Clean the pessary in warm, soapy water; rinse thoroughly; and reinsert.
   3. Irrigate the vagina using a 20-mL syringe with an irrigating tip using warm water. A weak solution of betadine or vinegar may be used.
   4. Document type and amount of solution used and note character of discharge.
   5. Replace the pessary if the old one shows signs of physical defects.
      a. It may become discolored but does not need to be replaced.

O. Complications
   1. Increase in vaginal discharge
   2. Odor
   3. Cytologic atypia from inflammatory changes that may occur
   4. Poorly fitted or improper schedule of cleaning may cause ulcerations and excoriation
   5. Incarceration: The cervix and uterus may herniate through the center of a poorly fitted ring pessary and become strangulated.
   6. Tissue may grow around a neglected pessary.
   7. There should be no evidence of serious problems with long-term wear of a well-maintained pessary.

P. Maintenance visits
   1. Slight bleeding may be seen during removal of pessary; question the client's compliance with estrogen therapy.
   2. If using the Estring, replace the ring every 3 months during the 3-month cleaning visit. Insert before the pessary.
   3. Refit pessary if there has been a gain or loss of 20 pounds or more.
   4. If heavy discharge
      a. Perform wet mount to check for infection.
   5. Reinforce use of Kegel exercises.
      a. Compliance is the key.
      b. Success rate of more than 80% resolution of incontinence can be achieved in 4 to 8 weeks.
   6. Offer use of support groups.

Q. Monitor urination
   1. Ask the woman to keep a voiding diary.

a. Keep the diary for 1 week.
b. Include frequency and quality of fluids.
c. Note quantity and frequency of urination.
d. Record which types of activities cause leaking.
2. Note use of pads.
a. Brand name
b. How often must wear (continuous vs. intermittent)
c. How often must change if continuous
3. Kegel exercises
a. Inquire whether the client has done them in the past.
b. Was she successful?
4. Kegel exercise cones
a. These cones were designed as an aid to locating and identifying the correct pelvic floor muscle.

DESCRIPTION OF THE VARIOUS TYPES OF PESSARIES

Vaginal pessaries are either space-occupying or support pessaries. Space-occupying pessaries are chosen for a capacious vagina where a support pessary may not support as well.

A. The ring pessary (the incontinence ring; Figure 53.2).
1. Indications
a. First choice for most providers regardless of prolapse
b. Considered a support pessary. Thus, when the vaginal introitus is too large, the pessary may not stay in.
c. The administration of estrogen is advocated to improve tissue circulation and regain vaginal mucosal integrity.
d. The folding-ring pessary is especially useful for a client who is sexually active because it can easily be inserted and removed, or it may remain in place during intercourse (as with a diaphragm).
2. **Description:** Comes with a porous diaphragm for additional support.
a. Diaphragm helps support a mild cystocele that accompanies other prolapses.
b. It is usually made of medical-grade silicone.

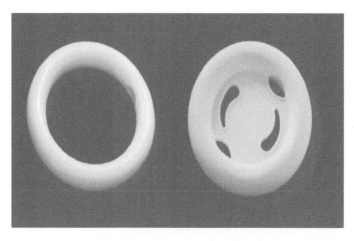

FIGURE 53.2 Ring with and without support.
Source: Photo courtesy of PersonalMed.

3. Insertion technique
   a. Fit like a diaphragm.
   b. Bend pessary in half at the notches.
   c. Insert the pessary with the folded arc concavity facing upward.
   d. Direct past the cervix into the posterior fornix.
   e. Place in the posterior fornix, allowing the ring to spring open once it is in the vagina.
   f. Give a quarter turn to secure in position to prevent the pessary from falling in on itself and coming out of the vagina.
   g. When the pessary is placed properly, it will take up redundant vaginal tissue and support and elevate the uterus or apex, to flatten and support the cystocele (Figure 53.3).
4. Removal
   a. Palpate the notch, and rotate a quarter turn, gently pulling down and out to remove.
   b. It is much easier to insert a pessary than to remove one.

B. Cube
   1. **Indications:** Third-degree prolapse, cystocele, or rectocele, with or without vaginal tone
      a. Often, this is the only satisfactory support with complete prolapse.
      b. It is excellent for vaginal wall prolapse in that it keeps the vaginal wall from collapsing by using six pressure points.
   2. Description
      a. Each side of cube has concave suction cups that adhere to the vaginal walls, helping to restore the anatomic vaginal support of the pelvic organs (Figure 53.4).
      b. Moist vaginal mucosa invaginates into the concavities owing to a slight negative pressure.
      c. Needs to be removed daily or requires regular follow-up care.
         (1) Requires highly motivated client with good dexterity.
         (2) Difficult to remove (action of suction), so it may not be possible to be removed by the older client.
         (3) Remember that the longer the cube is left in place, the stronger the negative pressure and thus the more difficult it is to remove.
         (4) The cube completely fills the vagina and blocks off drainage of any secretions.
   3. Insertion
      a. It requires the compression of the cube before placement in the vagina.

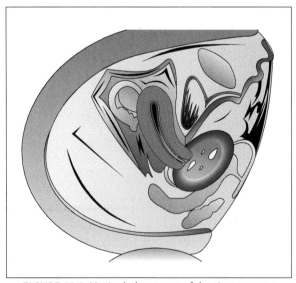

FIGURE 53.3 Vaginal placement of the ring pessary.

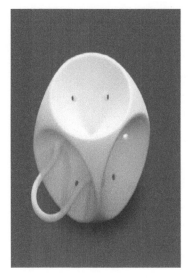

FIGURE 53.4 Cube pessary. Note the six concave sides. The holes are for drainage.

Source: Photo courtesy of PersonalMed.

    b. The string should be oriented toward the vagina.
      (1) It should never be used to pull the pessary out because it may cause vaginal tears of the fragile mucosa.
    c. Insert by compressing the cube as much as possible.
    d. Spread the labia with the nondominant hand.
    e. Push the compressed cube through introitus.
    f. Place as high in the vagina as possible.
  4. Removal
    a. Removal may be difficult because of the suction that has been created.
    b. Suction must be broken before removal.
    c. Do not pull on the string to remove. The string will break.
    d. Slide the fingertips between the vaginal mucosa and the pessary to break the seal.
    e. Compress the pessary and remove.
    f. If the woman is not able to remove the pessary, she needs to see her clinician immediately.
  5. Available sizes
    a. Eight sizes (0–7)
    b. Recommend stocking sizes 2 to 4; need a minimum of four sizes to fit a client properly
C. Gellhorn pessary (Figures 53.5 and 53.6)
  1. **Indications:** Provides support of a third-degree uterine prolapse and procidentia. (Note: Gellhorn comes with both a short and long stem.)
  2. Description
    a. Most used pessary for uterine prolapse (ring and doughnut pessaries also commonly used).
    b. Available
      (1) Flexible silicone
      (2) Ninety-five percent rigid acrylic
    c. Silicone can be boiled or autoclaved; acrylic should not be autoclaved or boiled because heat can alter the shape.
      (1) It needs to be disinfected in Cidex.
      (2) Never use alcohol because it will give the acrylic a shattered appearance.

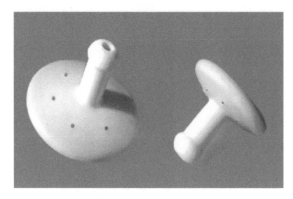

FIGURE 53.5 Gellhorn pessary. Note holes for drainage of vaginal discharge. The stem comes in two sizes, long and short. The disk compresses the urethra at the bladder neck and the stem helps anchor the pessary in place.

Source: Photo courtesy of PersonalMed.

    d. Provides less support for a rectocele because it fits superiorly and anteriorly, with less surface area to support the posterior segment

    e. Cervix rests against the flat base of the pessary, with the stem extending to the vaginal orifice.

        (1) The base of the pessary is large enough to support the tissue proximal to it, and rests above the levator muscles.

        (2) Its concave shape provides suction, helping to prevent spontaneous expulsion.

        (3) The stem fills the vagina, preventing the device from turning (requires a capacious vaginal vault).

    f. It is useful with intact (not lax) perineal body. If not successful for the patient, may progress to a cube.

3. Insertion

    a. The main method of determining the proper size of the Gellhorn pessary is by trial and error.

    b. Lubricate the edge of the round disc.

    c. Insert sidewise, with the disc portion held parallel to the introitus.

    d. Apply downward pressure on the perineum with the nondominant hand.

    e. Be careful to avoid the urethral opening while the perineum is pushed downward.

    f. Push the pessary into the vagina until the disc lies transversely beneath the cervix.

    g. Once the large disc is inside the vagina, push forward until the end of the stem slips within the orifice (see Figure 53.6).

4. Removal

    a. This is a two-handed removal. The clinician reaches behind the disc with the nondominant hand and bends the disc forward to break the seal caused by suction (may be difficult).

    b. Grasp the stem and pull out gently, slowly changing the angle of the disc parallel to the introitus for easy removal through the introital opening.

    c. Another option is to fill a 20-mL slip-tip syringe with warm water. Insert the tip through the hole in the stem of the Gellhorn. Flush the fluid through the hole to release the suction behind the Gellhorn.

    d. Grasp the knob and gently pull the disc toward the introitus.

    e. If it is difficult to grasp the knob, insert a clamp through the hole and gently pull downward.

    f. Follow steps a and b for removal.

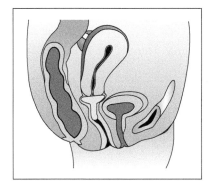

FIGURE 53.6 Gellhorn pessary (note the base holds up the cervix).

5. Available sizes
   a. It comes in varying sizes of disc diameter, from 1½ to 3½ inches, increasing in quarter-inch increments.
   b. Choose from sizes 1 to 9.
   c. The recommended fitting size includes 2½, 2¾, and 3.
D. Donut (Figure 53.7)
   1. **Indications:** Occludes upper vagina and supports a uterine prolapse
      a. Mass of the inflated pessary must be greater than the defect in the levator muscles.
      b. It provides no support for the proximal urethra and may increase incontinence.
      c. Good to use for prolapse of the vagina after hysterectomy.
   2. Description
      a. Useful for uterine prolapse, some recommend it for third- to fourth-degree cystocele or rectocele, and apical prolapse after a hysterectomy
      b. The hollow ring comes in two models of medical-grade silicone.
      c. Coitus is not possible with the pessary in place.
   3. Insertion technique
      a. Like the ring pessary, but there is no notch, so internal rotation is not necessary.
      b. Once the labia is separated with nondominant hand, compress the doughnut.

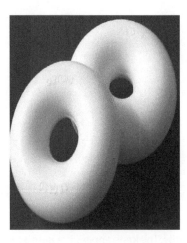

FIGURE 53.7 Donut pessary, which fills the vaginal space to support a prolapse.

Source: Photo courtesy of PersonalMed.

    c. With two fingers of the nondominant hand pressing down on the peritoneum, hold the pessary parallel, angle slightly, and slip past introitus into vagina.

  4. Removal technique

    a. Hook finger inside on the center of the pessary.

    b. Compress the doughnut using the thumb and middle finger and bring them parallel.

    c. Gently pull down and out through introitus. (The clinician may have to lubricate the pessary to remove it.)

    d. Depending on the introital opening, there may occasionally be perineal cutaneous lacerations with removal. This will self-heal.

  5. Available sizes

    a. Choice of six sizes, ranging in diameter from 2 to 3¾ inches

    b. Recommended stocking sizes: 2 and 3

E. Incontinence ring pessary (Figure 53.8)

  1. Description

    a. Designed to stabilize the urethra and the urethrovesical junction

  2. Indication

    a. Stress incontinence

  3. Insertion technique

    a. Like the ring pessary without support

    b. Must fit properly because if it is too small, the knob may not remain in proper position

    c. Fold the pessary in half. The knob is in the middle of the concave.

    d. Push the pessary up and behind the cervix.

    e. Insert a gloved hand into the vagina and rotate the knob from its position on the side of the vagina to the front of the vagina with the knob resting behind the pubic bone.

  4. Incontinence dish

    a. This is a variation of the incontinence ring.

    b. It is indicated for SUI associated with a mild first- or second-degree prolapse.

    c. It is available in sizes 55 to 85 mm, in increments of 5 mm.

    d. Insert end without knob first. It is fitted with the knob behind the pubic bone to further compress the urethra.

  5. Incontinence dish with support (Figure 53.9)

    a. This is a variation of dish with flexible diaphragm used to support a mild cystocele.

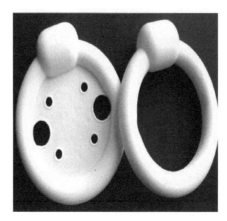

FIGURE 53.8 Incontinence ring pessary with knob. Note: It comes with or without support. The holes allow for drainage of vaginal discharge. The knob applies pressure against the bladder neck and compresses the urethra.

Source: Photo courtesy of PersonalMed.

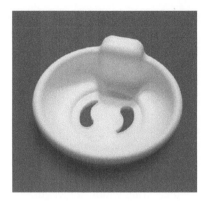

FIGURE 53.9 Incontinence dish.

Bowl shape allows for support of a cystocele. Has large holes for drainage of vaginal discharge.

Source: Photo courtesy of PersonalMed.

b. It is indicated for SUI in conjunction with a first- or second-degree prolapse, or a mild cystocele. (Some clinicians recommend this type of pessary for second- or third-degree cystocele because it provides additional support for the cystocele.)

c. It is available in sizes 55 to 85 mm, in increments of 5 mm.

d. Some clinicians recommend cube pessary for use in younger women who have incontinence with exercise.

(1) It can be inserted before vigorous exercise in young women to eliminate leakage.

(2) Other clinicians would recommend the ring with support for this condition.

F. The lever pessary, called *Hodge* or *Smith*

1. Indications

a. **Uterine retroversion:** Posteriorly displaces the cervix and the uterus is anteverted.

b. Incompetent cervix in pregnancy: To support an anterior-pointing cervix during pregnancy (Hodge pessary)

c. To support and correct retrodisplacement of the uterus in early pregnancy

d. Diagnostic evaluation of patients with large cystocele or urinary stress incontinence demonstrates support of the anterior vagina.

e. Provides support to the proximal urethra, promoting increase in urethral function length and closing pressure without causing obstruction.

f. Useful for stress urinary incontinence (SUI), with or without prolapse

g. If it is properly fitted, sexual intercourse is possible.

2. Insertion technique

a. First, manually elevate a retrodisplaced uterus.

b. Fold the device along the long axis, with the curved end oriented toward the vaginal introitus.

c. Push into the vagina with the index finger, advancing the posterior bar into the posterior vaginal fornix.

d. Keep pressure on the posterior bar during insertion.

e. Anchor the anterior bar under the symphysis pubis.

f. Note: The long arm of the pessary should face anteriorly, so that the device straddles the rectum.

3. The Smith pessary has a narrower anterior limb for use in a patient with a deep symphysis and a well-defined, narrow pubic arch.

4. The Hodge pessary

a. The border anterior limb prevents the pessary from turning.

    b. It is used when there is minimal pubic support and the symphysis is somewhat shallow.

    c. The anterior notch prevents urethral impingement and obstruction.

    d. It comes with a support for correction of a concomitant cystocele.

    e. It is especially useful for clients with stress incontinence.

    f. The Hodge pessary with support is indicated for women with SUI, with a mild cystocele, and a very small introitus.

   5. The Risser pessary

    a. Is a modification of the Hodge pessary.

    b. The Hodge pessary has a wider bar and a deeper notch, which allows a larger weight-bearing region with a lesser likelihood of soft tissue pressure necrosis.

   6. Available sizes

    a. Ten available sizes (0–9), measuring width and length

    b. Recommend stocking sizes: 2 through 4

G. The Gehrung pessary

   1. **Indications:** Correction of a cystocele and rectocele

   2. Description

    a. Provides support to the anterior vaginal wall; arms or heels rest flat on the posterior vaginal floor

    b. Avoids pressure on the rectum while supporting the bladder

    c. Does not interfere with coitus

    d. Arclike, flexible plastic

    e. Bars may also flatten out a rectocele

    f. May be underused

   3. **Insertion:** Creates a bladder bridge

    a. The unusual shape of the pessary may make the clinician uncomfortable with insertion.

    b. It is relatively simple to insert.

    c. Fold with the arch convexity oriented upward, with both heels parallel to the pelvic floor, left heel first.

    d. Hold the device on its side and insert the lateral bar over the perineum and into the vagina.

    e. When it is positioned intravaginally, push one heel back and the other forward to complete a 90° rotation, so that the convex curved portion lies against the anterior vaginal wall.

    f. The back arch should be positioned over the cervix in the anterior fornix, and the front arch should be positioned behind the symphysis.

    g. Both heels should be resting on the posterior vaginal wall, with the arches and cross-support forming a bridge to raise the bladder.

   4. Available sizes

    a. Choice of 10 sizes (0–9)

    b. Recommended stocking sizes: 3, 4, and 5

H. Inflatoball pessary

   1. Used to be made of latex but is now available in silicone

    a. Support is adjusted by varying air pressure via the two-way valve.

    b. The patient can easily remove and clean this device herself; even with a stenotic introitus, it can be inflated and reinflated.

   2. Indications

    a. Pelvic organ prolapse

    b. Extreme degrees of uterine prolapse

    c. Prolapse of the vagina following a total hysterectomy

   3. Insertion

    a. Approximate size by using fingers to determine vaginal vault width.

    b. With the pessary deflated, hold it compressed between the thumb and forefingers.

    c. While it is deflated, insert metal part of the inflation bulb into air vent.

   d. Insert the deflated pessary into the vaginal vault.
   e. Inflate the ball by squeezing the inflation bulb to the desired pressure.
   f. Inflate the ball to a diameter large enough so that one finger can pass around the pessary and the vaginal wall.
4. Removal
   a. Deflate the pessary.
   b. Gently pull the deflated pessary through the introitus (do not pull on the stem).
5. Available sizes
   a. Small, medium, large, and extra large
   b. Corresponding to ball diameter of 2 to 2.5 inches
   c. Recommended stocking sizes: medium and large

NONTRADITIONAL INSERTS

A. Vaginal inserts
   1. Poise Impressa bladder support
      a. An over-the-counter, nonabsorbent, disposable intravaginal device that physically supports the urethra to help prevent stress urinary incontinence (SUI) leaks.
      b. Inserted with an applicator and removed by the pull of a string.
      c. Women may wear it for up to 8 hours within a 24-hour time.
      d. Women can use the bathroom without having to remove the device.
      e. Provides support to the urethra whenever pressure is transferred from the abdomen to the pelvic floor.
      f. Normal urinary flow and vaginal secretions remain unaffected.
   2. Uresta
      a. Uniquely shaped pessary that allows a woman to self-manage; easy to remove and insert, like a tampon; removed in the evening.
      b. The tissues compress the urethra and may reduce leakage.
      c. FDA approved in America. May soon be available as an over-the-counter option. A starter kit comes with three sizes. Contact the manufacturer for prescription-ordering directions as the product is sold through Canada.
      d. Safe to use all day. Do not need to remove to void.
   3. Colpexin Sphere
      a. Round plastic sphere that is placed intravaginally above the levator ani muscle
      b. Space-occupying properties allow support of the prolapse.
      c. Reflectively causes contraction of the pelvic floor muscle to retain the slippery sphere.
      d. Polycarbonate sphere with nylon string of various sizes that supports the pelvic floor musculature
      e. Pelvic floor muscle exercises is facilitated with sphere in place.

BIBLIOGRAPHY

Abrams, P., Andersson, K. E., Apostolidis, A., Birder, L., Bliss, D., Brubaker, L., Cardozo, L., Castro-Diaz, D., O'Connell, P. R., Cottenden, A., Cotterill, N., de Ridder, D., Dmochowski, R., Dumoulin, C., Fader, M., Fry, C., Goldman, H., Hanno, P., Homma, Y., … members of the committees (2018). 6th International Consultation on Incontinence. Recommendations of the International Scientific Committee: Evaluation and treatment of urinary incontinence, pelvic organ prolapse and faecal incontinence. *Neurourology and Urodynamics, 37*(7), 2271–2272. https://doi.org/10.1002/nau.23551

Alperin, M., Khan, A., Dubina, E., Tarnay, C., Wu, N., Pashos, C. L., & Anger, J. T. (2013). Patterns of pessary care and outcomes for medicare beneficiaries with pelvic organ prolapse. *Female Pelvic Medicine & Reconstructive Surgery, 19*(3), 142–147. https://doi.org/10.1097/SPV.0b013e31827e857c

Al-Shaikh, G., Syed, S., Osman, S., Bogis, A., & Al-Badr, A. (2018). Pessary use in stress urinary incontinence: A review of advantages, complications, patient satisfaction, and quality of life. *International Journal of Women's Health, 10*, 195–201 https://doi.org/10.2147/IJWH.S152616

Brown, L. K., Fenner, D. E., DeLancey, J. O., & Schimpf, M. O. (2016). Defining patient knowledge and perceptions of vaginal pessaries for prolapse and incontinence. *Female Pelvic Medicine & Reconstructive Surgery, 22*(2), 93–97. https://doi.org/10.1097/SPV.0000000000000252

Cheung, R. Y., Lee, J. H., Lee, L. L., Chung, T. K., & Chan, S. S. (2016). Vaginal pessary in women with symptomatic pelvic organ prolapse: A randomized controlled trial. *Obstetrics and Gynecology, 128*(1), 73–80. https://doi.org/10.1097/AOG.0000000000001489

Coelho, S. C. A., Giraldo, P. C., Florentino, J. O., Castro, E. B., Brito, L. G. O., & Juliato, C. R. T. (2017). Can the pessary use modify the vaginal microbiological flora? A Cross-sectional study. *Revista brasileira de ginecologia e obstetricia, 39*(4), 169–174. https://doi.org/10.1055/s-0037-1601437

Collins, S., Beigi, R., Mellen, C., O'Sullivan, D., & Tulikangas, P. (2015). The effect of pessaries on the vaginal microenvironment. *American Journal of Obstetrics and Gynecology, 212*(1), 60.e1–60. e6. https://doi.org/10.1016/j.ajog.2014.07.024

Ding, J., Song, X. C., Deng, M., & Zhu, L. (2016). Which factors should be considered in choosing pessary type and size for pelvic organ prolapse patients in a fitting trial? *International Urogynecology Journal, 27*(12), 1867–1871. https://doi.org/10.1007/s00192-016-3051-3

Giri, A., Hartmann, K. E., Hellwege, J. N., Velez Edwards, D. R., & Edwards, T. L. (2017). Obesity and pelvic organ prolapse: A systematic review and meta-analysis of observational studies. *American Journal of Obstetrics and Gynecology, 217*(1), 11–26. e3. https://doi.org/10.2147/IJWH.S152616

Hagen, S., Stark, D., Maher, C., & Adams, E. (2006). Conservative management of pelvic organ prolapse in women. *Cochrane Database of Systematic Reviews,* (4), CD003882. https://doi.org/10.1002/14651858.CD003882.pub3

Harvey, M. A., Lemieux, M. C., Robert, M., & Schulz, J. A. (2021). Guideline No. 411: Vaginal pessary use. *Journal of Obstetrics and Gynaecology Canada: JOGC = Journal d'obstetrique et gynecologie du Canada: JOGC, 43*(2), 255–266. e1. https://doi.org/10.1016/j.jogc.2020.11.013

Hooper, G. L., Atnip, S., & O'Dell, K. (2017). Optimal pessary care: A modified Delphi consensus study. *Journal of Midwifery & Women's Health, 62*(4), 452–462. https://doi.org/10.1111/jmwh.12624

Iglesia, C. B., & Smithling, K. R. (2017). Pelvic organ prolapse. *American Family Physician, 96*(3), 179–185.

Jelovsek, J. E., Maher, C., & Barber, M. D. (2007). Pelvic organ prolapse. *Lancet, 369*(9566), 1027–1038. https://doi.org/10.1016/S0140-6736(07)60462-0

Li, B., Chen, Q., Zhang, J., Yu, C., Zhang, L., & Chen, L. (2020). A prospective study of pessary use for severe pelvic organ prolapse: 3-year follow-up outcomes. *Archives of Gynecology and Obstetrics, 301*(5), 1213–1218. https://doi.org/10.1007/s00404-020-05526-1

Lone, F., Thakar, R., Sultan, A. H., & Karamalis, G. (2011). A 5-year prospective study of vaginal pessary use for pelvic organ prolapse. *International Journal of Gynaecology and Obstetrics, 114*(1), 56–59. https://doi.org/10.1016/j.ijgo.2011.02.006

Meriwether, K. V., Rogers, R. G., Craig, E., Peterson, S. D., Gutman, R. E., & Iglesia, C. B. (2015). The effect of hydroxyquinoline-based gel on pessary-associated bacterial vaginosis: A multicenter randomized controlled trial. *American Journal of Obstetrics and Gynecology, 213*(5), 729.e1–729. e9. https://doi.org/10.1016/j.ajog.2015.04.032

Meriwether, K. V., Komesu, Y. M., Craig, E., Qualls, C., Davis, H., & Rogers, R. G. (2015). Sexual function and pessary management among women using a pessary for pelvic floor disorders. *The Journal of Sexual Medicine, 12*(12), 2339–2349. https://doi.org/10.1111/jsm.13060

Murray, C., Thomas, E., & Pollock, W. (2017). Vaginal pessaries: Can an educational brochure help patients to better understand their care? *Journal of Clinical Nursing, 26*(1–2), 140–147. https://doi.org/10.1111/jocn.13408

Newman, D. K., Wyman, J. F. & Welch, V. W. (Eds.). (2017). *Society of Urologic Nurses and Associates Core Curriculum for Urologic Nursing* (1st ed.). Anthony J. Jannetti, Inc.

Nygaard, I., Barber, M. D., Burgio, K. L., Kenton, K., Meikle, S., Schaffer, J., Spino, C., Whitehead, W. E., Wu, J., Brody, D. J., & Pelvic Floor Disorders Network (2008). Prevalence of symptomatic pelvic floor disorders in US women. *Journal of the American Medical Association, 300*(11), 1311–1316. https://doi.org/10.1001/jama.300.11.1311

Pair, L. S., & Somerall, W. E. Jr. (2018). Urinary incontinence: Pelvic floor muscle and behavioral training for women. *The Nurse Practitioner, 43*(1), 21–25. https://doi.org/10.1097/01.NPR.0000527571.66854.0d

Propst, K., Mellen, C., O'Sullivan, D. M., & Tulikangas, P. K. (2020). Timing of office-based pessary care: A randomized controlled trial. *Obstetrics and Gynecology, 135*(1), 100–105. https://doi.org/10.1097/AOG.0000000000003580

Robert, M., Schulz, J. A., Harvey, M. A., & Urogynaecology Committee (2013). Technical update on pessary use. *Journal of Obstetrics and Gynaecology Canada: JOGC = Journal d'obstetrique et gynecologie du Canada: JOGC, 35*(7), 664–674. https://doi.org/10.1016/S1701-2163(15)30888-4

Rockefeller, N. F., & Ninnivaggio, C. S. (2020). Treating POP and SUI with pessaries. *Contemporary OB/GYN, 65*(3), 8–12. https://www.contemporaryobgyn.net/view/treating-pop-and-sui-pessaries

Thys, S. D., Hakvoort, R. A., Asseler, J., Milani, A. L., Vollebregt, A., & Roovers, J. P. (2020). Effect of pessary cleaning and optimal time interval for follow-up: A prospective cohort study. *International Urogynecology Journal, 31*(8), 1567–1574. https://doi.org/10.1007/s00192-019-04200-8

Wolff, B., Williams, K., Winkler, A., Lind, L., & Shalom, D. (2017). Pessary types and discontinuation rates in patients with advanced pelvic organ prolapse. *International Urogynecology Journal, 28*(7), 993–997. https://doi.org/10.1007/s00192-016-3228-9

Index